T0345088

LOW VISION REHABILITATION

A Practical Guide for Occupational Therapists

SECOND EDITION

LOW VISION REHABILITATION

A Practical Guide for Occupational Therapists

SECOND EDITION

Stephen G. Whittaker, PhD, FAAO, OTR/L, CLVT
Outpatient Occupational Therapy
MossRehab Hospital
Elkins Park, Pennsylvania

Mitchell Scheiman, OD, FCOVD, FAAO
Professor
Dean of Research
Salus University
Elkins Park, Pennsylvania

Debra A. Sokol-McKay, OTR/L, SCLV, CDE, CVRT, CLVT
Consultant in Vision Rehabilitation and Diabetes Self-Management
Adjunct Faculty, College of Education and Rehabilitation, Salus University
Elkins Park, Pennsylvania
Consultant for BlindAlive LLC
Seminar Speaker for Cross Country Education, LLC
Contractor and Consultant at the Center for Vision Loss
Allentown, Pennsylvania

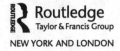

Routledge
Taylor & Francis Group

NEW YORK AND LONDON

First published 2016 by SLACK Incorporated

Published 2024 by Routledge
605 Third Avenue, New York, NY 10158

and by Routledge
4 Park Square, Milton Park, Abingdon, Oxon OX14 4RN

Routledge is an imprint of the Taylor & Francis Group, an informa business

Library of Congress Cataloging-in-Publication Data

Whittaker, Stephen, 1950- , author.
  Low vision rehabilitation : a practical guide for occupational therapists / Mitchell Scheiman, Stephen G. Whittaker, Debra A. Sokol-Mckay -- Second edition.
     p. ; cm.
  Includes bibliographical references and index.
  ISBN 978-1-61711-633-9 (alk. paper)
  I. Scheiman, Mitchell, author. II. Sokol-McKay, Debra A., 1957- , author. III. Title.
  [DNLM: 1. Vision, Low--rehabilitation. 2. Occupational Therapy--methods. 3. Optometry--methods. WW 140]
  RE91
  617.7'12--dc23
                              2015011173

ISBN: 9781617116339 (hbk)
ISBN: 9781003524915 (ebk)

DOI: 10.4324/9781003524915

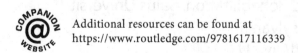

Additional resources can be found at
https://www.routledge.com/9781617116339

Dedication

I dedicate this book to my wife, my favorite and most influential teacher and best buddy, Jan Whittaker.

Stephen G. Whittaker, PhD, FAAO, OTR/L, CLVT

To Maxine, for her love, patience, and understanding

Mitchell Scheiman, OD, FCOVD, FAAO

To my husband and best friend, Joe, whose writing, photography, and computer skills were integral to putting my ideas into print and without whose patience, support, and assistance this book would not have been possible. To my father who taught me more about living with diabetes than any book could and gave me the ability to express myself. To my mother, from whom I inherited my attention to detail and for her listening ear when things got rough.

Debra A. Sokol-McKay, OTR/L, SCLV, CDE, CVRT, CLVT

Contents

Dedication...*v*
Acknowledgments...*ix*
About the Authors..*xi*
Contributing Authors...*xiii*
Foreword by Theresa M. Smith, PhD, OTR, CLVT...*xv*
Preface...*xvii*

Section I   **Introduction and Background Information** **1**

Chapter 1   Overview and First-Response Interventions 3

Chapter 2   Epidemiology, History, and Clinical Model for Low Vision Rehabilitation 19

Chapter 3   Review of Basic Anatomy, Physiology, and Development of the Visual System 39

Chapter 4   Eye Diseases Associated With Low Vision 47

Chapter 5   Optics of Lenses, Refraction, and Magnification..67

Chapter 6   Psychosocial and Cognitive Issues Related to Vision Disability 79

Section II   **Evaluation** **95**

Chapter 7   Overview and Review of the Optometric Low Vision Evaluation 97
               Paul B. Freeman, OD, FAAO, FCOVD

Chapter 8   Occupational Therapy Low Vision Rehabilitation Evaluation...........................107

Section III **Treatment** **141**

Chapter 9   Overview of Treatment Strategy...143

Chapter 10   Foundation Skills and Therapeutic Activities 161

Chapter 11   Managing Peripheral Visual Field Loss and Neglect 181

Chapter 12   Environmental Modifications 203

Chapter 13   Optical Devices and Magnification Strategies 219

Chapter 14   Computer Technology in Low Vision Rehabilitation 253

Section IV   **Occupational Performance** **279**

Chapter 15   Reading and Writing...281

Chapter 16   Basic Self-Care 301

Chapter 17   Home Management...309

Chapter 18   Leisure, Recreation, and Sports...323

Chapter 19   Community Activities and Mobility 335

Chapter 20   Managing Diabetes and Medications. 347
              Debra A. Sokol-McKay, OTR/L, SCLV, CDE, CVRT, CLVT

Chapter 21   Establishing a Low Vision Rehabilitation Specialty Practice. 379
              Maxine Scheiman, MEd, OTR/L, CLVT and
              Stephen G. Whittaker, PhD, FAAO, OTR/L, CLVT

Financial Disclosures 399
Index 401

Acknowledgments

I would like to acknowledge fellow faculty at the Pennsylvania College of Optometry, vision researchers, and clinicians for helping me develop a basic understanding of vision and low vision, especially Gale Watson, Roger Cummings, Rich Brilliant, and Georgia Crozier. Jan Lovie-Kitchin inspired my interest in the clinic service delivery and appreciation of clinical research during my sabbatical in Queensland, Australia, in 1990. The faculty at Thomas Jefferson Department of Occupational Therapy challenged me to broaden my perspective to understand that low vision rehabilitation was about so much more than vision. The staff at MossRehab hospital took a floundering therapist and patiently taught him so many basic skills, especially Mary Ferraro, OT; Joe Padova, OT; Alison Bell, OD; Janine Brodovsky, DPT; and Matt Vnenchak, DPT, to name a few. Early chapters of the book, especially Chapter 6 on psychosocial and caregiver issues, were written while I and a circle of family, friends, and professional caregivers provided hospice care for my mother, Trudy Whittaker, who taught us all so much about faith, hope, the power of occupation, good food, and that "living life to its fullest" can continue to the last few hours. I also learned from my sister, Kathy Whittaker, how to forge a bond of love from a team of helpers comprising of very different, often difficult, people.

Stephen G. Whittaker, PhD, FAAO, OTR/L, CLVT

My family, for their support, and for showing so much patience with me during the many months of writing. To Dr. Barbara Steinman, for her outstanding work in designing the illustrations for the second edition of this book.

Mitchell Scheiman, OD, FCOVD, FAAO

I want to thank my husband for the love, encouragement, and support that kept me focused on becoming the best that I could be in the field of low vision and diabetes. Maureen Duffy planted the seed and to this day nurtures my knowledge and development as a vision rehabilitation therapist, professional writer, and educator. Ann Williams has served as my guiding light in the field of diabetes and disability and always inspires me to be and do more. And last but not least, the many clients who probably taught me more than I taught them and who have given me the greatest joy and purpose in life.

Debra A. Sokol-McKay, OTR/L, SCLV, CDE, CVRT, CLVT

About the Authors

Stephen G. Whittaker, PhD, FAAO, OTR/L, CLVT, is an occupational therapist, certified low vision therapist and research Fellow of the American Academy of Optometry with a PhD in experimental psychology and post-doctoral training in visual science. For over 35 years, Steve has been teaching, doing research, and providing clinical services in low vision rehabilitation. He lectures internationally. Prior to becoming an occupational therapist, Steve was a member of the faculty at the Pennsylvania College of Optometry (now Salus University) during which time he was principal investigator on National Eye Institute-, NIDRR-, and NASA-funded research on low vision and visual enhancement devices. He switched careers, earned his Master's in Occupational Therapy from Thomas Jefferson University in 2002, and now practices as an occupational therapist at MossRehab Hospital and consults in area private practices where he provides low vision rehabilitation services. He has served on the low vision subject matter expert committee of the Academy of Certification for Vision Rehabilitation Professionals (ACVREP) and participated in the writing of the certification examinations. His broad training in occupational therapy enables Dr. Whittaker not only to treat visual impairment across the lifespan but also a variety of neurological conditions as well. From his unique background, Dr. Whittaker has built the pragmatic approach of an occupational therapist on a foundation of over 40 years of research from many disciplines.

Mitchell Scheiman, OD, FCOVD, FAAO, is a nationally known optometric educator, lecturer, author, and private practitioner. He is the author of *Understanding and Managing Visual Deficits: A Guide for Occupational Therapists.* Dr. Scheiman has a long and close relationship with occupational therapists. He works closely with occupational therapists in his practice co-managing patients and has presented post-graduate continuing education courses to over 6000 occupational therapists. Dr. Scheiman is currently Dean of Research and Professor of Optometry at Salus University. He has written three books for optometrists covering the topics of binocular vision and vision therapy, pediatric optometry, and learning related vision problems and he has published over 165 articles in the professional literature. He is a Diplomate in Binocular Vision and Perception and a Fellow in the College of Optometrists in Vision Development.

In the last 20 years he has spent the majority of his professional time as a researcher involved in randomized clinical trials. He was the national Study Chair of the Convergence Insufficiency Treatment Trial that was completed in 2008, and the recently NEI-funded follow-up Convergence Insufficiency Treatment Trial study investigating changes in reading and attention after treatment.

Debra Sokol-McKay, OTR/L, SCLV, CDE, CVRT, CLVT, is a licensed Occupational Therapist in the state of Pennsylvania. She has a specialty certification in Low Vision through the American Occupational Therapy Association (AOTA) and is a Certified Low Vision Therapist, Certified Diabetes Educator, and Certified Low Vision Rehabilitation Therapist. Ms. Sokol-McKay received her Bachelor of Science in Occupational Therapy from Temple University in Philadelphia, PA, and her Master's in Vision Rehabilitation Therapy from the Pennsylvania College of Optometry (now Salus University) in Elkins Park, PA.

Ms. Sokol-McKay has been a practicing occupational therapist for over 30 years and both a low vision therapist and a diabetes educator for over 15 years, is the second lead author of Disabilities Position Statement of the American Association of Diabetes Educator (AADE), and has presented at the AADE's national conference many times. Ms. Sokol-McKay wrote the Occupational Therapy and Diabetes Fact Sheet for AOTA and co-presented AOTA's podcast on diabetes. She has been a national speaker on low vision rehabilitation for Cross Country Education for the past 5 years.

Ms. Sokol-McKay was a member of the AOTA's National Expert Low Vision Practice Certification Panel, which wrote the AOTA's standards for specialty certification in low vision. Debbie is the current chairperson of the abstract reviewer committee of the national low vision Envision conference and a reviewer for the *Journal of Vision Impairment and Blindness.* Ms. Sokol-McKay is also the author of peer-reviewed professional articles on low vision rehabilitation and/or diabetes self-management and has presented more than 20 times at national/international conferences of AOTA, AADE, Envision Conference, and the Association for Education and Rehabilitation of the Blind and Visually Impaired.

Contributing Authors

Paul B. Freeman, OD, FAAO, FCOVD, is an internationally known lecturer, author, and private practitioner. He is the co-author of *The Art and Practice of Low Vision*. Dr. Freeman is chief of low vision services at Allegheny General Hospital in Pittsburgh, Pennsylvania and consults to a number of rehabilitation settings where he works closely with occupational and physical therapists, as well as others on the rehabilitative team. He has limited his practice to the care and rehabilitation of visually-impaired, brain-injured, and multi-handicapped individuals of all ages.

Maxine Scheiman, MEd, OTR/L, CLVT, decided to change careers, after working as a learning disabilities specialist for many years, and in 1988 graduated from Temple University in Philadelphia as an occupational therapist. She has been practicing as an occupational therapist for 27 years and has worked in many different settings including acute care and rehabilitation hospitals, school occupational therapy, early intervention, low vision rehabilitation, and remedial vision rehabilitation. In 2000, Dr. Scheiman became interested in low vision rehabilitation and she attended the Rehabilitation Teaching program at the Pennsylvania College of Optometry in Philadelphia. After becoming certified as a low vision therapist she has worked as a low vision rehabilitation therapist helping patients with visual impairment. She is currently providing remedial vision rehabilitation in the Salus University Vision Clinic at Magee Rehabilitation Hospital.

Foreword

Occupational therapists are in need of a comprehensive text on how to provide low vision rehabilitation. This text is suitable for educators, clinicians, and students alike to learn about eye diseases, optics, low vision evaluations, goal writing, treatment strategies, environmental modifications, nonoptical assistive devices, and software and technology for the visually impaired.

This text was written by low vision rehabilitation experts with many, many years of experience among them. In fact, you may have attended a workshop, used an assessment, or owned a previous text by one or more of the authors; I certainly have! The authors do not base the text just on their clinical skills but provide the reader with the knowledge needed to deliver evidence-based practice.

This second edition of *Low Vision Rehabilitation: A Practical Guide for Occupational Therapists* is a classic resource for any type of setting. It can be kept and referenced for years to come. In it you will find the information you need on how you can help your clients optimize performance of their desired occupations.

Theresa M. Smith, PhD, OTR, CLVT
Assistant Professor
Department of Occupational Therapy and Department of Rehabilitative Sciences
University of Texas Medical Branch
Galveston, Texas

Preface

When first published in 2007, *Low Vision Rehabilitation: A Practical Guide for Occupational Therapists* was written for practitioners who wished to specialize in low vision. The strength of the first edition was that the presentation was easy to understand. We organized a straightforward presentation of best practices, rich with excellent illustrations and photographs and based on evidence from multiple disciplines as well as occupational therapy. Rather than overwhelm the reader with several alternative evaluation and intervention techniques, we carefully selected 1 or 2 evaluation and treatment protocols that had both an evidence basis for inclusion and, from our personal experience, were found to be practical and effective in the clinic. Since most chapters were written by the same authors, the chapters meshed into a coherent approach.

The second edition is intended to broaden its appeal to general occupational therapy practitioners and students who have no immediate intention of specializing in low vision. The first chapter enables the reader to develop an empathetic understanding of different types of vision impairment using realistic simulations. This chapter describes how to screen for these vision impairments and apply first-response rehabilitation interventions that use generally available materials to enable a client to function while waiting for specialized low vision services. We added information on managing sensory and perceptual vision disability caused by neurological pathology or injury, including an entire chapter on treatment and conditions commonly encountered by the general occupational therapist. We also have incorporated extensive information on nonvisual compensatory strategies in evaluation, treatment, and outcomes definition and assessment. As occupational therapists, our focus is on participation with whatever means are available, not just visual interventions alone.

The book also is organized to combine a traditional approach with features available in an e-book presentation. In the age of Google, many therapists prefer "targeted learning," searching for specific answers rather than reading overall presentation of a topic from start to finish. We present the traditional organization of information that, so far, has been successful in the current first edition. For example, under this traditional structure, a therapist might read the book from start to finish, starting with background chapters on evaluation, pathogenesis, devices, therapeutic approaches, and finally occupational performance. The proposed new section on occupational performance will follow the background chapters and pull this information on various optical, electronic, and nonvisual strategies together as solutions to common problems encountered by people with low vision.

For those who prefer targeted learning, the therapist usually starts with a problem as it presents in the clinic. For example, a therapist may suspect a patient is unable to read because of low vision. For such targeted learning, the therapist should read the first chapter to learn basic concepts, terminology, and basic evaluation procedures. Then the reader should be able to go to any chapter, such as the chapter in the "Occupational Performance" section on reading. In this chapter, the reader would learn first-response interventions that are easily put together in any clinical situation without specialized training or equipment. This might satisfy the needs of a general therapist, who would then refer the patient for advanced treatment. Some would seek information beyond the first response and might follow the links or cross-references to other chapters to learn more sophisticated evaluation and treatment protocols. As a result, readers who use targeted learning will learn as they go. In an e-book presentation, links would cross-reference the information, so this skipping around would become seamless.

Major changes have occurred in blindness and low vision rehabilitation in the past 5 years. Chapters on evaluation and treatment of psychosocial complications of vision loss, environmental modification, and lighting and the chapter on diabetic management have been substantially revised. The latest developments in electronic readers, tablet computers, and smart phones are now so widely used, even among older adults, that references to these devices have been incorporated throughout the book. We have included the latest in electronic magnifiers that not only enlarge and enhance text, but read it aloud, as well as newer compact fluorescent lamp and light-emitting diode lighting, especially portable lighting.

Just as the most effective therapy involves a team approach, our team of authors represents complementary skills and backgrounds. An optometrist, Mitchell Scheiman contributes an in-depth understanding of pathology, optics, medical treatment, and interventions. Stephen G. Whittaker, one of the pioneer low vision researchers in the field, provided a critical review of the evidence, as well as his more recent experience as a general occupational therapist treating not only visual but all aspects of physical disability, especially neurological impairments. He also has treated people in a more traditional optometric low vision practice and as a computer technology specialist. Steve has experience establishing a low vision practice in these different settings as well. Debra Sokol-McKay is an occupational therapist with more than 30 years of practice experience with physical and vision-related disability, and holds certifications as a low vision therapist, a vision rehabilitation therapist, and diabetes educator. Debbie specializes in evaluation and treatment of a wide range of deficiencies in activities of daily living and instrumental activities of daily living client performance, including but not limited to those related to adaptive diabetes self-management. She has worked extensively in the blindness field and brings to the team extensive training in low vision, nonvisual, and "blind rehab" techniques. Together we have written and/or reviewed most chapters in this book, keeping our focus on combining our different approaches to enable people to recover and achieve valued occupations, roles, hopes, and dreams once again.

Recommended Curricula

For the generalist occupational therapist or occupational therapy assistants, we recommend starting by reading Chapter 1 for an overview of the conditions, evaluation, and treatment approaches. This chapter is packed with information, but with cross-links to other chapters that provide more explanation and additional illustrations as needed. From Chapter 1, the reader should be able to skip to any chapter in the book and understand much of it. Most will skip directly to the chapters in the last section on occupational performance that provide a mix of easily implemented interventions and interventions that require more advanced understanding. When advanced concepts and terminology are introduced, such as the use of magnification devices and adaptive techniques, links and cross-references direct the reader to chapters within the book for advanced instruction, as well as to blindness rehabilitation professionals who would have the advanced training and certification to complete a treatment plan.

For the occupational therapy student, the overview in Chapter 1 and Chapter 11 on neurological disorders should provide the basic information that you will need as a beginning therapist. This text is designed to be used as a reference and has extensive cross-links within the book and on the Web that will prove valuable as you begin your careers as occupational therapists or occupational therapy assistants.

For those seeking advanced training, we recommend the traditional approach, starting at Chapter 1 and then sequentially through the chapters. The content will cover most of the information required for Academy for Certification of Vision Rehabilitation & Education Professionals (ACVREP) certification as a certified low vision therapist or American Occupational Therapy Association (AOTA) specialty certification in low vision. The chapters in Section IV can supplement and update existing texts and readings assigned in a program for certification as a vision rehabilitation therapist or educator for the visually impaired, as well. This book is especially well suited for readers in clinical practice who can quickly locate information and references as needed to address the vision disability when encountered in the clinic. For advanced training, university-sponsored or other interactive courses of study are recommended because structured programs provide different perspectives from different instructors. However, a self-study is possible and continuing education credits can be earned inexpensively, a chapter at a time, by passing examinations on each chapter at http://elearning.visionedseminars.com. For those who choose self-study, we suggest finding a mentor through www.acvrep.org in your chosen field of study or the www.aota.org specialty certification program. These examinations often use clients from our "virtual clinic" and are written in the style of the ACVREP certification examination. Although written for occupational therapists, many who are not occupational therapists have used the first edition of this text in their courses of study from around the world. The text was written for an international readership. Only information on service delivery is specific to the United States. (Power point slides are available to faculty who wish to use this book in their educational programs. See www.routledge.com/9781617116339 for access.)

I

Introduction and
Background Information

I

1

Overview and First-Response Interventions

A MODEL OF CARE FOR A GENERAL REHABILITATION OR OTHER SETTING

This chapter provides an overview of the conditions that lead to low vision and more common disabilities, as well as an overview of the evaluation process and common interventions. Having read this chapter, the reader could read and understand most any other chapter in the book. Let's start with a case illustrating a typical first encounter with low vision.

Ms. Jones was admitted to a subacute rehabilitation facility with a diagnosis of recent left hemisphere stroke with hemiplegia, alexia (inability to read from a stroke), and dementia. Although her hemiplegia was resolving, she exhibited poor initiation and was very difficult to engage in therapy, forgot instructions and people's names, often ending sessions in tears. Although she said she was an avid reader, she could not read even enlarged text. She complained that things appeared and disappeared and reported vivid visual hallucinations of her deceased husband.

Actually, Ms. Jones did have mild vascular dementia. Most of her symptoms, however, were the result of vision impairment or of severe depression that often occurs in

people with macular degeneration who have not received low vision rehabilitation. If her therapists could identify and treat her vision disability, she would be more likely to successively progress through her rehabilitation program. As this case illustrates, vision disability is often hidden and may be confused with cognitive disability, perceptual, and even postural problems incorrectly attributed to other conditions.

These misdiagnoses can be prevented by establishing routine screening for vision disability. Rarely are people admitted for inpatient rehabilitation with a low vision diagnosis; however, low vision is a comorbidity common among the elderly that severely impacts the effectiveness of a rehabilitation treatment plan. In other settings, like schools or in community programs, again, vision disability will affect participation and needs to be identified and addressed. We cannot count on optometrists, ophthalmologists, and other physicians to refer patients in need of low vision rehabilitation services. Even in countries that have national health care systems, many, if not most, of those with significant vision disability who found their way to a rehabilitation service were not referred by a physician.[1-6] All professionals treating patients should accept responsibility to identify and properly refer patients or clients who are suspected of having a vision disability.

Whittaker SG, Scheiman M, Sokol-McKay DA.
Low Vision Rehabilitation: A Practical Guide for Occupational Therapists,
Second Edition (pp 3-18).
© 2016 Taylor & Francis Group.

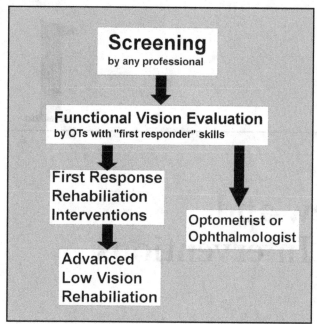

Figure 1-1. Model of care for low vision rehabilitation within a medical rehabilitation, education, other setting where vision disability is not the focus.

This chapter will enable the reader to start applying the material immediately. We will describe how any professional might screen for 6 different types of vision disability by using available materials and careful behavioral observation. The goal of this chapter is to provide the reader with the material to teach others how to recognize a possible vision disability, as well as to perform a basic functional vision assessment themselves. The evaluation will indicate appropriate "first-response interventions"—treatments that do not require special equipment or training.

First-response interventions are described in Chapter 12, and Chapters 15 through 20 on specific occupations. These chapters also include advanced treatments that require a more thorough reading of this book. Although considered a "stopgap," first-response interventions enable a person to continue with a rehabilitation program while waiting for treatment by a low vision rehabilitation specialist. These interventions by themselves can be highly effective. The chapters on advanced treatment describe how these first interventions are often the most effective interventions used by specialists.

THE MODEL OF CARE IN SETTINGS WHERE VISION IS NOT THE FOCUS

In an ideal model of low vision rehabilitation (Figure 1-1), the first step is to train all staff who treat patients to screen for vision disability by looking for behavioral signs of vision problems (Table 1-1). This screening has high sensitivity but lower specificity; that is, people may be referred who have other impairments but not a vision disability. When the staff member suspects a vision disability, he or she refers the patient to another staff member, usually an occupational therapist, who knows how to perform this "functional vision evaluation." The functional vision evaluation has high specificity. In the continuum of care, once a vision disability is identified, the treating team takes two actions: First, the treating team assures that the client is under the care of an optometrist or ophthalmologist and has seen one of these eye care physicians since a vision change or any major physical change has occurred. Second, the assessment results will lead the evaluator to the first-response intervention (examples are in Table 1-1). While waiting to be seen by an eye care physician, the vision disability can be addressed with these first-response interventions. Finally, but most importantly in this continuum of care, the treatment team must ensure that a client who has a vision disability has received vision rehabilitation from a qualified specialist who can provide advanced care. This book provides the reader with the basic information required for advanced certification as an Academy for Certification of Vision Rehabilitation & Education Professionals (ACVREP)–certified low vision therapist (www.acvrep.org) or for specialty certification in occupational therapy (www.aota.org).

To continue the example of Ms. Jones, the screening revealed, among other problems, that Ms. Jones could not read. The occupational therapist then performed a functional vision evaluation and found Ms. Jones could not read because she could not see the text as a result of low vision. This evaluation revealed 3 specific visual impairments that contributed to the reading disability. For first-response interventions, the reader could turn directly to Chapter 15 on reading. These interventions are appropriate for the visual impairments that were identified, such as enlarging the print to a specific size for a specific distance, and how to optimize lighting. Applying these interventions would allow Ms. Jones to more effectively undergo treatment for her admitting diagnosis. Later, in discharge planning, the patient would be referred for more advanced low vision rehabilitation.

Applying this continuum of care requires that someone provide education on screening for the entire professional staff of a service provider. Once the staff learns to screen for low vision, they will generate referrals that will help a specialist in low vision rehabilitation build a practice.

TYPES OF VISUAL IMPAIRMENT

Table 1-1 lists 4 sensory impairments commonly associated with low vision and oculomotor dysfunction. Another type of visual impairment is a perceptual impairment—a

TABLE 1-1: SUMMARY OF 5 KEY TESTS IN A VISUAL ASSESSMENT

The functional visual evaluation consists of 5 tests that evaluate different aspects of visual function

TEST	PERFORMANCE INDICATIONS	COMMON CAUSES	COMPENSATION
1. Visual acuity threshold: The smallest high-contrast shape someone can see.	• Difficulty reading • Holds material close • Difficulty seeing TV	• Needs new glasses • Macular degeneration • Untreated or advanced diabetic retinopathy • Advanced glaucoma • Optic atrophy	1. Enlarge the shape or print being viewed or write larger. 2. Use an optical or electronic magnification device (advanced technique). 3. Move object closer. 4. Improve lighting.
2. Contrast sensitivity: The lowest contrast shape someone can see. The shape is at least twice as large as the visual acuity threshold.	• Difficulty seeing spilled water • Glare sensitivity • Difficulty seeing faded print or print on colored backgrounds or carpeted steps	• Macular degeneration • Diabetic retinopathy • Advanced glaucoma • Optic atrophy • Optic neuritis • Multiple sclerosis	1. Enhance the contrast of shapes, usually color or light. 2. Change light so that it is from the side or above. Eliminate glare. 3. Adjust light intensity according to person's preference changing the distance of a task light. 4. Use an electronic contrast enhancement device or tinted lenses (advanced technique).
3. Central visual field loss: Blind areas where someone is trying to look.	• Missing words and letters • Difficulty finding place when scanning • Frustration	• Macular degeneration • Untreated diabetic retinopathy • Acquired brain injury (stroke)	1. Teach person to use side vision (advanced technique). 2. Magnification. 3. Use nonsighted techniques.
4. Peripheral visual field loss: Vision to the side, above, or below where someone is looking.	• Hesitation when reaching for objects • Trips, bumps, and not seeing objects to the side	• Optic atrophy • Treated diabetic retinopathy • Advanced glaucoma • Acquired brain injury (stroke)	1. Teach the person visual scanning strategies to compensate for field defects. 2. People might adopt head positions to compensate for field defects. 3. Prism glasses under the supervision of an eye doctor or certified low vision therapist.
5. Oculomotor function: Eye movement and eye teaming, nystagmus.	• Atypical head positions • Complaint of double vision, headaches or blurred vision at near	• Traumatic brain injury, especially closed head trauma	1. Train eyes to move in the direction of the impairment (advanced technique). 2. Use an eye patch to eliminate double vision. 3. Tracking activities with small, just visible targets.

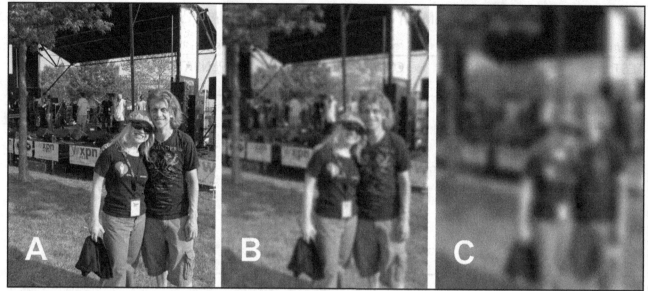

Figure 1-2. Photographs comparing (A) normal visual acuity with (B) a moderate loss in acuity (6/18 or 20/60) and (C) legal blindness (6/60 or 20/200).

disorder in the processing of sensory information, such as visual alexia (an acquired inability to recognize words even though the letters can be clearly seen). It is important to rule out the sensory impairment and oculomotor dysfunction before concluding that a patient has a perceptual impairment such as alexia from a brain injury. A person may not recognize words because some or all of the letters cannot be seen due to reduced acuity or contrast sensitivity, or central or peripheral field loss.

In addition to impaired visual acuity, contrast sensitivity, and central and peripheral visual field loss associated with low vision, another condition that may affect a client's ability to read, find, and recognize objects is oculomotor problems such as binocular vision (eye teaming), accommodative (focusing), and eye movement problems. These problems may affect the ability to see clearly and comfortably in certain directions or at a particular distance, and may be associated with visual symptoms and even double vision. Oculomotor symptoms may be relieved by eye patching. Otherwise, an optometrist or ophthalmologist must be involved in the diagnosis and treatment planning.

VISUAL ACUITY

Screening: Illustration and Behavioral Signs

Visual acuity, as the name suggests, describes a patient's ability to see high-contrast detail, such as the gap in a C, or the difference between a P and an F. Figures 1-2(B) and 1-2(C) illustrate two levels of visual acuity impairment: moderate and severe. Moderate visual impairment meets

minimum Centers for Medicare/Medicaid Services (CMS) criteria for reimbursable rehabilitation.[7] Someone with moderate impairment cannot read newsprint at a typical reading distance of 40 cm (16 inches) even with eyeglasses. The severe visual impairment in Figure 1-2(C) illustrates vision at the level of legal blindness, which traditionally has been the criterion for eligibility for rehabilitation services by educational, private, and state service providers. "Legal blindness" entitles the individual to a number of entitlements and benefits, such as property tax exemptions, an extra income tax exemption, reduced fares on public transportation, and access to Social Security disability. The definition of legal blindness is quite arbitrary, has no functional basis, and, fortunately, is being relaxed by most organizations in favor of the more functional "moderate" level of visual impairment. Surprising to many, a person who is "legally blind" usually has considerable functional vision, and many who receive advanced low vision rehabilitation recover the ability to read normally sized print. People experiencing impaired visual acuity often do not experience the blurriness illustrated in Figures 1-2(B) and 1-2(C). To experience a different type of acuity loss, instead of looking directly at Figure 1-2(A), look to the right or left edge of the photograph.

In screening for a possible loss in visual acuity, reading newspaper-size print at 40 cm (16 inches) is the most convenient and sensitive method to screen for acuity loss because a person with a functionally significant loss in visual acuity has difficulty reading newsprint-size text at this distance. Care must be taken to prevent a person from bringing the newspaper closer when it becomes difficult to see. Adults younger than about 40 years of age easily compensate by holding the material closer because they can focus at near. If a child or younger person holds material closer than

40 cm (16 inches), then acuity loss is indicated. Reading small print is the best screening method because it is sensitive to the other types of vision impairments as well.[8,9] To test for acuity loss at distance or in people who are not literate, the therapist can (assuming the therapist has normal vision) use his or her own vision to find something in the room—a sign, a distant clock on the wall, objects or words that are difficult to see—and then ask the client to describe or read it. If the therapist can read it but the client cannot, the client should be referred for a functional vision evaluation to determine if visual acuity is indeed impaired.

The most common cause of acuity loss is refractive error, that is, optical blur that requires correction by contact lenses or eyeglasses. The examiner, therefore, must be careful to make sure eyeglasses are current and are used correctly. A person over about 40 years of age usually needs reading glasses or to use bifocals to see closer because of age-related loss of focusing ability. With bifocal or progressive addition lenses (no-line bifocal), the reader must look through the bottom of the lenses to see clearly at near. Even if the only thing a client needs to see clearly is new eyeglasses, a referral for a first-response intervention that compensates for reduced acuity allows the course of treatment to continue while waiting for an eye examination by an optometrist or ophthalmologist.

Definition

Visual acuity is the measure of the smallest high-contrast detail that one can resolve. It usually is measured with letters or words: the detail is one-fifth the size of the letter, or about the stroke width or the gap in a C. Most people are familiar with the concept of 20/20 visual acuity, or in most countries who use metric measurements, 6/6 visual acuity. An individual with 20/20 (6/6) acuity is considered to have normal ability to see small detail at the distance tested. The numerator refers to the testing distance at which the subject recognizes the stimulus. The denominator refers to the letter size. Letter size is described as the farthest distance at which the letter being viewed could still be identified by a client with normal visual acuity. Since larger letters can be seen further away, a larger number in the denominator indicates a larger size letter on the eye chart. For example, we will use a client who has low vision with 20/100 (6/30) acuity. This indicates that the letter size that a client could barely see at 20 feet (6 meters) was large enough to been seen by someone with normal vision at 100 feet (30 meters). A letter that could be seen at 100 feet is 5 times larger than a letter seen at 20 feet. The client in our example could only see this letter at 20 feet, indicating that the visual acuity is reduced 5 times relative to the normal finding. This method of recording visual acuity is routinely used in the United States, and the units in feet are referred to as "imperial units." In other countries, in the research literature, and in some clinics in the United States, meters rather

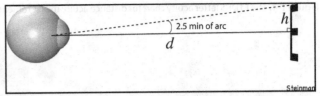

Figure 1-3. At 20/20 acuity (6/6), a letter size and distance are set so the image on the retina is 5 minutes of arc. A larger size or closer distance will increase the retinal image size. (Reprinted with permission from Barbara Steinman.)

than feet are used to express distance visual acuity using the M system described later. For example, 6/6 is equivalent to 20/20 acuity (6 meters is about 19 feet), 6/60 is equivalent to 20/200 acuity, and 6/30 is equivalent to 20/100 acuity.

The meaning of 20/20 visual acuity can also be expressed in angular units—the measure the occupational therapist uses to measure joint mobility. However, the measures of visual acuity are in minutes of arc, where 1 minute is 1/60th of a degree. Someone with 20/20 visual acuity is able to recognize a letter that subtends a visual angle of 5 minutes of arc at the eye (Figure 1-3); the critical detail is 1 minute of arc. A lowercase letter in newsprint is about 12 to 15 minutes of arc: 2.5 to 3 times normal visual acuity.

As illustrated in Figure 1-3, this means that if you draw a line from the top of a 20/20 letter to the eye and another line from the bottom of the letter to the eye, the size of the angle at the intersection of these two lines at the eye is 5 minutes of arc. When measuring near visual acuity, the convention is based on the "meter system," or "M" notation. In this system, a 1M letter will subtend 5 minutes of arc at 1 meter. Note in this diagram that changing either the size of the object or distance affects the angular size of the object and size of the image on the retina.

More conventional clinical measures of visual acuity always include specification of both test distance and print size. It is critical to carefully control and record a test distance during acuity measurement.

Evaluation

Optometrists and ophthalmologists measure visual acuity using individual, standardized letters (Figure 1-4) because letter acuity is sensitive to refractive error (need for eyeglasses) and the emergence and progression of eye diseases. In a functional vision evaluation, reading acuity (reading words instead of individual letters) is measured because reading is a common functional goal (Figure 1-5). To measure visual acuity, one first is careful that the patient is using the eyeglasses for the testing distance and that distance is kept constant and is recorded along with letter size. For reading, the typical test distance is about 40 cm (16 inches), but one must be careful to test at the distance appropriate for the eyeglasses worn, especially if someone is older and cannot focus at near (see Chapter 8).

Figure 1-4. The ETDRS letter acuity chart for distance acuity measurement.

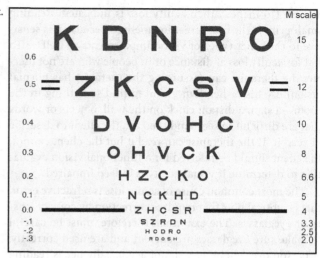

TABLE 1-2: STEPS FOR ASSESSMENT		
VISUAL READING ACUITY	**CONTRAST SENSITIVITY**	**LIGHTING**
1. Check correction.*	1. Check correction.	1. Measure contrast or acuity threshold.
2. Set and maintain test distance (40 cm for near, 2 to 4 meters for distance, specified by chart).*	2. Check that symbol size at the reading test distance is at least 2 times acuity threshold.	2. Vary distance of light to reading material and change illumination until lowest threshold and best reported comfort.
3. Test both eyes first.*	3. Test both eyes first.	
4. Carefully observe client reading from largest to smaller print, noting error patterns and hesitations.	4. Have client read down the chart.	3. Vary light position to increase or decrease glare and note effects on performance. Position light to minimize glare.
5. Record test distance and critical print size (eg, 2M at 40 cm).	5. Record contrast threshold and test distance.	4. Note best light position and range.
6. Record test distance and acuity threshold (eg, 0.4/0.8M).*	6. Test each eye or both eyes to determine which eye or if both eyes should be used.	5. Note glare sensitivity.
7. Test each eye to determine if one eye or both eyes should be used.*		
*Steps for measuring distance letter acuity.		

Critical Print Size and Reading Threshold Acuity

To test reading acuity (Table 1-2), the client reads down the chart from larger to smaller font sizes. The examiner uses a stopwatch to time reading and notes the range of font sizes where reading is fastest and records at what print size reading slows. The smallest font that produces the fastest and most comfortable reading is called *critical print size*. This is the most important measure for rehabilitation because this is the print size that will be best for reading. Reading acuity threshold is the smallest print someone can read and understand. At a given distance, critical print size is about 2 to 3 times larger than print size at reading acuity threshold. The examiner can estimate the best print size for reading critical print size 3 ways: the print size before reading slows; the print size that is 2 times the acuity threshold; or the examiner can just ask the client, "Where does reading become difficult?" and use the next larger print size as the estimate of critical print size. The examiner records the critical print size and reading acuity threshold print size, along with test distance, using critical print size to estimate how much magnification a person needs to read. The details and specifics of visual acuity measurement, as well as interpretation, are in Chapter 8, but for first-response interventions, one needs only to estimate critical print size and try to make sure the print size a person will be reading is about the same size as critical print size or larger. Although bigger is usually better, one cannot assume this is always the case. It is important to measure reading starting with the largest print size because, in some instances with a visual field restriction, larger print is harder to read because whole words cannot be seen at once.

Reading Speed

To get an accurate measure of reading speed, the length of each sentence and its difficulty need to be carefully controlled. The online appendix lists recommended assessment instruments, including standardized tests such as the MNREAD (see Figure 1-5), that are necessary for advanced treatment. Less expensive, nonstandardized tests are acceptable for first-response interventions as long as sentences are at about the same level of linguistic difficulty and length. For evaluating functional acuity for tasks other than reading—for example, a patient needs to see a TV or appreciate a family photograph—the examiner can vary the distance and size of the object until it is easily seen and then record the size of the object and distance. Many medical rehabilitation facilities have electronic magnifiers (see Chapter 14), as well as access to computers where the size of objects or pictures of objects can be easily changed.

Refractive Disorders

A common cause of reduced visual acuity is refractive error. Refractive error indicates that visual acuity is reduced because a person needs eyeglasses or some sort of optical correction that will focus the image of an object on the retina. Understanding refractive error is very important in advanced practice and is discussed in Chapter 5. Correction for refractive error includes eyeglasses or spectacles, contact lenses, refractive (laser) surgery, or lens implants. Low vision rehabilitation necessarily involves eye care practitioners because optometrists and ophthalmologists perform "refractions" to correct for refractive error. One can quickly check if acuity loss is due to refractive error. Acuity will improve if the client is looking through pinholes (see Chapter 5). The different types of refractive error are as follows:

- **Myopia, or nearsightedness.** People with myopia are able to see things in clear focus when they are closer, but not farther away. Through the corrective eyeglasses of someone with myopia, everything looks smaller.
- **Hyperopia, or farsightedness.** People with hyperopia can see things farther away better than at near. Looking through the eyeglasses of someone with hyperopia, everything looks a little larger and blurry. Milder hyperopia often does not affect visual acuity

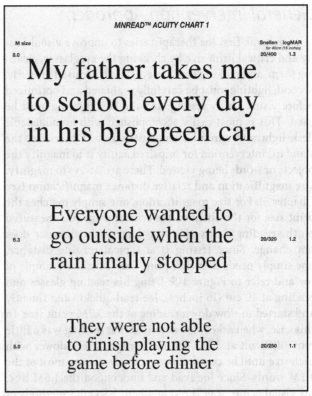

Figure 1-5. The MNREAD reading acuity chart for near reading acuity and critical print size measurement. Note that line lengths and reading difficulty are held constant so changes in reading performance can be attributed to changes in print size.

in children and young adults because they can refocus their eyes to compensate; however, this compensation can lead to eye strain and binocular problems at near.

- **Astigmatism.** If the optical elements of the eye, the lens, and cornea are not spherical in shape like a properly shaped lens, astigmatism results. If one looks through the eyeglasses of someone with astigmatism, the view is out of focus at any distance, and if you look through the top of the lenses, the shape warps as the lenses are rotated.
- **Presbyopia.** People over around 40 years of age have difficulty focusing at near because as someone ages, the lens in the eye loses its ability to focus at near. People with presbyopia usually have reading glasses or bifocals. Looking through the eyeglasses of someone with presbyopia, the bottom of the lenses will appear larger and more out of focus at distance than the top part.

Although acuity loss from refractive error can be easily fixed by a proper refraction and new eyeglasses, if a client has already started a rehabilitation program, the occupational therapist cannot wait for this to happen. In the meantime, the acuity loss still needs to be addressed with first-response interventions.

General Intervention Approach

In general, first the therapist tries to improve visual acuity and critical print size by checking the eyeglasses, cleaning them, and making sure the eyeglasses are used properly. Second, lighting must be carefully evaluated and optimized before visual acuity testing, and the best lighting must be used. This is most easily accomplished with an adjustable desk light and careful client instruction. Otherwise, the standard intervention for impaired acuity is to magnify the objects or words being viewed. There are 2 ways to magnify: size magnification and relative distance magnification (see Chapter 5). For size magnification, one simply matches the print size for the client to the critical print size measured on the reading acuity chart—as long as the distance does not change. Since testing is at typical reading distance, one simply needs to match print size. Take the example of Joe and refer to Figure 1-5. Using his reading glasses and reading at 40 cm (16 inches), Joe read quickly and fluently and started to slow down reading at the 3.2M print size. In this case, when asked, Joe admitted that reading was a little more difficult at 3.2M. He read progressively slower with each size until he could no longer read, missing most of the 1.2M words. Since Joe read and understood the 1.6M line, his visual acuity was "1.6M at 40 cm." So all 3 methods of determining critical print size indicated that the smallest print that could be read easily and comfortably was 4M. To convert the M size to more familiar "point size" used in word processors, multiply M times 8. For making notes to himself to compensate for memory loss and for all written directions, Joe would need larger than 4M (32 point) print size. Note also that critical print size is usually more than 2 times (3 lines on the acuity chart) acuity threshold of 2M[8], so if the print size is a bit smaller, he still will be able to see and read it, but it is usually better to overestimate print size unless someone has a visual field restriction.

Bringing an object closer produces relative distance magnification. Moving a television closer or standing closer to a patient to enable him to recognize a face exemplifies relative distance magnification. In addition, carefully position objects on a table so they are closer or use a reading stand. Younger people, under about 35 years of age, can focus closer than 40 cm. People who are over about 40 years of age require reading glasses to see closer than 40 cm, which can only be prescribed by an optometrist or ophthalmologist.

To keep an object at acuity threshold, the letter or print size changes proportionally to distance. If you change the distance, you must change the size of the object in direct proportion. For example, if you double the distance, you must double the size of the print or object. If you cut the distance in half, then you can reduce the size of the object being viewed by one half. For example, for Joe, critical print size was 4M (32 point) at 40 cm, so he could see regular-size playing cards when he was holding them at 40 cm (16 inches). To easily see playing cards on a table at twice the distance, the numbers and letters on the cards would need to be twice as large. The therapist would then use jumbo-size playing cards, which are large enough to see on the table. This is an example of size magnification. For objects of a fixed size, like a TV screen, the distance can be decreased; one-half of the original distance is equivalent to doubling the size of the TV. This very important and basic principle of magnification is discussed again in greater detail in Chapter 5.

With more severe loss in acuity, where, for example, critical print size is larger than 2M (16 point) and written materials are not as accessible (large-print books, electronic books, and computers can magnify text up to 16 to 18 point size), then first-response interventions should include non-visual compensatory options such as National Library Service (NLS) recordings for the blind (www.loc.gov/nls). More specialized devices, such as stronger magnifiers, reading glasses, and electronic devices, allow for much greater magnification and recovery of visual reading, but to evaluate and dispense these devices require learning the more advanced material in this book.

CONTRAST SENSITIVITY

Screening: Illustration and Behavioral Signs

An important topic related to visual acuity is contrast sensitivity. Visual acuity only allows us to evaluate one limited aspect of the person's ability to see. While visual acuity tests enable the therapist to estimate how well someone can see small, high-contrast objects, contrast sensitivity testing enables the therapist to estimate how well someone can see larger, low-contrast objects such as washed-out images on a light background, a carpeted step, or water on a floor. Contrast sensitivity is related to visual acuity, but provides information that is not described by visual acuity measurement.[10] Contrast sensitivity is associated with reading performance,[8,11,12] mobility,[13,14] driving,[15] and activities of daily living.[13,16]

Typically, people with impaired contrast sensitivity also have impaired visual acuity. It is possible, however, for a client to have reasonably good visual acuity but still complain of problems such as dim, foggy, or unclear vision or sensitivity to bright light. People with reduced contrast sensitivity often are very particular about lighting. They usually are glare sensitive or can see best over only a very narrow range of light intensity. Everyday examples of reduced contrast sensitivity might include driving in the fog or with a cloudy windshield, trying to see a projected image on a screen with a lot of stray light in a room, or seeing in very bright light such as on the water or in snow on a very bright sunny

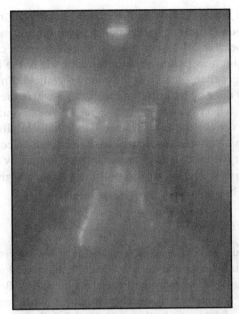

Figure 1-6. A simulated loss in contrast sensitivity due to a cloudy cornea or lens. Note acuity would also be impaired and the variable effects of lighting and increased light down the hall made features of a scene easier to see (the walls in the hallway) and others harder to see (the exit signs).

TABLE 1-3: CONTRAST OF COMMON EVERYDAY OBJECTS	
CONTRAST (%)	**OBJECT**
5	Maroon chair on maroon carpet
74	Maroon chair on gray carpet
80	Illuminated red exit sign
82	Black automobile on sunny street
32	Gray automobile on shady street
55 to 60	U.S. currency
71 to 75	Daily newspaper
76 to 80	Paperback books
88 to 93	Glossy periodicals

Adapted from Brilliant RL. *Essentials of Low Vision Practice.* Boston, MA: Butterworth-Heinemann; 1999:48-49, based on measurements by S. Whittaker.

day. Figure 1-6 illustrates how impaired contrast sensitivity might affect someone's view of a hallway. Note the variable effects of lighting.

Usually, a person with impaired contrast sensitivity will fail the screening because of poor visual acuity as well, but not always. In a visual screening, behavioral indicators of a contrast sensitivity problem include 1) difficulty reading faded print or advertisements where dark print is on a dark background, maybe of another color; 2) difficulty recognizing faces; 3) difficulty seeing the TV in a bright room; and 4) glare or light sensitivity (photophobia). If a client squints both eyes in bright light, a referral for a vision evaluation is indicated, even if other aspects of vision are fine. Glare sensitivity and problems with contrast sensitivity often may be solved by teaching someone how to optimize lighting as a first-response intervention. People sometimes complain of variable vision. If careful questioning indicates that vision depends on a person's location or lighting, this may suggest poor contrast sensitivity. For example, a person might reveal that he or she sees the TV better in the evening (after dark) than during the day, presumably when light from a bright window washes out the picture on the screen.

Definition

Contrast sensitivity determines the lowest contrast level that can be detected by a client for a given size target. Contrast can vary from no contrast (0%) to highest contrast (100%). For example, high-quality print has 85% to 95% contrast, while paper currency has only

55% to 60% contrast. Another term that is used is *contrast threshold*. Contrast threshold is defined as an object with the lowest contrast that a client can recognize. A client with normal vision can usually see objects with as little as 2% to 3% contrast. If the contrast of an object is less than the contrast threshold of the client, the object cannot be seen. Table 1-3 shows the contrast of some common everyday objects. This table indicates that the contrast of most objects is considerably higher than the normal contrast threshold of 2% to 3%. The difference between the contrast of objects and a client's contrast threshold is contrast reserve, expressed as a ratio of object contrast divided by contrast threshold. For fluent reading and presumably quick identification of objects, contrast must be greater than 10 times threshold and ideally greater than 20 times the threshold.[8,11]

Contrast sensitivity is the reciprocal of the contrast at threshold, 1/CT, where CT is the lowest contrast at which forms or lines can be recognized. If a person can see details at very low contrast, his or her contrast sensitivity is high, and vice versa. A client with a contrast threshold of 2% has higher contrast sensitivity (1/2 = 50) than a client with a contrast threshold of 10% (1/10 = 10).

Examples of Low Contrast in Activities of Daily Living

- **Communication:** The faint shadows on people's faces carry the visual information related to facial expressions.
- **Orientation and mobility:** We need to see low-contrast forms such as water on a floor, an unmarked

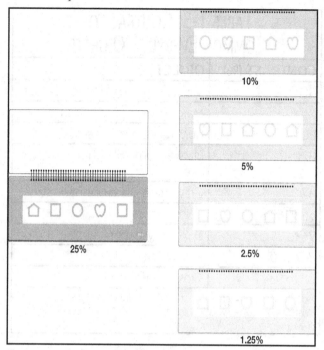

Figure 1-7. The Lea symbol contrast sensitivity booklet. The symbol sizes should be more than twice the acuity letter size at a given distance. This test and near acuity are used for lighting evaluation. (Reprinted with permission from Lea Hyvärinen [www.lea-test.fi].)

curb, faint shadows, and the last step of carpeted stairs when walking. When driving, seeing in dusk, rain, fog, snowfall, and at night are challenging tasks requiring good contrast sensitivity.

- **Reading and writing:** This includes poor-quality copies, newsprint, or an old Bible. People with vision that was normal when tested with a high-contrast letter chart in a doctor's office have lost interest in reading. The poor lighting in their living room disabled reading because of typical age-related loss in contrast sensitivity.

- **Kitchen tasks:** Cutting chicken, onions, or other light-colored objects on a white or light-colored cutting board may be difficult, as is seeing blemishes on vegetables and fruit or pouring a glass of water.

- **Self-care:** Seeing early stages of wound development, soiled skin, and soiled clothing may be problematic.

Evaluation of Contrast Sensitivity

One administers a letter contrast sensitivity test much like a visual acuity test (see Table 1-2). Be certain that the client is using the appropriate eyeglasses for near and that the symbols or numbers on the chart are large enough at a given working distance (at least 2 times acuity threshold). The client is instructed to read from higher to lower contrast on the chart much like he or she reads an acuity chart from larger to smaller font (Figure 1-7).

Both visual acuity and contrast sensitivity involve instructions to test at a set distance based on near-normal vision (see Table 1-2). For low vision, one must be careful that testing was performed at a distance where the letters were larger than the size at the acuity threshold. This can be easily done by first finding the distance where the high-contrast letters on the chart are barely visible and then making certain the test distance is one-half the distance where the high-contrast letters are barely seen. A contrast chart may be used in a lighting evaluation to quickly determine glare sensitivity and an optimum range of light (see Chapter 8).

Interventions

As indicated earlier, contrast sensitivity testing provides us with information about the client's visual function that is not available from standard visual acuity testing. Because contrast sensitivity is closely associated with reading, mobility, driving, and other activities of daily living, it is particularly important that occupational therapists know if a person has impaired contrast sensitivity. In vision rehabilitation, occupational therapists can help clients with contrast sensitivity problems by increasing the contrast of objects being viewed. Methods of modifying contrast include the environmental modifications that enhance contrast or add color contrast, lighting modifications that eliminate glare, mobility instruction, and the use of electronic magnification and viewing devices. These interventions are described in detail in Chapters 10 and 14.

VISUAL FIELD DISORDERS

Definition

The term *visual field* describes how much of the visual world an individual can see while looking straight ahead at a point of fixation. When a client has a normal visual field, he or she can see everything from the fixation point superiorly about 50 degrees, inferiorly about 70 degrees (Figure 1-8[A]), temporally (toward the ear) about 90 degrees, and nasally (toward the nose) about 60 degrees (Figure 1-8[B]). Thus, with only one eye open, a client has a horizontal visual field of about 150 degrees and vertically about 120 degrees. This is true for each eye. Note that with both eyes open, the horizontal field only increases by about 30 degrees so a person has a horizontal field of view that is 180 degrees. While only the object being viewed directly is seen clearly, the client is able to see this entire area peripherally and can perceive movement and the presence of objects or other players in the entire visual field while looking at a small object like a ball. The CMS definition of low vision is the minimum eligibility for Medicare and Medicaid reimbursement and includes not only visual acuity, but visual field as well. A person is said to be legally blind if the visual field is 20 degrees or less in the better-seeing eye. For CMS, a diagnosis of any significant visual field deficit would qualify the client for low vision rehabilitation even if visual acuity is normal. Although visual requirements for driving vary from state to state, in most states, the field requirement for driving is 120 degrees horizontally through the fixation target.

Central Versus Peripheral Field Loss

Visual field loss is usually classified as central versus peripheral. As described earlier and in Figures 1-8(A) and 1-8(B), the visual field is 150 degrees horizontally and about 120 degrees vertically. The central 10 to 20 degrees are referred to as the *central visual field*. Outside this central 20 degrees is referred to as the *peripheral visual field*. These two different patterns of visual field loss have very different functional effects as well as evaluation and treatment.

Central Visual Field Loss

Screening: Illustration and Behavioral Signs

The opening clinical scenario in this chapter, the case of Ms. Jones, had the most common visual field loss among the elderly: a central visual field loss associated with diseases of the macula, such as macular degeneration or maculopathy. This type of visual field loss is referred to as a *central scotoma*. A scotoma is defined as an island of absent or reduced vision in the visual field surrounded by an area of better vision. An example of a central scotoma is illustrated in Figure 1-9. Note that unlike many published simulations of field loss, people do not experience areas of blackness, light, or gray. The visual system just fills in the scotoma, usually with some vision that resembles the surroundings. As a result, people with central scotoma often are not even aware they have a blind area in the center of their visual field; rather, they experience everything as "being unclear" (impaired acuity) and they report objects just appear and disappear. To further confuse these individuals, the visual system sometimes fills the central scotoma with formed hallucinations such as images of people or things. This condition is called *Charles Bonnet syndrome* (see Chapter 4). Because the scotoma is central, the visual phenomena move to wherever the person is looking. One can easily appreciate how this visual confusion might exacerbate the symptoms of a milder dementia.

People with central field loss all have reduced acuity; some have reduced contrast sensitivity as well. As mentioned, other behavioral signs of central field loss include the client reporting that suddenly things appear and disappear. Indeed, the hallmark of central field loss is inconsistent vision. The signs of central vision loss most clearly emerge

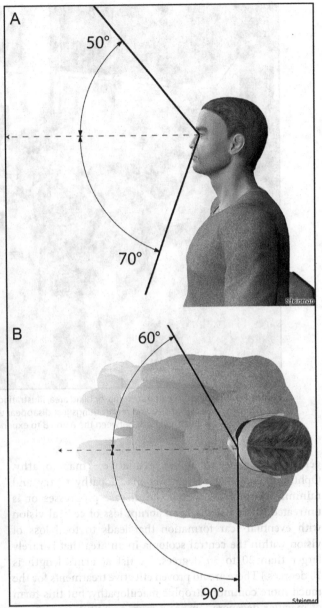

Figure 1-8. The (A) vertical and (B) horizontal visual field of one eye. Note that limitations in the monocular field of view depend on facial features like the nose and depth of the eye socket. (Reprinted with permission from Barbara Steinman.)

during reading. Even when print is enlarged to compensate for impaired acuity, words or parts of words will not be seen and will be skipped. A person with central field loss might read "somewhere" as "some" or "where" and completely miss shorter words. People who have adapted somewhat to central field loss may turn their head or move their eyes so they are not looking directly at a person's face. Also, those who have not been treated can suffer from depression and may be more confused than expected. Visual hallucinations occur when the central field loss is complete.

The 2 most common types of macular degeneration among the elderly include dry, or atrophic, macular

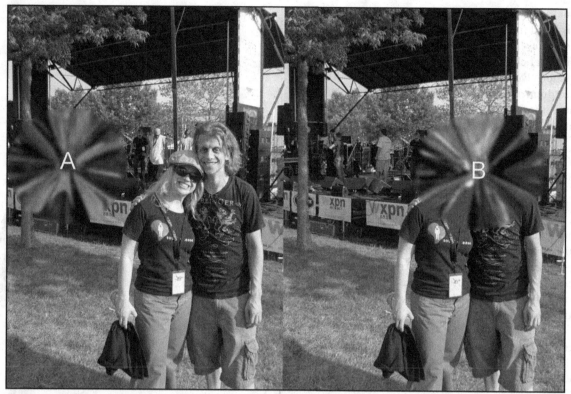

Figure 1-9. A simulated central scotoma, or blind area, illustrating how the visual system fills in the blind area. Often, people cannot experience this blind area and report things just disappear when in fact the retinal image of the object is projecting within the scotoma. Look back and forth between the A and B to experience the effect.

generation and wet, or exudative, maculopathy. Ophthalmologists can treat wet maculopathy to try and minimize visual loss, but if the disease progresses or is untreated, there usually is an abrupt loss of central vision with eventual scar formation that leads to total loss of vision within the central scotoma in an area that is rarely larger than 20 to 30 degrees. (A fist at arm's length is 10 degrees.) There are no proven effective treatments for the much more common atrophic maculopathy, but this form of macular degeneration has a more merciful progression because vision gradually deteriorates. The deterioration in vision starts at the center, but can be patchy or leave someone with a central island of better vision. Most people with the dry type of macular degeneration still have some central vision with reduced visual acuity and impaired contrast sensitivity.

Assessment and First-Response Interventions

Field testing requires a person to maintain steady fixation. Detecting a central scotoma using formal field testing is very difficult and considered a more advanced skill because people with central loss have unreliable fixation (Chapters 8 and 10). They are looking around or to the side of a target to try to see it because, as illustrated in Figure 1-9, the faces disappear when looking straight at

them. Evaluation is similar to screening: the evaluator is looking for evidence of reduced vision at the point of fixation. To detect a central scotoma, one first determines a print size at which at least some letters can be seen and notes the number of reading errors, looking for omitted words or parts of words. One test involves a simple drawing of a clock. The examiner can view the patient's eyes from behind the drawing through a peephole in the center. When asked to look at the word in the center so it is clearest, sometimes the person looks at the word and sometimes around the target. The therapist determines if words in the center or clock numerals fade if the person is looking directly at it. The Amsler grid (Figure 1-10) is another common method to identify central field loss, especially if there are distortions associated with this loss. When the client is asked to look at the center of this grid pattern, he may report some of the squares are missing or distorted, indicating a central field loss. As will be discussed in Chapter 8, evidence indicates that the Amsler grid is not a sensitive screening procedure because a central scotoma is often missed—a person's visual perception just fills in the blind area.

Low vision rehabilitation after central field loss requires advanced techniques. First-response interventions for central field loss primarily involve patient education and nonvisual interventions. The therapist demonstrates and explains to the client that the vision loss is limited to the

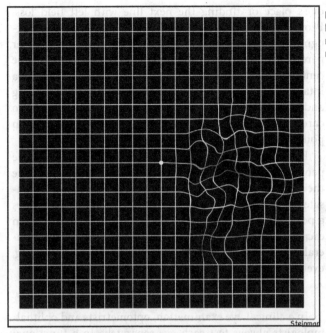

Figure 1-10. Amsler grid testing for central visual field loss. Central field loss is indicated by wavy or missing squares. Central scotomas are often missed with this technique, but are detected as missing letters during reading. (Reprinted with permission from Barbara Steinman.)

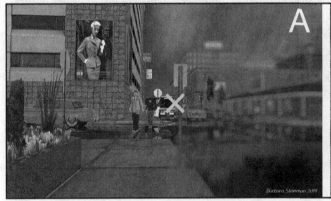
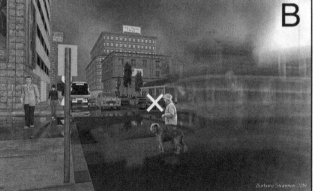

Figure 1-11. A simulation of peripheral field loss, a homonymous hemianopsia, or "field cut," common with stroke, as it might be experienced as someone (A) looks straight ahead or (B) toward the field loss. Even though vision loss is total, a person does not visualize the area of vision loss, but rather fills it in with a visual memory and is sometimes unaware of the extent of vision loss. (Reprinted with permission from Barbara Steinman.)

center of vision. Because central vision has the best vision, people with central loss often report "going blind." The therapist should carefully demonstrate using confrontation field testing (see later) how much vision a person has that is intact and the importance of using side vision to see. The client learns the reason why things disappear and that hallucinations are just a symptom of central field loss, not of mental illness. Reading is often difficult, even with considerable magnification, but can improve with training using more advanced techniques. For leisure reading, the best first-response intervention would be having someone read aloud to the client or using recorded books even for less severe vision loss (see Chapter 15). For TV, one uses relative distance magnification. For dry macular degeneration in particular, a lighting evaluation and interventions are usually very important (see Chapter 12). Otherwise, a combination of visual and nonvisual options is often used for first-response interventions (see Chapter 12).

Peripheral Field Loss

Screening: Illustration and Behavioral Signs

Peripheral field loss affects vision above, below, or to the side of where the client is looking. Figures 1-11(A) and 1-11(B) illustrate a type of vision loss associated with a cerebrovascular accident (CVA) or traumatic brain injury (TBI) that affects one side of the brain. When approximately one-half of the visual field is affected in both eyes, the right field, or the left field, the result is called a *homonymous hemianopia*, sometimes more casually referred to as a *field cut*. Note in this illustration that in our clinical experience,

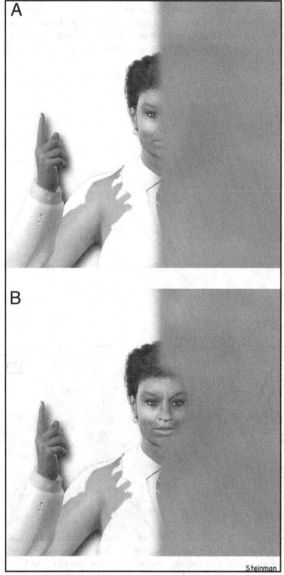

Figure 1-12. Confrontation field testing from the patient's point of view. In the gray area on the right, the client cannot see the examiner's finger wiggle and will not respond. Illustrated is a visual field loss with (A) central sparing and (B) the more debilitating split central visual field loss. (Reprinted with permission from Barbara Steinman.)

one's place or finding the next line with left field loss. People with central field loss may have object and face recognition problems that can be mistaken for higher-order perceptual problems. If the peripheral field loss spares the central visual field, leaving both sides of the macular area intact, then clients will rarely have problems with reading and object recognition. It becomes important therefore to carefully assess the extent of field loss around the fixation point.

People with field loss might bump into objects, not see people approach, have difficulty finding things, or lose their place when reading. Since one can quickly compensate by looking in the direction of the field loss, sometimes a peripheral field loss, especially with central sparing, can escape notice. The best way to test for a significant peripheral field loss is by performing confrontation field testing, even for screening.

Evaluation

In a clinical eye examination, optometrists and ophthalmologists always test each eye separately. In a functional vision evaluation, however, clients are tested under natural viewing conditions with both eyes open. If one suspects damage to the eye, optic nerve, or optic chiasm disease or damage, then it becomes necessary to test each eye separately because the field loss may differ in each eye, called a *heteronymous field loss*. Confrontation field testing is part of both the screening and more formal evaluation for first-response interventions. Since the visual field is always defined relative to where a patient is looking, it is imperative that the examiner carefully note where the client is looking during testing. To do this, the examiner "confronts," or sits in front of, the client and carefully observes the eye to see where the client is looking (see Figures 1-12[A] and 1-12[B]). The examiner asks the client to look at the examiner's nose during testing with both eyes. For functional testing, both of the client's eyes are open. The examiner asks the client to point or otherwise indicate when a finger moves. The examiner then holds his or her hands to either side and wiggles a finger on one side, always carefully watching where the client is looking. After the client shows he or she can respond reliably when the examiner places his or her hand where the client can see it, the examiner then moves his or her fingers in an attempt to find a blind area. If the client consistently fails to respond when the finger is wiggled in a particular area of the visual field, then a field loss is indicated.

When performing confrontation field tests on patients unable to follow directions or maintain fixation, the examiner can be creative with what to use as a fixation target or target in the periphery. Often with confrontation field tests, the client is asked to count fingers rather than simply detect when they wiggle. With clients who have attention problems, field testing becomes an art. With these individuals, they might tend to look at the fingers immediately

people with a field loss do not actually see a gray or black area where vision has been lost. Most commonly, the visual system fills in the blank area with remembered or expected vision as illustrated in Figure 1-11, so the person can be unaware that half of his or her visual field is missing and might try to drive. As a result, when peripheral field loss occurs, the person experiences people and objects unexpectedly "popping" into view. Often, a peripheral field loss might extend into and split the central field, sometimes splitting it in half (Figure 1-12[A]). These individuals will have functional problems similar to central field loss such as missing the ends of words with right field loss or losing after they see them. This quick glance can be the response indicating intact vision. Confrontation field testing usually does not provide a very accurate map of the seeing and nonseeing areas, but with skill and the right targets, a therapist may improve on the accuracy of this technique (see Chapter 8).

Interventions

Advanced treatment for field loss (see Chapter 12) should be part of the repertoire of any occupational therapist treating people with brain injury. In summary, the practice standard for peripheral field loss is to teach compensatory scanning, that is, to teach a client to look in the direction of the field loss. With quick, repeated habitual scanning in the direction of the loss, the client will fill in the blind area with a visual working memory of his or her surroundings. People may learn to do this without instruction, but may not look far enough to fully fill in the missing visual field. Another problem is that the client may not scan frequently enough. Thus, a person might walk up to the client on the blind side and the client may not see the person, causing a startle response. Another approach is to use other sensory cues, such as the sounds of people walking, cars driving, or smells. To teach a person to look far enough, he or she can be taught to look for "anchors," or reference points in the periphery, such as the edge of a tabletop or wall on the blind side. A person's shoulder on the blind side is a good reference point that may be used for first-response interventions, as this "anchor" is always available.

A patient with near-normal cognitive function will quickly learn these strategies; the challenge is to embed compensatory scanning as a habit so that the person will always keep scanning to the blind side, even when performing another task. Teaching habitual compensatory scanning requires repeated practice in a variety of situations and eventually when the client does not expect it. Laser tag and a progression of other suggested interventions, including the use of prisms, are detailed in Chapter 12.

SUMMARY

Vision disability is often hidden and misdiagnosed as a cognitive or perceptual impairment. In the case of Ms. Jones in the opening scenario, a nurse noticed that she could not read the menu even when enlarged, complained when the sun came through her window, and seemed not even to look at the TV when it was on. Having been taught how to screen for vision disability, the nurse alerted her therapists. The occupational therapist performed a functional vision evaluation and performed first-response interventions using materials available in her facility. The therapist found that Ms. Jones needed very large print, about 6M or 50-point font, to read comfortably but could read print as small as 3.2M (20 point) and only with light carefully positioned

from the side because Ms. Jones was quite glare sensitive. The occupational therapist advised the nursing staff, who drew the shades to reduce glare and brought in a table task light so she could see things on her table better. For written instructions, the occupational therapist employed size magnification by simply typing instructions with a greatly enlarged 50-point font using a word processor. A TV on a cart was obtained so that it could be moved close enough to see, employing the principle of relative distance magnification. The occupational therapist also educated Ms. Jones and her family about her condition, helping her understand that when she looked at objects, they "disappeared" into a central scotoma and that this condition often had hallucinations associated with it. They were greatly relieved. She also advised her family members to read to her daily, and as a result, they felt a bit more helpful during visitation. The therapist who performed the functional vision evaluation also advised all therapists involved in the case—the speech therapist was told about the best print size and the physical therapists was told how to teach her to avoid tripping hazards. Thus, because her vision disability was properly evaluated and first-response interventions were provided, Ms. Jones progressed through her therapy in an acute rehabilitation setting. Most importantly, the occupational therapist who was managing her vision interventions ensured that her discharge plan included treatment by an optometrist specializing in low vision, a certified low vision therapist who was also an occupational therapist, and a psychiatrist to manage her depression.

REFERENCES

1. Southall K, Wittich W. Barriers to low vision rehabilitation: a qualitative approach. *J Vis Impairment Blindness.* 2012;106:261-274.
2. O'Connor PM, Mu LC, Keeffe JE. Access and utilization of a new low-vision rehabilitation service. *Clin Exp Ophthalmol.* 2008;36:547-552.
3. Owsley C, McGwin G, Jr, Lee PP, Wasserman N, Searcey K. Characteristics of low-vision rehabilitation services in the United States. *Arch Ophthalmol.* 2009;127:681-689.
4. Stelmack JA, Massof RW, Stelmack TR. Is there a standard of care for eccentric viewing training? *J Rehabil Res Dev.* 2004;41:729-738.
5. Nia K, Markowitz SN. Provision and utilization of low-vision rehabilitation services in Toronto. *Can J Ophthalmol.* 2007;42:698-702.
6. Massof RW, Lidoff L. *Issues in Low Vision Rehabilitation.* New York: AFB Press; 2000:354.
7. Anonymous. *Vision Rehabilitation for Elderly Individuals with Low Vision and Blindness.* Rockvile, MD: National Institutes of Health; 2004.
8. Whittaker SG, Lovie-Kitchin JE. Visual requirements for reading. *Optom Vis Sci.* 1993;70:54-65.
9. Legge GE. *Psychophysics of Reading in Normal and Low Vision.* Mahwah, NJ: Lawrence Erlbaum Associates; 2007.
10. Haegerstrom-Portnoy G, Schneck ME, Lott LA, Brabyn JA. The relation between visual acuity and other spatial vision measures. *Optom Vis Sci.* 2000;77:653-662.
11. Crossland MD, Rubin GS. Text accessibility by people with reduced contrast sensitivity. *Optom Vis Sci.* 2012;89:1276-1281.

12. Haegerstrom-Portnoy G. The Glenn A. Fry Award Lecture 2003: Vision in elders: summary of findings of the SKI study. *Optom Vis Sci.* 2005;82:87-93.

13. West SK, Rubin GS, Broman AT, Munoz B, Bandeen-Roche K, Turano K. How does visual impairment affect performance on tasks of everyday life? The SEE Project. Salisbury Eye Evaluation. *Arch Ophthalmol.* 2002;120:774-780.

14. Hassan SE, Lovie-Kitchin JE, Woods RL. Vision and mobility performance of subjects with age-related macular degeneration. *Optom Vis Sci.* 2002;79:697-707.

15. McGwin G, Jr, Chapman V, Owsley C. Visual risk factors for driving difficulty among older drivers. *Accident Anal Prev.* 2000;32:735-744.

16. Haymes SA, Johnston AW, Heyes AD. A weighted version of the Melbourne Low-Vision ADL Index: a measure of disability impact. *Optom Vis Sci.* 2001;78:565-579.

Epidemiology, History, and Clinical Model for Low Vision Rehabilitation

2

The objectives of this chapter are to establish the importance of low vision rehabilitation for the practice of occupational therapy and to review the definitions, epidemiology, and history of low vision and low vision rehabilitation in the United States. We will also present a model of clinical care with suggested roles for the various professions involved with low vision rehabilitation.

WHY SHOULD OCCUPATIONAL THERAPISTS BE INTERESTED IN THE FIELD OF LOW VISION REHABILITATION?

Effect of Visual Impairment on Occupation

Mrs. Smith is a 75-year-old woman who recently developed age-related macular degeneration (AMD). Other than her vision problem, she has no other significant medical conditions. She has always been an active woman, working until age 67 as a real estate agent and raising her family of three children. After retirement, Mrs. Smith became active as a volunteer in both her church and local civic organizations. She has been an avid recreational tennis player and continued to play tennis twice a week with friends. Thus, she was involved in many activities, looking after herself and her family, enjoying life, and woven into the social and economic fabric of her community—that is, until AMD started slowly eating away at her lifestyle.

Mrs. Smith's vision deteriorated, and this impairment affected almost every aspect of her life. She could no longer safely drive, which created difficulty in many everyday activities, such as shopping, doctors' visits, visiting her grandchildren, maintaining her role as a volunteer at church, and playing tennis. Because of her vision impairment, she had trouble taking care of her personal needs as well. Household tasks such as cooking, thoroughly washing dishes, and finding ingredients for recipes had become frustrating and difficult to perform. After some mistakes, Mrs. Smith had to ask her son to manage the monthly task of paying bills and balancing the checkbook. Of course, she also had stopped reading for pleasure as well as everyday, essential reading tasks. Her color perception and vision had deteriorated, so she was deeply embarrassed on some occasions to discover she had mismatched clothes and

Whittaker SG, Scheiman M, Sokol-McKay DA.
Low Vision Rehabilitation: A Practical Guide for Occupational Therapists,
Second Edition (pp 19-37).
© 2016 Taylor & Francis Group.

applied her makeup incorrectly. As a result, she began to decline social invitations.

Mrs. Smith also hesitated to go to meetings, parties, and other social events because she was unable to identify people's faces. Even if she could identify a person by his or her voice, she was unable to see facial expressions, and this made it challenging to interact in a meaningful manner. This devastating combination of loss of so many specific activities of daily living (ADL), along with the negative impact on her social life, led to secondary depression and lack of desire and motivation. Not understanding what was happening, her family and friends did not make appropriate accommodations, and a handicap developed.

This case history exemplifies the effects of AMD on the life of a client with this common ocular disease. With early intervention, as each problem arose, low vision rehabilitation could have quickly and easily addressed most of the disabled activities: reading, applying makeup, playing tennis, paying bills, cooking, and participating in various social functions. Specific disabled activities are but weakened or broken threads in the fabric of a person's life. With a bit of mending, the fabric can be restored. When combined, however, these specific disabilities will unravel the fabric of a person's life, at which point restoration becomes multifaceted and complex.

This book will describe how to address many specific disabilities through a process called *low vision rehabilitation*. Using largely compensatory techniques, low vision rehabilitation restores a person's ability to perform specific activities—the "threads." This book also describes low vision rehabilitation provided by an occupational therapist that goes well beyond more traditional low vision rehabilitation service delivery to help a person restore the fabric of his or her life. The occupational therapist must be able to identify and address not only visual disabilities, but other physical disabilities and psychosocial limitations as well. Since its inception, the focus and mission of the profession of occupational therapy have been to care for people with specific needs but from a much broader perspective. The American Occupational Therapy Association (AOTA) published the second edition of the *Occupational Therapy Practice Framework*, to reaffirm and articulate occupational therapy's focus on "occupation," a term that captures the objective and subjective dimensions of everyday activities as well as the context in which the occupations are performed.[1]

From the perspective of an occupational therapist, the goals are not just to maximize vision, compensate for vision loss, or even promote independence. The occupational therapist must evaluate and possibly develop treatments that address several domains, including areas of occupation (activities), client factors (visual, other sensory, cognitive and motor functioning), performance skills, performance patterns (roles and routines), and context (social, physical, and activity demands). *The Occupational Therapy Practice Framework* outlines the language and constructs that define the profession's focus. This framework states that "all aspects of the domain are of equal value and together they interact to influence the client's engagement, participation and health."

Given this framework, it is clear that the client described earlier, and others with low vision, often require occupational therapy services. It is also clear that the occupational therapist cannot address all of the domains of practice without careful coordination with other practitioners who provide specialized services within a particular domain. The occupational therapist must understand the specific service that involves other practitioners within the context of the life of a person when the disabilities begin to emerge, and at various stages in the progression of a disease or untreated disability. The following discussion of the definition, prevalence, and incidence of low vision and the availability of resources will provide the basic information required to perform a needs analysis and even develop a proposal to provide low vision rehabilitation services. To provide low vision services, the occupational therapist must network with other professionals, who will be described toward the end of this chapter.

DEFINITIONS AND EPIDEMIOLOGY

Definition of Blindness and Low Vision

A commonly quoted prevalence figure for vision impairment in the United States is that 1 in 6 adults (17%) age 45 and older, representing 13.5 million Americans, report some form of visual impairment.[2] Massof[3] argues that this figure is inaccurate and a significant overestimation of the prevalence of low vision in the United States. There are a number of problems with determining the prevalence of blindness and visual impairment.[3,4] These problems include differences in criteria to define visual impairment, differences in study methodology, variation in methods of assessing visual acuity, and differences in the age range of the oldest category.

Differences in Criteria to Define Visual Impairment

The criteria used to define blindness and low vision vary from study to study. In the United States, the standard definition of legal blindness is nominally 20/200 or worse in the better eye and a visual field less than 20 degrees.[5] The criteria of legal blindness used for eligibility for the substantial Social Security Administration benefits use a visual efficiency score that allows some with between 20/100 and 20/200 acuity and irregular visual field loss to qualify as well,[5] but the standard definition is used most consistently in epidemiological research. There is much more variability, however, in the definition of low vision. The World Health

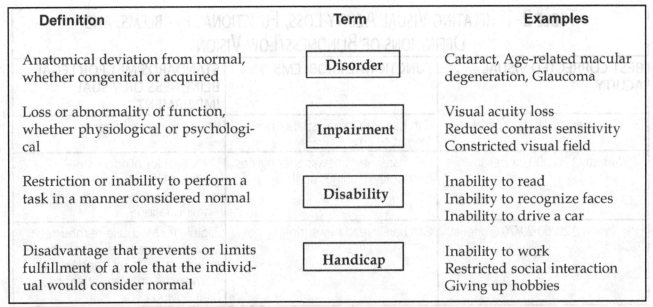

Definition	Term	Examples
Anatomical deviation from normal, whether congenital or acquired	**Disorder**	Cataract, Age-related macular degeneration, Glaucoma
Loss or abnormality of function, whether physiological or psychological	**Impairment**	Visual acuity loss Reduced contrast sensitivity Constricted visual field
Restriction or inability to perform a task in a manner considered normal	**Disability**	Inability to read Inability to recognize faces Inability to drive a car
Disadvantage that prevents or limits fulfillment of a role that the individual would consider normal	**Handicap**	Inability to work Restricted social interaction Giving up hobbies

Figure 2-1. World Health Organization terminology for impairment and disability. (Reprinted with permission from the WHO. *International Classification of Impairments, Disabilities, and Handicaps: A Manual of Classification Relating to the Consequences of Disease.* Geneva: WHO; 1980.)

Organization (WHO) proposed a classification system that is now accepted as the international standard (Figure 2-1). The definition of blindness is a visual acuity of worse than 20/400 in the better eye with best correction or a visual field diameter of less than 10 degrees in the widest meridian in the better eye. The WHO definition for low vision is worse than 20/60 in the better eye with best correction.[6] Another commonly used criterion by epidemiologists is to define low vision as corrected visual acuity worse than 20/40 in the better eye with correction.[7] This criterion is based on the ability to obtain an unrestricted driver's license. Finally, Medicare carriers have adopted the International Classification of Diseases, Clinical Modification (ICD-9, ICD-10-CM) coding system definition of low vision, which is worse than 20/60 visual acuity in the better-seeing eye, as the eligibility criterion for coverage of low vision services. Because different authors have used varying definitions of blindness and low vision, it is easy to understand the difficulty in establishing the prevalence of these conditions. The practitioner needs to be vigilant to changing definitions of low vision and blindness because this debate will lead to changes in the criteria Medicare, Medicaid, government payers, and insurance companies use for reimbursable rehabilitation services.

Table 2-1 is an attempt to help the reader appreciate the relationship among visual acuity loss, functional visual problems, and definitions of blindness and visual impairment. In this book, we define low vision as a condition caused by eye disease in which the vision is worse than 20/60 in the better eye (nominally 20/70), the vision cannot be improved with eyeglasses, and there is a loss in the central or peripheral visual fields that affects both eyes. It is important to remember that this is not necessarily

the definition that has been used in prevalence studies. However, it is a definition that makes sense in the everyday practice of low vision rehabilitation by occupational therapists because people with this level of acuity cannot read normal newsprint. This also is the definition that is currently used by Medicare to establish medical necessity for low vision rehabilitation.

The use of this definition does not preclude treating clients with visual acuity better than 20/70. Mild acuity loss—20/40, for example—can create significant disability for a client who values reading or occupations that require detail vision, such as fine needlepoint. If there are no other impairments, vision disability at this level usually can be referred to and be easily addressed by optometrists and ophthalmologists with stronger reading glasses or weak magnifiers. These services are often not covered as well. Early intervention is critical for success. Once a patient's visual acuity deteriorates to 20/70, he or she may have already started to disengage from many ADL, leading to potential depression. We feel that the primary impediment to routinely initiating therapy when visual acuity is better than 20/70 is lack of reimbursement and an eye doctor telling someone "nothing more can be done."

Differences in Study Methodology

The 2 main study methods to evaluate prevalence of low vision have been self-assessment surveys and population-based vision screening studies. The Lighthouse study quoted earlier was a telephone survey of 1219 people over the age of 45 years.[2] Data were not available about refractive error (nearsightedness, farsightedness, or astigmatism) or eye disease for the people surveyed. Massof[3] argues that some of the criteria used in the survey to determine

TABLE 2-1: RELATING VISUAL ACUITY LOSS, FUNCTIONAL PROBLEMS, AND DEFINITIONS OF BLINDNESS/LOW VISION

BEST CORRECTED VISUAL ACUITY	FUNCTIONAL PROBLEMS	STANDARDS MET FOR LEGAL BLINDNESS OR VISUAL IMPAIRMENT
6/120 (metric) 20/400 (Imperial)	Can barely read newspaper head-lines at 40 cm	WHO criteria for blindness
6/60 (metric) 20/200 (Imperial)	Can barely read newspaper bylines or chapter headings at 40 cm	US criteria for blindness, eligible for all services by state, federal agencies and Veterans Administration
6/18 (metric) 20/60-20/70 (Imperial)	Can barely read newsprint	Eligible for Medicare-reimbursed services and receive limited services from state, federal and Veterans Administration. Many states prohibit driving
6/12 (metric), 20/40 (Imperial)	Reading normal print and street signs is slower and more difficult	Impaired visual acuity becomes disabling. Legal criteria for unrestricted driving in most states

if a person had low vision could simply reflect inadequate eyeglass correction at the time of the survey. For example, the Baltimore Eye Study found that if they used presenting visual acuity only as a criterion for defining low vision, they found a prevalence of about 10.25 million people. However, 7.5 million people in this group would not actually have low vision because with new eyeglasses, their visual acuity reached normal levels. Thus, the main problem with estimating low vision prevalence from self-assessment surveys is that the cause of the reduced visual acuity is unknown.

In contrast to the self-assessment methodology, a number of population-based prevalence studies have been performed in the United States.[7-11] All of these studies measured visual acuity with refractive errors corrected and determined if eye disease was present. The results of these studies indicate that the prevalence of low vision is much lower than the estimate based on self-assessment surveys. However, even among these studies, there are differences in estimates because the studies differ in their definitions of low vision (visual acuity cutoff that determines if the client has low vision) and methodology of performing the visual acuity assessment.

Variation in Method of Assessing Visual Acuity

Generally, measures of distance visual acuity have been used to define significant vision loss, and there are 2 important sources of variation in the current literature when trying to categorize persons into affected and nonaffected groups. These include the type of acuity chart used

and the visual acuity criteria used to define the condition.[4] There is no standardized method of assessing visual acuity in clinical practice. Various charts, such as Landolt C, Snellen charts, and Sloan letters, are commonly used. In recent years, a standardized visual acuity chart was developed for research studies called the Early Treatment of Diabetic Retinopathy Study (ETDRS) acuity chart and is now the standard for research involving visual acuity measurements.[12] However, this chart has not been widely used in the literature on low vision prevalence. Only 3 of the 5 population-based studies of low vision in the United States referred to earlier used the ETDRS chart as the method for assessing distance visual acuity. Even in those studies using the ETDRS chart, the distance at which testing occurred and the method for determining the final visual acuity differed among the studies.

Differences in the Age Range of the Oldest Category

All studies, regardless of methodology, agree that the prevalence rate of low vision and blindness increases sharply with age. Various studies, however, have categorized the age brackets differently. This creates difficulty in comparing one study to another.

Prevalence of Low Vision and Blindness in the United States

In this section, we review the prevalence and incidence of low vision and blindness in the United States. This research is important to someone planning to develop a new low vision service. The planner combines these statistics with published census data to estimate the potential need for services in a given area. Prevalence refers to the current number of people suffering from an illness in a given year. This number includes all those who may have been diagnosed in prior years, as well as in the current year. For example, if the prevalence of a disease is 80,000, it means that there are 80,000 people living in the United States with this illness.

Incidence refers to the frequency of development of a new illness in a population in a certain period of time, normally 1 year. When we say that the incidence of a disease has increased in past years, we mean that more people have developed this condition year after year (eg, the incidence of some type of cancer has been rising, with 13,000 new cases diagnosed this year).

While many studies have used less than 20/40 visual acuity in the better-seeing eye as the criterion for low vision, from a practical standpoint, it is reasonable for occupational therapists to be interested in the 20/70 or worse criterion that has been adopted by Medicare carriers. Medicare is the main source of reimbursement for low vision rehabilitation for occupational therapists, and the ICD-9-CM coding system definition of low vision is worse than 20/60 visual acuity in the better-seeing eye.

Massof[3] analyzed the data from all 5 population-based studies of vision impairment in the United States. He used the 20/70 or worse criterion as the definition of low vision, along with the 2000 census data. Based on these parameters, he estimated that 1.3 million Whites and 230,000 Blacks over age 45 have low vision. Looking only at the Medicare-eligible population (65 years and older), he estimates that 1.12 million Whites and 135,000 Blacks have low vision. It is important to note that even these numbers are an overestimation because they include many potentially correctable cases of cataract (about 15% to 20%). Although these prevalence rates are certainly significant, they are only about one-tenth the number cited by other authors.[2,13]

The Eye Diseases Prevalence Research Group published data on the prevalence of visual impairment in the United States in 2004.[14] Because of the difficulty and expense of implementing an appropriate sampling scheme, few population-based studies of a national scope have been carried out in the United States to estimate the prevalence of visual impairment.[13] To meet this need for prevalence data, principal investigators from 8 population-based vision studies agreed to standardize definitions and methodology so that their data could be analyzed together. Age- and race/ethnicity-specific prevalence of blindness and low vision were calculated based on these 8 different studies. These estimates were then applied to the population of the United States as reported in the 2000 census to estimate the number of visually impaired persons nationally. Projections of

prevalence in 2020 were also made based on census projections for the US population in that year. The definition of blindness used was 20/200 or worse in the better-seeing eye, and for low vision 20/40 or worse in the better-seeing eye.

Using this approach, the authors found that in 2000 there were an estimated 937,000 blind Americans older than age 40, a prevalence of 0.78%. The number of persons with low vision was estimated to be 2.4 million (1.98% prevalence). This number is significantly higher than the estimate from Massof of about 1.5 million. The main reason for the difference is likely the definition of low vision used in each study. Massof[3] used 20/70 or worse in the better-seeing eye as the criterion, versus 20/40 or worse in the better-seeing eye used in this recent study. Because occupational therapists in the United States function within the health care system and depend primarily on Medicare funding for reimbursement of low vision rehabilitation, the lower estimate is more representative of the need for occupational therapy services for low vision rehabilitation in the United States.

More recently, a consensus meeting was convened by the National Eye Institute at which many of the world's leading ophthalmic epidemiologists created standard case definitions for the eye conditions (www.nei.nih.gov/eyedata). Data were obtained from a review of the major epidemiological studies with the cooperation of their authors. In collaboration with Prevent Blindness America, the prevalence rates have now been applied to the 2010 US Census population. Vision impairment was defined as the best-corrected visual acuity <20/40 in the better-seeing eye. Figure 2-2 illustrates the age-specific prevalence rates for vision impairment by age and race/ethnicity. The rates for all race/ethnicity groups increase dramatically in every 5-year category from age 70 and up, with the highest prevalence rates in Whites. These data show that in the >80-year-old category about 1 out of 4 people are visually impaired. The report showed that females make up 64% of visual impairment. The authors also projected that the prevalence rates would rise from about 4 million in 2010 to ~7 million in 2030 and ~13 million by 2050.

Incidence of Low Vision and Blindness

The only published incidence data (new cases of low vision each year) for the United States are from the Beaver Dam Eye Study.[15] The number of new cases of low vision and blindness is greatest for people over the age of 65 years. Based on the Beaver Dam Eye Study data, Massof[3] estimated the incidence to be about 250,000 cases per year in 2000 and 500,000 new cases per year in 2025.

The prevalence and incidence of low vision in the United States are high, and experts predict a large increase over the next 2 decades because the prevalence of low vision increases sharply in persons older than 65. In the study by Congdon et al, persons older than 80 years made up only 7.7% of the population, but accounted for 69% of the severe visual impairment.[14] It is this group

Figure 2-2. 2010 US age-specific prevalence rates for vision impairment by age and race/ethnicity. (Reprinted with permission from the National Eye Institute and Prevent Blindness America, 2010.)

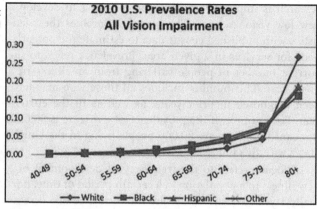

TABLE 2-2: CAUSES OF BLINDNESS (VISUAL ACUITY < 20/200) BY RACE/ETHNICITY					
	AGE-RELATED MACULAR DEGENERATION	CATARACT	GLAUCOMA	DIABETIC RETINOPATHY	OTHER
White Persons	54.4%	8.7%	5.4%	6.4%	9.7%
Black Persons	4.4%	36.8%	7.3%	26%	25.6%
Hispanic Persons	14.3%	14.3%	28.6%	14.3%	28.6%
Adapted from Congdon N, O'Colmain B, Klaver CC, et al. Causes and prevalence of visual impairment among adults in the United States. *Arch Ophthalmol.* 2004;122:477-485.					

that is the fastest-growing segment of the US population. Prevalence and incidence clearly depend on ethnicity, age, and socioeconomic variables. Someone planning to develop services should look to the most recent published research and census data to develop more precise estimates of need by considering age, ethnic, and socioeconomic composition of the region being studied.

LEADING CAUSES OF VISUAL IMPAIRMENT IN THE UNITED STATES

The leading cause of severe visual impairment among White Americans in 2000 was AMD, which accounted for 54% of visual impairment with cataract (9%). Diabetic retinopathy (6%) and glaucoma (5%) were the next most common causes[14] (Table 2-2). These conditions are described in detail in Chapter 4.

The leading causes of severe visual impairment in black persons were cataract (37%), diabetic retinopathy (26%), glaucoma (7%), and AMD (4%). Among Hispanic individuals, glaucoma was the most common cause (29%), followed by AMD (14%), cataract (14%), and diabetic retinopathy (14%).

It is surprising that there is such a high prevalence of low vision due to cataract, since it is generally a treatable condition. Surgical treatment of cataract has been shown to

be a very effective procedure. A national study of cataract surgery investigators found that 96% of the clients were improved based on Snellen visual acuity, and 89% reported improvement and satisfaction based on a 14-item instrument designed to measure functional impairment. Since cataract surgery is so successful, it is questionable whether it should even be included as a cause of low vision, because low vision is defined as a loss of vision that cannot be treated with lenses or any other medical/surgical treatment. There are, of course, some situations in which cataracts cannot be treated surgically because of other coexisting medical or ocular conditions. In such cases, cataracts could indeed be a cause of low vision. Evans and Rowlands[16] reviewed the literature to determine the prevalence of correctable visual impairment in the United Kingdom. Many of their findings apply to the United States. They reported that between 20% and 50% of older people have undetected reduced vision and the majority of these had correctable vision problems such as refractive error and cataracts. The Baltimore Eye Study found that almost 70% of people reporting low vision based on reduced visual acuity alone would not actually have low vision because with new eyeglasses, their visual acuity reaches normal levels.[7] Correctable vision impairment is associated with poorer general health, living alone, and lower socioeconomic status.[16] Often, the therapist becomes the first person to identify correctable impairment and initiate appropriate referral to an ophthalmologist or optometrist. In the meantime, when correctable vision

TABLE 2-3: LOW VISION PROFESSIONALS AND THEIR ROLES

PROFESSION	ROLE
Ophthalmologists	• Examination and diagnosis of eye disease • Treatment of eye disease • Medication • Surgery
Optometrists	• Low vision examination • Treatment of refractive error • Eyeglasses • Contact lenses • Treatment of low vision • Optical magnification • Modification of lighting and contrast
Occupational therapists	• Low vision rehabilitation examination • Low vision rehabilitation • Management of multiple disabilities
Vision rehabilitation therapists (formerly rehabilitation teachers)	• Low vision rehabilitation examination • Low vision rehabilitation, braille reading instruction
Orientation and mobility specialists	• Orientation and mobility examination • Orientation and mobility
Teachers of the visually impaired	• Special education of children with low vision and blindness
Low vision therapist	• Low vision rehabilitation examination • Low vision rehabilitation
Social worker	• Individual and group counseling, facilitate access to resources and support services

loss is encountered, the therapist needs to have available relatively inexpensive, short-term interventions that enable clients to maintain their occupations and routines until the underlying problem is corrected.

Most studies have indicated that AMD is the leading cause of low vision in developed countries.[17,18] The prevalence of AMD in low vision clinics has been reported to be between 23% and 44%.[19] Warren[20] reported on her experience as an occupational therapist working in a low vision program in an ophthalmology department. Thirty-seven percent of the clients referred for occupational therapy (low vision rehabilitation services) had AMD, 9% had diabetic retinopathy, 7% had glaucoma, 3% had neurological problems, and 44% had other miscellaneous conditions. Thus, low vision caused by AMD is the condition that occupational therapists will be most likely to treat. Note that because people with stroke and resulting hemianopia or oculomotor problems do not meet the criteria for low vision, the current estimates of low vision associated with neurological problems likely are underestimated. In these cases, the underlying condition can still be treated by an occupational therapist using the neurological diagnostic codes.

PROFESSIONS INVOLVED WITH LOW VISION CARE

Low vision rehabilitation is a relatively young, developing discipline, and occupational therapy is the newest professional addition to this field. The various professions and their roles are listed in Table 2-3. At the end of this chapter, we present our ideas about the roles and relationships for these various professions in the field of low vision rehabilitation.

Ophthalmologists

Ophthalmologists are physicians who, after graduating from medical school, specialize in the diagnosis and treatment of eye disease by completing a residency in ophthalmology. Many ophthalmologists also complete a fellowship program to further specialize in an area of ophthalmology. A number of specialty areas exist, including cataract, glaucoma, retina, cornea, pediatric ophthalmology, and neuro-ophthalmology. Considering that the most common causes of low vision are retinal and neurological pathology, the main sources of potential referrals for low vision rehabilitation are ophthalmologists specializing in retinal disease and neuro-ophthalmologists. There is no specific subspecialty of low vision in the profession of ophthalmology. Occasionally, ophthalmologists specialize in low vision rehabilitation. There are currently about 16,000 practicing ophthalmologists in the United States.

Typically, the primary areas of interest and responsibility of ophthalmologists are the diagnosis and treatment of eye disease. Treatment modalities generally involve the use of medication and surgery. Thus, clients often see the ophthalmologist first because of a perceived significant change in vision. The ophthalmologist attempts to restore normal visual function by treating the eye disease. In some cases, this fails; in other cases, the vision can never be restored to normal and the client is now faced with permanent low vision. It is at this point that the ophthalmologist should refer the client with low vision to other professionals for further evaluation and rehabilitation.

Optometrists

After graduating from a 4-year college program, optometrists complete 4 years of additional education at one of the 17 colleges of optometry in the United States. During this 4-year program, optometry students learn to diagnose and treat vision and eye health problems. Treatment modalities include the use of eyeglasses, contact lenses, eye drops and other medication, vision therapy, and low vision rehabilitation. After graduating from optometry school, some optometrists complete residency programs in specialty areas such as low vision, vision therapy, pediatrics, contact lenses, and primary care optometry.

Trying to locate a qualified low vision optometrist for a client can be challenging because the profession of optometry does not recognize specialties. Therefore, any optometrist can provide low vision services, regardless of his or her experience in this area. However, the American Academy of Optometry Low Vision Section has a diplomate program for interested optometrists. To become a diplomate in low vision, an optometrist must pass a written test, an oral examination, and a practical low vision examination. As of 2014, there were only about 60 practicing low vision diplomats worldwide. A current list of optometrists that have successfully completed this process can be found at the website for the American Academy of Optometry (www.aaopt.org).[21] The American Optometric Association also has a Low Vision Section. Although no testing program is required to become a member of this section, optometrists who have joined are likely to have a strong interest in the area of low vision. Some low vision optometrists have completed a residency program and/or a master's degree in low vision rehabilitation, while others have chosen to specialize in this area and have acquired additional knowledge and clinical skills through continuing education and independent learning. Currently there are about 36,000 optometrists in the United States, and there are about 1000 members in the Low Vision Section of the American Optometric Association.

Optometrists who specialize in low vision help those with vision problems see better, even if surgery, medications, and conventional glasses can no longer improve sight. They design and prescribe low vision devices (eg, optical, nonoptical, electronic) and make recommendations about lighting, contrast, and other environmental factors that influence vision. Low vision optometrists often work along with low vision therapists such as occupational therapists, vision rehabilitation therapists, and orientation and mobility specialists who teach clients how to use these assistive devices in ADL and assist with orientation and mobility issues.

Occupational Therapists

According to the AOTA's *Practice Framework*, occupational therapists focus on assisting people to engage in ADL or occupations that they find meaningful and purposeful. Occupational therapists' expertise lies in their knowledge of occupation and how engaging in occupations can be used to affect human performance and the effects of disease and disability.[1] Occupational therapists work with individuals who have conditions that are mentally, physically, developmentally, or emotionally disabling, including low vision.

Occupational therapists may work exclusively with individuals in a particular age group or with particular disabilities. In schools, for example, they evaluate children's abilities, recommend and provide therapy, modify classroom equipment, and help children participate as fully as possible in school programs and activities. Occupational therapy also is beneficial to the elderly population. Therapists help the elderly lead more productive, active, and independent lives through a variety of methods, including the use of adaptive equipment.

Occupational therapists in mental-health settings treat individuals who are mentally ill, developmentally disabled, or emotionally disturbed. To treat these problems, therapists choose activities that help people learn to engage in and cope with daily life. Activities include time management skills, budgeting, shopping, homemaking, and the use of public transportation. Occupational therapists also may work with individuals who are dealing with alcoholism, drug abuse, depression, eating disorders, or stress-related disorders.

Currently, a master's degree or higher is the minimum educational requirement. All states and the District of Columbia regulate the practice of occupational therapy. To obtain a license, applicants must graduate from an accredited educational program and pass a national certification examination. The National Board for Certification in Occupational Therapy, Inc (NBCOT) is a not-for-profit credentialing agency that provides certification for the occupational therapy profession. Those who pass the exam are awarded the title Occupational Therapist Registered (OTR).

As of 2013, entry-level education was offered in about 155 master's degree programs (with 4 more programs in development) and 6 entry-level doctoral programs (with 4 more programs in development).

Occupational therapists have been peripherally involved in the rehabilitation of clients with low vision since the early days of the profession in 1917.[20] Their involvement, however, was never as the main caregiver for low vision clients. Rather, if a client with other disabilities also happened to have low vision, the occupational therapist would attempt to take care of these needs as well. Until recently, low vision rehabilitation was rarely the primary focus of occupational therapists. This all changed in 1990, when the Health Care Finance Administration (HCFA) expanded the definition of physical impairment to include low vision as a condition that can benefit from rehabilitation. With this change, physicians could specifically refer clients with only low vision to occupational therapists for low vision rehabilitation services.[20]

Occupational therapists are currently the only therapists among the group described in this chapter that are licensed and can function independently in the Medicare reimbursement program. Thus, occupational therapists have a unique opportunity to make an impact as providers for the older client with low vision in the United States. Three other professions have been providing rehabilitation services for people with low vision for decades.

In 2006, the AOTA introduced a program in which an occupational therapist or occupational therapy assistant who has substantial clinical experience may achieve Specialty Certification in Low Vision rehabilitation (SCLV). Occupational therapists are eligible and often pursue additional education and clinical experience and become certified as any of the other mentioned low vision and blindness professionals. Certification for these other professions is provided by the Academy for Certification of Vision Rehabilitation and Education Professionals (ACVREP).

Vision Rehabilitation Therapists

Once called rehabilitation teachers, certified vision rehabilitation therapists (CVRTs)[22] constitute a cadre of university-trained professionals who address the broad array of skills needed by individuals who are blind and visually impaired to live independently at home, to obtain employment, and to participate in community life. As a discipline, vision rehabilitation therapy combines and applies the best principles of adaptive rehabilitation, adult education, and social work to the following broad areas: home management, personal management, communication and education, ADL, leisure activities, and indoor orientation skills.

Vision rehabilitation therapists provide instruction and guidance in adaptive independent living skills, enabling individuals who are blind and visually impaired to confidently carry out their daily activities. Historically, vision rehabilitation therapists have emphasized use of nonvisual strategies, although they have certainly employed low vision techniques as well. Vision rehabilitation therapists are also qualified to teach braille. They are active members of multidisciplinary and interdisciplinary service teams and provide consultation and referrals through the utilization of community resources. Vision rehabilitation therapists provide services in a variety of settings: agencies serving people who are blind and visually impaired, community-based rehabilitation teaching services, centers for people with developmental disabilities, state vocational rehabilitation services, hospital and clinic rehabilitation teams, residential schools, and local school districts.[23]

There are currently about 10 colleges and universities in the United States, Canada, central Europe, and New Zealand that provide either a bachelor's or master's degree or a certificate in vision rehabilitation therapy. Six of these universities are located in the United States.[23]

There is currently no state licensing for vision rehabilitation therapists; however, a national certification process is administered by ACVREP. When a vision rehabilitation therapist becomes certified, he or she can use the initials CVRT with his or her signature.

Certified vision rehabilitation therapists are currently not eligible Medicare providers. A recent policy change by the Centers for Medicare & Medicaid Services (CMS) also prevents ophthalmologists and optometrists from billing for services provided by vision rehabilitation therapists who are salaried to work with their clients.

Orientation and Mobility Specialists

Certified orientation and mobility specialists (COMSs) are professionals who specialize in teaching travel skills to persons who are visually impaired, including the use of a sighted guide, a long mobility cane, and a variety of electronic travel devices. They teach route planning, analysis of street crossings, and use of public transportation. They will help to determine if their clients are suitable candidates for use of a guide dog, and can refer them to a nearby guide dog school. The goal of orientation and mobility instruction is to enable individuals with visual impairments to become familiar with new environments and travel safely, efficiently, confidently, and independently throughout their environment. Certified orientation and mobility specialists are prepared to work with individuals of all ages, including young children.

To become a COMS, one must attend an undergraduate or graduate program accredited by the Association for Education and Rehabilitation of the Blind and Visually Impaired (AER), although certification programs may be developed for people with undergraduate degrees. At present, there are approximately 19 programs that prepare COMSs.[23] The majority of COMS programs are at the graduate level and attract students with diverse backgrounds, including the social and physical sciences, art and music therapy, and general education.

Certified orientation and mobility specialists are also currently not eligible Medicare providers, but were part of the CMS Low Vision Rehabilitation Demonstration Project that began in April 2006.

Teachers of the Visually Impaired

The profession that takes care of the needs of children with low vision is the teacher of children with visual impairments (TVI). These individuals generally acquire the common core of knowledge and skills essential for all beginning special education teachers in addition to the specialized body of knowledge required for teachers of students with visual impairments.[22] Teachers of children with visual impairments work with blind and visually impaired infants, children, and youth of all ages, including those with multiple disabilities. They apply low vision and blindness adaptive equipment and strategies and, like vision rehabilitation therapists, are qualified to teach braille. Teachers of children with visual impairments often operate as itinerant teachers, traveling from school to school to serve children where they are located. They serve as the child's primary case manager in school, and may solicit the expertise of additional therapists to develop specific goals and objectives that comprise the child's Individualized Education Plan (IEP).

Teachers of children with visual impairments are prepared in accredited higher education programs in the United States and Canada recognized by the AER. At present, there are approximately 40 institutions of higher learning offering special education programs for teacher preparation in the area of blindness and low vision.[22] Teacher of children with visual impairments programs

often recommend or require prior degrees or certification in elementary, secondary, or special education. Teachers of children with visual impairments are certified through their appropriate state's Department of Education.

Low Vision Therapists

Therapists engage in low vision rehabilitation and have been certified by the ACVREP as certified low vision therapists (CLVTs). This term is actually trademarked and can only be used by someone who has been certified by the ACVREP. An individual who has been certified as a low vision therapist by the ACVREP will have the initials CLVT after his or her name and degree. Two universities currently offer graduate-level programs in low vision therapy. Salus University offers both a master's degree and certificate, while the University of Alabama, Birmingham offers a certificate. There are ACVREP-approved providers of online educational programs as well. However, the term "low vision therapist" is also being used in the low vision field to describe any therapist engaged in low vision rehabilitation. To become a low vision therapist, one must pass a national certification examination administered by the ACVREP. To be eligible for this examination, one must possess a bachelor's degree. Thus, a vision rehabilitation therapist, a COMS, a TVI, an occupational therapist, a physical therapist, and a nurse would all be qualified to take this examination. There is no licensure for low vision therapists, and such a person would not be eligible for Medicare reimbursement as an independent practitioner, with the exception of the occupational or physical therapist. These 2 professionals would be eligible because they are already part of the health care and Medicare systems. Many occupational therapists also have become CLVTs with additional continuing education, by passing a certification exam, and also completing supervised clinical training.

Social Workers

Social workers help people function optimally in their environment, deal with their relationships, and solve personal and family problems. Social workers often see clients who face a life-threatening disease or a social problem, such as inadequate housing, unemployment, a serious illness, a disability, or substance abuse. Social workers also assist families that have serious domestic conflicts, sometimes involving child or spousal abuse. Social workers often provide social services in health-related settings that now are governed by managed care organizations.

In regard to low vision rehabilitation, social workers provide individual and group counseling and facilitate consumer access to appropriate community-based services, including public assistance programs, rehabilitation programs, senior centers, hospitals, and clinics.[24] They use self-help techniques to assist blind and visually impaired adults who may be economically, physically, mentally, or socially in need of vision-related rehabilitation services.[24] Because of the significant psychosocial problems related to vision impairment, social workers play a key role in the field of vision rehabilitation.

Although a bachelor's degree is sufficient for entry into the field, an advanced degree has become the standard for many positions. A master's degree in social work (MSW) is typically required for positions in health settings and is required for clinical work as well. As of 2004, the Council on Social Work Education (CSWE) accredited 442 bachelor's degree in social work (BSW) programs and 168 MSW programs. All states and the District of Columbia have licensing, certification, or registration requirements regarding social work practice and the use of professional titles. Most states require 2 years (3000 hours) of supervised clinical experience for licensure of clinical social workers. In addition, the National Association of Social Workers (NASW) offers voluntary credentials. Social workers with an MSW may be eligible for the Academy of Certified Social Workers (ACSW), the Qualified Clinical Social Worker (QCSW), or the Diplomate in Clinical Social Work (DCSW) credential, based on their professional experience.

HISTORY OF LOW VISION

General History

Eye care professionals have been treating correctable vision problems such as myopia (nearsightedness), hyperopia (farsightedness), and astigmatism for centuries using eyeglasses and, more recently, contact lenses and refractive surgery. Blindness teaching and rehabilitation, a profession as old as occupational therapy, initially emphasized use of the other senses. However, attempts to help people with permanent vision loss secondary to eye disease make best use of their remaining vision is a relatively new phenomenon.[25] Earlier in this chapter, we demonstrated that the incidence and prevalence of low vision are currently quite high, and as the population ages, these numbers are expected to grow significantly. However, until the mid-20th century, the prevalence of low vision was not significant and most of the care provided was for children with blindness and visual impairment. We know that the most common causes of low vision—macular degeneration, diabetic retinopathy, glaucoma, and cataract—are all diseases related to the aging process. Given the fact that age is the single best predictor of low vision[25] and that longer life expectancy has characterized the 20th century, it is not surprising that more attention has been given to low vision rehabilitation in the past 50 years.

Goodrich has written extensively about the history of low vision[25-29] and divided low vision history into a number of stages that are summarized in Table 2-4.[26] In the following summary, we have modified his 5 stages into 4.

Pre-1950

This was a time period during which low vision rehabilitation for adults essentially did not exist. Most services were provided for blind children, and little distinction was made between those children who were blind and those who had low vision. A common belief at the time was that it was important to prevent further loss of vision in these children by restricting the use of their eyes. By the end of the 1940s, about 17 residential schools for the blind had been established with specially equipped classrooms for children with low vision. While some schools began to question whether blind children should be separated from those with low vision, the principle of sight conservation prevailed in the majority of schools.[26] This was the era in which the rehabilitation teachers and TVIs became defined as professions.

In 1934, the American Medical Association (AMA) defined legal blindness as visual acuity 20/200 or worse in the better-seeing eye. This definition was adopted for establishing eligibility for special services and benefits for the blind in the Social Security Act of 1935. This stage of low vision history was also the era in which William Feinbloom, an optometrist and pioneer in low vision, began to develop numerous optical devices for people with low vision. Some of the earliest journal articles about low vision were written by William Feinbloom.[30,31] Nevertheless, the field of low vision rehabilitation was in its infancy.

1950s to 1970s

From the 1950s to 1970s, low vision rehabilitation for adults finally became a priority for the various professions involved in low vision care. With the return of veterans from World War II and with the increasing life expectancy of the population, the number of people with "low" but usable vision increased, leading to a greater demand for low vision services. This led to the development of a low vision service delivery system that has been called the *blindness system*, the educational rehabilitation model, or the nonmedical vision rehabilitation system.[29] This system is a comprehensive nationwide network of services consisting of state, federal, and private agencies serving children and adults with blindness and low vision.[32] Table 2-5 lists the 4 components of the blindness or nonmedical rehabilitation system in the United States.

One of the key components in this system of care has been the Veterans Administration (VA). In the 1950s, the VA was among the first organizations to establish comprehensive low vision care and has served as a model for others.[33] Two well-known private agencies also started comprehensive low vision programs in the 1950s. The Industrial Home for the Blind began in 1953, and the Lighthouse (New York Association for the Blind) in 1955. The professionals working in the blindness system included

TABLE 2-4: HISTORY OF LOW VISION—FIVE STAGES

STAGE	KEY ISSUES/DEVELOPMENTS
Stage 1: Pre-1950	• No distinction between blindness and low vision • Almost all services provided to children • Commonly believed that children with poor vision needed to restrict the use of their eyes to prevent further loss (sight-saving programs) • Residential schools for the blind established (by the end of the 1940s, 17 schools established) • In 1934, the AMA defined legal blindness • 1930s William Feinbloom (optometrist) began developing optical devices for people with low vision
Stage 2: 1950s to 1970s	• Various professional disciplines developed knowledge bases for treating people with low vision • Beginning of "blindness system" for low vision rehabilitation with adults • Emphasis on sight-saving for children replaced by concept of low vision rehabilitation • Optometrists and ophthalmologists developed reliable tools for assessment of vision and new optical devices for the treatment of low vision • Optometrists and ophthalmologists develop low vision practices
Stage 3: Mid-1970s to mid-1980s	• Concept of team approach to low vision care developed • Low vision becomes more prevalent as life expectancy increases • Expansion of low vision rehabilitation programs • Significant increase in low vision research
Stage 4: Mid-1980s to mid-1990s	• Significant increase in low vision research continues • Significant expansion of the interdisciplinary approach • Professionals of each discipline become more familiar with philosophies, skills, and techniques of associated disciplines
Stage 5: Present	• Important changes in Medicare lead to changes in delivery system for low vision rehabilitation, including occupational therapists for the first time • Significant increase in low vision research continues

Adapted from Goodrich GL, Sowell V. Low vision: a history in progress. In: Corn AL, Koenig AJ, eds. *Foundations of Low Vision: Clinical and Functional Perspectives.* New York: American Foundation for the Blind; 2000.

TABLE 2-5: FOUR MAJOR SUBSYSTEMS OF BLINDNESS SERVICES IN THE UNITED STATES

1. Federal and state vocational rehabilitation system administered by the Rehabilitation Services Administration (RSA) of the US Department of Education, Office of Special Education and Rehabilitative Services, which serves primarily adults

2. The US Department of Veterans Affairs

3. The private nonprofit sector, which serves both children and adults

4. The Office of Special Education Programs, which primarily serves children through its educational services

Adapted from Ponchillia PE, Ponchillia SV. *Foundations of Rehabilitation Teaching with Persons Who Are Blind or Visually Impaired.* New York, NY: American Foundation for the Blind; 1996:3-21.

optometrists, ophthalmologists, rehabilitation teachers, COMSs, and TVIs. The blindness system is separate from the traditional health care system in the United States, and services provided are not reimbursed by Medicare or any other type of health insurance. Occupational therapists have generally not been part of this system of care.

The blindness system has been chronically underfunded. As a result, agencies have had to prioritize their services, generally favoring children and young adults of working age. In addition, the limited number of rehabilitation professionals in the blindness system primarily work in metropolitan areas. Thus, for many older clients and for those not living in large metropolitan areas, low vision rehabilitation has not been readily available through the blindness system.[13]

This is also the time period in which educators developed new methods for teaching children with low vision how to more effectively use their vision, rather than trying to conserve their vision. This movement was led by Natalie Barraga, who developed a visual efficiency scale and a set of sequential learning activities designed to develop "visual efficiency" in children with low vision.[34,35]

Finally, this was the era in which a number of influential books on low vision care were published, when a variety of professional organizations devoted significant time at conferences to low vision, and new testing equipment and optical devices, including the first video magnification units, were developed.

1970s to 1990s

From the 1970s to the 1990s, the team approach to low vision care gained momentum as professionals from various disciplines became more familiar with the philosophies, skills, and techniques of associated disciplines.[26] As life expectancy continued to increase, the prevalence of low vision in the elderly population grew and fueled the expansion of low vision programs. This era also saw a significant increase in the quantity and quality of research on low vision. This started with a National Eye Institute initiative in the mid-1980s, and the growth in low vision research continues to grow today with publications in major vision and vision rehabilitation journals throughout the world. Starting with maybe a dozen publications before 1950, the number of publications has doubled every decade to approximately 3700 between 1990 and 2000.[29]

1990s to Present

"The last decade of the twentieth century produced what is perhaps the greatest change in vision rehabilitation since the 1950s."[25] Beginning in the late 1980s, the federal government dramatically reduced funds for programs that provided services to individuals who were blind or visually impaired. Subsequently, in 1991, the HCFA, which administered Medicare, amended its definition of physical impairment to include visual impairment. This change allowed Medicare coverage for the first time by licensed health care providers for low vision rehabilitation with vision loss as the primary diagnosis when prescribed by a physician. This amendment also set the stage for the involvement of occupational therapy in the field of low vision rehabilitation.

This delivery system of low vision rehabilitation service is sometimes referred to as the "health care system" in contrast to the blindness system described earlier. Because Medicare does not recognize vision rehabilitation therapists or COMSs as licensed health care providers, these professionals are not reimbursed for their services through Medicare. While these changes were certainly welcomed by occupational therapists, other professionals such as rehabilitation therapists, COMSs, and low vision therapists were concerned about being left out of this alternative system for providing low vision rehabilitation. In addition, some vision rehabilitation therapists even expressed concern about the ability of occupational therapists to provide low vision rehabilitation care, as indicated in the following statement from a report of the American Foundation for the Blind's National Task Force on General and Specialized Services, Working Group on Allied Health Professional Relationships:

> Professionals in the vision field are demonstrating a heightened awareness of a concern about the increasing number of allied health professionals (ie, occupational therapists) who are providing vision-related services that have been traditionally administered by trained and certified rehabilitation teachers, teachers of students with visual impairments, O&M specialists, and low vision therapists.[36]

Orr and Huebner go on to state that "the concern of professionals in the vision field is that allied health professionals may not have the specialized knowledge base and skills needed to work with this population because they have not received university training in rehabilitation teaching and/ or O&M."[37]

There have been several failed attempts to introduce legislation to the US Congress that provides Medicare coverage for vision rehabilitation professionals other than occupational therapists. The Medicare Low Vision Demonstration Project was a most recent attempt started in April 2006. It was designed as a 5-year project to help deliver services in a new manner and evaluate the utilization of Medicare funding for vision rehabilitation services by a new set of providers who had not previously been covered by Medicare: CLVTs, COMSs, and vision rehabilitation therapists. In order to participate, service providers had to be certified by the ACVREP. Under this demonstration project, these professionals were supposed to provide training to persons with a documented visual impairment under the "general supervision" of an optometrist or ophthalmologist (in which the supervising physician does not need to be present), rather than "incident to" supervision (in which the supervisor does need to be present). The advantage of general supervision is that vision rehabilitation services may be provided in a patient's home or assisted living center, where the supervising physician would not be present. This new model of service delivery was the thrust of the demonstration project; however, the demonstration project also covered vision rehabilitation training that may be provided in the eye care specialist's office or at a qualified agency. This project was not managed well and had inconclusive results. The topic of Medicare coverage for low vision rehabilitation will be covered in detail in Chapter 21.

History of Occupational Therapy Involvement in Low Vision Rehabilitation

The impetus for occupational therapy's involvement in the area of low vision rehabilitation was the 1991 amendment by the HCFA that allowed Medicare coverage for the first time for licensed health care providers for low vision rehabilitation. Since that time, efforts have been made at the national, state, and local levels to enable occupational therapy to play a primary role in low vision rehabilitation.

Mary Warren has been a strong advocate of occupational therapy involvement in low vision rehabilitation. She has led the way with significant publications,[13,20,36-41] national leadership,[41] presentation of many continuing education courses, clinical work as an occupational therapist treating clients with low vision,[20] and helping to establish a university-based training program in low vision rehabilitation for occupational therapists at the University of Alabama, Birmingham. In 1995, she stated, "Although occupational therapists have been involved in the rehabilitation of persons with vision loss since the inception of the profession in 1917, we never played an extensive role in low vision rehabilitation."[36] Occupational therapists have indeed always played a role in low vision rehabilitation because nearly two-thirds of older adults with low vision have at least one other chronic medical condition that may interfere with ADL and require occupational therapy.[42] Thus, in the context of providing care for other chronic conditions, occupational therapists routinely manage issues related to low vision to some degree in their elderly clients.

However, with the inclusion of low vision as a disability under Medicare guidelines in the early 1990s, occupational therapists now have a primary role to play in this field. This sudden involvement by occupational therapists in low vision rehabilitation has led to some controversy. The primary basis for this controversy was a perception that the impetus for occupational therapy's entrance into the low vision arena was not a change in education and preparation of its practitioners. Rather, it was purely based on reimbursement issues. Thus, other vision rehabilitation therapists have raised questions about occupational therapists' qualifications, education, and clinical experience in

the area of low vision. For example, Lambert[42] raised the following concerns about occupational therapists:

- They may be unfamiliar with the various disciplines in the field, and thereby fail to appropriately refer clients for other needed services.

- They may have inadequate knowledge or specialized training in low vision.

- Clinics may favor occupational therapy in the delivery of low vision services even though more disability-specific professionals may be the most appropriate provider.

As discussed earlier, similar concerns were raised by Orr and Huebner in 2001[37] when they expressed their unease about occupational therapists' lack of specialized knowledge base and skills needed to work with the low vision population.

Others have argued that there are a number of important reasons why the occupational therapist should play a primary role in low vision rehabilitation.[36,43] These reasons include the following:

- Although the elderly comprise the majority of the low vision population, they are the most underserved by existing state, charitable, and private programs. Because of the lack of availability of services through the blindness system, rehabilitation may be delayed, and these individuals are likely to become socially isolated, depressed, and dependent. Involvement of occupational therapists through the health care system provides significantly greater access to low vision rehabilitation for the elderly.[43]

- Two-thirds of older persons have at least one other chronic condition, in addition to low vision, that limits their independent functioning. Occupational therapists are already primary providers for older clients with other chronic conditions.[36,43] Occupational therapists are trained in the physical, cognitive, sensory, and psychological aspects of disability and aging and, therefore, may be the natural choice of professionals to work with older persons whose limitations in ADL are a result of a combination of deficits.[36]

- Occupational therapists are more evenly distributed throughout the United States than COMSs and vision rehabilitation therapists, who tend to be located in larger metropolitan areas. Low vision services can be more widely disseminated through the health care delivery system.[36]

Occupational therapy as a profession, as well as individual therapists, has reacted in a positive way to this debate. In the past 15 years, many occupational therapists have gained the knowledge base and clinical skills necessary to provide excellent care to clients requiring low vision rehabilitation. Low vision rehabilitation is now being included in the curricula of a number of occupational therapy programs.[44]

This has been accomplished through a variety of learning formats, including independent study, continuing education courses, clinical internships, and university-based training. In addition, many occupational therapists have completed the same national certification programs that other low vision rehabilitation professionals must complete. This certification process is run by the ACVREP, which was established in January 2000. It is an independent and autonomous legal certification body governed by a volunteer board of directors. The mission of ACVREP is to offer professional certification for vision rehabilitation and education professionals in order to improve service delivery to persons with vision impairments.

In 1995, the AOTA devoted its entire October issue to the topic of low vision, and in 1998 developed the *Occupational Therapy Practice Guidelines for Adults with Low Vision*, which was recently updated in 2013 under the title *Occupational Therapy Practice Guidelines for Older Adults with Low Vision*. In recent years, the AOTA has listed low vision rehabilitation as one of the "10 emerging areas" of clinical practice for occupational therapists. The AOTA also created a low vision panel to develop a set of competencies by which occupational therapists and occupational therapy assistants can achieve specialty certification from the AOTA, indicating that they have acquired the knowledge and skills to be specialists in low vision intervention.[45]

About 20 years in the history of a profession is a relatively short time. Yet within this time frame, occupational therapy has made dramatic strides toward becoming a primary care provider in the area of vision rehabilitation. With the need for these services growing significantly as the US population grows older, there is a need for many more occupational therapists to become involved in this exciting area of practice. As occupational therapists become involved, it is critical to be aware of the history of low vision rehabilitation in the United States, the various professions involved, and some of the sensitivities and important political issues described earlier.

CLINICAL MODEL

Although the blindness system, or educational model of low vision rehabilitation, has been the dominant system since the 1950s, the 4 factors listed next challenge the continued viability of this model of care:

1. Growing demand for low vision services: The demand for low vision services is expected to grow rapidly in the next decade. The population of the United States is aging, and the prevalence of eye disease that causes low vision is greatest in people 65 years of age and older. More therapists are needed to meet this demand.

2. Poor distribution of vision rehabilitation providers: Vision rehabilitation therapists and COMSs are not well distributed throughout the country and number under 4000. They tend to be located in larger metropolitan areas. As a result, large numbers of people requiring low vision rehabilitation could not be served within this model.

3. Decrease in funding for the blindness system: There have been significant budget cuts, creating funding problems and limited availability of services for the older population.

Changes in Medicare: Changes in Medicare policy over the past decade now allow occupational therapists to provide low vision rehabilitation in medical settings such as hospitals, outpatient clinics, nursing homes, and clients' homes. There about 115,000 occupational therapy jobs and another 35,000 occupational therapists in the United States.

Massof[46] proposed a practice model for standardizing low vision rehabilitation as a health care service (Table 2-6). He and others have emphasized the similarities between physical medicine and rehabilitation (PM&R) and low vision rehabilitation.[46-48]

According to Fishburn,[48] the aims of PM&R are to prevent injury or frailty, minimize pathology, prevent secondary complications, enhance function of involved systems, and develop compensatory strategies. She argues that these are essentially the same aims of low vision rehabilitation. In addition, many clients now being served within the PM&R system have low vision as a secondary disability. The primary reason for their rehabilitation might be physical, neurologic, or cognitive impairments caused by stroke, diabetes, brain injury, or demyelinating disease.[48] Thus, low vision rehabilitation should be part of the larger rehabilitation system. We agree with this approach and believe that this model addresses each of the 4 issues listed earlier.

When designing a model for vision rehabilitation, it is also important to review the WHO vocabulary defining impairment and disability. In 1980, the WHO proposed 4 terms that should be used when defining impairment and disability.[5] This terminology is illustrated in Figure 2-1.

- A *disorder* is an anatomical deviation from normal and can be congenital or acquired. Examples of visual disorders causing low vision are AMD, diabetic retinopathy, glaucoma, and cataract.

- *Impairment* is a loss or abnormality in function. The impairment can be either physiological or psychological. Visual impairments include decreased visual acuity, reduced contrast sensitivity, central scotomas (blind spots in the center of the visual field), and constricted visual fields.

- *Disability* refers to a restriction or an inability to perform a task in the normal way. Examples are difficulty reading newspaper print, recognizing faces, and driving a car.

TABLE 2-6: LOW VISION REHABILITATION IN THE US HEALTH CARE SYSTEM SERVICE DELIVERY MODEL

PHYSICAL MEDICINE AND REHABILITATION PROFESSIONAL	ROLE	LOW VISION REHABILITATION PROFESSIONAL
Physiatrist	Responsible for evaluating the client, diagnosing functional disabilities, planning therapy, coordinating health care, and performing procedures that are within the purview only of a licensed physician	Ophthalmologist Optometrist
Occupational therapist	Specializes in the rehabilitation of daily living and other functional activities	Occupational therapist Vision rehabilitation therapist
Physical therapist	Specializes in mobility training, joint mobilization, and muscle-strengthening exercises	Orientation and mobility specialist
Social worker	Helps the client and family cope with psychosocial issues related to disabilities and to identify and use resources	Social worker

Based on model proposed by Massof RW, et al. Low vision rehabilitation in the U.S. health care system. *J Vis Rehab.* 1995;9(3):3-31.

- *Handicap* is a disadvantage that prevents or limits the fulfillment of a role that is normal for the client. Examples are the inability to work or engage in hobbies, and restricted social interactions. A handicap results from a failure by a community or society to provide accommodation.

In the model presented next, the ophthalmologist and optometrist are primarily interested in the disorder and impairment, while the occupational therapist manages the disability and handicap, although there may be overlap in some areas.

Role of the Ophthalmologist

The role of the ophthalmologist is to diagnose and treat the eye disease. This might involve the use of medication or surgery. When it is clear that vision has been permanently impaired due to the eye disease, the ophthalmologist refers the patient to a low vision optometrist for evaluation and treatment.

Role of the Low Vision Optometrist

The optometric low vision examination is described in detail in Chapter 7. The evaluation includes the components listed in Table 2-7.

Although occasionally ophthalmologists specialize in low vision rehabilitation, typically, optometrists specialize in low vision rehabilitation. The role of the low vision optometrist is to evaluate the patient and determine whether a change in the traditional eyeglass prescription might be of benefit. The optometrist also performs a detailed

TABLE 2-7: OPTOMETRIC LOW VISION EVALUATION

- Case history
- Distance visual acuities
- Near visual acuities
- Central visual field testing
- Color vision testing
- Visual/mobility field testing
- Contrast sensitivity testing
- Refraction
- Eye health evaluation
- Magnification evaluation

evaluation of distance and near visual acuity, contrast sensitivity, assessment of central scotomas, and peripheral visual field. Based on the results of this evaluation and the case history, the optometrist begins the process of determining the magnification needs of the client and recommends devices and treatments, much like a physiatrist would be involved in a medical rehabilitation setting. The occupational therapist works with the optometrist to evaluate and recommend devices and develop a treatment plan. The low vision optometrist is then the physician to approve the treatment plan, which prescribes appropriate low vision optical aids. In an older model of service delivery, the optometrist would prescribe devices and the occupational therapist would provide training with these devices. Under the newer model presented in this book, the process of selecting devices and development of a treatment plan require consideration of all domains and should be a collaborative effort.

Role of the Occupational Therapist

The role of the occupational therapist is to determine the cognitive, psychosocial, and physical needs of the client to resume meaningful roles, routines, and occupation. The occupational therapist performs a comprehensive evaluation of the client's performance areas such as ADL and instrumental activities of daily living (IADL), education, work, play, leisure, and social participation.[1] According to the AOTA *Practice Framework*, ADL refers to activities that are oriented toward taking care of one's own body, such as bathing, bowel and bladder management, dressing, eating, feeding, functional mobility, personal device care, and personal hygiene.[1] Instrumental activities of daily living refer to activities that are oriented toward interacting with the environment and are generally optional in nature, such as care of others, child rearing, communication device use, community mobility, financial management, health management, and meal preparation.[1] The occupational therapy low vision evaluation includes review of the reports from the ophthalmologist and low vision optometrist, and further evaluation of the impairment as needed to identify what client and contextual factors might present barriers to performance. This evaluation is described in detail in Chapter 8.

Based on the results of the optometric low vision evaluation and the occupational therapy evaluation, the therapist designs a vision rehabilitation treatment program to enable the client to achieve the established performance goals. The rehabilitation program should include education about the functional implications of visual impairment; management of psychosocial issues; referral to community resources; teaching the client visual scanning skills that optimize the use of remaining vision; the use of both optical and nonoptical assistive devices in ADL; and environmental modifications, including management of lighting, contrast, and glare. In most states, a physician must approve and periodically review the occupational therapy treatment plan. In our model of care, ideally the physician approving the plan should be a low vision optometrist even in states in which approval is not required. Low vision rehabilitation is more effective with the specialized expertise of a low vision optometrist because rehabilitation requires integrated management of the visual effects of the disease, refractive error, and the optical demands of a task. Because there are so few optometrists who specialize in low vision, the occupational therapist may need to work with a general optometrist. Other potential referrals include orientation and mobility, vision rehabilitation therapy (depending on the depth of expertise of the occupational therapist and the time constraints of the reimbursement party), and social work.

An important issue is how the occupational therapist interacts with eye care providers. In the earlier sections, we described a typical model where the ophthalmologist will generally refer the client to a low vision optometrist for further evaluation and treatment. Then the optometrist refers to the occupational therapist. There are exceptions to this standard of practice. When an ophthalmologist has advanced training in low vision, a direct referral might be made to the occupational therapist, along with collaboration with the occupational therapist in evaluation and treatment of the visual impairment. Many occupational therapists practice in educational, home care, or other settings in which a low vision optometrist is not physically present. In these settings, eye care providers not specializing in low vision rehabilitation or other physicians may refer clients directly to the occupational therapist. In such cases, we propose that following the initial occupational therapy evaluation, ideally, the occupational therapist refer the patient to a low vision optometrist before implementation of the treatment plan.

We believe that the ideal practice situation would be for an occupational therapist to play a role in the final determination of the appropriate optical devices. In this model, after the optometrist performs the optometric low vision examination and determines the approximate ideal magnification based on visual acuity, the client would be examined by the occupational therapist. The role of the occupational therapist would be to assess the client's occupational goals and to determine the physical, cognitive, and other sensory capabilities and limitations that context and activity demand, all of which impact the optometrist's final decision about optical aids and magnification selection. The therapist would convey this information to the optometrist, who would then determine and write the final prescription. Of course, to be effective, this would have to be an ongoing and interactive process in which the optometrist and occupational therapist work together to determine the appropriate optical devices for a client. Under either model, ultimately, the optometrist would formally prescribe all recommended optical devices as he or she would prescribe eyeglasses.

In every other area of practice, occupational therapists routinely include measurement of client factors as part of the evaluation. When an occupational therapist with advanced training in low vision rehabilitation works with a low vision optometrist, an occasion may present in which the occupational therapist may be asked to measure acuity, visual fields, and contrast sensitivity. Optometrists, with their specialized understanding of optics, refractive error, and the functional effects of disease and progression of disease, must ensure that all optical device options are considered and that the optical devices and prescribed eyeglasses work together. This model highlights the strengths of each profession and allows both the occupational therapist and low vision optometrist to provide complementary and essential components of the rehabilitation process. This model would also be a cost-effective collaboration, with the occupational therapist performing many of the time-consuming procedures typically required in a low vision evaluation, thereby decreasing the time required by the eye care provider.

SUMMARY

This chapter was designed to establish the importance of low vision rehabilitation for the practice of occupational therapy and to review the definitions, epidemiology, and history of low vision and low vision rehabilitation in the United States. We also presented a model of clinical care with suggested roles for the various professions involved with low vision rehabilitation.

REFERENCES

1. Amini DA, Kannenberg K, Bodison S, et al. Occupational therapy practice framework: domain & process, 3rd edition. *Am J Occup Ther.* 2014;S1-s48.

2. Lighthouse. *The Lighthouse National Survey on Vision Loss: The Experience, Attitudes, and Knowledge of Middle-Aged and Older Americans.* New York: The Lighthouse; 1995:11.

3. Massof RW. A model of the prevalence and incidence of low vision and blindness among adults in the U.S. *Optom Vis Sci.* 2002;79:31-38.

4. Tielsch JM. The epidemiology of vision impairment. In: Silverstone B, Lang MA, Rosenthal BP, Faye EE, eds. *The Lighthouse Handbook on Vision Impairment and Vision Rehabilitation.* New York: Oxford University Press; 2000:5-17.

5. Rondinelli RD. *Guides to the Evaluation of Permanent Impairment*: American Medical Association; 2007.

6. World Health Organization. *International Classification of Impairment, Disabilities, and Handicaps: A Manual of Classification Relating to Consequences of Disease.* Geneva, Switzerland: World Health Organization; 1980.

7. Tielsch JM, Sommer A, Witt K, Katz J, Royall RM. Blindness and visual impairment in an American urban population. The Baltimore Eye Survey. *Arch Ophthalmol.* 1990;108:286-290.

8. Kahn HA, Leibowitz HM, Ganley JP, et al. The Framingham Eye Study. I. Outline and major prevalence findings. *Am J Epidemiol.* 1977;106:17-32.

9. Klein R, Klein B, Linton K, DeMets D. The Beaver Dam Eye Study: visual acuity. *Ophthalmology.* 1991;98:1310-1315.

10. Dana MR, Tielsch JM, Enger C, Joyce E, Santoli JM, Taylor HR. Visual impairment in a rural Appalachian community. Prevalence and causes. *JAMA.* 1990;264:2400-2405.

11. Rubin GS, West SK, Munoz B, et al. A comprehensive assessment of visual impairment in a population of older Americans: The SEE study. *Invest Ophthalmol Vis Sci.* 1997;38:557-568.

12. Ferris FL, Kassof A, Bresnick GH, Bailey I. New visual acuity charts for clinical research. *Am J Ophthalmol.* 1982;94:91-96.

13. Warren M, Barstow E. *Occupational Therapy Interventions for Adults with Low Vision* 2nd ed. Bethesda, MD: AOTA Press; 2011.

14. Congdon N, O'Colmain B, Klaver CC, et al. Causes and prevalence of visual impairment among adults in the United States. *Arch Ophthalmol.* 2004;122:477-485.

15. Klein R, Klein B, Lee KE. Changes in visual acuity in a population:the Beaver Dam Eye Study. *Ophthalmology.* 1996; 103:1169-1178.

16. Evans BJ, Rowlands G. Correctable visual impairment in older people: a major unmet need. *Ophthalmic Physiol Opt.* 2004;24:161-180.

17. Schwartz SD. Age-related maculopathy and age-related macular degeneration. In: Silverstone B, Lang MA, Rosenthal BP, Faye EE, eds. *The Lighthouse Handbook on Vision Impairment and Vision Rehabilitation.* New York: Oxford University Press; 2000.

18. Schmidt EU, Miller JW, Sickenberg M, et al. Photodynamic therapy with verteporfin for choroidal neovascularization caused by age-related macular degeneration: results of treatments in a phase 1 and 2 study. *Arch Ophthalmol.* 1999;117:1177-1187.

19. Lovie-Kitchin J, Bowman KJ. *Senile Macular Degeneration: Management and Rehabilitation.* Boston: Butterworth; 1985.

20. Warren M. Providing low vision rehabilitation services with occupational therapy and ophthalmology: a program description. *Am J Occup Ther.* 1995;49:877-883.

21. American Academy of Optometry. American Academy of Optometry Low Vision Section List of Low Vision Diplomates. 2005.

22. Crews JE, Luxton L. Rehabilitation teaching for older adults. In: Orr AA, ed. *Vision and Aging.* New York, NY: American Foundation for the Blind; 1992:233-253.

23. Duffy MA, Huebner K, Wormsley DP. Activities of daily living and individuals with low vision. In: Scheiman M, ed. *Understanding and Managing Vision Deficits: A Guide for Occupational Therapists.* Thorofare, NJ: Slack, Inc; 2002:289-304.

24. Graboyes M. Psychosocial implications of visual impairment. In: Brilliant RL, ed. *Essentials of Low Vision Practice.* Boston, MA: Butterworth-Heinemann; 1999:12-17.

25. Goodrich GL, Bailey IL. A history of the field of vision rehabilitation from the perspective of low vision. In: Silverstone B, Lang MA, Rosenthal BP, Faye EE, eds. *The Lighthouse Handbook on Vision Impairment and Vision Rehabilitation.* Oxford: Oxford University Press; 2000:675-715.

26. Goodrich Gl, Sowell V. Low vision: a history in progress. In: Corn AL, Koenig AJ, eds, *Foundations of Low Vision: Clinical and Functional Perspectives.* New York, NY: American Foundation for the Blind; 2000.

27. Goodrich GL, Arditi A. An interactive history: the low vision timeline. In: Stuen C, Arditi A, Horowitz A, et .al., eds. *Proceedings of the Vision '99 Conference, Vision Rehabilitation: Assessment, Intervention and Outcomes.* Lisse: Swets & Zeitlinger; 2000:3-9.

28. Mogk L, Goodrich G. The history and future of low vision services in the United States. *J Vis Imp Blind.* 2004;98:585-600.

29. Goodrich GL, Arditi A. A trend analysis of the low-vision literature. *Br J Vis Impair Blind.* 2004;22:105-196.

30. Feinbloom W. Introduction to the principles and practice of subnormal vision correction. *J Am Optom Assoc.* 1935;6:3-18.

31. Feinbloom W. Report of 500 cases of subnormal vision. *Am J Optom Arch Am Acad Optom.* 1938;22:238.

32. Ponchillia PE, Ponchillia SV. *Foundations of Rehabilitation Teaching with Persons Who Are Blind or Visually Impaired.* New York, NY: American Foundation for the Blind; 1996:3-21.

33. Goodrich GL. Low vision services in the VA: an "aging" trend. *J Vis Rehab.* 1991;5:11-17.

34. Barraga NC. *Increased Visual Behavior in Low Vision Children (Research Series No. 13).* New York, NY: American Foundation for the Blind; 1964.

35. Barraga NC. Learning efficiency in low vision. *J Am Optom Assoc.* 1969;40:807-810.

36. Warren M. Including occupational therapy in low vision rehabilitation. *Am J Occup Ther.* 1995;49:857-860.

37. Orr AL, Huebner K. Toward a collaborative working relationship among vision rehabilitation and allied health professionals. *J Vis Imp Blind.* 2001;95:468-482.

38. Warren ML, Lampert J. Assessing daily living needs. In: Fletcher DC, ed. *Ophthalmology Monographs: Low Vision Rehabilitation: Caring for the Whole Person.* San Francisco: American Academy of Ophthalmology; 1999:89-125.

39. Warren M. An overview of low vision rehabilitation and the role of occupational therapy. In: Warren M, ed. *Low Vision: Occupational Therapy Intervention with the Older Adult.* Bethesda, MD: American Occupational Therapy Association; 2000:3-21.

40. Warren M. *Low Vision: Occupational Therapy Intervention with the Older Adult.* Bethesda, MD: American Occupational Therapy Association; 2000.

41. Warren M. Occupational therapy practice guidelines for adults with low vision. In: Lieberman D, ed. *The AOTA Practice Guidelines Series.* Bethesda, MD: American Occupational Therapy Association; 2001:1-25.

42. Elliott DB, Trukolo-Ilic M, Strong JG, Pace RJ, Plotkin AD, Bevers P. Demographic characteristics of the vision-disabled elderly. *Invest Ophthalmol Vis Sci.* 1997;38:2566-2575.

43. McGinty Bachelder J, Harkins D. Do occupational therapists have a primary role in low vision rehabilitation? *Am J Occup Ther.* 1995;49:927-930.

44. Deacy R, Yuen H, Barstow EA, Warren M, Voqtle L. Survey of the low vision rehabilitation currciula in occupational therapy and occupational therapy assistant programs. *Am J Occup Ther.* 2012;66:114-118.

45. Sokol-McKay DA. Facing the challenge of macular degeneration: therapeutic interventions for low vision. *OT Pract.* 2005;10:10-15.

46. Massof RW, Dagnelie G, Deremeik JT, DeRose JL, Alibhai SS, Glasner NM. Low vision rehabilitation in the U.S. health care system. *J Vis Rehab.* 1995;9:3-31.

47. Wainapel SF. Low vision rehabilitation and rehabilitation medicine: a parable of parallels. In: Massof RW, Lidoff L, eds. *Issues in Low Vision Rehabilitation.* New York, NY: AFB Press; 2001:55-60.

48. Fishburn MJ. Overview of physical medicine and rehabilitation. In: Massof RW, Lidoff L, eds. *Issues in Low Vision Rehabilitation.* New York, NY: AFB Press; 2001:61-70.

3

Review of Basic Anatomy, Physiology, and Development of the Visual System

BASIC ANATOMY AND PHYSIOLOGY

This chapter is designed to provide an overview of the basic anatomy and physiology of the visual system that is sufficient enough to get started with low vision therapy. Readers requiring more in-depth information about these topics should review the texts listed in the bibliography of this chapter.

Orbit, Eyelids, and Eyeball

A traditional method of describing the anatomy of the eye is to begin with the outermost structures and move inward. The orbit of the eye, which is a bony recess in the skull, contains a number of major structures, including the eyeball, the optic nerve, the muscles of the eye, and their nerves and blood vessels. The eyeball, which is about 2.5 cm long, is suspended in the orbital cavity in such a way that the 6 extraocular muscles can move it in all directions.

The eyelids protect the eyes from injury and excessive light and keep the cornea moist. As illustrated in Figure 3-1, the upper eyelid partially covers the iris, whereas the entire inferior half of the eye is normally uncovered. The eyelids are covered internally by the highly vascular palpebral conjunctiva. The palpebral conjunctiva continues onto the

eyeball and is called the *bulbar conjunctiva*. Inflammation of either the bulbar or palpebral conjunctiva is referred to as conjunctivitis, commonly called *pink eye*. Conjunctivitis can be secondary to bacterial, viral, or allergic etiology. Infection of the conjunctiva is generally self-limiting, but occasionally conjunctivitis can lead to inflammation of the cornea as well.

The bulbar conjunctiva covers the white portion of the eye called the *sclera*. The sclera is the external coat of the eye and is a white tissue covering the posterior five-sixths of the eye. The anterior one-sixth of the outer coat of the eye is the transparent structure called the *cornea* (Figure 3-2). The cornea is an extremely important structure of the eye because it is the key optical component responsible for refraction of light that enters the eye. It is an unusual tissue because it is clear and has no blood vessels. The cornea is susceptible to infection from bacterial, viral, fungal, or allergic causes, and inflammation of the cornea is referred to as keratitis. Severe inflammation, a corneal burn due to exposure to toxic substances, or trauma to the cornea can all lead to scarring and loss of transparency of the cornea. This can then lead to loss of vision if the scarring is located in the central portion of the cornea. Reduced visual acuity secondary to central corneal scarring is a condition that may be encountered by occupational therapists in clients

Whittaker SG, Scheiman M, Sokol-McKay DA.
Low Vision Rehabilitation: A Practical Guide for Occupational Therapists,
Second Edition (pp 39-45).
© 2016 Taylor & Francis Group.

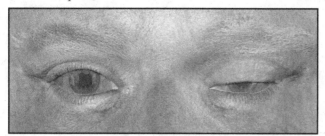

Figure 3-1. The upper eyelid partially covers the iris, whereas the entire inferior half of the eye is normally uncovered. (Reprinted with permission from Barbara Steinman.)

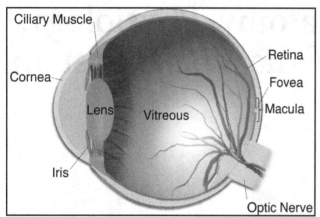

Figure 3-2. Cross-section of the eye. The anterior one-sixth of the outer coat of the eye is the transparent structure called the cornea. (Reprinted with permission from Barbara Steinman.)

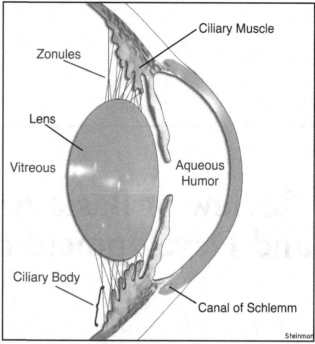

Figure 3-3. Directly behind the cornea is a clear, watery fluid called the aqueous humor. Aqueous is drained off through the canal of Schlemm. (Reprinted with permission from Barbara Steinman.)

who have experienced head trauma. Other common age-related problems of the anterior part of the eye that affect vision and cause discomfort include blepharitis (chronic inflammation of the lids) and dry eye. These can be managed medically, but with varying success.

Directly behind the cornea is a clear, watery fluid called the *aqueous humor*, which is produced in the posterior chamber and fills the anterior chamber of the eye (Figure 3-3). The aqueous is continuously produced by the ciliary body and provides nutrients for the avascular cornea and lens. After passing through the pupil from the posterior chamber into the anterior chamber, the aqueous is drained off through canal of Schlemm (see Figure 3-3).

Lens

The lens is a transparent, flexible structure that is held in position by zonular fibers (see Figure 3-3). It is located posterior to the iris and anterior to the vitreous humor. Like the cornea, the lens is both transparent and avascular and is another key part of the refractive system of the eye. To accommodate, or focus, on objects, the lens must change shape. The ciliary muscle contracts, and this allows the lens to thicken, enabling the individual to focus. As an object moves away, the ciliary muscle relaxes, the lens becomes thinner, and the focusing system relaxes. The lens of the

eye is the structure that gradually loses its transparency as a person ages. This loss of transparency and development of opacities is referred to as cataracts.

Vitreous

The vitreous body is located behind the lens (see Figure 3-3). It consists of a jellylike substance called *vitreous humor*, in which there is a meshwork of collagen fibrils. Vitreous humor is a colorless, transparent gel. It consists of 99% water and forms four-fifths of the eyeball. In addition to transmitting light, it holds the retina in place and provides support for the lens. Unlike the aqueous humor, it is not continuously replaced.

Choroid

The eyeball has 3 concentric coats. The first, or outermost, coat, the sclera, was described earlier. The middle coat is a heavily pigmented, vascular layer consisting of the iris, ciliary body, and the choroid. The iris, which is the colored portion of the eye (Figure 3-4), is located between the cornea and the lens. The eye color depends on the amount and distribution of pigment in the iris. The iris is a contractile diaphragm that has a central, circular aperture for transmitting light called the *pupil*. The size of the iris continually varies to regulate the amount of light entering the eye through the pupil. The ciliary body lies between the iris and the choroid (see Figure 3-3). This structure secretes aqueous humor. The ciliary body also contains

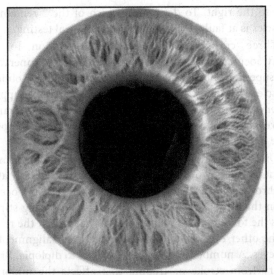

Figure 3-4. The iris is the colored portion of the eye located between the cornea and the lens. (Reprinted with permission from Barbara Steinman.)

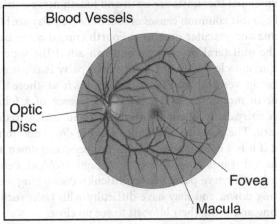

Figure 3-5. The retina as viewed through the dilated pupil: the optic disc is a circular depression in the posterior portion of the retina. This is where the optic nerve enters the eye, and its fibers spread out in the neural layer of the retina. The fovea is lateral to the optic disc. (Reprinted with permission from Barbara Steinman.)

the ciliary muscle, which can contract or relax to permit accommodation, or focusing, of the eye. The choroid is a dark-brown membrane and is also part of this middle coat of the eye. It continues from the ciliary body and covers the entire posterior portion of the eye. The choroid attaches firmly to the retina and contains the venous plexus and layers of capillaries that are responsible for nutrition of the retina.

Retina

The most internal coat of the eye is the retina, which is a thin, delicate membrane. The retina is the posterior portion of the eye, and there is a circular depressed area called the

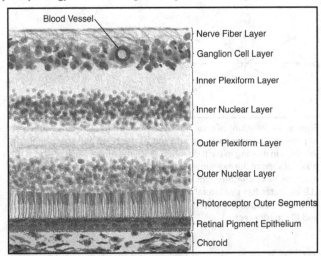

Figure 3-6. Ten layers of the retina. (Reprinted with permission from Barbara Steinman.)

optic disc (Figure 3-5). This is where the optic nerve enters the eye, and its fibers spread out in the neural layer of the retina. Because it contains nerve fibers and no photoreceptor cells, the optic disc is insensitive to light. For this reason, it is sometimes referred to as the blind spot. Another very important structure just lateral to the optic disc is the fovea (see Figure 3-5). The fovea is the part of the eye that contains the area of most acute vision. Whenever we look at an object, we must aim the eye so that the image of the object is focused on the fovea. Smooth eye movements, called *pursuits*, move the eye to keep a moving target in the fovea so that it can be most clearly seen. Jump eye movements, called *saccades*, very quickly move the eye toward a target so that the target lands in the fovea.

The retina is composed of 10 layers, including the pigmented epithelium, which is closest to the choroid and the photoreceptors (cones and rods).

Beneath the pigmented epithelium of the retina are these 4 layers (Figure 3-6), from the outside (furthest from the retina) to the inside (closest to the retina):

1. Sclera (white part of the eye)

2. Large choroidal blood vessels

3. Choriocapillaris

4. Bruch's membrane (separates the pigmented epithelium of the retina from the choroid)

Note that light must pass through all layers of the retina to reach the photoreceptors, where the visual process begins. Diseases such as macular degeneration or diabetic retinopathy that affect the clarity of retina, or swelling that affects the shape of the retina, will have a profound effect on vision.

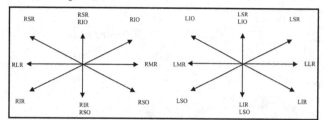

Figure 3-7. Positions of gaze that are evaluated by clinicians when testing the extraocular muscles and the extraocular muscles principally involved in moving in each direction. Note the movements are from the point of view of the examiner. The first letter indicates right (R) or left (L) eye. The next 2 letters indicate the extraocular muscle. For example, LLR indicates left eye lateral rectus. Other muscles include MR (medial rectus), SO (superior oblique), IO (inferior oblique), SR (superior rectus), and IR (inferior rectus).

Photoreceptors (Cones and Rods)

Light causes a chemical reaction in cones and in rods, beginning the visual process. Activated photoreceptors stimulate bipolar cells, which in turn stimulate ganglion cells. The impulses continue into the axons of the ganglion cells, through the optic nerve, and to the visual cortex at the occipital lobe of the brain.

There are about 6.5 to 7 million cones in each eye, and they are sensitive to bright light and to color. The highest concentration of cones is in the macula. The center of the macula contains only cones and no rods. The highest concentration of rods is in the peripheral retina, decreasing in density up to the macula. Rods are used for night vision and do not detect color, which is the main reason it is difficult to tell the color of an object at night or in the dark. Defective or damaged cones result in color deficiency. Defective or damaged rods result in problems seeing in the dark and at night.

Muscles of the Orbit and Their Innervation

Six extraocular muscles attach to each eye and allow movement in all directions of gaze. There are 4 rectus muscles—the superior, inferior, lateral, and medial recti muscles—and 2 oblique muscles called the *inferior and superior oblique muscles.*

Each of the 6 muscles has one position of gaze in which it exerts the main influence on eye position. Figure 3-7 illustrates the various positions of gaze that are evaluated clinically. The diagram also displays the muscle that is primarily responsible for movement into each position of gaze. This diagram is the basis for the clinical evaluation of eye muscle problems. For example, if a client has difficulty moving his eyes down and to the right, the 2 possible muscles involved are the right inferior rectus and the left superior oblique. The left superior oblique moves the left eye down and to the right, and the right inferior rectus moves the right eye down

and to the right. To determine which of the 2 remaining muscles is at fault requires additional clinical testing.

Three cranial nerves supply innervation to the 6 extraocular muscles. The third cranial nerve innervates the superior, inferior, medial recti, and the inferior oblique muscle. The fourth cranial nerve (trochlear nerve) supplies innervation to the superior oblique, and the sixth cranial nerve (abducens nerve) innervates the lateral rectus responsible for abducting the eye.

Diplopia, or double vision, is a common symptom of clients treated by occupational therapists, particularly after cerebrovascular accident or head trauma. Diplopia occurs when the object at which the individual is looking stimulates the fovea of one eye and a nonfoveal part of the retina of the other eye. Thus, diplopia suggests misalignment of the eyes. A number of disorders can lead to diplopia. Brain injury from stroke or trauma that affects the midbrain or cerebellum area often affects both balance and eye movements. Among the more common problems are cranial nerve palsies. The most common nerve palsies seen by occupational therapists are sixth and fourth nerve palsies.

The most common causes of fourth nerve palsy are head trauma and vascular problems. Fourth cranial nerve palsy can be unilateral or bilateral and can affect the superior oblique muscle. Bilateral fourth nerve palsy is often seen following vertex blows to the head, such as those that occur in motorcycle accidents. The presence of a fourth nerve palsy causes the eye with the affected muscle to drift upward. The client has difficulty looking down and to the right if it is a left superior oblique problem, and down and to the left if it is a right superior oblique problem. People with fourth nerve palsies have difficulty converging while looking down, and may have difficulty with tasks such as reading and using their bifocals to see up close.

Sixth cranial nerve palsies are the most frequently reported ocular motor nerve palsies. The nerve has the longest intracranial course of any nerve and is often subject to damage with raised intracranial pressure and even the natural course of aging. The causes include vascular disease, trauma, elevated intracranial pressure, and neoplasm. The sixth nerve innervates the lateral rectus. A sixth nerve palsy will interfere with the client's ability to abduct the eye (move the eye away from the nose).

Anatomy/Physiology of Binocular Vision

Binocular vision is the ability of the visual system to fuse or combine the information from the right and left eyes into one image. Visual information that enters the right and left eyes remains monocular as it passes from the optic nerve through the chiasm, the optic tract, the lateral geniculate body, and the optic radiation. At the level of the visual cortex (area 17), the information finally reaches cortical cells capable of binocular processing. For binocular vision to occur, the information arriving from each eye must be identical and approximately equal in clarity and size. To satisfy these requirements, the 2 eyes must be aligned so that they point at the same object at all times, and the optics or refractive error of the 2 eyes must be approximately equal. Problems with either alignment or refractive equality will cause binocular vision disorders. The hallmark symptom of a binocular vision disorder is double vision (diplopia).

The 2 primary categories of binocular vision problems are referred to as strabismic and nonstrabismic (phoria) binocular vision disorders. When the 2 eyes actually lose alignment, it is referred to as strabismus. When strabismus occurs and the eyes drift in, out, up, or down, each eye views a different part of the environment and sends different information to the visual cortex. The result is visual confusion, with each eye seeing something different. In addition, the same object in the environment, like a penlight, will be seen in different positions by each eye, resulting in the perception of diplopia (double vision). Usually, diplopia and visual confusion occur together, but people with a visual field loss in one or both eyes may have visual confusion without diplopia and complaints of double vision.

Because diplopia and visual confusion are intolerable, the visual system attempts to eliminate the problem through one of two mechanisms: by trying to overcome the problem and restore normal alignment using muscular effort or by adapting to the misalignment of the eyes. In some cases, the tendency for the eye to turn can be overcome with muscular effort. In such cases, patients often successfully eliminate double vision and experience binocular vision, but may be uncomfortable. They report eyestrain, headaches, an inability to sustain attention for long periods of time, intermittent blurred vision, and occasional diplopia. The other option is to allow the eye to turn, but to eliminate diplopia by either ignoring the information coming from the eye that turns (suppression) or by altering the neurophysiology at the level of the visual cortex (anomalous correspondence). Until the age of about 6 years, the human visual system has been shown to have an extraordinary plasticity and ability to adapt to strabismus. Age affects adaptation; generally, younger children adapt more quickly than do older children and adults. Suppression often is believed to be unlikely to occur after early childhood, but does occur in adults. It is also more likely to occur if the eye turn is a constant, rather than an intermittent, problem.

A nonstrabismic binocular vision problem, also referred to as a phoria, is a condition in which the eyes have a tendency to drift in, out, up, or down, but the visual system is able to control the tendency using excessive neuromuscular effort. While the eyes always look straight in cases of phoria, the condition can cause eye fatigue, blurred vision, and discomfort. The most common binocular vision problem after traumatic brain injury or concussion, for example, is a phoric condition called *convergence insufficiency*. This

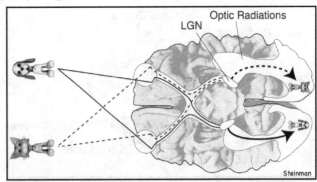

Figure 3-8. The right visual cortex receives information from the left visual field, and the left visual cortex receives information from the right visual field. (Reprinted with permission from Barbara Steinman.)

is a condition in which the eyes have difficulty converging accurately during near visual activities. Although the eyes have a strong tendency to drift outward in this condition, with effort, the person often can control this tendency, but will complain of headaches and double vision when fatigued.

Visual Pathways

One of the most common vision problems occupational therapists encounter after acquired brain injury is visual field deficits. A right or left field loss is referred to as a homonymous hemianopsia. To understand why a client would lose vision on one side in both eyes, it is necessary to understand how visual information travels from the retina to the visual cortex. Vision begins with the capture of images focused by the optical media on photoreceptors of the retina. The fibers from the upper half of each retina enter the optic nerve above the horizontal meridian, and those from the lower half enter below the horizontal meridian. Fibers from the periphery of the retina lie peripherally in the optic nerve, and fibers from the fovea lie centrally. In other words, you can map an image of most of a person's visual field on the retina of each eye. A retinotopic map and map of a person's visual field persists throughout the entire course of the visual pathways from the optic nerve through the chiasm, the optic tracts, and visual cortex optic radiations.

Visual information from the right field strikes the nasal half of the retina of the right eye and the temporal half of the retina of the left eye. Similarly, visual information from the left field strikes the nasal half of the retina of the left eye and the temporal half of the retina of the right eye (Figure 3-8). When the fibers from each optic nerve reach the optic chiasm, a semidecussation, or partial crossing, takes place. The fibers from the temporal part of the retina remain on the temporal or outside aspect of the chiasm and are called *uncrossed fibers*. The nasal fibers of the retina cross over in the chiasm and are called *crossed fibers*. After leaving the chiasm, the fibers form the optic tract. Thus, all

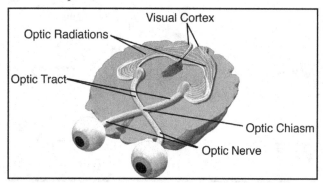

Figure 3-9. Visual pathway from the optic nerve to the visual cortex. (Reprinted with permission from Barbara Steinman.)

visual information originating from the right field travels in the left optic tract, and all visual information originating from the left field travels in the right optic tract. The fibers in the upper half of the tract originate from the upper half of the two retinas, and the fibers from the lower half of the tract come from the lower half of the two retinas. The fibers from the optic tract synapse in the lateral geniculate body. The cells of the lateral geniculate body give rise to new fibers, which form the optic radiation. These fibers then proceed to the cells of the visual cortex (Figure 3-9). Any lesion that affects the visual pathway on only the right or left side after this decussation takes place will affect either the left visual field or right visual field. Given the architecture of the visual pathway posterior to the optic chiasm, a common result of an insult to the brain is a complete or partial loss of sensitivity to one-half of the visual field in each eye. The vertical midline constitutes the boundary between the seeing and unseeing fields. The individual with a left field loss or hemianopia is responsive to objects to the right of fixation, but not to the left. This condition is then called a *left hemianopia*. A similar problem occurs with injury to the left side of the brain and is referred to as a *right hemianopia*. This is a bit of an oversimplification. Actually, projections from the fovea actually protrude to both halves of the brain. For this reason, people with a hemianopia often have central sparing—that is, the central part of the affected visual field is spared and a person can see both sides of an object or word being viewed.

Vision Areas of the Brain

The brain is divided into several different lobes. Starting anteriorly are the frontal lobes, which are responsible for decision making, planning ahead, emotional tone, abstract thinking, and carrying out intentions. Attention to one side, planning, and initiating eye movements to scan the visual environment take place in the frontal cortex. Immediately behind them and in front of the motor area is the prefrontal cortex, which is involved in organizing and sequencing complex motor behavior and processing spatial information and responding to stimuli. The temporal lobes

are associated with hearing, object recognition, and at the temporal-parietal-occipital junction, reading. The parietal lobes are responsible for tactile recognition, spatial perception, and responding to stimuli. Parietal lobe injury results in perceptual deficits that disrupt ambulation and self-care activities. Hemisensory neglect is a common problem in clients with a lesion in the posterior parietal cortex that affect their ability to respond to stimuli on one side (unilateral inattention) and estimate distances and the relative positioning of objects (see Chapter 11).

The occipital lobe contains the visual cortex, with nerve pathways leading to higher centers in the parietal and temporal lobes, where visual sensations acquire meaning. Lesions in the visual cortex and in associated areas can produce visual and perceptual problems.

Nearly all of the visual fibers end in the striate area of the cortex, which is called *area 17*. Area 17 is considered the primary visuosensory area in man. Outside of area 17 and closely following its contours are 2 other areas that are concerned with visual reactions as well. These are called *area 18* and *area 19*. Most physiologists agree that vision is a function of higher parts of the brain than just the visual cortex. The message relayed to area 17 enables a person to see. It does not enable a person to recognize what he or she sees or to recall things that have been seen. These functions are dependent on other parts of the brain. In order for a person to be able to interpret the sensory information reaching area 17, the message must be sent on to the two secondary visual areas and areas 18 and 19. Area 18 is concerned exclusively with the recognition of objects, animate or inanimate, but is not concerned with the recognition of written or printed symbols of language. Area 19 is concerned with the recall of visual memory relating to objects, but not to language symbols. In general, parietal-occipital areas are involved with spatial relations, while temporal-occipital areas are involved with object and letter recognition.

Two parallel routes carry visual information from the occipital lobe to the prefrontal lobe and the frontal eye fields. Fibers from these 2 routes distribute fibers to many other areas along each route before terminating in the prefrontal cortex and in the frontal eye fields. The first route, the dorsal stream, is the superior route via the parietal and frontal lobes and, if damaged, affect attention and spatial perception, sometimes called the *where system*. The other route, the ventral stream, (the "what system") is the inferior route via the temporal and frontal lobes and affects the face, and object and word recognition.

The cerebellum integrates the smooth coordination of muscular activity. If it is damaged, general motor clumsiness occurs. This may interfere with manual dexterity and other forms of fine muscular performance, as well as eye movement control. Dysfunction within the cerebellum yields problems with equilibrium, motor control, body image, laterality, and sometimes with reading and speech.

SUMMARY

Low vision has historically been associated with damage to primary visual processing systems, from the cornea to and including the striate or primary visual cortex. Functional vision, a person's ability to use visual information to engage in visual activities, depends on the integrity of "higher order" processing that occurs in other areas of the brain. These other areas often are damaged in people with stroke and other acquired brain injury who are treated by occupational therapists working in medical rehabilitation settings. As a result, the influence of occupational therapists has broadened the definition of low vision to include these higher-order perceptual deficits. Accordingly, rehabilitation of disability due to impairments in perceptual function has been included in the second edition of this book.

BIBLIOGRAPHY

1. Moore KL. *Clinically Oriented Anatomy.* Baltimore, MD: Williams and Wilkins; 1980.
2. Moses RA. *Adler's Physiology of the Eye.* 7th ed. St. Louis, MO: CV Mosby Co; 1981.
3. Scheiman M. *Understanding and Managing Visual Deficits: A Guide for Occupational Therapists.* 3rd ed. Thorofare, NJ: SLACK Incorporated; 2011.
4. Solomon H. *Binocular Vision: A Programmed Text.* London: William Heinemann Medical Books Ltd; 1978.

Eye Diseases Associated With Low Vision

This chapter reviews the eye diseases that are the leading causes of low vision in the adult population and includes description, prevalence, risk factors, effect on vision, and treatment of each condition. In addition, oculomotor vision disorders, visual field loss, and visual perceptual disorders associated with acquired brain injury are reviewed in this chapter. Although some of these conditions have historically been associated with vision impairment/low vision, they may be present in patients being treated for low vision. Therefore, therapists working with visually impaired patients may encounter some of these other problems.

The leading causes of severe visual impairment among white Americans in 2000 were age-related macular degeneration (AMD), accounting for 54% of visual impairment, with cataract (9%), diabetic retinopathy (6%), and glaucoma (5%) the next most common causes.[1] The leading causes of severe visual impairment in black persons were cataract (37%), diabetic retinopathy (26%), glaucoma (7%), and AMD (4%). Among Hispanics, glaucoma was the most common cause (29%), followed by AMD (14%), cataract (14%), and diabetic retinopathy (14%).[1] Therefore, while the relative prevalence may differ depending on race and ethnicity, the primary eye diseases that the occupational therapist will encounter when dealing with adult patients in a low vision clinic are AMD, diabetic retinopathy, glaucoma, and cataract. In many cases, the therapist must be the one

to educate the patient regarding the condition and treatments. For this reason, this information about the pathology is considered part of the core knowledge base for a low vision therapist. This chapter also describes more common visual impairments and low vision treatments associated with these pathologies, again information that is part of the core knowledge requirements for low vision therapists.

AGE-RELATED MACULAR DEGENERATION

Description

Age-related macular degeneration is a degenerative, acquired disorder of the central retina called the *macula*, which usually occurs in patients over age 55, and results in progressive, sometimes significant, irreversible loss of central visual function from either fibrous scarring or atrophy of the macula. It is the leading cause of vision loss in the adult population.

The macula is located roughly in the center of the retina and is a small and highly sensitive part of the retina responsible for detailed central vision. The fovea is the very

Whittaker SG, Scheiman M, Sokol-McKay DA.
Low Vision Rehabilitation: A Practical Guide for Occupational Therapists,
Second Edition (pp 47-66).
© 2016 Taylor & Francis Group.

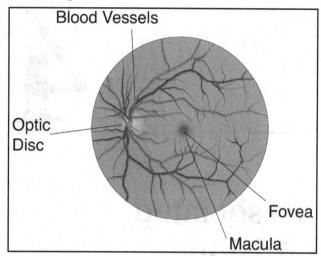

Figure 4-1. The normal macula has a characteristic appearance and is more heavily pigmented than the surrounding retina. (Reprinted with permission from Barbara Steinman.)

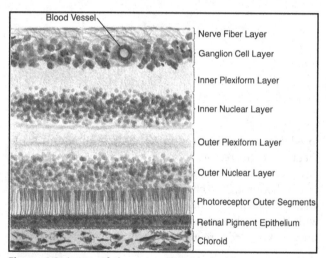

Figure 4-2. Layers of the retina. (Reprinted with permission from Barbara Steinman.)

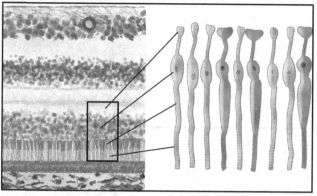

Figure 4-3. Photoreceptors. (Reprinted with permission from Barbara Steinman.)

2. Large choroidal blood vessels

3. Choriocapillaris

4. Bruch's membrane (separates the pigmented epithelium of the retina from the choroid)

The underlying etiology of AMD is poorly understood, and no cure currently exists. The International ARM Epidemiological Study Group defined AMD in 1995.[2] Age-related macular degeneration typically occurs in adults over the age of 50 and is characterized by any of the following problems:

- Drusen: Drusen are discrete, round, slightly elevated whitish-yellow spots in the macular area and elsewhere in the retina. Drusen are one of the earliest signs of AMD and are typically clustered in the macular area. They may change in size, shape, color, and distribution over time.

- Hyperpigmentation: Hyperpigmentation refers to areas of increased pigmentation and may not be associated with drusen.

- Hypopigmentation: Hypopigmentation refers to depigmentation and is typically associated with drusen.

Age-related macular degeneration is classified as either dry (nonexudative) or wet (exudative).

Dry Age-Related Macular Degeneration

Dry (nonexudative or atrophic) AMD accounts for 90% of all patients with AMD in the United States.[3] The disorder results from a gradual breakdown of the retinal pigment epithelium (RPE), the accumulation of drusen deposits, and loss of function of the overlying photoreceptors (Figure 4-3). Most patients with dry AMD experience gradual, progressive loss of central visual function, often with more reduced vision surrounding some central vision in the earlier stages. This loss of vision is more noticeable during near tasks, with smaller, lower-contrast objects and

center of the macula. The normal macula has a characteristic appearance and is more heavily pigmented than the surrounding retina (Figure 4-1). The macula allows us to appreciate detail and perform tasks that require central vision, such as reading, writing, recognizing faces, and driving.

To understand this disease, it is important to have an understanding of the anatomy of the retina and adjacent structures of the eye, which was reviewed in Chapter 3. As a brief review, the retina is composed of 10 layers. Two of the important layers that become an issue in AMD are the retinal pigment epithelium that is closest to the choroid, and the photoreceptors (cones and rods) (Figure 4-2). Beneath the retinal pigment epithelium of the retina are 4 additional layers (see Figure 4-2), ranging from the outside (furthest from the retina) to the inside (closest to the retina):

1. Sclera (white part of the eye)

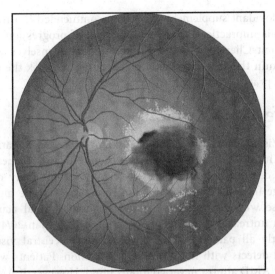

Figure 4-4. Wet AMD. (Reprinted with permission from Barbara Steinman.)

TABLE 4-1: RISK FACTORS ASSOCIATED WITH AGE-RELATED MACULAR DEGENERATION
• Age
• Smoking
• Genetics
• Female gender
• Race (higher prevalence in whites)
• High intake of fats
• Elevated levels of serum cholesterol
• Hypertension
• Cardiovascular disease
• Ultraviolet light exposure
• Obesity
• Cataract surgery

print under dimmer illumination, especially in the early stages of the disease. In an estimated 12% to 21% of patients, dry AMD progresses to vision levels of 20/200 or worse.[4,5] Neovascularization is not present in dry AMD. Sometimes after long periods of time, the retinal changes associated with dry AMD can spread outside of the macula, a condition called *geographic atrophy.*

Wet Age-Related Macular Degeneration

Although wet (exudative) AMD accounts for only 10% of patients with AMD, 90% of the AMD patients with significant vision loss have this form of the disease.[4,6] Wet AMD is characterized by the development of neovascularization in the choroid, leading to leakage of blood and subsequent elevation of the RPE (Figure 4-4). Patients with wet AMD tend to notice a more profound and rapid decrease in central visual function or distortions in shape. The leakage of blood from the new choroidal vessels causes distorted vision, central scotoma, and blurred vision.[7] As the blood in the vitreous dissipates, vision might improve somewhat.

Prevalence

Most studies have indicated that AMD is the leading cause of low vision in developed countries.[8,9] The prevalence of AMD increases with age, and about 30% of patients 75 years of age and older are affected.[3,10] While AMD is the leading cause of visual impairment among white Americans (54%), it is less prevalent in Blacks (4%) and Hispanics (14%).[1] Warren[11] reported on her experience as an occupational therapist working in a low vision program in an ophthalmology department. Thirty-seven percent of the patients referred for occupational therapy (low vision

rehabilitation services) had AMD. Thus, low vision caused by AMD is the condition that occupational therapists working in eye clinics will most likely treat.

Risk Factors

Table 4-1 lists the risk factors associated with AMD. Age is the most significant risk factor and clearly increases the risk of both developing AMD and of progressing to the late stages of the disorder.[12] Although age is a strong risk factor, AMD and vision loss do not inevitably occur with advancing age. People with an AMD-affected first-degree relative have a 50% lifetime risk of experiencing advanced AMD and vision loss, and tend to develop it earlier than those without a family history.[13] Smoking is associated with a fourfold increase in the risk of AMD and visual loss and, again, tends to promote earlier occurrence.[14] Studies have consistently implicated female gender as a risk factor. In the Framingham Eye Study, females with AMD outnumbered males by 50%, but this may have reflected the increased proportion of women in the older age groups. In the Beaver Dam Study, results controlling for age showed a twofold higher incidence of AMD in women than in men in the 75-year and older group.[15] A relationship seems to exist between increased cumulative exposure to sunlight and ultraviolet radiation and wet AMD.[16] However, strong epidemiologic evidence is lacking. Weaker associations have been found with obesity, hypertension, macrovascular disease, raised cholesterol, and cataract surgery.

Dietary associations have also been found both with the signs of AMD and with progression to vision loss.[17-19]

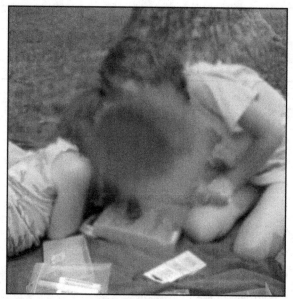

Figure 4-5. The effect of macular scotoma in AMD degeneration. (Reprinted with permission from Barbara Steinman.).

In a well-conducted prospective study, dietary fat intake was systematically analyzed after correcting for other risk factors.[18] Vegetable fat intake had the strongest relationship with AMD progression, with a relative risk of 3.82 for the highest fat-intake quartile compared with the lowest quartile. Higher intakes of total fat and of saturated, monounsaturated, polyunsaturated, and trans fats all raised the relative risk of AMD progression about twofold. Weekly fish intake and eating nuts 2 to 3 times a week were mildly protective. The implication is that a large shift away from vegetable oils, margarine, and fat-containing processed foods might reduce this epidemic of blindness in the elderly.

There is also evidence from a randomized controlled trial that high-dose dietary supplements of the antioxidants vitamin C, vitamin E, beta-carotene, and zinc can reduce the risk of progression from large or soft drusen to advanced AMD and visual loss by about 20% compared with controls over 6 years.[20] However, high-dose zinc can cause gastric irritation or anemia, and beta-carotene may possibly be associated with an increased risk of lung cancer among smokers. Uncontrolled studies suggest the antioxidants selenium, lutein, and zeaxanthin, which localize in the normal macula, may also help. There are as yet no studies to show whether dietary supplements are protective in patients in the early stages of dry AMD or in the 20% of patients who are at genetic risk.

It is not yet known whether major dietary adjustment and/or introduction of dietary supplements for large numbers of elderly people will be justified in terms of preventing blindness. On present evidence, we should identify people at increased risk of AMD; encourage them to stop smoking; and promote a diet that includes vegetables, fish, and nuts and reduces fatty foods laced with vegetable oils.

Antioxidant supplements may be recommended if a fresh diet is impractical and if retinal signs of progression are present. Clients should not attempt to treat themselves with vitamin therapy and should be encouraged to ask the eye care practitioner who is treating the retinal disease.

Effect on Vision

Visual acuity varies with the extent of the degeneration and includes distortion, blurred vision (especially at near), and central scotoma. With dry AMD, visual acuity can range from 20/20 to 20/400, but sometimes can be much worse with advanced geographic atrophy. Visual acuity with untreated wet AMD is generally worse than 20/400. Nearly all patients with only AMD have central visual field defects with normal peripheral vision. Patients with only AMD almost never go totally blind. However, if AMD occurs in both eyes, the visual acuity loss, along with the central scotoma, significantly impair a person's ability to engage in activities of daily living (ADL) and quality of life. High-resolution tasks such as reading, writing, sewing, telling time, taking care of financial issues, driving, and distinguishing colors and facial expressions usually become severely impaired. A hallmark of dry AMD is specific lighting requirements; usually more light is needed. The consequences of AMD lead to loss of independence, lowered self-esteem, decreased mobility, increased risk of injury due to falls,[21, 22] and depression.[23]

Figures 4-5 and 4-6 are schematics of the vision loss with AMD and a macular scotoma; people do not actually see the gray area, but tend to fill in the missing area with an unclear visual memory (see Figure 1-9). Some patients with absolute scotomas from AMD have a phenomenon called *Charles Bonnet syndrome*, or visual hallucinations.[24] This is an occasional complaint of patients with bilateral AMD and may occur spontaneously with no known external cause.

Treatment

Treatment of AMD includes various medical procedures to slow the progression of the disease; low vision rehabilitation, including optical and nonoptical devices to compensate for impaired visual acuity; environmental changes, especially changes in lighting; education; support groups; and training in eccentric viewing, scanning, and reading.

Dry Age-Related Macular Degeneration

There is no medical treatment for dry AMD that can restore vision loss. Patients who have early retinal changes, such as small drusen or mild pigmentation changes, may experience no symptoms or may notice slowly progressive changes in visual function. These patients are generally seen by an eye doctor every 6 months. The eye doctor should educate the patient to look for signs of decreased vision, scotoma, and distortion by covering each eye and

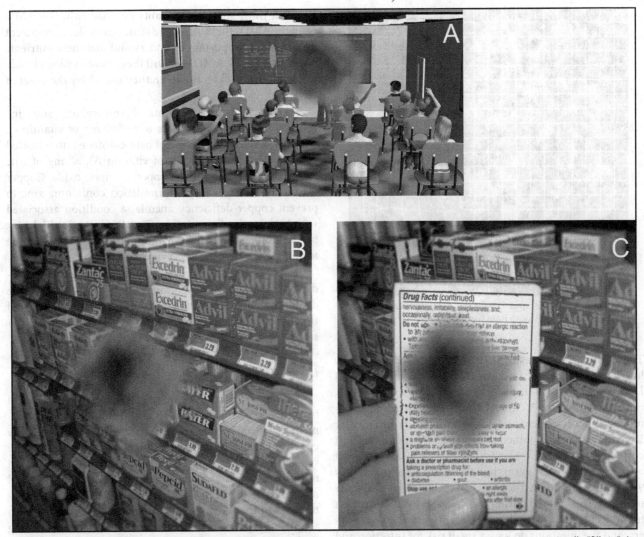

Figure 4-6. (A-C) The effect of macular scotoma in age-related macular degeneration. The person with a central scotoma visually "fills in" the gray area so that it blends into the visual scene and cannot be easily distinguished. (Reprinted with permission from Barbara Steinman.)

assessing visual function monocularly. The technical term for the distortion is *metamorphopsia* which is an indicator of retinal edema. Some eye doctors give the patient an Amsler grid (Figure 4-7) for self-assessment at home. The patient is able to see changes in the pattern of blur, distortion, and scotoma using the Amsler grid. Patients are instructed to return for further examination within 24 hours of the onset of new symptoms because 10% of patients with dry AMD progress to wet AMD. Studies have shown that early treatment of wet AMD may limit the extent of damage and vision loss.

Wet Age-Related Macular Degeneration

The principal aim of treatment of wet AMD is to preserve visual acuity and reduce the risk of additional severe vision loss for as long as possible. This goal can be accomplished by destroying the choroidal neovascularization without causing serious damage to the retina. Several treatments for wet AMD have proven effective in large-scale randomized clinical trials. These involve injection of drugs that inhibit vascular endothelial growth factor (VEGF). These treatments are not a cure for wet AMD, but may slow the rate of vision decline or stop further vision loss and in some cases even improve up to 3 lines, but visual impairment usually persists.

Injections

Injections of anti-VEGF drugs have revolutionized the treatment of wet AMD in recent years. Anti-VEGF injection therapy has largely supplanted older, less effective wet AMD therapies, including ocular photodynamic therapy and laser photocoagulation.[25] The 2 primary anti-VEGF agents approved by the US Food and Drug Administration (FDA) for wet AMD are Lucentis (ranibizumab) and Eylea (aflibercept). Another drug, Avastin (bevacizumab), has only been approved as an antiangiogenic cancer agent, but it has been successfully used off-label to treat wet AMD.[25]

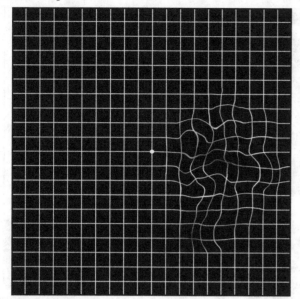

Figure 4-7. Amsler grid. Distortion reported by patient. (Reprinted with permission from Barbara Steinman.)

The advantage of Avastin is that the cost is dramatically lower than the cost of Lucentis. The safety and efficacy of Lucentis for wet AMD was demonstrated in 2 prospective, randomized, phase 3 clinical trials. In both studies, significantly more patients treated with monthly intraocular Lucentis either maintained vision (< 15 letters lost in best corrected visual acuity) or had improved vision (gain of >15 letters) versus sham injections.[26,27] Approximately 95% of Lucentis-treated patients had their vision stabilize or improve. The original dosing that was approved was once a month. But this is a burden for patients and their caregivers, and the injections do have a small risk for infection and endophthalmitis, a potentially devastating complication.[28] A number of studies have been done to compare monthly to quarterly dosing of the injections. All studies to date show that monthly dosing is superior.[28] While acknowledging that monthly injections of Lucentis is still considered the "gold standard" in wet AMD therapy, many retinal specialists use a treat-and-observe strategy to try to maximize intervals between injections.[29] Patients may defer treatment because they fear having injections directly into the eye, usually with devastating consequences.

Antioxidants

In a clinical trial called the Age-Related Eye Disease Study (AREDS), researchers found that high levels of antioxidants and zinc significantly reduce the risk of advanced AMD and its associated vision loss.[20] In this study, patients at high risk of developing advanced stages of AMD lowered their risk by about 25% when treated with a high-dose combination of vitamin C, vitamin E, beta-carotene, and zinc. In the same high-risk group, the nutrients reduced the risk of vision loss caused by advanced AMD by about 19%. For those study participants who had either no AMD or early AMD, the nutrients did not provide an apparent benefit.[20] It is important to understand that these nutrients are not a cure for AMD, nor will they restore vision already lost from the disease. However, they may delay the onset of advanced AMD.

The specific daily amounts of antioxidants and zinc used by the study researchers were 500 mg of vitamin C, 400 IUs of vitamin E, 15 mg of beta-carotene (often labeled as equivalent to 25,000 IUs of vitamin A), 80 mg of zinc as zinc oxide, and 2 mg of copper as cupric oxide. Copper was added to the AREDS formulation containing zinc to prevent copper-deficiency anemia, a condition associated with high levels of zinc intake. People who are at high risk for developing advanced AMD should consider taking the formulation under the supervision of a retinal specialist.

It is also important to understand that there is no evidence that this AREDS formulation is effective for those diagnosed with early-stage AMD. The study did not find that the formulation provided a benefit to those with early-stage AMD.

Low Vision Rehabilitation

Although vision loss cannot be restored with medical treatment, low vision rehabilitation is an effective treatment that enables patients with dry AMD to function more effectively in ADL and regain independence in spite of the visual deficit. The occupational therapist's role in low vision rehabilitation includes instruction in the use of optical and nonoptical assistive devices; modification of lighting, contrast, and other environmental factors; treatment to learn adaptive eye movement patterns, scanning, and reading skills; education; and involvement in support groups.

Many patients with AMD may not have had a recent examination and may benefit from a change in eyeglass prescription. Although new eyeglasses rarely restore vision, vision can significantly improve. Thus, a refraction is the starting point in low vision rehabilitation. This is especially true with people who have the dry type of AMD. If prescribed in conjunction with low vision rehabilitation in the early stages, most patients with AMD respond well to magnification at both distance and near (see Chapter 9). If they have absolute central scotoma, they often benefit from eccentric viewing instruction as well. With dry AMD, where the loss of vision is gradual, individuals with milder vision loss may disengage from occupations such as reading for pleasure or sewing because the tasks become difficult, and are often not referred because the condition has not stabilized. Left untreated, clients may develop clinically significant depression (see Chapter 6), yet early interventions that could avert serious disability may be as simple as instruction about lighting (see Chapter 10), use of contrast-enhancing e-readers (see Chapter 14), and a new set of stronger reading glasses (see Chapter 7).

DIABETIC RETINOPATHY

Description

Diabetic retinopathy is the most serious vision-threatening complication of chronic diabetes mellitus. Although there has been extensive research over several decades, knowledge about the etiology of diabetic retinopathy is still incomplete. Diabetes mellitus is a chronic, incurable disease with major medical and social implications. It occurs when the pancreas does not produce enough insulin or when the body cannot effectively use the insulin it produces. This results in high blood glucose levels in the body that can cause significant damage when levels are chronically high. The vascular complications of diabetes involve all organ systems, including the eye. Diabetes is a heterogeneous group of diseases with different etiologies and clinical features. The 2 major categories of diabetes are type 1 diabetes and type 2 diabetes.

Type 1 Diabetes

Type 1 diabetes occurs at any age, but most often before the age of 30 years. It has an abrupt onset. Those with type 1 diabetes are dependent on an exogenous, or outside, source of insulin. Only approximately 10% of the patients with diabetes have type 1 diabetes, and the remaining 90% have type 2 diabetes.

Type 2 Diabetes

Type 2 diabetes occurs at any age, but most often in adults over 30. It has an insidious onset and a subtle progression of symptoms. Those with type 2 diabetes are treated with diet, exercise, oral medications, and in some cases, an external source of insulin. People with type 2 diabetes are frequently obese and sedentary.

Diabetes can affect the retinal blood vessels and cause hemorrhaging and abnormal growth of new blood vessels into the vitreous (Figure 4-8).

Diabetic retinopathy has 4 stages:

1. Mild nonproliferative retinopathy: At this earliest stage, microaneurysms occur. They are small areas of balloonlike swelling in the retina's tiny blood vessels.

2. Moderate nonproliferative retinopathy: As the disease progresses, some blood vessels that nourish the retina are blocked.

3. Severe nonproliferative retinopathy: Many more blood vessels are blocked, depriving several areas of the retina of their blood supply. These areas of the retina send signals to the body to grow new blood vessels for nourishment.

The symptoms of nonproliferative diabetic retinopathy may be observed by the eye care practitioner, but individuals may not detect changes in vision.

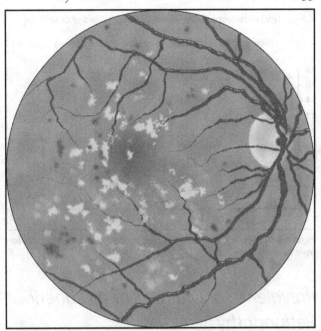

Figure 4-8. Diabetes can affect the retinal blood vessels and cause hemorrhaging and abnormal growth of new blood vessels into the vitreous. (Reprinted with permission from Barbara Steinman.)

4. Proliferative retinopathy: At this advanced stage, the signals sent by the retina for nourishment trigger the growth of new blood vessels. These new blood vessels are abnormal and fragile. They grow along the retina and along the surface of the clear, vitreous gel that fills the inside of the eye. By themselves, these blood vessels do not cause symptoms or vision loss. However, they have thin, fragile walls. If they leak blood, severe vision loss and even blindness can result. Proliferative diabetic retinopathy is the more advanced form of the disease, and in this condition the new blood vessels hemorrhage and grow into the vitreous. The vitreous may then pull away from the retina, causing additional hemorrhage into the vitreous. The hemorrhaging blocks transmission of the light through the normally transparent vitreous, causing significant vision loss. Floaters or debris in the vitreous may follow, along with retinal tears and detachment and additional loss of vision. Fluid can also leak into the center of the macula, the part of the eye where sharp, straight-ahead vision occurs. The fluid makes the macula swell, blurring vision. This condition is called *macular edema*. It can occur at any stage of diabetic retinopathy, although it is more likely to occur as the disease progresses. About half of the people with proliferative retinopathy also have macular edema. Macular edema can cause significant loss of vision along with distortion of vision.

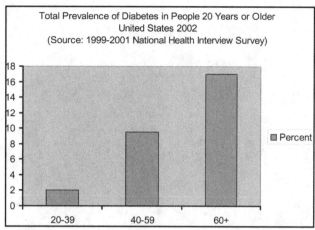

Figure 4-9. Prevalence of diabetes by age. (Reprinted with permission from Barbara Steinman.)

Prevalence of Diabetes and Diabetic Retinopathy

Diabetes affects 29.1 million people (about 9.3% of the population) in the United States.[30] An estimated 8.1 million people in the United States have diabetes and do not know it.[30]

Diabetes is the third leading cause of death in the United States after heart disease and cancer.[31] The prevalence of diabetes varies by age, as indicated in Figure 4-9. Men and women are equally affected. About 1.7 million people aged 20 years or older are diagnosed per year with new cases of diabetes.[30]

Diabetic retinopathy is the leading cause of new blindness in the 20- to 64-year-old population in the United States. It accounts for about 12% of all new cases of blindness each year. In a recent study of US adults 40 years and older known to have diabetes, the estimated prevalence rates for retinopathy and vision-threatening retinopathy were 40.3% and 8.2%, respectively.[1] The estimated US general-population prevalence rates for retinopathy and vision-threatening retinopathy were 3.4% (4.1 million persons) and 0.75% (899,000 persons respectively).[1] Future projections suggest that diabetic retinopathy will increase as a public health problem, both with aging of the US population and increasing age-specific prevalence of diabetes over time.[1] The prevalence of diabetic retinopathy among patients with diabetes is more dependent on the duration of the disease than the patient's age.[32]

Risk Factors

Having diabetes (whether type 1 or type 2) puts an individual at risk of retinopathy. The risk increases the longer the person has the disease. The Wisconsin Epidemiologic Study of Diabetic Retinopathy found that after having diabetes for 20 years, almost all people with type 1 diabetes

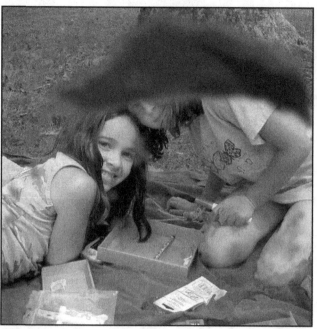

Figure 4-10. Illustration of visual problems of a client with diabetic retinopathy. (Reprinted with permission from Barbara Steinman.)

and more than 60% of those with type 2 diabetes have some degree of retinopathy.[32] The duration of the diabetes is also a major determinant of the severity of retinopathy and its progression. Other risk factors for diabetic retinopathy include poorly controlled blood glucose levels, high blood pressure, high blood cholesterol, pregnancy, obesity, and kidney disease.

Effect on Vision

Patients with diabetic retinopathy experience decreased, fluctuating, or distorted vision; focusing problems; loss of color vision; and floaters.[33] They frequently have impaired contrast sensitivity (because of cataracts), cloudy vitreous and retinal edema, are very glare sensitive, and are particular about lighting. They may also have a central scotoma due to effects the diabetes has on the macular area (maculopathy), loss of peripheral vision, and difficulty in dim light. Treatments (described next) often leave clients with a small island of good vision. They may see individual numbers or letters but not words. The treatments also produce scotomas in the periphery, or "Swiss cheese" vision. Figure 4-10 illustrates a schematic of the visual problems of a patient with diabetic retinopathy. Note once again that they do not see the scotomas as gray spots, but perceptually fill in the missing spaces.

Treatment

During the first 3 stages of diabetic retinopathy, no medical treatment is needed, unless macular edema is present. The current approach in these early stages emphasizes the early recognition of retinopathy, vigorous control of blood glucose, and direct therapy with laser photocoagulation and vitreous surgery. Rehabilitation interventions focus on lighting and glare control (see Chapter 10) and other compensations for mild acuity loss. Although the Centers for Medicare/Medicaid Services (CMS) criterion low vision diagnostic codes required for occupational therapy treatment are rarely met at these stages, occupational therapists can treat them in general rehabilitation if they are admitted under different diagnostic codes for conditions related to diabetes. Typically, these individuals will be seeing an ophthalmologist who specializes in treating the eye diseases. The most valuable intervention at this stage would be for the occupational therapist to make certain the client is under the care of an optometrist or general ophthalmologist who is paying close attention to functional issues such as refraction, tinted lenses for glare control, and possible need for extra-reading addition for mild acuity loss.

Proliferative retinopathy has been traditionally treated with laser surgery. This procedure is called *laser photocoagulation treatment*. Laser photocoagulation treatment helps to shrink the abnormal blood vessels. The ophthalmologist places 1000 to 2000 laser burns in the areas of the retina away from the macula, causing the abnormal blood vessels to shrink. Because a high number of laser burns are necessary, 2 or more sessions usually are required to complete treatment. Although the patient may lose some peripheral vision, scatter laser treatment can save central vision.

Laser photocoagulation treatment works better before the fragile new blood vessels have started to hemorrhage. Thus, patients with diabetic retinopathy should be seen frequently for follow-up appointments. Even if hemorrhaging has begun, laser treatment may still be possible, depending on the amount of bleeding.

With the development of anti-VEGF drugs, these medications are now being used to treat diabetic retinopathy as well. Lucentis has been shown to be effective for the treatment of diabetic macula edema. In the Restoring Insulin Secretion study of patients with type 1 and 2 diabetes and vision loss, 18.1% of those in the placebo group gained at least 15 letters of visual acuity vs 44.8% in the Lucentis group.[34]

If the hemorrhaging is severe, the patient may need a surgical procedure called a *vitrectomy*. During a vitrectomy, blood is removed from the vitreous of the eye. The ophthalmologist inserts a small instrument into the vitreous of the eye and removes the vitreous that is clouded with blood. The vitreous is replaced with a saline solution. The improvement in vision can be dramatic.

Effectiveness of Treatment

Both laser surgery and vitrectomy are effective in preventing additional vision loss.[35,36] People with proliferative retinopathy have less than a 5% chance of becoming blind within 5 years when they get timely and appropriate treatment. Although both treatments have high success rates, they do not cure diabetic retinopathy. Once a patient has proliferative retinopathy, he or she will always be at risk for new hemorrhages and should be carefully monitored by an eye care provider.

Low Vision Rehabilitation

The first step in low vision rehabilitation is an accurate refraction by the low vision optometrist and modification of the patient's eyeglasses, if required. One of the unique problems that occurs with diabetes is fluctuation of vision due to changes in refractive error and vitreous debris. This examination may need to be repeated if blood sugar levels are unstable. Visual acuities should be frequently remeasured. Because diabetes is often associated with other conditions treated by occupational therapists, the occupational therapist should routinely screen for vision loss (see Chapter 8), screen for the onset of retinal edema with an Amsler grid (see Chapter 8), and ensure the patient has a thorough retinal examination by an eye care practitioner at least every 6 months. In managing any client with diabetes, even those without a diagnosis of low vision, the occupational therapist should always be vigilant for visual changes and frequent eye examinations.

A hallmark of diabetic vision changes is impaired contrast sensitivity and glare sensitivity. The low vision optometrist may prescribe special tinted lenses that block blue wavelengths in an attempt to improve contrast, eliminate glare, and reduce sensitivity to light (photophobia) (see Chapter 10 and Chapter 12).[33] Patients often require multiple optical devices for various ADL (see Chapter 13). Because of their fluctuating vision, these individuals usually respond well to electronic magnification (see Chapter 14), where contrast can be enhanced and magnification varied. The occupational therapist must often work with the patient to improve eccentric viewing (see Chapter 10) if the macula is involved in the disease. Nonoptical devices, such as a talking glucose monitor and insulin-syringe aids, are helpful to the patient. Chapter 20 covers the rehabilitation of the diabetic patient in detail.

GLAUCOMA

Description

Glaucoma is not a single clinical entity, but a group of ocular diseases with various etiologies that cause an elevation of pressure in the eye (intraocular pressure [IOP]), ultimately leading to progressive optic nerve damage and loss of peripheral visual function.

Figure 4-11(A) is an illustration of the front of the eye, called the *anterior chamber*. The ciliary body is the

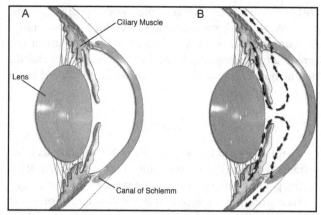

Figure 4-11. (A) Illustration of the front of the eye called the anterior chamber. (B) Aqueous fluid flowing into anterior chamber. (Reprinted with permission from Barbara Steinman.)

structure that produces *aqueous fluid*. This fluid is produced on a daily basis and flows to the front of the eye as illustrated in Figure 4-11(B). Because the eye is a closed structure, if new fluid is produced on a daily basis, an equal amount of fluid must drain out of the eye to maintain the proper IOP. Under normal conditions, the amount of aqueous fluid that is produced is equivalent to the amount that drains out on a daily basis, maintaining equilibrium and normal IOP. In glaucoma, this equilibrium is disrupted. There are a number of reasons why a person may develop glaucoma; however, regardless of the cause, the ultimate problem is loss of this equilibrium, which causes a rise in IOP. When the IOP rises, the nerve fibers exiting the eye through the optic nerve are compressed and damaged. The fibers that are generally affected in the beginning of the disease are those that carry information about our side vision (peripheral vision). Thus, in the initial stages of the disease, glaucoma leads to a gradual loss of peripheral vision. In most cases, the disease is painless because the rise in pressure is very gradual. As a result, a person with glaucoma may be unaware of the problem until the loss of vision is advanced. Thus, routine eye examinations are important to rule out this disease, and are the best way to avoid the consequences of glaucoma.

Glaucoma is classified as *primary* open-angle glaucoma when it is not related to another underlying condition, and *secondary* when the cause of the glaucoma is another ocular or systemic disease, trauma, or the use of certain drugs. Primary open-angle glaucoma represents about 70% of all glaucoma and is a chronic, progressive disease causing optic nerve damage and subsequent visual field loss. It occurs primarily in adults and generally affects both eyes, although one eye can have more advanced disease than the other. The majority of persons with primary open-angle glaucoma have elevated IOP. As described earlier, the elevated IOP observed in primary open-angle glaucoma usually results from decreased outflow of aqueous fluid from the eye. The cause of this decreased outflow is not well understood, but may be due to acceleration and exaggeration of normal aging changes in the area of the eye responsible for drainage of aqueous fluid (anterior chamber angle).[37,38]

How Is Glaucoma Diagnosed?

Several tests can help the eye care professional detect glaucoma. Individuals at high risk for the condition should have a dilated-pupil eye examination at least every 2 years. High-risk factors for glaucoma include being Black over 40, having a family history of the disease, or, for the general population, being over age 60. Those who are very nearsighted, have a history of diabetes, have experienced eye injury or eye surgery, or take prescription steroids also have an increased risk of developing glaucoma. Japanese ancestry is a risk factor for normal-tension glaucoma. Tests involved in the diagnosis of glaucoma include:

- Tonometry: Measures the fluid pressure inside the eye. There are several methods for measuring eye pressure. The Schiøtz and applanation tonometer measure eye pressure by directly applying pressure on the cornea. The tonometer is gently placed against the eyeball, and a pressure reading is then taken from the instrument. These methods require anesthetic drops in both eyes. Eye pressure can also be measured by sending a puff of air onto the eyeball. No anesthetic eye drops are required for this method.

- Pupil dilation: Special eye drops are used to temporarily enlarge the pupil so that the eye care specialist can obtain a better view of the inside of the eye.

- Visual field or perimetry: This measures the entire area that can be seen when the eye is looking forward to document straight-ahead (central) and/or side (peripheral) vision. The test measures the dimmest light that can be seen at each spot tested. The test consists of responding by pressing a button every time a flash of light is perceived.

- Visual acuity: This measures how well the person sees at various distances. While seated 20 feet away from an eye chart, the person is asked to read standardized visual charts with each eye. The test is performed with and without corrective lenses.

- Pachymetry: This procedure uses ultrasonic waves to help determine corneal thickness.

- Optical coherence tomography (OCT): This procedure is a noncontact, noninvasive imaging technique that can reveal layers of the retina by looking at the interference patterns of reflected laser light. Optical coherence tomography can detect problems with the retinal nerve fiber layer axons that cause the characteristic visual field defects and corresponding optic nerve head anatomical changes in glaucoma.

TABLE 4-2: RISK FACTORS FOR PRIMARY OPEN-ANGLE GLAUCOMA		
GENERAL	**OCULAR**	**NONOCULAR**
Age	Elevated or asymmetric levels of IOP	Diabetes Race Diffuse or focal enlargement of cup Vasospasms
Family history	Portion of optic nerve	Systemic hypertension
	Diffuse or focal narrowing of neuroretinal rim	
	Asymmetry of cup-to-disc ratio >0.2	
	Myopia	

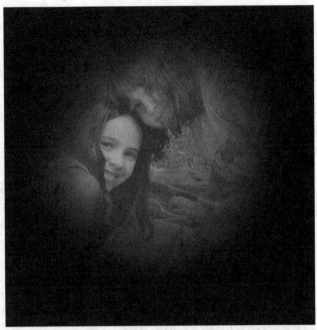

Figure 4-12. Reduction in visual field caused by glaucoma. (Reprinted with permission from Barbara Steinman.)

Prevalence

Glaucoma is an incipient disease and can progress to significant loss in peripheral visual function before the patient is aware that there is a problem. An estimated 2.5 million Americans have open-angle glaucoma,[39] although at least half of all cases may be undiagnosed.[40] Primary open-angle glaucoma represents about 70% of all adult glaucoma cases.[41] The Baltimore Eye Survey estimated the prevalence of glaucomatous blindness to be 1.7 per 1000 in the general population, of which more than 75% was due to primary open-angle glaucoma.[42] Over 11% of all blindness and 8% of all visual impairment may be due to glaucoma.[41] Primary open-angle glaucoma is 6.6 to 6.8 times more prevalent and accounts for about 19% of all blindness among Blacks, compared with 6% of blindness in Whites.[42]

Risk Factors

Risk factors for glaucoma include general and ocular factors (Table 4-2). Age is a major risk factor. The prevalence of glaucoma is 4 to 10 times higher in the older age groups than in persons in their 40s.[43,44] Race is another major risk factor for primary open-angle glaucoma. Blacks develop the disease earlier, do not respond as well to treatment, are more likely to require surgery, and have a higher prevalence of blindness from glaucoma than Whites.[44] Finally, a family history of glaucoma is also a significant risk factor. Ocular factors include high IOP, thinness of the cornea, and abnormal optic nerve anatomy.

Effect on Vision

Left uncorrected, glaucoma causes a reduction in the visual field (Figure 4-12), which may progress to total blindness. Central vision is generally unaffected until the end stage of the disease.[33]

Treatment

Treatment of glaucoma usually begins with medications (pills, ointments, or eye drops) that help the eye either drain fluid more effectively or produce less fluid. Patient adherence to glaucoma medications is a significant problem. Studies show that patients with glaucoma take 70% or less of the prescribed medications.[28] Several forms of laser surgery can also help fluid drain from the eye. There are assistive devices ("eye drop guides") available from vendors of low vision products and adaptive techniques to facilitate self-administration of eye drops.

Laser Trabeculoplasty

In this procedure, a high-intensity beam of light is aimed at the area of the anterior chamber of the eye responsible for drainage of the aqueous fluid. Several evenly spaced burns are used to stretch the drainage holes and allow the fluid to drain better. Laser trabeculoplasty is a common treatment if topical medication is not effective. The long-term benefits remain controversial because its effectiveness diminishes over time.[45]

Conventional Surgery

Conventional surgery makes a new opening for the fluid to leave the eye. This often is done after medicines and laser surgery have failed to control pressure.

Conventional surgery is about 60% to 80% effective at lowering eye pressure. If the new drainage opening narrows, a second operation may be needed. Conventional surgery works best if the patient has not had previous eye surgery, such as a cataract operation.

Surgical intervention, the third level of treatment for primary open-angle glaucoma, is required in many moderate or advanced glaucoma patients to lower the pressure if other treatments have not been successful. This surgery is also designed to improve the drainage of aqueous fluid from the eye. Filtration surgery usually results in a dramatic and stable reduction in IOP.[46] Although long-term control of IOP is often achieved, many patients must remain on medications and may require additional surgery.

Low Vision Rehabilitation

The hallmark of vision loss associated with glaucoma is night blindness and a need for more-than-typical amounts of light to see clearly. They are often glare sensitive and thus need a careful lighting evaluation (see Chapter 8) and management (see Chapter 10 and Chapter 12). For patients with intact central visual acuity and peripheral visual field loss, minification optical devices that expand the visual field are sometimes (but rarely) used. This is the opposite approach used for macular degeneration where visual acuity is impaired but peripheral fields are intact and magnification optics are used. Visual scanning strategies to compensate for an overall field loss, similar to techniques used with field cuts associated with stroke, are used as well. Severe visual field loss and impaired nighttime/low light vision associated with end-stage glaucoma can create problems with orientation and mobility (O&M), and referral to an O&M specialist is often required.[33] One problem in treating advanced glaucoma is that magnification to compensate for impaired visual acuity is contraindicated because of the small visual field. Many patients benefit from a change in eyeglass prescription to maximize visual acuity and reduce the need for magnification. Electronic magnification is often useful because it allows for improved visibility of text by increasing contrast and brightness rather than size of the text.[33] The occupational therapist's role in low vision rehabilitation includes techniques for medication management, especially if eye drops are used; instruction in the use of optical and nonoptical assistive devices; modification of lighting, contrast, and other environmental factors; referral for O&M; education; and involvement in support groups. Chronic glaucoma usually responds well to treatment if the patient consistently administers eye drops. For this reason, the occupational therapist should carefully evaluate

medication management if a patient experiences vision loss with chronic glaucoma.

CATARACT

Description

A cataract is an opacification or clouding of the lens in the eye that affects vision. Cataracts are very common in older people and can occur in either or both eyes. Figure 4-13 is an illustration of a cataract.

Age-related cataracts develop in 2 ways:

1. *Clumps of protein reduce the sharpness of the image reaching the retina.* The lens consists mostly of water and protein. When the protein clumps up, it clouds the lens and reduces the light that reaches the retina. The clouding may become severe enough to cause blurred vision. Most age-related cataracts develop from protein clumpings. When a cataract is small, the cloudiness affects only a small part of the lens. Over time, the cloudy area in the lens may get larger, and the cataract may increase in size.

2. *The clear lens slowly changes to a yellowish/brownish color.* The clear lens slowly changes color with age. At first, the amount of tinting may be small and may not cause a vision problem. Over time, increased tinting may make it more difficult to read and perform other routine activities. This gradual change in the amount of tinting does not affect the sharpness of the image transmitted to the retina. With advanced lens discoloration, a person may have difficulty identifying colors.

How Is a Cataract Diagnosed?

A cataract is easily detected in the course of any routine eye examination. The eye care provider finds reduced visual acuity that cannot be improved by modifying the patient's prescription. After dilating the pupil, the eye doctor uses instruments that provide views of the lens under a variety of magnified conditions. This direct examination of the lens allows the eye care provider to detect and diagnose the condition.

Prevalence

The Eye Diseases Prevalence Research Group completed a research study in 2004 designed to determine the prevalence of cataract in the United States and to project the expected change in these prevalence figures by 2020.[47] They collected data from major population-based studies in the United States and found that an estimated 20.5 million (17.2%) Americans older than 40 years have a cataract in either eye. Women have a significantly higher age-adjusted

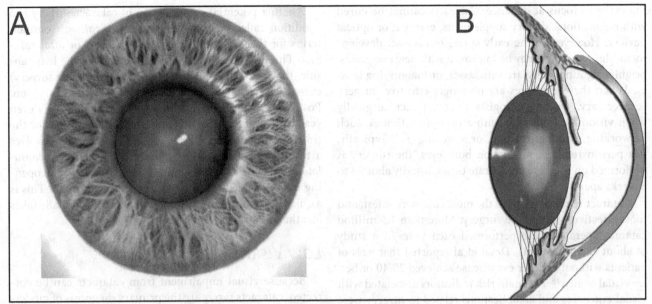

Figure 4-13. Illustrations of a cataract (A,B). (Reprinted with permission from Barbara Steinman.)

prevalence of cataract than men in the United States. The total number of persons who have a cataract is estimated to rise to 30.1 million by 2020. They concluded that the number of Americans affected by cataract and undergoing cataract surgery will dramatically increase over the next 20 years as the US population ages.[47]

Risk Factors

The main risk for developing cataracts is aging. By age 65, about half of all Americans have developed some degree of lens clouding, although it may not impair vision significantly. Other significant risk factors are diabetes, a family history of cataracts, previous eye injury or inflammation, previous eye surgery, prolonged use of corticosteroids, excessive exposure to sunlight, and smoking.

Effect on Vision

A cataract usually develops slowly and causes no pain. As a result, most people are unaware of its development until it begins to interfere with everyday activities. Symptoms of a cataract include the following:

- Blurry vision
- Increasing difficulty with vision at night
- Sensitivity to light and glare
- Poor contrast sensitivity
- Halos around lights
- The need for brighter light for reading and other activities
- Frequent changes in eyeglass or contact lens prescription

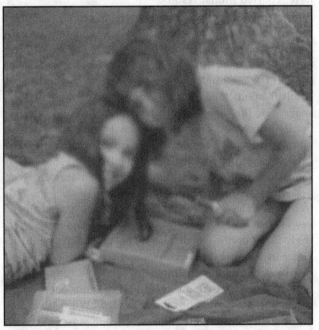

Figure 4-14. Illustration of visual problems of a client with a cataract. (Reprinted with permission from Barbara Steinman.)

- Fading or yellowing of colors
- Double vision in a single eye

Figure 4-14 illustrates the effect of a cataract on vision.

Treatment

The only effective treatment for a cataract is surgery to remove the clouded lens and replace it with a clear lens implant. The lens implant can correct refractive error as well. In some cases, one eye is corrected to focus at near and the other to focus at distance. Cataracts cannot be cured with medications, dietary supplements, exercise, or optical devices. However, in the early stages of cataract development, the symptoms may be improved with new eyeglasses, brighter lighting, antiglare sunglasses, or magnifying lenses. When these measures are no longer effective, surgery is necessary. Ophthalmologists treat cataract surgically when vision loss interferes with a person's activities, such as working, driving, reading, or watching TV. Typically, if a person requires surgery on both eyes, the surgery is performed on each eye at separate times, usually about 4 to 8 weeks apart.

Cataract removal is one of the most common, safest, and most effective types of eye surgery. More than 1.5 million cataract operations are performed each year. In a study of about 18,000 patients, Desai et al reported that 92% of patients without another eye disease achieved 20/40 or better visual acuity.[48] The main risk indicators associated with visual outcomes and complications related to surgery were age, other eye diseases, diabetes, and stroke. Other studies have reported similar results.[49,50]

There are 2 types of cataract surgery. The most common procedure is called *phacoemulsification*. During this procedure, the surgeon removes the cataract but leaves most of the outer layer (lens capsule) in place. The capsule helps support the lens implant when it is inserted. During phacoemulsification, the ophthalmologist makes a small incision where the cornea meets the conjunctiva and inserts a needle-thin probe. The surgeon then uses the probe, which vibrates with ultrasound waves, to break up (emulsify) the cataract and suction out the fragments. This procedure is sometimes referred to as *small-incision cataract surgery*. The other procedure is called *extracapsular surgery*. This technique is generally used if the cataract has advanced beyond the point where phacoemulsification can effectively break up the clouded lens. This procedure requires a larger incision where the cornea and sclera meet. Through this incision, the ophthalmologist opens the lens capsule, removes the nucleus in one piece, and vacuums out the softer lens cortex, leaving the capsule in place. With either procedure, after the lens has been removed, it is replaced with an artificial lens, called an *intraocular lens* (IOL). An IOL is a clear, plastic lens that requires no care and becomes a permanent part of the person's eye. If a person cannot have an IOL because of some other eye disease or problems during surgery, a soft contact lens or glasses that provide high magnification would be required to obtain clear vision.

Although cataract surgery is one of the most effective surgical procedures, there are potential risks, including inflammation, infection, bleeding, swelling, retinal detachment, and glaucoma. Occasionally, cataract surgery fails to improve vision because of conditions such as glaucoma or macular degeneration.

Another potential complication of cataract surgery is a condition called *posterior capsule opacification*. Common terms for this condition are *second cataract* or *after cataract*. This condition occurs when the back of the lens capsule (the part of the lens that isn't removed during surgery) eventually becomes cloudy and blurs the patient's vision. Posterior capsule opacification can develop months or even years after cataract surgery and occurs about 25% of the time. Treatment for posterior capsule opacification involves a technique called *yttrium-aluminum-garnet laser capsulotomy*, in which a laser beam is used to make a small opening in the clouded capsule to let light pass through. This is a quick and painless outpatient procedure that usually takes less than 5 minutes.

Low Vision Rehabilitation

Because visual impairment from cataracts can be corrected, cataracts rarely are the primary diagnosis of moderate or severe vision loss. Because normal lens changes in the eyes of patients over 80 years old involve mild cataracts, in most cases, low vision rehabilitation involves managing the mild impairment in contrast sensitivity, light sensitivity, and visual acuity in older patients with a nonvisual primary diagnosis. In some cases, especially when other visual pathologies are present, if a patient is medically fragile or refuses surgery, more severe cataracts are not removed. When moderate cataracts are involved, treatment focus is on management of glare, careful control of lighting, and environmental interventions and electronic devices to maximize contrast of reading material and objects with good results. Severe cataracts left untreated will result in profound vision loss and remain a major cause of blindness in underdeveloped countries.

DEMYELINATING DISEASE

Description

The term *demyelination* refers to a loss of myelin with relative preservation of axons. This results from diseases that damage myelin sheaths or the cells that form them. Demyelinating diseases of the central nervous system (CNS) can be classified according to their pathogenesis into several categories: demyelination due to inflammatory processes, demyelination caused by acquired metabolic derangements, hypoxic-ischemic forms of demyelination, and demyelination caused by focal compression.[51-53] Multiple sclerosis (MS) is the most common demyelinating disease and often is associated with numbness or weakness throughout the body, vision impairment, lack of balance, and fatigue.

How Is Multiple Sclerosis Diagnosed?

There are no specific diagnostic protocols for this disease. Rather, a series of tests is typically run to rule out other reasons for the patient's symptoms. The current diagnosis of MS involves a comprehensive history and neurological exam, along with a magnetic resonance imaging (MRI); spinal tap; and visual, auditory, and somatosensory evoked potential testing. The MRI is performed to detect areas of demyelination. Evoked potential testing is used to determine where delays in nerve transmission occur. The spinal tap is performed to rule out other conditions that can masquerade as MS.

Signs and symptoms suggesting a diagnosis of MS include the following:

- Age of onset between 20 and 50 years
- Evidence of 2 or more lesions in the brain from an MRI scan
- Objective evidence of disease of the brain or spinal cord on doctor's exam
- Two or more episodes lasting at least 24 hours and occurring at least 1 month apart
- No other explanation for the symptoms

Prevalence

Multiple sclerosis is the most common demyelinating disease and is an example of demyelinating disease due to inflammatory etiology.[54] It is the leading cause of neurological disability in young adults. Approximately 300,000 individuals in the United States are affected. It affects primarily young adults between 20 and 40 years of age. Multiple sclerosis is a major chronic disabling disease of young adults, affecting women more often than it does men.[55] A rare autoimmune disease that is often misdiagnosed as MS is neuromyelitis optica (NMO). This condition often quickly leads to total blindness and produces neuropathies and weakness because the spinal cord is involved.

Risk Factors

Several different genetic, sociodemographic, and environmental factors have been explored to determine who is more likely to get MS.[56] Some of the risk factors associated with MS include the following:

- Age: MS can occur at any age, but most commonly affects people who are ages 20 to 40.
- Gender: Women are about twice as likely as men to develop MS.
- Family history: If a parent or sibling has MS, the chance of developing it is 1% to 3% compared with the risk in the general population, which is just one-tenth of 1%.

- Ethnicity: White people, particularly those whose families originated in northern Europe, are at highest risk of developing MS. People of Asian, African, or Native American descent have the lowest risk.
- Environmental factors: Smoking has been found to be a risk factor for MS.
- Geographic regions: MS is far more common in areas such as Europe, southern Canada, northern United States, New Zealand, and southeastern Australia.

Effect on Vision

The human visual system relies on the constant transmission of information along myelinated pathways, and is therefore quite vulnerable to the effects of demyelinating disease.[57] Visual symptoms are common and may be transient or become permanent. If symptoms become permanent, they may become a source of significant disability among client rehabilitation services.[58] The visual pathways (retina, optic nerves, chiasm, and tracts) are often targets of inflammation, demyelination, and axonal degeneration. Nearly half of MS patients develop optic neuritis.[59] Optic neuritis may be the first indication of MS in 15% to 20% of patients. It can cause reduced visual acuity, difficulty with contrast sensitivity, and color vision anomalies. Other vision problems such as nystagmus, saccadic disorders, and binocular vision disorders with diplopia are commonly associated with MS.[57]

Treatment

There is no cure for MS. Rather, treatment focuses on strategies to treat attacks, manage symptoms, and reduce the progression of the disease. Pharmacological management of relapses involves the use of corticosteroids, while approved long-term treatments (disease-modifying treatments) aim to decrease the clinical relapse rate and concomitant inflammation within the CNS.[54,60] First-line disease-modifying treatments glatiramer acetate (GA) and interferon β (IFNβ) have been shown to be safe, but they are only moderately effective, and up to 40% of MS patients continue to show disease activity on these treatments. So far, no drug is available that can completely halt the neurodegenerative changes associated with MS.[61] New disease-modifying treatments are being developed and studied with the hope of improving the effectiveness of slowing progression and preventing relapses.[60,61]

Low Vision Rehabilitation

Patients with MS may not have had a recent examination and may benefit from a change in eyeglass prescription. For patients with diplopia and intact central visual acuity, vision therapy to restore normal binocular function may be useful. A common binocular vision condition that may be responsible for double vision in MS is convergence insufficiency.[62] Vision therapy has been found to be an effective treatment strategy for this condition.[63] Another potential treatment for diplopia due to a binocular vision disorder is the use of prism incorporated into the client's eyeglasses.[62] Both vision therapy and prism would have to be prescribed and administered by an optometrist. For patients with visual acuity, contrast, and visual field loss, the occupational therapist's role in low vision rehabilitation includes instruction in the use of optical (see Chapter 13) and nonoptical assistive devices (see Chapter 14); modification of lighting, contrast, and other environmental factors (see Chapter 12); referral for O&M; education; and involvement in support groups. Because these individuals often have hand tremor, weakness, and tactile impairments, they often respond especially well to electronic devices (see Chapter 14), which can be adapted for multiple impairments.

VISUAL FIELD AND RELATED DISORDERS

Description

The term *visual field* describes how much of the visual world an individual can see while looking straight ahead at a point of fixation. When a client has a normal visual field (see Chapter 3), he or she can see everything from the fixation point superiorly about 50 degrees, inferiorly about 70 degrees, temporally (toward the ear) about 90 degrees, and nasally (toward the nose) about 60 degrees. Thus, with only one eye open, a client has a horizontal visual field of about 150 degrees and vertically about 120 degrees. This is true for each eye. Note that with both eyes open, the horizontal field only increases by about 30 degrees. While only the object being viewed directly is seen clearly, the client is able to see this entire area peripherally and can perceive movement and the presence of objects in the entire visual field. The definition of low vision includes not only visual acuity, but visual field as well. A person is said to be legally blind if the visual field is 20 degrees or less in the better-seeing eye. Therefore, an individual could have perfect 20/20 visual acuity and still have low vision or even be legally blind. For Medicare using ICD9 codes, a diagnosis of a significant binocular visual field deficit would qualify the client for low vision rehabilitation even if visual acuity is normal. Although visual requirements for driving vary from state to state, in most states, the field requirement for driving is 120 degrees horizontally.

Visual field loss is usually classified as central vs peripheral visual field loss. As described earlier, the visual field is 150 degrees horizontally and about 120 degrees vertically. The central 10 to 20 degrees are referred to as the *central*

visual field. Outside this central 20 degrees is referred to as the *peripheral visual field*.

Another vision condition often confused with field loss is spatial neglect. This is a condition in which the client does not attend to stimuli on one side of the body, typically contralateral to the side of the cortical lesion. The term *visual inattention*, one component of the visual/spatial neglect syndrome, is also referred to as hemispatial neglect or unilateral neglect (see Chapter 11).

Peripheral Visual Field Loss

Peripheral visual field problems are associated with many eye diseases and diseases that affect the brain, such as glaucoma, retinitis pigmentosa, and acquired brain injury. One of the most common peripheral visual field disorders encountered by the occupational therapist in medical rehabilitation settings is a right or left field loss, referred to as a *homonymous hemianopsia* or *quadrantopia*. To understand why a patient would lose vision on just one side, it is necessary to understand how visual information travels from the retina to the visual cortex (see Chapter 3). Vision from the visual field on one side projects to the cortex on the opposite side of the brain. Vision begins with the capture of images focused by the optical media on photoreceptors of the retina. The fibers from the upper half of each retina enter the optic nerve above the horizontal meridian, and those from the lower half enter below the horizontal meridian. Fibers from the periphery of the retina lie peripherally in the optic nerve, and fibers from the fovea lie centrally. This arrangement persists throughout the entire course of the visual pathways from the optic nerve through the chiasm, the optic tracts, and optic radiations.

Any damage to the eye or optic nerve will affect one eye. Any damage beyond the optic chiasm will cause peripheral visual field loss in approximately the same place in both eyes. Brain injury associated with trauma or stroke often leads to this type of visual field loss and may require vision rehabilitation by occupational therapists.

Traumatic brain injury with a frontal or rear impact that damages the visual cortex may create tunnel vision because the cortical representation of the macular area is buried in a fissure and is somewhat protected. As described earlier, glaucoma is a disease that causes progressive peripheral field loss that leads to overall field loss.

Central Visual Field Loss

As discussed earlier, the most common visual field loss that an occupational therapist is likely to encounter is central visual field loss associated with diseases of the macula, such as macular degeneration. This type of visual field loss is referred to as a *central scotoma*. A scotoma is defined as an island of absent or reduced vision in the visual field, surrounded by an area of normal vision. These can occur with acquired brain injury as well.

Visual Inattention

Neglect can be divided into sensory (input) and premotor (output) neglect. Sensory neglect is characterized by unawareness of sensory stimuli of different modalities—including vision and tactile/somatosensory hemispace. Premotor neglect is described as failure to orientate the limbs toward contralesional hemispace despite awareness of the stimulus.

How Are Visual Field Disorders and Visual Inattention Diagnosed?

Peripheral visual field testing is generally performed in the office of the optometrist or ophthalmologist who refers the client for low vision rehabilitation. Standardized and more expensive computerized visual field testing is typically only available in the office of an eye care provider. Standard field testing requires that a client maintain a steady-fixation eye position. With people who have gaze instability or severe attention deficits, visual field testing becomes more of an art. As a therapist teaches a client to function with gaze instability, he or she often combines field testing with instruction on controlling gaze position and may provide critical data on a client's visual fields. Central field testing is best performed using a simple screen set at 1M (tangent screen) or in a less standardized fashion by an occupational therapist using a light-colored wall with a laser pointer (see Chapter 8). Unless one has a bowl perimeter, testing can be done using confrontation field testing methods described in Chapter 8. This requires no special equipment and can easily be performed by an occupational therapist.

Central visual field testing can be performed using a device called the *Amsler grid* test. The standard Amsler grid consists of a square grid of white horizontal and vertical lines on a black background. The client views this target with one eye open at a distance of about 13 inches. The client is asked to fixate on the central dot and report if all the corners are visible, if the grid is uniform, and if any areas of the grid are distorted or missing. Although easy to administer and interpret, the Amsler grid will miss scotomas. Other more reliable methods are discussed in Chapter 8.

Central field testing becomes more difficult to administer and interpret if people have central field loss because when they attempt to look directly at the fixation target in the center of the field test, the target disappears from view. As a result, people may look to the side of a target to see it, or some with recent vision loss just keep generating random searching eye movement, trying to look at a fixation target. With central field loss, sometimes functional tests such as reading can be sensitive to scotoma and informative to the practitioner. By adapting the standardized procedure, the eye care practitioner or low vision therapist can not only

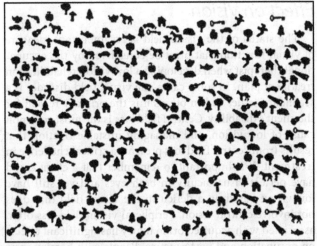

Figure 4-15. Illustration of a cancellation test for assessment of visual inattention.

describe a client's central fields, but also his or her fixation eye movements (see Chapter 8).

Visual inattention is typically assessed using pencil-and-paper tests, behavioral assessments, or clinical observation (see Chapter 11). A commonly used paper-and-pencil test is the cancellation test illustrated in Figure 4-15. The cancellation task requires the client to delete multiple identical visual target symbols on a sheet of paper. Incomplete or disproportionate deletion on one side indicates visual inattention. The Behavioral Inattention Test (BIT) and the Catherine Bergego Scale (CBS) are 2 of the most frequently used behavioral assessments and have been shown to have much higher sensitivity than pencil-and-paper tests (96% vs 65%).[64] A skilled clinician can observe a client engaged in ADL and, based on observations, make a tentative diagnosis of visual inattention.

Prevalence

Peripheral visual field loss has been found to be prevalent after acquired brain injury. Recent studies have found prevalence rates from 14% to 32% after stroke and traumatic brain injury.[65-69] A US study of 1281 stroke patients reported a prevalence rate of visual/spatial neglect (VN) of 43% and 20% following right and left hemispheric stroke, respectively.[70] This asymmetry in prevalence of VN probably occurs because the right hemisphere tends to allocate attention to both hemispaces, but the left hemisphere accords attention more selectively to the right hemispace.[71]

Risk Factors

Any brain injury affecting the visual pathways may have an adverse effect on visual fields. Injury to the right hemisphere is more likely to cause left visual inattention.

Effect on Vision

The status of the visual field is an important measure of visual function that must be considered by the occupational therapist when developing a low vision rehabilitation treatment plan. In some cases, the visual field disorder is a secondary issue, and in others it is the primary reason for the client's disability. Central field loss is the most common cause of low vision, and managing unstable fixation that results from central field loss presents a critical challenge in treatment. It is important to remember that a client could have perfect visual acuity in both eyes and yet still have low vision based on a deficit in the visual field that does not involve central vision. Peripheral vision field loss often associated with acquired brain injury has significant effects on occupation and performance. People with hemianopsia may have difficulty with any ADL that requires scanning the environment. A hemianopsia may be one of the reasons why a client experiences difficulty with grooming, eating, reading, cooking, finances, etc, after a stroke.

The effects of visual inattention are typically more serious than those of a hemianopsia because in visual inattention, the client is essentially unaware of the problem. In a recent review of visual inattention, Ting et al[71] reported some of the common problems reported with visual inattention, including difficulty with the following:

- Personal space (the space occupied by one's body): Combing, grooming, shaving, recognizing the right half of the body only, and anosognosia (a feature in which the patient is unable to recognize his or her own deficit)
- Peripersonal space (the space surrounding one's body within arm's reach): Eating food from the right half of the plate and neglecting the food on the left, reading the right half of the two pages of an open book, or missing the first couple of words in a sentence.
- Extrapersonal space (the space surrounding one's body beyond arm's reach): Failing to identify meaningful stimuli and people on the left, colliding into objects on the left while mobilizing or using a wheelchair.
- Allocentric space: Not attending to the left side of objects being viewed, such as the first couple of letters of a word being viewed to the right or left. This can be confused with field loss.

Treatment

There is no proven, effective treatment to restore normal visual fields (see Chapter 11). Once loss occurs, it becomes a chronic condition, and the only management is referred to as compensatory vision rehabilitation.

Low Vision Rehabilitation

Compensatory rehabilitation for visual field defects/inattention involves a number of steps, including awareness training, scanning practice and eye movement training, retraining reading skills, and the prescription of field expansion prism (see Chapter 11). The first goal is to increase the client's awareness and recognition that there is indeed a problem. If this can be accomplished, the therapy is often successful. Once the client understands the nature of the vision loss and accepts the idea that compensation is required, the therapists can teach the client how to safely scan the environment when engaged in ADLs. Additional rehabilitation to improve eye movement skills and reading training can then occur. In patients with hemianopsia without inattention visual field, expansion prism can be used to expand the visual field by up to 30 degrees.[72]

SUMMARY

It is important for the occupational therapist specializing in low vision rehabilitation to keep updated about the latest research regarding eye pathology and treatment. In a multidisciplinary low vision rehabilitation setting, the occupational therapist often is involved in helping clients with medication management. With clients who have active pathology, a treatment plan usually includes instructing the client about how to self-monitor for vision changes and educating the client regarding the cause, treatment, and prognosis associated with eye diseases. In home care, general outpatient, or inpatient setting where the occupational therapist does not practice with eye care providers, the occupational therapist who specializes in low vision plays an active role in ensuring that patients are receiving appropriate eye care and in ensuring appropriate referrals. In inpatient settings with older persons who typically also have nonvisual primary diagnoses, the occupational therapist often is the first to identify the need for a referral to a low vision optometrist. In these settings, the occupational therapist may provide the stopgap, nonoptical, low vision interventions necessary to maintain a rehabilitation program while the patient is waiting for an eye examination.

REFERENCES

1. Congdon N, O'Colmain B, Klaver CC, et al. Causes and prevalence of visual impairment among adults in the United States. *Arch Ophthalmol.* 2004;122:477-485.
2. Bird AC, Bressler NM, Bresler SB, et al. An international classification and grading system for age-related maculopathy and age-related macular degeneration. *Surv Ophthalmol.* 1995;39:367-374.

3. Klein R, Klein BEK, Linton K. Prevalence of age-related maculopathy. The Beaver Dam Study. *Ophthalmology*. 1992;99:933-943.

4. Hyman LG, Lilienfeld AM, Ferris FLI, Fine SL. Senile macular degeneration: a case control study. *Am J Epidemiol*. 1983;118:213-227.

5. Murphy RP. Age-related macular degeneration. *Ophthalmolog.y* 1986;93:969-971.

6. Ferris FLI, Fine SL, Hyman LA. Age-related macular degeneration and blindness due to neovascular maculopathy. *Arch Ophthalmol*. 1984;102:1640-1642.

7. Fine AM, Elman MJ, Ebert JE, et al. Earliest symptoms caused by neovascular membranes in the macula. *Arch Ophthalmol*. 1986;104:513-514.

8. Schmidt-Erfurth U, Hasan T. Mechanisms of action of photodynamic therapy with verteporfin for the treatment of age-related macular degeneration. *Surv Ophthalmol*. 2000;45:195-214.

9. Schwartz SD. Age-related maculopathy and age-related macular degeneration. In: Silverstone B, Lang MA, Rosenthal BP, Faye EE, eds. *The Lighthouse Handbook on Vision Impairment and Vision Rehabilitation*. New York: Oxford University Press; 2000.

10. Leibowitz HM, Krueger DE, Maunder LR, et al. The Framingham Eye Study monograph: an ophthalmological and epidemiological study of cataract, glaucoma, diabetic retinopathy, macular degeneration, and visual acuity in a general population of 2631 adults, 1973-1975. *Surv Ophthalmol*. 1980;24:335-610.

11. Warren M. Providing low vision rehabilitation services with occupational therapy and ophthalmology: a program description. *Am J Occup Ther*. 1995;49:877-883.

12. Hirvela H, Luukinen H, Laara E, Sc L, Laatikainen L. Risk factors of age-related maculopathy in a population 70 years of age or older. *Ophthalmology*. 1996;103:871-877.

13. Klaver CC, Wolfs RC, Assink JJ, et al. Genetic risk of age-related maculopathy. *Arch Ophthalmol*. 1998;116:1646-1651.

14. Klein R, Klein BE, Franke T. The relationship of cardiovascular disease and its risk factors to age-related maculopathy. The Beaver Dam Eye Study. *Ophthalmology*. 1993;100:406-414.

15. Klein R, Klein BE, Jensen SC. The relation of cardiovascular disease and its risk factors to the 5-year incidence of age-related maculopathy: the Beaver Dam Eye Study. *Ophthalmology*. 1997;104:1804-1812.

16. Newsome D. Medical treatment of macular diseases. *Ophthalmol Clin North Am*. 1993;6:307-314.

17. Cho E, Hung S, Willett WC, et al. Prospective study of dietary fat and the risk of age-related macular degeneration. *Am J Clin Nutr*. 2001;73:209-218.

18. Seddon JM, Cote J, Rosner B. Progression of age-related macular degeneration: association with dietary fat, transunsaturated fat, nuts, and fish intake. *Arch Ophthalmol*. 2003;121:1728-1737.

19. Seddon JM, Rosner B, Sperduto RD, et al. Dietary fat and risk for advanced age-related macular degeneration. *Arch Ophthalmol*. 2001;119:1191-1199.

20. Age-Related Eye Disease Study Research Group. A randomized, placebo-controlled, clinical trial of high-dose supplementation with vitamins C and E, beta carotene, and zinc for age-related macular degeneration and vision loss: AREDS report no. 8. *Arch Ophthalmol*. 2001;119:1417-1436.

21. Ivers RQ, Cumming RG, Mitchell P. Visual impairment and risk of falls and fracture. *Inj Prev*. 2002;8:259.

22. de Boer MR, Pluijm SM, Lips P, et al. Different aspects of visual impairment as risk factors for falls and fractures in older men and women. *J Bone Miner Res*. 2004;19:1539-1547.

23. Brody BL, Gamst AC, Williams RA, et al. Depression, visual acuity, comorbidity, and disability associated with age-related macular degeneration. *Ophthalmology*. 2001;108:1893-1900; discussion 1900-1891.

24. Siatkowski RM, Zimmer B, Rosenberg PR. The Charles-Bonnet syndrome. *J Clin Neuroophthalmol*. 1990;10:215-218.

25. Jager RD, Mieler WF, Miller JW. Age-related macular degeneration. *N Engl J Med*. 2008;358:2606-2617.

26. Brown DM, Kaiser PK, Michels M, et al, ANCHOR Study Group. Ranibizumab versus verteporfin for neovascular age-related macular degeneration. *N Engl J Med*. 2006;355:1432-1444.

27. Rosenfeld PJ, Brown DM, Heier JS, et al, MARINA Study Group. Ranibizumab for neovascular age-related macular degeneration. *N Engl J Med*. 2006;355:1419-1431.

28. Akpek EK, Smith RA. Current treatment strategies for age-related ocular conditions. *Am J Manag Care*. 2012;19:S76-S84.

29. Stewart MW. Aflibercept (VEGF Trap-eye): the newest anti-VEGF drug. *Br J Ophthalmol*. 2012;96:1157-1158.

30. American Diabetes Association. *Statistics about Diabetes*. Alexandria, VA: American Diabetes Assn; 2014.

31. National Institute of Diabetes and Digestive and Kidney Diseases. National Diabetes Statistics Fact Sheet: general information and national estimates on diabetes in the United States, 2003. In: Services UDoHaH, ed. Bethesda, MD: National Institutes of Health; 2003.

32. Klein R, Klein BEK, Moss SE, Davis MD, DeMets DL. The Wisconsin Epidemiologic Study of Diabetic Retinopathy. X. Four-year incidence and progression of diabetic retinopathy when age at diagnosis is 30 years or more. *Arch Ophthalmol*. 1989;107:244-249.

33. Brilliant RL. *Essentials of Low Vision Practice*. Boston: Butterworth-Heinemann; 1999.

34. Nguyen QD, Brown DM, Marcus DM, et al, RISE and RIDE Research Group. Ranibizumab for diabetic macular edema: results from two phase III randomized trials: RISE and RIDE. *Ophthalmology*. 2012;119:789-801.

35. Early Treatment Diabetic Retinopathy Study Research Group. Photocoagulation for diabetic macular edema. Early Treatment Diabetic Retinopathy Study report number 1. *Arch Ophthalmol*. 1985;103:1796-1806.

36. Smiddy WE, Feuer W, Irvine WD, Flynn HW Jr, Blankenship GW. Vitrectomy for complications of proliferative diabetic retinopathy. Functional outcomes. *Ophthalmology*. 1995;102:1688-1695.

37. Alvarado J, Murphy C, Juster R. Trabecular meshwork cellularity in primary open-angle glaucoma and nonglaucomatous normals. *Ophthalmology*. 1984;91:564-579.

38. Grierson I. What is open angle glaucoma? *Eye*. 1987;1:15-28.

39. Quigley HA. Models of open-angle glaucoma prevalence and incidence in the United States. *Invest Ophthalmol Vis Sci*. 1997;38:83-91.

40. Prevent Blindness America. *Vision Problems in the U.S.* Schaumburg, IL: Prevent Blindness America; 1994.

41. Leske MC, Rosenthal J. The epidemiologic aspects of open-angle glaucoma *Am J Epidemiol*. 1979;109:250-272.

42. Sommer A, Tielsch JM, Katz J, et al. Racial differences in the cause-specific prevalence of blindness in East Baltimore. *N Engl J Med*. 1991;325:1412-1417.

43. Hollows FC, Graham PA. Intraocular pressure, glaucoma, and glaucoma suspects in a defined population. *Br J Ophthalmol*. 1966;50:570-586.

44. Tielsch JM, Sommer A, Katz J, et al. Racial variations in the prevalence of primary open-angle glaucoma. The Baltimore Eye Survey. *JAMA*. 1991;266:369-374.

45. Baez K, Spaeth GL. Argon laser trabeculoplasty controls one third of patients with progressive, uncontrolled open-angle glaucoma for five years. *Trans Am Ophthalmol Soc*. 1991;84:47-58.

46. Werner EB, Drance SM, Schulzer M. Trabeculectomy and the progression of glaucomatous visual field loss. *Arch Ophthalmol*. 1977;95:1374-1377.

47. Congdon N, Vingerling JR, Klein BE, et al. Prevalence of cataract and pseudophakia/aphakia among adults in the United States. *Arch Ophthalmol.* 2004;122:487-494.

48. Desai P. The National Cataract Surgery Survey: II. Clinical outcomes. *Eye.* 1993;7(Pt 4):489-494.

49. McGwin G Jr, Scilley K, Brown J, Owsley C. Impact of cataract surgery on self-reported visual difficulties: comparison with a no-surgery reference group. *J Cataract Refractive Surg.* 2003;29:941-948.

50. Desai P, Reidy A, Minassian DC, Vafidis G, Bolger J. Gains from cataract surgery: visual function and quality of life. *Br J Ophthalmol.* 1996;80:868-873.

51. Hirtz D, Thurman DJ, Gwinn-Hardy K, Mohamed M, Chaudhuri AR, Zalutsky R. How common are the "common" neurologic disorders? *Neurology.* 2007;68:326-337.

52. Poser CM, Brinar VV. The accuracy of prevalence rates of multiple sclerosis: a critical review. *Neuroepidemiology.* 2007;29:150-155.

53. Graves J, Balcer LJ. Eye disorders in patients with multiple sclerosis: natural history and management. *Clin Ophthalmol.* 2010;4:1409-1422.

54. Tanasescu R, Ionete C, Chou IJ, Constantinescu CS. Advances in the treatment of relapsing-remitting multiple sclerosis. *Biomed J.* 2014;37:41-49.

55. Haberland C. *Clinical Neuropathology: Text and Color Atlas.* New York, NY: Demos Medical Publishing; 2007.

56. Finlayson M. *Multiple Sclerosis Rehabilitation: From Impairment to Participation.* Boca Raton, FL: CRC Press; 2013:247-271.

57. Nastasi JA, Krieger S, Rucker JC. Visual impairments. In: Finlayson M, ed. *Multiple Sclerosis Rehabilitation: From Impairment to Participation.* Boca Raton, FL: CRC Press; 2013:247-271.

58. McDonald WI, Barnes D. The ocular manifestations of multiple sclerosis. *J Neurol Neurosurg Psychiatry.* 1992;55:747-752.

59. Arnold AC. Evolving management of optic neuritis and multiple sclerosis. *Am J Ophthalmol.* 2005;139:1101-1108.

60. Nicholas J, Morgan-Followell B, Pitt D, Racke MK, Boster A. New and emerging disease-modifying therapies for relapsing-remitting multiple sclerosis: what is new and what is to come. *J Cent Nerv Syst Dis.* 2012;16:81-103.

61. Castro-Borrero W, Graves D, Frohman TC, et al. Current and emerging therapies in multiple sclerosis: a systematic review. *Ther Adv Neurol Disord.* 2012;5:205-220.

62. Scheiman M, Wick B. *Clinical Management of Binocular Vision: Heterophoric, Accommodative and Eye Movement Disorders.* 4th ed. Philadelphia: Lippincott, Williams and Wilkins; 2014.

63. Scheiman M, Gwiazda J, Li T. Non-surgical interventions for convergence insufficiency. *Cochrane Database Syst Rev.* 2011;CD006768.

64. Azouvi P, Samuel C, Louis-Dreyfus A, et al. Sensitivity of clinical and behavioural test of spatial neglect after right hemisphere stroke. *J Neurol Neurosurg Psychiatry.* 2002;73:160-166.

65. Brahm KD, Wilgenburg HM, Kirby J, Ingalla S, Chang CY, Goodrich GL. Visual impairment and dysfunction in combat-injured servicemembers with traumatic brain injury. *Optom Vis Sci.* 2009;86:817-825.

66. Goodrich GL, Kirby J, Cockerham G, Ingalla SP, Lew HL. Visual function in patients of a polytrauma rehabilitation center: a descriptive study. *J Rehabil Res Dev.* 2007;44:929-936.

67. Stelmack JA, Frith T, Van Koevering D, Rinne S, Stelmack TR. Visual function in patients followed at a Veterans Affairs polytrauma network site: an electronic medical record review. *Optometry.* 2009;80:419-424.

68. Ciuffreda KJ, Kapoor N, Rutner D, Suchoff IB, Han ME, Craig S. Occurrence of oculomotor dysfunctions in acquired brain injury: a retrospective analysis. *Optometry.* 2007;78:155-161.

69. Suchoff IB, Kapoor N, Waxman R, Ference W. The occurrence of ocular and visual dysfunctions in an acquired brain-injured patient sample. *J Am Optom Assoc.* 1999;70:301-308.

70. Ringman JM, Saver JL, Woolson RF, et al. Frequency, risk factors, anatomy, and course of unilateral neglect in an acute stroke cohort. *Neurology.* 2004;63:468-474.

71. Ting DSJ, Pollock A, Dutton GN, et al. Visual neglect following stroke: current concepts and future focus. *Surv Ophthalmol.* 2011;56:114-134.

72. Peli E. Field expansion for homonymous hemianopia by optically induced peripheral exotropia. *Optom Vis Sci.* 2000;77:453-464.

5

Optics of Lenses, Refraction, and Magnification

Optical devices are an important part of low vision rehabilitation, as they are used to compensate for impaired visual acuity by magnifying objects to enable a person to see objects more effectively at near, intermediate, and far distances. These optical devices include handheld magnifiers, spectacle magnifiers, stand magnifiers, and telescopes. An optometrist or ophthalmologist ultimately prescribes these devices. The occupational therapist contributes to the selection of the device, evaluates these devices with the tasks the client wishes to perform, often problem solves when the devices do not work as predicted, and plays the key role in teaching the client how to use the optical aids in various activities of daily living (ADL). To teach a client how to effectively utilize these devices, however, requires an understanding of the basic principles of lenses, optics, accommodation, and refraction. In this chapter we have carefully selected information that forms the core knowledge base for an occupational therapist providing low vision rehabilitation. This chapter provides the foundation for Chapter 8, the functional vision evaluation, and Chapter 13, where we describe details about the devices and instructional methods that can be used to select and teach clients how to use optical aids.

LENSES

Three types of lenses are used for eyeglass prescriptions and low vision optical devices: convex, concave, and cylindrical.

Convex Lens (Plus Lens)

A convex lens is thicker in the middle and thinner at the edges (Figure 5-1) and is also referred to as a plus lens, because when an optometrist writes a prescription for a convex lens, the + symbol is used. Convex lenses are used by eye doctors when prescribing glasses for hyperopia (farsightedness), as described in Chapter 2.

A typical prescription for a client with hyperopia (farsightedness) would look like this:

OD: +1.50

OS: +1.50

In this case, the acronym OD is used to designate the right eye, or oculus dextrus, and OS is the acronym for the left eye, or oculus sinister. Occasionally, you will see the acronym OU used. This is used to refer to both eyes, or oculus uturque.

Whittaker SG, Scheiman M, Sokol-McKay DA.
Low Vision Rehabilitation: A Practical Guide for Occupational Therapists, Second Edition (pp 67-77).
© 2016 Taylor & Francis Group.

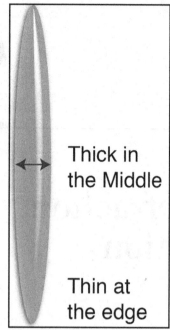

Figure 5-1. A convex lens is thicker in the middle and thinner at the edges. (Reprinted with permission from Barbara Steinman.)

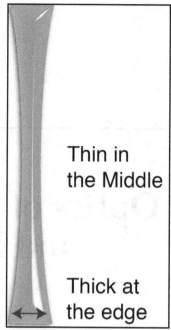

Figure 5-2. A concave lens is thicker at the edges and thinner in the middle. (Reprinted with permission from Barbara Steinman.)

Convex lenses are also used in most low vision optical devices such as handheld magnifiers, stand magnifiers, spectacle magnifiers, and telescopes (see Chapter 13). The therapist can quickly check to see if a client has been prescribed a plus lens for hyperopia by looking through it. If distance objects are blurred and near objects are clear, it is a convex lens. Note that because the lens compensates for hyperopia, it will have an effect opposite to the refractive error, making objects clear at near.

Concave Lens (Minus Lens)

A concave lens is thinner in the middle and thicker at the edges (Figure 5-2) and is also referred to as a minus lens. When an optometrist writes a prescription for a convex lens, the symbol (–) is used. Concave lenses are used by eye doctors when prescribing glasses for myopia (nearsightedness), as described in Chapter 2.

A typical prescription for a client with myopia (nearsightedness) would look like this:

OD: –1.50

OS: –1.50

The therapist can quickly check to see if a client has been prescribed a concave lens for myopia by looking through it. If distance objects look smaller and are clear, it is a concave lens, opposite to the effect of myopia.

Cylindrical Lens (Astigmatic Lens)

While a convex or concave lens has only one uniform power throughout the lens, a cylindrical lens has 2 powers and is used for the treatment of astigmatism. Most clients have a combination of hyperopia and astigmatism or myopia and astigmatism. The occupational therapist can easily determine if a client has astigmatism by looking at his or her eyeglass prescription. A typical prescription for a client with astigmatism and myopia (nearsightedness) would look like this:

OD: –1.50 –1.25 × 180

OS: –1.50 –1.50 × 180

This would be read as "Right eye, minus 1.50 with minus 1.25 axis 180 and left eye, minus 1.50 with minus 1.50 axis 180."

An example of a prescription for a client with astigmatism and hyperopia (farsightedness) would look like this:

OD: +2.50 –2.25 × 180

OS: –2.00 –1.75 × 180

The therapist can quickly check to see if a client has been prescribed a cylindrical lens for astigmatism by looking through it and slowly turning the lens clockwise or counterclockwise. If the object being viewed changes shape as it is rotated, the correction has a cylindrical component to correct for astigmatism.

ACCOMMODATION

Definition and Description

Assuming that any refractive error has been corrected with eyeglasses, the human visual system is physiologically focused for objects at distances of 20 feet and greater. If an object is brought closer than 20 feet, a focusing adjustment must be made or the object will appear blurred. This focusing adjustment is referred to as accommodation. Accommodation is the ability to change the focus of the eye so that objects at different distances can be seen clearly. Accommodation occurs by stimulating the smooth muscle of the ciliary body in the eye to contract, thereby enabling the lens to change its shape to become more convex. Optically, therefore, accommodation is identical to putting a variable plus-lens in front of the eye. Figure 5-3(A) is a cross-section of the human eye showing the lens and the ciliary muscle in its relaxed state. The light rays entering the eye are focused behind the retina, which would cause blurred vision. In Figure 5-3(B), the ciliary muscle has contracted and allows the light rays to focus on the retina.

The accommodative ability of an individual is inversely related to age. We use the term *accommodative amplitude* to refer to the total amount of accommodation available for a particular client. Young children have very large amplitudes of accommodation, and this declines with age. This relationship between age and accommodative amplitude is so consistent across the population that it is possible for an optometrist to predict a client's age within several years simply by measuring the amplitude of accommodation. The accommodative amplitude declines gradually with age, and by 40 to 45 years of age, the decline is significant enough to interfere with the ability to see small print held at a normal reading distance of 40 cm (16 inches). This is referred to as presbyopia.

Presbyopia is a condition in which near visual acuity is decreased because of an age-related decline in accommodative ability. All adults after the age of 45 or so have this condition and require reading glasses or some modification of their eyeglasses to account for it. Reading glasses that supplement accommodation position plus lenses in front of each eye. Bifocals are lenses that add extra plus to a person's distance prescription, referred to as reading addition or by the shorthand term *add*. Since most clients will be older, occupational therapists working in the field of low vision rehabilitation of adults usually deal with clients who have presbyopia and require a reading addition to focus at near.

In the report from an eye care practitioner, the reading addition is specified as the number at the end of the prescription for refractive error. It always follows a plus sign, but should not be confused with the correction for

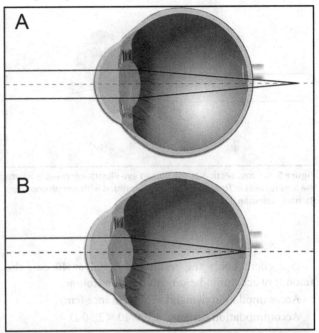

Figure 5-3. (A) Cross-section of the human eye illustrating hyperopia where the lens, when relaxed, focuses behind the retina. (B) Ciliary muscle around the lens has contracted, increasing the thickness and power of the lens so the light rays focus on the retina. (Reprinted with permission from Barbara Steinman.)

hyperopia. An example for a correction for 1 diopter (D) of hyperopia, 2.25 D of astigmatism, with 2.50 D of reading addition to compensate for presbyopia would be as follows:

OD: +1.00 –2.25 × 180, +2.50

OS: +1.00 –2.25 × 180, +2.50

Significance of Accommodation for Low Vision Rehabilitation

When working with optical aids, it is important to consider accommodation and how it may impact the client's ability to use the device. With some optical devices, the client is required to accommodate; with others, accommodation is not required. To determine if a client must use accommodation, one must consider a number of factors, including the working distance, or the distance from the eye to the material being viewed. The working distance is the distance at which the object being viewed is held from the eye, always specified in metric units. If an object is held at 20 feet (~6 meters), no accommodation is required. As the object is brought closer, more and more accommodation is required. We determine the amount of accommodation required by using the following formula:

Accommodation demand = 100(cm)/working distance in centimeters (sometimes if distance is specified in meters, the formula used is 1/working distance in meters)

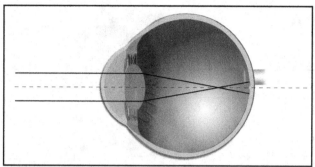

Figure 5-4. Cross-section of the human eye illustrating myopia where the lens focuses in front of the retina. (Reprinted with permission from Barbara Steinman.)

Example 1

If a client holds the reading material at 40 cm, the amount of accommodation required is as follows:
Accommodation demand = 100/distance (cm)
Accommodation demand = 100/40 = 2.50 D

Example 2

If a client holds the reading material at 10 cm, the amount of accommodation required is as follows:
Accommodation demand = 100/distance (cm)
Accommodation demand = 100/10 = 10 D

Thus, close working distances require a considerable amount of accommodation. In the adult population over the age of 40 years, the ability to accommodate has declined significantly. The optometrist must consider this when prescribing the optical aid, and the occupational therapist must always be aware of the issue of accommodation when instructing clients in the use of optical devices.

If a client is experiencing difficulty using an optical device, one of the issues to consider is accommodation. This will be reviewed in detail in Chapter 13.

REFRACTIVE DISORDERS

Definition

Refraction is the term used to describe the evaluation of the optical system of the eye. We use the term *refractive error* to describe any disorder of refraction. When the optometrist performs the refraction, he or she determines whether the individual is emmetropic (absence of refractive error), myopic (nearsighted), hyperopic (farsighted), or astigmatic. The refraction is the examination procedure used to determine if a client will benefit from glasses and the exact prescription that is appropriate.

Classification of Refractive Conditions

Emmetropia

This term is used to describe the condition in which there is an absence of refractive error. In *emmetropia*, the light rays entering the eyes focus right on the retina. Figure 5-3(B) illustrates how the light rays entering the eye are perfectly focused on the retina. With emmetropia, this focus is achieved without any accommodation. In such a case, the client is neither nearsighted nor farsighted and does not have astigmatism. Emmetropia is not necessarily considered normal, expected, or desirable. In fact, the average person is slightly hyperopic.

Myopia (Nearsightedness)

Myopia is a condition in which the light rays entering the eye focus in front of the retina. In myopia, the vision is blurred at distance but clear at near. Figure 5-4 shows why a client with myopia experiences blurred vision. The light rays entering the eye are focused in front of the retina because the optics of the eye are too strong relative to the length of the eye. The myopic eye has a longer axial length than the emmetropic or hyperopic eye. The human eye can make no internal adjustment to overcome the optical problem associated with myopia. An individual with myopia can squint, which actually does allow improved vision, but this is generally considered an unacceptable way to regain clarity because it can cause discomfort and is cosmetically unacceptable. Squinting helps compensate for the blur associated with myopia because it creates a pinhole effect. A pinhole effect occurs when an individual views an object through a small opening in front of the eye. This setup will bring an object into focus on the retina, regardless of refractive error. Any attempted focusing adjustment by the lens of the eye (accommodation) will simply make the blurred vision worse. Thus, a client with myopia will have to move closer to the object he or she is trying to view. A person who has myopia ("nearsightedness") will have better visual acuity at near than at distance if he or she is not wearing correction.

Hyperopia (Farsightedness)

Hyperopia is a condition in which light rays entering the eye focus behind the retina and the individual must accommodate to see clearly. This need to accommodate requires the use of muscular effort. The amount of effort necessary is greater when the individual looks at near. Figure 5-3(A) and Figure 5-3(B) illustrate that to see clearly, a person with hyperopia must contract the ciliary muscle to change the shape of the lens in the eye to focus the image on the retina and regain clarity. Contraction of the ciliary muscle leads to a change in focus and is referred to as *accommodation*. The effort that is necessary to accommodate is directly related to the degree of hyperopia. A very high degree of hyperopia requires so much muscular effort that it cannot be overcome and results in blurred vision. Moderate degrees of hyperopia can be overcome using accommodation. The constant need for accommodation, however, requires the use of muscular effort and leads to signs and symptoms such as blurred vision, eyestrain, tearing, burning, inability to concentrate and attend, avoidance of visual tasks, and the need to move the object of interest closer or farther away. In younger people, small degrees of hyperopia are generally successfully overcome without symptoms. Remember that a low degree of hyperopia is considered normal, expected, and desirable. An older person with hyperopia (older than 45 to 50 years of age) cannot accommodate well enough to compensate for the hyperopia and will, therefore, have better acuity at distance than at near. A younger person with hyperopia who can compensate with accommodation might have normal acuity at near but complain of eyestrain or blurry vision at near when tired.

Astigmatism

Astigmatism is a condition in which vision is blurred and distorted at both distance and near. An astigmatic eye is not spherical. Rather, it has an oval shape, and this causes the light rays entering the eye to focus at 2 different points. Figure 5-5(A) illustrates the effect that astigmatism has on the light rays focusing on the retina and the effect on image perception (Figure 5-5[B]). In order to see clearly, a person with astigmatism will attempt to accommodate. While accommodation may improve clarity in one direction (eg, vertical lines), accommodation never completely clears an image with astigmatism, and the effort that is necessary to accommodate may lead to discomfort. As discussed earlier for hyperopia, the degree of accommodation necessary is related to the degree and type of astigmatism. In some cases of astigmatism, accommodation has no beneficial effect on clarity. A very high degree of astigmatism generally cannot be overcome and results in blurred vision. If not corrected early, such problems can lead to amblyopia (loss of vision) and difficulty interacting with the environment. Moderate degrees of astigmatism can sometimes be overcome using accommodation. The constant need for accommodation, however, requires the use of muscular effort and leads to signs and symptoms such as blurred vision, eyestrain, tearing, burning, inability to concentrate and attend, avoidance of visual tasks, and the need to move the object of interest closer or farther away. Small degrees of astigmatism are common and are generally successfully overcome without symptoms. A person with astigmatism will have reduced acuity at both distance and near, and may see stripes in one direction more clearly than stripes in another, so some letters may be easier to see than others.

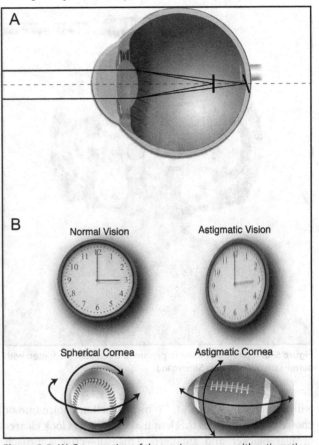

Figure 5-5. (A) Cross-section of the eye in someone with astigmatism. Asymmetry in the cornea and lens focuses lines at 2 points depending on the orientation of orthogonal lines (90 degrees different orientation). In this case, the vertical lines focus in front of the horizontal lines. (B) How objects appear with a symmetrical and astigmatic lens. (Reprinted with permission from Barbara Steinman.)

Clinical Assessment of Refractive Error

Refraction is a test that is performed by all eye care professionals. There are 2 general methods of evaluating the refractive status of the eye: objective and subjective. Subjective tests can only be successfully performed with cooperative, attentive clients with reasonable cognitive ability. Objective testing, however, can be successfully performed at any age and for virtually any client.

Subjective Refraction Techniques

Most adults have had an eye examination at least once in their lives, and, if so, they are likely to remember the subjective refraction portion of the examination. The instrumentation used is illustrated in Figure 5-6. This instrument, called the *phoropter*, contains numerous lenses and allows the optometrist to find the combination of lenses that will provide the best possible vision for any client being examined. The procedure is very subjective, and the optometrist

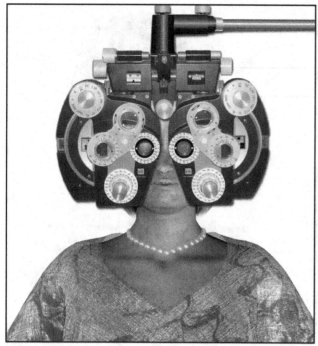

Figure 5-6. A phoropter used to perform a refraction. (Reprinted with permission from Barbara Steinman.)

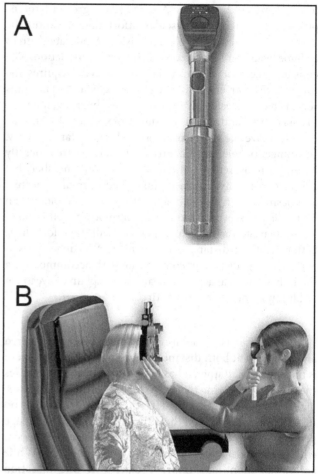

Figure 5-7. (A) A retinoscope used for an objective refraction. (B) An objective refraction involves the examiner using a retinoscope to look through lenses at the eye to determine refractive error. (Reprinted with permission from Barbara Steinman.)

will ask questions such as, "Which is better, choice one or choice two?" or "Does this lens make the letters look clearer or just blacker and smaller?" This subjective approach works well for most of the population, but is generally not used with children under the age of 6 or 7 or with clients who have attention problems, perceptual and cognitive disorders, or other special needs.

Objective Refraction Techniques

Using objective refraction, the optometrist or ophthalmologist is able to identify and correct refractive error in infants and patients who are unable to communicate. The instrument illustrated in Figure 5-7(A) is called a *retinoscope*. This instrument permits the optometrist to accurately and objectively assess refractive status in virtually any client by directing the light from the retinoscope into the client's eye and viewing the light that is reflected out of the eye (Figure 5-7[B]). As the optometrist moves the retinoscope from side to side, he or she interprets the movement of the reflected light. Lenses are used to alter the movement of light and help the clinician determine the refraction and necessary eyeglass prescription. The procedure generally requires less than 1 minute per eye. It can be performed with or without eye drops.

Screening for Refractive Error

A therapist can quickly screen for potential problems with refractive error when glasses are not available by having the patient look through a pinhole. The therapist asks the client to view a chart through a pinhole (a pinhole occluder can be purchased inexpensively). The pinhole bypasses the optics of the eye and focuses an image on the retina, regardless of refractive error. The pinhole will greatly reduce the amount of light, but will improve acuity regardless of the refractive error if the chart is illuminated enough. If reduced visual acuity improves with a pinhole, vision can usually be improved with eyeglasses.

Significance of Refractive Disorders for Occupational Therapy

It is important that significant refractive errors be treated by an eye care practitioner before low vision rehabilitation is initiated. Some might feel that a small amount of refractive error might not significantly affect functional vision in someone who has severe vision loss. However, a good refraction should always be the very first step in the treatment of any low vision client, even with severe vision loss. Researchers have been surprised at the high prevalence of uncorrected refractive errors in the elderly population. The Baltimore Eye Study found that almost 70% of people

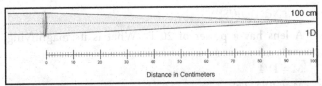

Figure 5-8. A 1-diopter lens will focus parallel light rays entering the lens from a distant object to a point of focus 100 cm away. (Reprinted with permission from Barbara Steinman.)

reporting low vision based on reduced visual acuity alone actually only needed new eyeglasses.[1] Correctable vision impairment is associated with poorer general health, living alone, and lower socioeconomic status.[2]

OPTICS OF LENSES

Manufacturers use 2 different methods to label the power or magnifying capability of optical devices. Some designate the device or lens by its actual power, while others label the device using the term *magnification*. This information, in whichever format provided, tells the therapist how to position the device and how to instruct the client to use the optical device. It is, therefore, important to understand various parameters of lenses, such as focusing power, focal distance, and magnification.

Focusing Power of a Lens

The unit of measurement of the focusing power of a lens is called a *diopter* (D). The definition of a 1-D lens is one that will focus parallel light rays entering the lens from a distant object to a point of focus 100 cm away (Figure 5-8). We refer to this as a 1-D lens. As the power of a lens increases, it focuses parallel rays of light closer and closer to the back surface of the lens.

We use the following formula to determine the power of a lens:

D = 100/d (cm)

Examples

1. A lens focuses parallel light at 1 meter: D = 100/100 = 1 D

2. A lens focuses parallel light at 50 cm: D = 100/50 = 2 D

3. A lens focuses parallel light at 33 cm: D = 100/33 = 3 D

4. A lens focuses parallel light at 25 cm: D = 100/25 = 4 D

5. A lens focuses parallel light at 10 cm: D = 100/10 = 10 D (Figure 5-9)

Many of the optical devices that the occupational therapist will use with clients will have the power of the device designated in diopters. Note that the formula for accommodative demand is the same because it measures the required

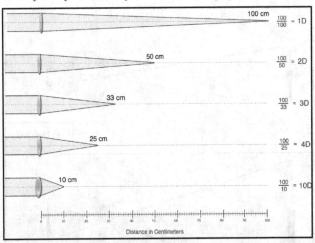

Figure 5-9. Five examples of convex lenses of varying power. (Reprinted with permission from Barbara Steinman.)

focusing power. Both indicate magnification because bringing something closer to the eye magnifies the object.

Focal Distance (Length) of a Lens

Another important term used in optics is the *focal distance* of a lens. The focal distance of a lens is the distance at which the lens brings parallel rays to a sharp focus. It is the distance between the lens and the point of focus. The point or plane at which the lens focuses light is called the focal point of the lens. The focal distance of the lens is determined by the power of the lens in diopters.

The focal distance of a lens is computed using the following formula:

Focal distance (cm) = 100/D

Thus, the focal distance of a lens is the reciprocal of the dioptric power. The greater the power of the lens, the closer the image is focused to the back of the lens.

Examples

1. The focal length of a 1-D lens: 100/1 = 100 cm

2. The focal distance of a 2-D lens: 100/2 = 50 cm

3. The focal distance of a 3-D lens: 100/3 = 33 cm

4. The focal distance of a 4-D lens: 100/4 = 25 cm

5. The focal distance of a 10-D lens: 100/10 = 10 cm

Knowledge of the focal distance is critical for the occupational therapist because it determines the distance at which the client needs to hold the optical device from the working material. We will refer to this distance as the lens-to-object distance.

For example, a client is using a 10-D handheld magnifier to read a label on a can of soup. How far from the can of soup should the client hold the magnifier to achieve the most magnification with a sharp focus? To determine lens-to-object distance of this magnifier, use the following formula:

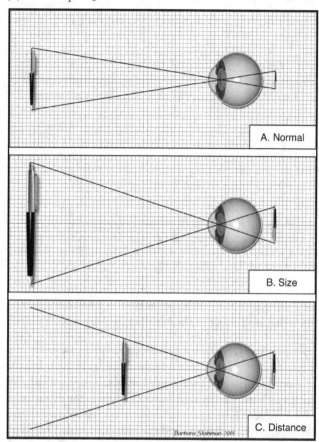

Figure 5-10. Size magnification (middle) and relative distance magnification (bottom) both have the same effect—to increase the size of the image on the retina. Doubling the size is equivalent to halving the distance. (Reprinted with permission from Barbara Steinman.)

Lens-to-object distance = 100/D = 100/10 = 10 cm

In this case, the occupational therapist would instruct the client to hold the magnifier 10 cm from the can of soup. Thus, if the dioptric power of the lens is known, the therapist can determine the appropriate lens-to-object distance of the optical device.

Optics of Magnification

One method of describing a low vision optical device lens is by its dioptric power as described earlier. For example, a handheld magnifier may have a power of 6, 10, or 20 D. Another method used by manufacturers to describe an optical device is by its degree of magnification. A device might be labeled as a 5× or 10× magnifier, for example. Unfortunately, the convention used to calculate magnification is inconsistent.

The most common formula used to relate the power of a lens to its magnifying ability is as follows:

M = D/4

where M = magnification

Examples

A lens has a power of 20 D. What is its magnifying power?

M = D/4

M = 20/4 = 5×

Other manufacturers may use the formula:

M = D/4 +1

Others may use the formula:

M = D/2.5

Thus, the actual magnification of a device marked as 4× may differ between manufacturers depending on the definition used to determine the magnification. In addition, for other devices such as telescopes and video magnifiers, magnification is described as how much the image viewed through the optical device is enlarged. For example, a 4× telescope implies that the object size as viewed through the telescope is 4 times larger than the same object viewed without the telescope. This inconsistency in terminology is a source of great confusion for therapists. Because of this inconsistency, in this text, we use the term *magnification* only in a general qualitative sense, as in "to make something appear larger."

Fortunately, one general convention has emerged in low vision care that helps resolve this problem. The magnification of any near device can be described as the power "equivalent" to the power of the near reading addition. This is referred to as equivalent power (EP).[3] All major manufacturers now list the EP of their devices. This is the standard used for the Academy for Certification of Vision Rehabilitation & Education Professionals (ACVREP) certification examination for low vision therapists as well. In order to understand how EP relates to magnification, one must first understand the various ways that an object can be magnified to compensate for impaired visual acuity. We will use terms such as *2×* and *4×*, but only to describe how many times something is enlarged.

Methods of Achieving Magnification

One of the primary ways to compensate for impaired visual acuity is to magnify the object of interest. All methods of magnification enlarge the retinal image of an object. There are 4 methods of achieving this goal. These 4 methods are actually variations of either relative distance or relative size magnification (Figure 5-10). The relationship between relative size and relative distance magnification forms the foundation for understanding all interventions, optical and nonoptical, that involve magnification of the object of interest to compensate for inadequate visual acuity.

Relative Size Magnification

In relative size magnification, the actual size of the object is increased (see Figure 5-10). To avoid confusion with the many other definitions of magnification, the convention is to call a size magnification an "enlargement ratio." The concept is quite simple. If the size of the object is doubled, the size of the retinal image is doubled. To achieve a 2× enlargement ratio, therefore, we simply enlarge the object twofold. If a client has trouble reading 8-point font but can fluently read the 16-point font typical of large-print books, the therapist could print a document on the computer using 16-point font or use large-print books typically printed with 16-point letters, as long as the eye-to-object distance remained the same.

This approach is relatively easy and can be an inexpensive option that is generally well accepted because the client does not require any optical aids and can read at a normal distance. However, as the magnification demands grow and the print size for books is increased, size and weight become issues. This method of magnification, therefore, is generally best suited for clients with mild to moderate loss of vision. It is also used in combination with other methods of magnification.

Relative Distance Magnification

Another simple means of achieving magnification of an object is to move closer to it (see Figure 5-10). As an object is moved closer to the eye, the retinal image of the object increases. If the distance is halved, the retinal image size doubles and 2× magnification is achieved. To achieve 4× magnification, the therapist would decrease the distance by one-fourth. If a client is having trouble seeing a 20-inch television at a distance of 12 feet, the therapist can suggest that the client move to 6 feet away. This would double the size of the retinal image of the television and magnify the image twofold.

If a client is having difficulty reading a newspaper at 40 cm, bringing the newspaper closer to 10 cm would magnify the print 4×. However, moving the newspaper this close creates another problem. Recall the discussion earlier about accommodation. The closer an object is brought to the eye, the more accommodation is required. Although decreasing the working distance from 40 cm to 10 cm achieves 4× magnification, the client would experience blurred vision if he or she is unable to accommodate for that distance. While a young child would be able to accommodate even at 25 cm, this would not be possible for an adult, particularly an adult age 40 and older. To solve this problem in adult clients with limited accommodation, the eye care practitioner prescribes a reading addition or other optical device that focuses the light on the retina. In this example, the amount of additional plus required to read at 25 cm can be calculated using the formula described earlier:

Power (D) = 100/D (cm) = 100/25 = 4 D

The amount of relative distance magnification can, therefore, be described in terms of the additional plus power required to see something at a given distance, otherwise called *equivalent power*.

Angular Magnification

Angular magnification is the magnification experienced when a person looks through a device like a telescope. Angular magnification also increases the size of the retinal image, just like relative size and relative distance magnification. The advantage of angular magnification is that it can be used when moving closer to an object or if enlarging the object is impractical or impossible. Viewing a sporting event is an example of such a situation. If an individual sits far from the action, neither relative distance nor relative size magnification is possible. However, the use of a telescope or binoculars will magnify the object of interest. When viewing objects further than 20 feet, angular magnification is an optical method of achieving size magnification, and the magnification specification can be described as an enlargement ratio. Indeed, for practical purposes and in calculations, angular magnification can be treated just like size magnification. A 4× telescope produces the same effect as enlarging an object 4×. The difference is that with a telescope, the field of view is much smaller.

Projection Magnification

Projection magnification refers to enlarging an object by projecting it on the screen of an electronic device. This is exactly the same as size magnification; the different terminology is simply the result of convention. Electronic devices like closed circuit televisions (CCTV) increase the size of the image to be viewed through the projection process, and like size and angular magnification, may be described as an enlargement ratio. A 4× enlargement on a CCTV screen means that the 1.5-mm-high (8-point) newsprint being viewed under the camera of the CCTV will be enlarged 8× to 12 mm (32-point) on the screen. A CCTV can be used to project printed and graphic materials to increase their size. Since electronic devices like electronic magnifiers (CCTVs) are usually viewed at 40 to 50 cm (16 to 18 inches), practically speaking, magnification is a combination of size and relative distance magnification expressed as an equivalent power.

In low vision care rehabilitation, the type of magnification used is dependent on many factors that will be discussed in Chapter 13. It is not unusual to use a combination of magnification systems. For example, the eye doctor may prescribe a magnifier, and the therapist may suggest the use of larger print. How to combine size and relative distance magnification will be discussed in Chapter 13.

Lovie-Kitchin and Whittaker compared the effect on reading rates of adults using relative distance versus relative size magnification.[4] They found that the reading rates of the subjects with low vision did not differ significantly between the 2 methods of providing magnification if the magnification provided was adequate. They also concluded that at that time for most tasks optics are used because an optical device is more practical than to enlarge the reading material physically.[4] In the age of e-readers and tablet computers, however, size magnification is easily achieved. Because therapists must now combine size and distance magnification, the formula for equivalent power has become a bit more complicated.

Equivalent Power

One very important role of the low vision therapist is to compare devices. To do this, the therapist must be able to select devices that have equivalent magnification. Although older methods to specify magnification are still widely used (and confused), the emerging standard has been to characterize near magnification as "equivalent power." Note that with many magnifiers, equivalent power is not always the actual power of the lens that is used. For those who have some accommodation or use a different device as at near, "equivalent power" means that whatever near device is used, it is "equivalent," or provides the same magnification produced by a single lens that focuses at a given distance. It is the closer distance that actually results in the magnification of the image on the retina, not the lens; the lens simply focuses the image. The distance is called "equivalent viewing distance" (EVD), and the power of the lens, EP = 100/EVD, using the formula described earlier.

For example, in order to read normal 8-point (1M) size print, a person who has reduced acuity requires the print to be magnified by moving the page of text to a distance of 10 cm to read it. A child could accommodate 10 D to focus print at a 10-cm eye-to-object distance without reading glasses. An older person who could not accommodate would need a 10-D lens in front of their eye as strong reading glasses (called a *reading addition*) to focus the print. For comfortable reading, most young adults would need a combination of a reading addition and use their own accommodation to make up the difference. In all three cases, as long as the viewing distance is 10 cm, the equivalent power would be 10 D. Now if the person had a handheld magnifier that had an equivalent power of 10, the lens might actually be a higher power, but if calculated magnification is 10 D of equivalent power, then it would be the same as reading at 10 cm.

The formula for equivalent power also takes size magnification (enlargement ratio, or ER) into account. The full formula is EP = 100/distance (cm) × ER. If, for example, a person read large print (16-point font) on an e-reader that is twice the size of normal 8-point font (ER = 2) at 20 cm, then the equivalent power would be calculated as EP = 100/20 × 2 = 10 D. Thus, the magnification that results from doubling the print size at 20 cm with 5 D of reading addition is "equivalent" to reading 8-point font at 10 cm. Both conditions have an EP = 10.

A situation often encountered in the clinic is that a client is prescribed stronger reading glasses and can read fluently with them, but dislikes the close reading distance. In such a case, the therapist might use the formula for equivalent power to quickly calculate that by doubling or even tripling the print size on an e-reader, the person could read most books more comfortably at a greater distance. In Chapter 8, the optimum print size for reading is measured by simply changing print size. At a given test distance (usually 40 cm), the examiner can use the formula for EP to quickly estimate the required magnification in terms of equivalent power and thus predict which device magnifications should produce the same reading performance as enlarging the print.

FIELD OF VIEW

Field of view refers to the size of the area that can be viewed through a lens, magnifier, or telescope. Typically, when we are reading a book, we are able to see the entire page at once. Although only the words we are looking at are clear, the rest of the sentence, paragraph, and page are visible in our peripheral vision. This is important because it is this peripheral vision that helps us know where to move our eyes next to continue to effectively gather visual information. When introduced to an optical device for the first time, clients often are pleased that they can now see detail better, but complain about the reduced field of view. A common question is, "Can I find a magnifier with a larger field of view?" The answer, unfortunately, is simple. When a client uses an optical device, the field of view will always be smaller; the stronger the magnification, the smaller the field of view. Magnification is like enlarging on a copy machine when the paper size cannot be changed. If the page is doubled in size, only half the original page will fit onto the copy. At times, a client may only be able to see a few words or even just a few letters at a time. This, of course, makes reading difficult, interfering with speed, fluency, and comprehension. The reason that larger size handheld magnifiers enable people to see with a larger field of view is generally because larger-diameter lenses generally have less magnification.

When using optical devices, a number of factors affect the field of view through the device. These are listed in Table 5-1. Stronger magnifiers have smaller fields of view because they must be made with smaller diameters and must be held closer to the material being viewed. The field of view also becomes smaller if the client moves his or her eyes away from the magnifier.

SUMMARY

The use of optical devices is an integral part of low vision rehabilitation. Occupational therapists will routinely need to educate and instruct clients about the use of these devices in ADL. In this chapter, we reviewed the basic principles of optics a low vision therapist needs to understand to instruct

TABLE 5-1: FACTORS AFFECTING THE FIELD OF VIEW

FACTOR	EFFECT ON FIELD OF VIEW
Diameter of the magnifier	A wider diameter lens will have a wider field of view. The diameter is related to the power of the lens. Stronger lenses have smaller diameters.
Power of the magnifier	The greater the power, the smaller the field of view.
Distance between eye and lens	The field of view becomes larger the closer the client is to the lens.
Type of optics	Defraction optics result in a larger field of view than traditional refraction optics.

people how to use optical devices and to problem solve when they are not working as predicted. Images can be enlarged on the retina by size or relative distance magnification according to a simple formula. For near magnification, equivalent power is central to understanding magnification at near and selecting devices that have equivalent magnification and has become the new convention for describing magnification.

REFERENCES

1. Evans BJ, Rowlands, G. Correctable visual impairment in older people: a major unmet need. *Ophthalmic Physiol Opt.* 24:161-180.
2. Tielsch, J. M., Sommer, A., Witt, K., Katz, J., Royall, R. M. Blindness and visual impairment in an American urban population. *Archives of Ophthalmology.* 108:286-290
3. Bailey IL. Equivalent viewing power or magnification? Which is fundamental? *The Optician.* 1984;188:14-18.
4. Lovie-Kitchin J, Whittaker S. Relative-size magnification versus relative-distance magnification: effect on the reading performance of adults with normal and low vision. *J Vis Impairment Blind.* 1998;16:433-446.

6

Psychosocial and Cognitive Issues Related to Vision Disability

Once the evaluation is complete, if the only impairment found is vision related, treatment usually proceeds quickly and effectively—often in just a few sessions. Most clients require some assistance by the therapist to identify achievable goals because they do not realize how effective low vision techniques and devices can be. Suggestion and demonstration of devices and interventions may be required. A person with typical cognition may have accepted the vision changes, successfully adjusted his or her lifestyle, and incorporated effective adaptations him- or herself. The therapist may simply need to describe, demonstrate, and briefly instruct on the use of devices and provide a list of home modifications, including a lighting demonstration. This allows the client to implement the changes him- or herself or direct a sighted assistant in doing so. If possible, clients should solve problems on their own, and many prefer to set the treatment agenda with minimal direction from the therapist. However, epidemiological research has found that many with low vision have depression, and low vision aggravates cognitive impairments. These are the people who are in most need of more prolonged, skilled occupational therapy.

An enduring irony of low vision rehabilitation often perplexes therapists. Once clients discover that interventions do not restore vision, they drop out of treatment, even though compensatory low vision devices and adaptive techniques may restore nearly all independent living skills and most leisure activities. Some practitioners may characterize these clients as "difficult" or "uncooperative." In fact, this resistance occurs because of other nonvisual barriers to performance, such as cognitive, psychological, or social problems. To be effective, therefore, low vision rehabilitation must include evaluation and treatment of the cognitive and emotional consequences of vision disability. Indeed, various studies have found a higher prevalence of depression, cognitive, and psychosocial problems associated with vision impairment and disability,[1-8] even after optical devices are prescribed.[1] The lack of initiation, memory impairment, and decreased activity level associated with depression present major impediments to a successful outcome with low vision rehabilitation.[9] Moreover, the symptoms of depression[10] exacerbate cognitive impediments.[5,7,8,10] We developed the "success-oriented" treatment approach (Table 6-1) because of the high prevalence of depression and age-related cognitive impairment encountered in low vision rehabilitation. This resembles a treatment approach termed *behavioral activation* that was found in 2014 to ameliorate the symptoms of depression in people with macular degeneration in a multicentered, prospective, randomized trial led by Barry Rovner and Robin Casten.[11]

Whittaker SG, Scheiman M, Sokol-McKay DA.
Low Vision Rehabilitation: A Practical Guide for Occupational Therapists,
Second Edition (pp 79-93).
© 2016 Taylor & Francis Group.

TABLE 6-1: THE SUCCESS-ORIENTED TREATMENT APPROACH WITH ADULTS WITH COGNITIVE AND EMOTIONAL IMPAIRMENTS

1. All sessions: **Client feels in control**

   a. Include the client in all conversations.

   b. Evaluation and treatment with caregivers involves the client.

   c. Review goals and treatment with client and proceed only with his or her approval.

   d. Encourage performance goals rather than visual goals.

2. Evaluation

   a. Predict what will be successful from evaluation. Avoid trial and error with devices.

3. Treatment

   a. Always start with devices or interventions that are easy and enable performance of high-value goals (eg, recorded books or a closed-circuit television for reading even if an optical device might work).

   b. Use reading materials or activities that interest the client for demonstration.

   c. When introducing a device or technique, set it up and provide enough assistance for immediate success. Never let the client struggle or fail.

   d. Try more difficult but more practical and affordable devices after successful performance has been achieved. Again, provide as much assistance as necessary for immediately successful performance.

   e. Encourage consideration of more than one option; have client choose and control treatment.

   f. In training with the selected devices, gradually withdraw assistance using shaping or reverse-chaining until a person can perform the task independently and solve problems with setup assist only.

   g. Encourage exploration of the device; instruct on setup, maintenance of devices, and troubleshooting last.

Occupational therapists typically address multiple disabilities, not just vision disability, and are aware that engagement in occupations and in daily life activities can be influenced by cognitive and psychosocial factors.[12] Not only must someone with low vision learn to reinterpret his or her visual experience, but rehabilitation involves the use of devices and learning new strategies, including the use of scanning and nonvisual compensatory strategies that, by themselves, present additional cognitive demands. As with other disabilities, occupational therapists address all aspects of performance (physical, cognitive, psychosocial, and contextual) when providing low vision intervention, and this includes consideration of the psychosocial problems commonly associated with vision impairment. This chapter is designed to provide background information about the psychosocial issues related to vision impairment.

FACTORS AFFECTING ADJUSTMENT TO VISION IMPAIRMENT

Clinical reports and descriptive research (mostly retrospective in nature) indicate a number of factors[13] that affect the client's adjustment to vision loss and suggest that information about these factors should be gathered during the history and while watching the client engaged in occupation and activities.[13,14] These factors, listed in Table 6-2, are briefly explained here and should be considered in every evaluation. Issues related to any of these factors have the potential to limit the overall positive outcome for a client. Evaluation of these factors would be based on careful questioning and formal assessment (see Chapter 8).

Type of Loss and Stages of Acceptance

A client's acceptance of a vision loss and prognosis impacts treatment. Acceptance of vision loss depends, in part, on whether the vision loss is congenital and long-standing or adventitious and recently acquired. Tuttle and Tuttle's review[14,15] uncovered a sequential pattern of coping with vision loss (Table 6-3). A review of phenomenological studies revealed that these stages often overlap and may occur in a different sequence.[16] Clients with a suddenly acquired vision loss from such conditions as untreated wet macular degeneration, acute glaucoma, proliferative diabetic retinopathy, or episodic demyelinating disease (multiple sclerosis) often are in denial and may defer rehabilitation

TABLE 6-2: COMMON IMPEDIMENTS TO A CLIENT'S ADJUSTMENT TO VISION LOSS

1. The type of vision loss and stage of coping
2. Cultural and family reaction: caregiver dependence
3. The life stage
4. Other significant life events
5. Patient's expectations and the stigma of blindness
6. Self-concept
7. Personality

Adapted from Graboyes M. Psychosocial implications of visual impairment. In: Brilliant RL, ed. *Essentials of Low Vision Practice*. Boston, MA: Butterworth-Heinemann; 1999:2-17.

TABLE 6-3: TUTTLE AND TUTTLE'S STAGES OF COPING

STAGE OF COPING	INTERVENTIONS
Trauma: physical and social	• Provide support and understanding
Shock and denial	• Be available • Permit time
Mourning and withdrawal	• Allow grieving/be a good listener • Introduce easily mastered practical solutions • Provide activities to redirect thinking away from self
Succumbing and depression	• Graded instruction on activities of high interest • Encourage involvement in support groups and cognitive behavioral therapy • Problem-solving therapy
Coping and mobilization	• Help to broaden scope of values (what defines independence) • Emphasize greater importance/control over personality than physical abilities • Assist to perceive that many areas of life are unrelated to disability • Help to assess/build on assets rather than focus on what cannot be done
Self-acceptance and self-esteem	• Reinforce that successful accomplishment of task is more important than the way it was completed • Introduce visually impaired role models • Involve in self-help and life skills groups • Incorporate role playing

because they may still be hopeful for a cure that will restore their vision. Many will also be in stages of mourning or depression and if "stuck" in this stage, this normal response deteriorates into a clinically significant depression. Gradual loss of vision caused by dry macular degeneration or congenital progressive disease may be easier to adapt to than the sudden loss of vision, especially if early rehabilitation intervention enables a client to maintain habits, routines, and occupations.[17,18] Not well documented is the influence of types of vision loss on denial of the condition. In our clinical experience, people with peripheral vision loss often are unaware of the extent of the loss. For example, after a few fender benders, a retired teacher, who was certainly intact cognitively, was discovered driving with approximately 20-degree visual fields. She was aware of a loss, but was in denial of the extent of the loss. When the extent of her vision loss was demonstrated, she acknowledged the impairment and stopped driving, but many are much more reluctant to give up this valued occupation. As will be discussed in Chapter 11, "denial" of impairment may be the direct result of brain damage such as spatial neglect syndrome, which results in anosognosia, an unawareness of impairment or sense of causality.

Denial and "unrealistic" hope are not necessarily problems; indeed, hope becomes a driving force in the arduous task of recovering a valued occupation. It is said that denial can be described as "the shock absorber for the soul." One clinical example was a jazz drummer who was told by his neurologist to stop driving because of a rather recent right field loss. He presented during an initial evaluation with a hope that the field loss would eventually resolve and he could drive again. His only impairment was a field loss; his motor function and ability to play the drums apparently were unchanged. After looking at a neuro-ophthalmological report that indicated extensive left occipital damage, his occupational therapist told him that it was unlikely he would be legal or safe to drive again. The man's response was to immediately stand up and leave the examination room. His parting words were, "No one will drive a drummer, too much equipment. I'm finished." In this case, a little denial and unrealistic hope would have enabled this gentleman to continue exploring transportation options and would likely have led to his playing again. An honest response to questions about prognosis is: "I don't know." Then the therapist should teach clients how to test their own visual fields (described in Chapter 11) that allows them to measure changes in vision so the client can determine for themselves when they may be "legal" to drive and are likely to pass the field test that must be given by an optometrist or ophthalmologist (see Chapter 11). This takes time, however, so even if recovery of vision does not occur, the client now has time to accept this and to benefit from compensatory therapy.

To determine the stage of acceptance, before discussing prognosis with a patient, ask the patient to "please describe your vision problem." If you get a general answer, like, "I have bad vision in this eye" (often, this is how a person describes a field loss) or "on this side," this indicates some level of acceptance. Listen carefully to the answer. If the client says, "*They say* I don't see on one side," this indicates denial.

Intervention Strategies

The best initial approach is not to correct denial or unrealistic expectations. Hope for recovery or denial of a poor prognosis will keep the client going as the reality of the situation slowly settles in and he or she explores compensatory options. However, denial can have another effect. While waiting and expecting recovery, a person might reject any compensatory interventions, especially devices, in the hopes that they will not be necessary. When this happens,

one might suggest, "Let's hope for the best but prepare for the worst." Plant a seed and encourage a person to try a compensatory device or strategy without pressuring for acceptance or confronting the person with a poor prognosis. This strategy will educate the client about options. After such instruction, when a person finally accepts the prognosis, he or she will recall devices or strategies that have been demonstrated and will return for treatment later. Often, during the course of therapy, clients will express interest in something they had vigorously rejected earlier. For this reason, when resistance is encountered, gently introduce some options as "something to think about" and then schedule follow-up visits and wait. Family members should be encouraged to take this approach as well. Nagging and pushing a person leads to oppositional behavior, anger, and delayed acceptance.

The success-oriented approach (see Table 6-1) focuses rehabilitation on a valued activity and activities that are relatively easy to accomplish at first. Nonsighted options should be introduced early, even before the vision evaluation, so the client does not have the impression that a nonvisual intervention is a last resort because visual solutions are not possible. Demonstrating an activity using nonvisual or simple visual techniques might engage and encourage a client. Examples might be sitting closer to a TV and removing glare sources to see the TV better before trying optical devices, demonstrating tactual techniques identifying coins, and demonstrating the free National Library Service (www.loc.gov/nls) program that provides recorded books and magazines before any visual reading devices are introduced. If the evaluation indicates reading can be easily accomplished, one might then demonstrate reading on an electronic magnifier so that the client can be reassured "reading is at least possible." The focus can then become "how to read," not "if reading is possible." Once a person's attention is drawn to performing a valued activity, often concern about a poor prognosis of improved vision fades into the background. This success-oriented approach contrasts with a somewhat traditional approach we have observed where a clinician responds to a client saying, "I want glasses to see again" by beginning treatment by showing the client optical devices. With more severe vision loss, optical devices are usually more difficult to learn to use than nonvisual and electronic devices. As a result, when the focus is on visual devices rather than performance we observed that clients often left treatment discouraged.

Cultural and Family Reactions

Vision impairment often leads to social problems such as nonacceptance, difficulty sustaining relationships, and attitudes of pity and overprotection by family members.[19-21] The family's reaction to the person's vision loss can have a significant effect on the client's adjustment. This reaction will vary with different cultures. For example, vision loss may cause role changes within the household, leading to anger and resentment. Stigmas associated with vision loss, perceptions of disability, and family expectations of recovery of roles and functions also vary with different cultures.[22] Cultural tendencies to care for "sick" family members may lead to overprotection, caregiver dependence, and ultimately, a significant loss in function.[20,21] "Caregiver burnout" can be equally deleterious to progress. The spouse of an older individual with low vision often is struggling with his or her own age-related disability.[19] Because caregivers, family, and loved ones are so important for success, it is important that the client consent to have caregivers participate in evaluation and be included in treatment.

Since cultural diversity exists even within broad ethnic groups, we find the best strategy is to try to understand such expectations by carefully interviewing the client *and* the family—and to listen carefully to their comments and answers. Again, open-ended questions like "What happened?" and "Why do you think this happened?" will reveal the cultural perspective, as well as provide the language that the therapist should use for instruction. Language interpreters help not only with translating language, but also in handling cultural differences.

Intervention Strategies

Some therapists find it difficult to accept a person's beliefs regarding locus of control, gender roles, and dependence. These patterns have been embedded in the client's culture and lifestyle and are unlikely to change. Within some cultures, for example, older people are expected to become more dependent and cared for. In other cultures, individualism, independence, and self-reliance are synonymous with selfishness, especially for women expected to be content in a subservient role. Within certain cultures or religions, admitting to and seeking treatment for psychological problems such as depression might further stigmatize people. If an attitude comes from religious beliefs, spiritual advisors might be consulted as well. If psychological problems are encountered, often, certain clergy are able to provide pastoral counseling.

An essential part of the success-oriented approach includes family and other supportive individuals in treatment sessions and implementation of a rehabilitation program appropriate for a person's culture (see Table 6-1). The only way to address overprotection and caregiver dependence is with full cooperation and involvement of caregivers. It is important to listen carefully and ask the caregiver to describe what has happened to the individual, why, and what could be done to help that person get better. The caregiver's answer will reveal the family and cultural expectations and fears, and will become the framework for addressing the caregiver's role in rehabilitation. For example, a person who wants to help out of a sense of devotion can be convinced that "helping" involves "therapeutic assistance," gradually withdrawing assistance when

independence is possible. Another caregiver who helps out of fear for her mother's safety can be taught to observe for herself that her mother can perform an activity safely. By standing behind the client while she prepares his meal, the caregiver is in a position to intervene if safety is in question, but since the caregiver is not visible, the client will be less likely to ask for help. Many clients who have been receiving help will continue to expect help and become quite upset with a caregiver who does not provide help when asked. In some cultures, or if the caregiver is an employee, the client is in a position of authority. In such cases, the therapist needs to meet with both the client and caregivers, who must explicitly agree to a plan for withdrawing assistance, often in writing.

Loneliness often emerges as one of the most disabling sequelae of chronic disability,[23-25] especially when a person is socially isolated by a co-morbid hearing loss, which is often common among the elderly. Fatigued, and sometimes underappreciated, caregivers and friends may withdraw from interacting with a person, creating a hole in the social fabric of the client's life. The client becomes angry and more depressed, and these behaviors further drive people out of his or her life. This vicious cycle represents a challenging situation. Caregiver education and client education can help if the people involved are able to develop insight into the problem. It often takes a group of committed, understanding, and tolerant people; a religious congregation; or social group to break this cycle of anger and isolation.

Life Stage

The life stage of the client at the onset of the visual impairment and at the time of intervention has implications for psychological adjustment. When confronted with vision impairment, one expects a younger adult, who was already committed to a family and a challenging career, to be receptive to challenging devices and compensatory strategies that enable continuation of these roles. One might expect the older adult to be less likely to undertake another arduous program like low vision rehabilitation if that person was already tired and discouraged from other challenges related to aging. Low vision rehabilitation often involves hard work and stress. Many older individuals consider themselves as having retired from this. Vision loss may interfere with many of the leisure activities that a retiree expected to enjoy, and for an elderly person living alone, vision impairment can lead to increased dependence. These are common expectations and stereotypes. In this author's opinion, more important than age is a client's focus on something outside of him- or herself and whether the client has been a role model. Regardless of their age, people focused on "getting jobs done" tend to be more open to new devices and compensatory strategies that will enable them to perform the goal activities. Their focus could be leisure activity, an upcoming trip, a vocational activity, or a general desire to live by themselves. Their focus could also be on a service commitment or religious activity.

Intervention Strategies

These stereotypes of aging will depend on a person's interests and overall health, and should never replace a careful interview to learn of a person's expectations, mood, history, and interests. With either younger or older individuals, the therapist should carefully explore interests, roles and routines, and dreams and aspirations before the vision loss and most recently after the vision loss, turning past aspirations into future clinical goals and a treatment plan. Ideally, rehabilitation would involve items related to current interests, such as cards, menus, bingo, spiritual materials, family photographs, and travel brochures. With some who have enjoyed competitive games, the process of rehabilitation can almost be approached as a challenging game by itself. With this approach, the therapist sets specific objective goals and objective performance measures so the client can "keep score" of his or her success. For those who are feeling overwhelmed, the therapist should develop the success-oriented approach with a focus on using familiar activities and strategies with which a person is already comfortable rather than try to introduce devices and new techniques that are difficult to learn.

Even at the end of life, when people naturally drop activities and social involvement and withdraw, the therapist still plays an important role in helping the person to focus on meaningful activity that improves the quality of the life that remains. For example, a person may use a low vision assistive device to read spiritual materials or keep in touch with loved ones by phone or e-mail. Independence and social involvement are not always appropriate goals at the end of life, as often it is easier or more meaningful for a friend or relative to read to the client, catch him or her up on news, or help perform activities of daily living (ADL). In these cases, the therapist would teach a caregiver the communication and listening skills necessary for the client to receive such assistance without losing control. This is another reason for family and caregiver involvement in the therapeutic process.

Significant Life Events

Older age involves many stresses, especially the loss of loved ones, other illnesses, and dependence on others. Interestingly, older adults appear more resilient than their younger counterparts in adapting to stressful events, a resilience that appears to relate to social support.[16] It is important to determine if there have been recent stressful life events, such as loss of a loved one. A client who has recently been challenged to deal with other stressful situations may not have the energy to adjust to the vision impairment and embark on a vision rehabilitation program.[26] The intervention strategy for people overwhelmed by life events would be similar to the treatment strategy when someone is clinically depressed, which is reviewed later.

Patient Expectations

During the occupational profile/case history, the occupational therapist should ask about the client's goals and expectations from vision rehabilitation (see Table 6-1). Clients who have good insight and who have advanced to later stages of coping (see Table 6-2) begin to understand the nature of their problem, often develop good problem-solving skills, and will have realistic goals and expectations. For these individuals, the success-oriented approach and involvement of others may not be necessary. One might help a person identify specific skills and needs associated with an overall goal, such as a reading speed, or an endurance goal for a person who wishes to return to college full time. Indeed, many who have accepted their condition have been actively problem solving on their own and may be more satisfied if they are in control of the treatment program. Often, therapists are put off by clients who feel that they know it all and deny the need for help. However, this presentation is an excellent sign, and the therapist should accept direction from their clients. For example, a client may wish to evaluate a specific type of device that he or she has heard about, such as strong reading glasses. Then, the treatment plan should start with the device the client wants to evaluate. The therapist would introduce other, possibly more effective devices for comparison later and avoid "I told you so." Rather than gradually introducing the complexity of a device and setup, as suggested by the success-oriented approach, the therapist might start by just handing the device to the client to explore and "play with." On the other hand, clients still in denial, who have not fully accepted the vision loss, may expect the special pair of glasses to suddenly restore their vision. Then, the therapist might need the success-oriented approach to introduce easier-to-use devices before the spectacle devices are introduced. If the client presents with unrealistic objectives, it is important to accept the need to advance through the stages of coping, to not take a person's hope and denial away, and to place more of an emphasis on valued activities and involvement by caregivers and family.

Self-Concept or Perceived Locus of Control

A person's self-concept may be impacted in a negative way by vision impairment.[13] It is not unusual for a person with vision impairment to get the message from others that he or she is unable to perform certain activities, which implies that the person is unable to be independent anymore. People differ in their perceptions of their ability to control outcomes, and these differences affect quality of life and are associated with overall health, but not necessarily with the outcome of treatment.[25,27] A loss of self-esteem and loss of sense of control is observed behaviorally as lack of initiation, especially when problem solving is required. For example, a client may "give up" when a handheld magnifier that has enabled reading does not seem to work, rather than try different magnifier positions or experiment with lighting. Self-perception and self-concept often are altered by a disability. Locus of control or hardiness can be learned and so can helplessness.[16,28,29] Caregiver dependence often leads to learned helplessness.

The success-oriented treatment approach is designed to restore a person's "hardiness" by providing positive feedback when the individual exhibits a successful attempt at adaptation, even if a better solution to the problem might exist from the viewpoint of the therapist. The teaching of problem-solving strategies, which has been shown to affect depression, may also affect a person's perception of his or her ability to control the future. Avoid negative, corrective feedback and attention to errors by focusing on easily attained goals at first. A therapist also can guide withdrawal of caregiver dependence (discussed earlier).

Personality

Even with similar visual function, culture, and family situations, a client will react to vision loss in a different manner. As will be discussed later, older individuals with vision loss are at high risk for depression. Any other factor that predisposes a person to depression or helplessness, therefore, would also have an impact on low vision rehabilitation outcomes. By asking family members as well as the client, the therapist can determine if certain characteristics occurred before the vision loss, such as depression or distractibility. Occupational therapists should evaluate the 7 factors listed in Table 6-2, and this information should be considered when developing a treatment plan.

VISION IMPAIRMENT AND COGNITIVE FUNCTION

People who initially present as "more difficult," in that they are prone to missing appointments and prone to anger, actually may have a comorbid cognitive impairment that can be effectively treated by a knowledgeable therapist. Treatment planning to address disability from visual impairment should involve consideration of cognition as either a support or barrier to a successful performance outcome. Evaluation and treatment of cognitive and emotional impairments should be part of the repertoire of skills an occupational therapist brings to any rehabilitation team.[12] Although critical for success, a review of cognitive evaluation and treatment is beyond the scope of this book, and these topics have been covered elsewhere.[30-32] Low vision

and blindness present some unique cognitive demands, including dependence on higher-order processing of other senses, auditory localization and processing, and hepatic processing and stereognosis. Comorbid visual and cognitive impairment is strongly associated with greater disability.[5,8-10,33-39] Indeed, in a typical rehabilitation setting, visual impairment with a mild cognitive deficit can be confused with more severe cognitive impairment, as described in the first paragraph of this book. For example, a person who has severe depression associated with macular degeneration can have short-term memory deficits, decreased initiation, and emotional volatility that may appear like dementia, even to professionals. Charles Bonnet syndrome (CBS), where a person with visual field loss experiences hallucinations—sometimes quite vivid and realistic—might be confused with symptoms of more advanced dementia. With purely visual hallucinations, a person is aware that the hallucinations are not real and expresses great relief when a therapist educates them about this condition.

Because many of the standardized tests of cognition require visual processing, our approach involves some screening, such as the mini-mental status examination,[40,41] and careful interview, but we favor evaluation that emphasizes careful observation in the context of an activity with which the client is familiar (discussed later). In Cicerone's reviews of the cognitive rehabilitation literature,[42,43] his team has found that occupation-centered treatment produces outcomes that are generally successful with the task used in treatment. The approach presented here is based on the development of more activity-specific skills. With those who have cognitive impairments, treatment usually requires the participation of a caregiver, who should attend all sessions and help with carryover into the home or work environment. The success-oriented treatment approach (see Table 6-1) incorporates a "shaping" methodology from the behavioral approach, where the client experiences positive reinforcement in the form of "success" from the start, and assistance is withdrawn with care to maintain a successful outcome. Another effective approach with sequential activity is "reverse chaining" where ther therapist provides necessary assistance through all but the last step and a behavioral sequence, then at the end withdraws assistance. When the step is mastered, then assistance is withdrawn on the previous step and so forth until the client performs the first step in the sequence without assistance. This withdrawal of assistance can be slowed and the task broken into smaller steps to address more severe cognitive impairment.

Memory

There are several neurological systems for consolidating and recalling memories.[31,32] Long-term memory refers to information that has already been stored, or "consolidated." This includes events from a person's more distant past. Explicit memory refers to conscious recall of events or things seen. Implicit memory, or procedural memory, usually refers to the process of motor learning. Short-term, or working, memory is like a person's mental "scratch pad." Short-term memory involves recall of learned images, sounds, and words combined with information that is flowing into the brain at a given moment in time. Indeed, visual short-term memory may compensate for low vision, filling in where visual information is lost. With CBS, the "perceptual completion" of a blind area includes visual hallucinations. Since we have found formed hallucinations often include people, objects, or pets from a person's experience, long-term memory may be filling in for the absence of immediate visual information, although the mechanism of CBS is not well understood. A person's ability to follow multistep instructions, do mental math, and recall directions reflect short-term memory. On the other hand, as someone loses short-term memory, that person becomes more dependent on sensory information to orient to the environment. This interaction of working visual memory and sensory function may be a possible explanation for why low vision is associated with increased severity of dementia symptoms.[8,10,39]

The process of consolidating memory refers to how efficiently a person stores information into long-term memory for recall—what we refer to here as "learning." Important to note is that there are several task-specific memory systems. One person might more easily remember names and faces than directions around a building. Another person with motor disorders such as apraxia may have more difficulty learning a movement pattern, such as how to hold a device (implicit memory) than in recalling current events. People with dementia may have better motor learning, and thus learn how to use a device, but be less able to recall verbal instructions. For this reason, the therapist must also take care to observe actual performance rather than depend on a client's verbal report.

Although formal testing can be informative, evaluation of memory should include observation of performance of an activity required in the treatment plan or through casual conversation. Since remembering depends on attention, the therapist can test memory while developing a good rapport with a client by talking about something of interest to the client. To quickly evaluate storage and recall of explicit memory, one could discuss a recent sports event, news item, a recipe someone might have recently learned, or a TV show that the client finds interesting. The therapist should routinely test and document a person's ability to store information in both explicit and implicit memory by having the client both verbalize and demonstrate a skill taught earlier in the session or from prior sessions.

Intervention Strategies

In cases of impaired ability to learn, repetition of new tasks and avoidance of new learning become more important. It is not surprising that people with impaired learning

or short-term memory will tend to avoid change in general and will resist new devices and treatments. It is essential to carefully listen to and observe these individuals before interventions to discover already established skills on which to build treatment. For example, a person may have substantial experience with computers and more easily adopt computer-based adaptations to read and write than use an optical device. People who are highly myopic are familiar with holding reading material close to their face and may be good candidates for strong reading glasses. The success-oriented approach (see Table 6-1) incorporates the behavioral method of "shaping" or "reverse chaining." One starts with a task or device and provides enough assistance so the person will be successful, establishing positive reinforcement, and then gradually increases task difficulty and withdraws assistance while maintaining positive outcomes and avoiding failures. In cases of severely impaired learning, the therapist might focus on environmental adaptions, such as lighting, positioning a TV so that it can be better seen, placing more visible markers on appliances, and emphasizing previously learned skills rather than learning how to use new assistive devices or tactual strategies. In such cases, minimal adaptation is better (mark one setting on an appliance). The client should be given a choice when possible, but options should be limited to 2 choices.

An example that I often use when providing ADL adaptations to be persons with cognitive loss is to stay with what is familiar to them if possible. For telling time, for example, a person can get close to a large, high-contrast numbered wall clock or watch instead of introducing something new like a talking watch.

Self-Awareness and Insight

Self-awareness, or "insight," is an executive cognitive function that characterizes the ability of someone to view oneself and any disability from the viewpoint of others, as well as to monitor one's own behavior.[31,32] Often in the progression of cognitive impairment with conditions such as dementia, a person may lose awareness of his or her own cognitive disability and even some aspects of vision disability, such as peripheral field loss, and may, for example, try to drive again or engage in other unsafe activities. Anosognosia-associated spatial neglect syndrome is a lack of insight into the extent of an impairment and may occur as a complete lack of awareness or misperception of a problem.[31,32] For example, a person with impaired self-awareness whose disability might be attributable to social situations, multiple impairments, and depression might attribute the entire disability to his or her "blindness." With more generalized cognitive dysfunction such as dementia, impaired self-awareness and anosognosia are associated with impaired verbal reasoning and short-term memory, problem-solving, and attention deficits. However, with psychiatric illness or brain injury localized to certain parietal and frontal areas of the cortex, a person may lose insight into a specific condition, such as a left paresis, field loss, or a psychiatric illness, without losing general verbal reasoning ability. The best way to evaluate insight is by asking a person to "describe his or her vision." Before evaluating performance, ask if the client thinks he or she can perform the task and, if not, why. People with good insight and reasoning will describe the vision loss in detail; those with impaired insight might give general descriptions, such as "blurry vision," deny, or exaggerate vision problems. With field loss, a person will tend to fill in the area of loss perceptually so that even someone with good insight may not be aware of a scotoma or peripheral field loss. This in not necessarily lack of insight. A person with the capability of insight quickly develops such awareness with instruction.

Intervention Strategies

The initial evaluation and each session should always begin by asking the client to describe his or her vision or why some task is difficult to perform. Clients' description of their vision and why the vision loss occurred will provide a framework for explanations and instructions. During the functional vision evaluation (see Chapter 8), the therapist often will ask for a patient's subjective impressions and perceptions and also provide an explanation of the vision loss. After the evaluation and explanation, during the following session, the therapist should ask the client the same general questions. A person who has a better prognosis for recovering insight will develop insight as they learn about their condition during the evaluation. Those with lack of insight into a field loss may be taught to recognize and verbalize their visual and physical impairments by conducting self-testing. For example, a treatment for a peripheral field loss involves patients administering visual field testing themselves, using their own hand to demonstrate a loss in visual field (see Chapter 11). People with intact cognitive function will quickly develop an awareness of the extent of the field loss, whereas those with impaired cognition will take longer. Impaired self-awareness will affect problem solving because one must recognize a problem to solve it.

The client with impaired self-awareness and problem solving will require assistance for setup or establishment of a "structured environment" where schedules, setup location, devices, rules of conduct, and environment are consistent and change little so problems are avoided. These individuals will require distance supervision—some way to easily call on someone for help when they encounter a problem.

Problem Solving

Problem solving results from an integration of several cognitive functions.[31] It refers to someone's ability to maintain sustained attention on an activity with distraction, develop goals, plan actions, evaluate outcomes of those actions, and learn from those outcomes.[31] In addition to trial-and-error problem solving, higher-order problem solving involves reasoning and the ability to test options mentally, or "ideational" problem solving. Therefore, a person may still be taught to solve problems, and this has been effective in preventing geriatric depression,[44] although the finding was just found short of statistical significance with the depression associated with macular degeneration.[3] Problem solving with macular degeneration is likely much more difficult. A person with low vision must be able to detect when an error occurs, such as blur through a magnifier, and initiate a correction, such as changing the distance of the magnifier. Error detection is an important prerequisite skill. A decrease in error detection might not only result from low vision; some individuals with more severe cognitive impairment from brain injury may tend to "perseverate," or repeat the same movement over and over, even after an error is detected. Like memory deficits, problem-solving ability depends on prior experience. A person who had been a skilled cook prior to a cognitive and vision deficit might more easily solve a problem cutting vegetables by feel, but have considerable difficulty using a new mobile phone with adapted features.

Intervention Strategies

The interventions for impaired problem solving are identical to the strategy used for impaired memory and self-awareness noted earlier. In addition, one might use "errorless" learning strategies to teach a new task based on a gradual withdrawal of assistance in the success-oriented approach until a rather stereotypic movement pattern is learned. Generalization of learned strategies and use of devices might remain a problem if someone lacks problem-solving ability.

Attention

Attention is a complex and multifaceted aspect of executive functioning and is often decreased with cognitive decline and brain injury.[32] Attention refers to the brain's ability to select stimuli or activate processes of working memory that create "mental images."[32] This discussion will focus on 2 important aspects of attention. Sustained attention refers to the length of time a person can sustain a task before stopping. What, in part, limits sustained attention is distractibility—a person's susceptibility to other environmental stimuli, including visual or other sensory events. Individuals can be "internally distracted"—that is, they spontaneously might start talking about something in the past that is irrelevant to the task at hand, even in the absence of external stimuli. Attention is the cornerstone of executive function. Orientation, self-awareness, and the components of problem solving require controlled shifts in attention to stimuli, and motor processes to solve problems, learn new information, and complete tasks.

Intervention Strategies

Evidence supports the use of metacognitive strategies to help a person avoid distraction and sustain attention.[42,45] This involves teaching a person to recognize and remove distractions, both external and internal, as well as avoid "multitasking," or attempting multiple activities at the same time. One should have a quiet, distraction-free room in which to work with a client with any cognitive impairment. Attention deficits may be managed or inadvertently affected by medication as well. If cognitive deficits are identified, the treatment team should include a neurologist or internist specializing in geriatrics.

Emotional Volatility and Frustration Tolerance

Although not often discussed as a part of executive brain functioning, people with impaired executive functioning not only may experience more frustrations, especially with new information and devices, but damage to the frontal lobes tends to disinhibit emotion,[46,47] compounding this frustration. These individuals might be more prone to cry or get angry when encountering difficulty or if some verbal instruction is difficult to understand (see Table 6-1). The success-oriented approach was developed to address this challenge to effective treatment.

VISUAL IMPAIRMENT AND DEPRESSION

There is a significant body of literature demonstrating a relationship between visual impairment and depressive illness in adulthood and later life.[5,48-54] of nearly epidemic proportions, with prevalence of comorbid depressive symptoms in about 1 in 4 clients with macular degeneration.[4,55,56] Horowitz and Reinhardt suggest 2 possible reasons for this relationship.[57] The first factor is the relationship between chronic illness of any type and functional disability. This concept suggests that it is not the chronic illness itself that causes the depression; rather, it is the loss of independence in ADL caused by the chronic illness that leads to depression. Studies have demonstrated that adults with visual impairment are more functionally disabled in ADL than those without vision impairments.[1,2,6,24,55,56,58,59]

For example, Williams et al interviewed 86 patients with age-related macular degeneration (AMD) and found severe, disabling effects of the disease.[47] Patients rated their quality of life substantially lower than did people with intact vision. These patients were 8 times more likely to have trouble shopping, 13 times more likely to have difficulty managing finances, 4 times more likely to have problems with meal preparation, 9 times more likely to have difficulty with light housework, and 12 times more likely to have trouble using the telephone. Rovner et al found that depressive symptoms are more prevalent and persistent among low vision patients and appear more highly correlated to the disability than to the actual visual acuity loss.[60] Brody et al also found that in the group of patients they studied, visual acuity had little correlation with the severity of the depressive symptoms.[61] In a study of 144 subjects, Tolman et al examined psychological adaptation to vision loss and its relationship to depressive symptomatology in older adults. Their findings support the contention that depressive symptomatology is mediated by one's perceived sense of individual control as it relates to intrapersonal factors underlying adaptation to vision loss.[62]

Thus, there is convincing evidence demonstrating that vision impairment interferes with occupational performance, causing loss of independence. It is this loss of independence that may be a key factor in explaining the high prevalence of depression in clients with visual impairment.

The second factor that may explain the relationship between visual impairment and depressive illness is in the subjective characteristics of vision impairment. Horowitz and Reinhardt[63] suggest that the most unique characteristic of vision impairment is that it is a particularly feared disability. In 1995, the Lighthouse surveyed adults age 45 and older and found that blindness was more feared than other disabilities.[64] A public opinion poll found that blindness ranks fourth, following only HIV, cancer, and Alzheimer's disease, as the illness most feared by Americans.[65] The results of a Gallup survey in 1988 showed that blindness was the most feared disability by 42% of adults polled.[66] These are older studies. We have often encountered this fear in the clinic, but hopefully this attitude has been changing.

Another important issue is that vision impairment has a negative impact on driving and reading, 2 activities that are very highly valued by most people.[57,67-69] For older adults, the inability to drive affects their sense of autonomy, self-worth, and independence.[57] Losing the ability to drive has been identified as one of the most feared aspects of vision impairment.[68]

Thus, the emotion elicited by vision impairment, plus the relationship between vision loss and functional disability, combine to increase the client's susceptibility to develop clinically significant depression.

MEASURES OF DEPRESSION

Often, older individuals with low vision present with what most might consider lack of initiation, a common symptom of depression. Lack of initiation might reflect depression, cognitive impairment, or neither. It is, therefore, important to perform screenings for depressive illness.

TABLE 6-4: THE PROBLEM-SOLVING THERAPEUTIC APPROACH

1. Problem orientation

    a. Assess client's capacity and best style for problem solving

    b. Present easier problems first

    c. Teach client to avoid negative thinking; instead, focus on solutions

2. Problem recognition and breaking big problems into smaller problems

3. Problem definition

4. Generating and testing alternative solutions

    a. Develop an action plan

    b. Evaluate outcomes

    c. Perform by trials or, if able, mentally (ideational)

5. Guided practice solving similar problems

Adapted from D'Zurilla TJ, Nezu AM. Problem-solving therapy. In: Dobson KS, ed. *Handbook of Cognitive Behavioral Therapies.* New York: Guilford Press; 2009.

The Beck Depression Inventory

The Beck Depression Inventory (BDI) is a list of 21 symptoms and attitudes that are each rated in intensity.[70] Examples include mood, pessimism, sense of failure, lack of satisfaction, feelings of guilt, self-dislike, etc. It is scored by summing the ratings given to the 21 items. Although originally designed to be administered by trained interviewers, it is most often self-administered and takes 5 to 10 minutes.

The Geriatric Depression Scale

The Geriatric Depression Scale (GDS) is a self-reporting scale designed to be simple to administer and does not require the skills of a trained interviewer.[54,71] Each of the 30 questions has a yes/no answer, with the scoring dependent on the answer given. A shorter 15-item version of the GDS has been devised and is probably the most common version currently used. This is preferred as a screening instrument because it screens for "psychological stress" in general.

Because depression responds well to medication and counseling, if an occupational therapist suspects a client is depressed, the client should be referred to a mental health professional for treatment, and this professional should collaborate in treatment planning.

Rehabilitation and Depression

Depressed clients may be less likely to use optical devices and less likely to benefit from vision rehabilitation.[72] It is, therefore, important to try and address the psychosocial needs of clients as well as intervention aimed at improving occupation and ADL. Davis et al reported that despite vision rehabilitation, persons with long-standing AMD are likely to still show psychosocial dysfunction well after the onset of vision loss.[73] They recommend that therapists continue to assist clients with their psychosocial adjustment as a follow-up to previous intervention because vision rehabilitation at the time of vision loss does not fully meet the client's needs. Clients with depressive symptoms should be referred to a psychologist. Cognitive behavioral approaches,[74] specifically a self-management approach,[38] has a strong evidence base for effectiveness. In a randomized trial, Brody et al found a significant, long-lasting amelioration of depressive symptoms with a self-management therapy.[75] In self-management therapy, the therapist helps a client direct thoughts away from negative thoughts and events and toward positive events, and is quite compatible with the success-oriented approach (see Table 6-1). Indeed, low vision rehabilitation involving instructional sessions does relieve depression symptoms and improve quality of life.[3,53,76] Another psychological approach that actually incorporates low vision rehabilitation instruction as part of the treatment plan is problem-solving therapy[77] (Table 6-4), where patients are taught general problem-solving strategies to apply to specific problems relating to vision loss. This is the last step in the success-oriented approach. Implementing the problem-solving therapy is complicated, but can be adapted to a variety of disabilities; collaboration with a psychologist or psychiatrist is recommended, especially if signs of severe depression are evident. The chapter by D'Zurilla and Nezu, the architects of this approach, in *Dobson's Handbook of Cognitive Psychology*[77] is recommended. When compared to an active control treatment, quality-of-life measures improved and depressive symptoms were ameliorated.[3,44] The therapist should be careful to evaluate cognition to make sure the patient

TABLE 6-5: INTERVENTION STRATEGIES FOR DEPRESSION
Use the success-oriented treatment approach.
In cases of depression, refer for counseling to a therapist who uses cognitive behavioral and self-management therapy. Work with this therapist.
If the client is cognitively able, use problem-solving therapy.
Recommend resumption of premorbid routines, especially spiritual activities.
Let people have hope and denial, even if unrealistic.
Speak with family with the client present and included.
Provide family instruction on "courtesies" with people with low vision: • Always speak directly to the client. • Do not raise your voice. • Always ask before helping and accept "no" for an answer. • Do not leave without telling someone you are leaving. • Describe your feelings; do not use gestures or facial expressions to communicate. • Always introduce yourself and any people who arrive.
Provide family instruction in using proper human guide (sighted guide) techniques.
Provide family instruction to praise success and initiation of activity and to avoid any negative feedback, comments, or reference to premorbid activities.
Recommend specific activities that a person can resume, encourage family to gently encourage resumption of these activities and roles at home.
Encourage friend and family involvement in a shared activity, reading aloud, family members describing a TV show, games that all can play like Bingo.
Smile, joke, and tease. Encourage the family to do the same.

has the ability to perform these activities. This is actually a higher-level "ideational approach"; a less complex approach is simple trial-and-error problem solving. Most recently, Rovner and Casten found an approach closely resembling the success-oriented approach that significantly reduced depressive symptoms in people who had both vision loss from macular degeneration and signs of depression.[11]

Finally, Horowitz found that if older people with acquired vision loss use visual devices, depressive symptoms were less than if they used nonvisual devices.[78] If the evaluation predicts visual strategies and devices are relatively easy to use, then visual interventions would be a better starting place. People differ considerably in their acceptance of vision loss vs performing a task, whether visually or nonvisually. In our experience, people will tell you if their expectation is for a visual approach, and the therapist should take this into account when deciding where to start treatment. In addition to interventions that specifically address an underlying depression, Table 6-5 lists several general treatment strategies we have found help clients continue to participate in a rehabilitation program until performance goals are attained. In general, we have found that a good strategy to encourage resumption of

activity is to ask the patient to start an activity according to a routine but stop anytime when tired or feeling frustrated. Remember, low vision rehabilitation presents considerable challenges if someone has even mild cognitive limitations.

SUMMARY

People with low vision are like everyone else, except they happen to have "atypical" vision. Some may have developed adaptations and a satisfactory lifestyle. Some are content sitting in front of the TV, depending on others and doing little by themselves. If the client is not dissatisfied, then there may be no cause for treatment, other than encouraging enough activity to maintain wellness. If, however, a person with low vision is inactive and also feeling trapped, angry, frustrated, or sad, then there is reason for treatment. Like people with typical vision, many with low vision also have cognitive and psychosocial problems or are having problems adjusting to a major life change. These are the people who are in most need of occupational therapy. This chapter focuses on what we have found to be the major barriers to success in low vision rehabilitation: the psychosocial, cognitive, and adjustment issues related to vision impairment. This book can only outline intervention strategies that we have found effective clinically to "get started." The therapist should continue to search for and learn more advanced evaluation and treatment techniques of these complex and difficult conditions. Goals, the treatment team, and the treatment plan should address cognitive and psychosocial issues as well as vision impairment. The success-oriented treatment approach to low vision rehabilitation was designed for people who present with significant cognitive impairment or depressive symptoms.

REFERENCES

1. Renieri G, Pitz S, Pfeiffer N, Beutel ME, Zwerenz R. Changes in quality of life in visually impaired patients after low-vision rehabilitation. *Int J Rehabil Res Internationale Zeitschrift Für Rehabilitationsforschung Revue Internationale De Recherches De Réadaptation.* 2013;36:48-55.
2. Zhang X, Bullard KM, Cotch MF, et al. Association between depression and functional vision loss in persons 20 years of age or older in the United States, NHANES 2005-2008. *JAMA Ophthalmology.* 2013;1-9.
3. Rovner BW, Casten RJ, Hegel MT, et al. Improving Function in Age-Related Macular Degeneration: A Randomized Clinical Trial. *Ophthalmol.* 2013;120:1649-1655.
4. Casten RJ, Rovner BW. Update on depression and age-related macular degeneration. *Curr Opinion Ophthalmol.* 2013;24:239-243.
5. Whitson HE, Ansah D, Whitaker D, et al. Prevalence and patterns of comorbid cognitive impairment in low vision rehabilitation for macular disease. *Arch Gerontol Geriatr.* 2010;50:209-212.
6. Popescu ML, Boisjoly HLN, Schmaltz H, et al. Explaining the relationship between three eye diseases and depressive symptoms in older adults. *Invest Ophthalmol Vis Sci.* 2012;53:2308-2313.
7. Tay T, Wang JJ, Kifley A, Lindley R, Newall P, Mitchell P. Sensory and cognitive association in older persons: findings from an older Australian population. *Gerontology.* 2006;52:386-394.
8. Reyes-Ortiz CA, Kuo Y, DiNuzzo AR, Ray LA, Raji MA, Markides KS. Near vision impairment predicts cognitive decline: data from the Hispanic Established Populations for Epidemiologic Studies of the Elderly. *J Am Geriatr Soc.* 2005;53:681-686.
9. Whitson HE, Whitaker D, Sanders LL, et al. Memory deficit associated with worse functional trajectories in older adults in low-vision rehabilitation for macular disease. *J Am Geriatr Soc.* 2012;60:2087-2092.
10. Whitson HE, Malhotra R, Chan A, Matchar DB, Ostbye T. Comorbid visual and cognitive impairment: relationship with disability status and self-rated health among older Singaporeans. *Asia-Pacific J Public Health/Asia-Pacific Academic Consortium for Public Health.* 2012;26:310-319.
11. Rovner BW, Casten RJ, Hegel MT, et al. Low vision depression prevention trial in age-related macular degeneration: a randomized clinical trial. *Ophthalmology.* 2014;121:2204-2211.
12. Amini DA, Kannenberg K, Bodison S, et al. Occupational Therapy Practice Framework: Domain & Process, 3rd Edition. *Am J Occup Ther.* 2014;S1-s48.
13. Graboyes M. Psychosocial implications of visual impairment. In: Brilliant RL, ed. *Essentials of Low Vision Practice.* Boston, MA: Butterworth-Heinemann; 1999:12-17.
14. Tuttle DW, Tuttle NR. *Self-esteem and Adjusting with Blindness.* 2nd ed. Springfield, IL: Charles Thomas; 1996.
15. Overbury O, Wittich W. Barriers to low vision rehabilitation: the Montreal Barriers Study. *Invest Ophthalmol Vis Sci.* 2011;52:8933-8938.
16. Ringering L, Amaral P. The role of psychosocial factors in adaptation to vision impairment and rehabilitation outcomes for adults and older adults. In: Silverstone B, Lang MA, Rosenthal BP, Faye E, E, eds. *The Lighthouse Handbook on Vision Impairment and Vision Rehabilitation.* Oxford: Oxford University Press; 2000:1029-1048.
17. Horowitz A, Reinhardt JP. Mental health issues in vision impairment: research in depression, disability and rehabilitation. In: Silverstone B, Lang MA, Rosenthal BP, Faye EE, eds. *The Lighthouse Handbook on Vision Impairment and Vision Rehabilitation.* Oxford: Oxford University Press; 2000:1089-1109.
18. Southall K, Wittich W. Barriers to low vision rehabilitation: a qualitative approach. *J Vis Impairment Blindness.* 2012;106:261-274.
19. Bambara JK, Owsley C, Wadley V, Martin R, Porter C, Dreer LE. Family caregiver social problem-solving abilities and adjustment to caring for a relative with vision loss. *Invest Ophthalmol Vis Sci.* 2009;50:1585-1592.
20. Cimarolli VR. Perceived overprotection and distress in adults with visual impairment. *Rehabil Psychol.* 2006;51:338-345.
21. Cimarolli VR, Reinhardt JP, Horowitz A. Perceived overprotection: support gone bad? *J Gerontol Series B: Psychol Sci Soc Sci.* 2006;61B:S18-23.
22. Lee EO, Brennan M. I am the fighter until the last moment: the relation of race/ethnicity and education to self-reported coping strategies among older adults with visual impairment. *J Soc Work Disability Rehabil.* 2003;2:3-28.
23. Loh KY, Ogle J. Age related visual impairment in the elderly. *Med J Malaysia.* 2004;59:562-568, quiz 569.
24. Chou KL. Combined effect of vision and hearing impairment on depression in older adults: evidence from the English Longitudinal Study of Ageing. *J Affective Disord.* 2008;106:191-196.
25. Girdler S, Packer T, Boldy D. The impact of age-related vision loss. *OTJR.* 2008;28:110-120.
26. Kobasa SCO, Puccetti MC. Personality and social resources in stress resistance. *J Pers Soc Psychol.* 1983;45:839-850.
27. Reinhardt JP, Boerner K, Horowitz A. Personal and social resources and adaptation to chronic vision impairment over time. *Aging Ment Health.* 2009;13:367-375.
28. Shafer SW, Stephens MW. Emotionality, conditioned helplessness, and escape conditioning. *Psychol Rep.* 1974;35:1051-1056.
29. Camacho EM, Verstappen SMM, Chipping J, Symmons DPM. Learned helplessness predicts functional disability, pain and fatigue in patients with recent-onset inflammatory polyarthritis. *Rheumatology.* 2013;26:310-319.
30. Gillen G. *Cognitive and Perceptual Rehabilitation: Optimizing Function.* St. Louis, MO: Mosby Elsevier; 2009:xi, 308.
31. Zoltan B. *Vision, Perception, and Cognition : A Manual for the Evaluation and Treatment of the Adult with Acquired Brain Injury.* 4th ed. Thorofare, NJ: SLACK, Inc; 2007:338.
32. Kolb B, Whishaw IQ. *Fundamentals of Human Neuropsychology.* 6th ed. New York: Worth Publishers; 2009.
33. Wahl H-W, Heyl V, Drapaniotis PM, et al. Severe vision and hearing impairment and successful aging: a multidimensional view. *The Gerontologist.* 2013;53:950-962.

34. O'Malley PG. Evolving insights about the impact of sensory deficits in the elderly: comment on "the prevalence of concurrent hearing and vision impairment in the Uni ted States" and "hearing loss and cognitive decline in older adults." *JAMA Intern Med.* 2013;173:299-299.

35. Goldstein JE, Massof RW, Deremeik JT, et al. Baseline traits of low vision patients served by private outpatient clinical centers in the United States. *Arch Ophthalmol.* 2012;130:1028-1037.

36. Cimarolli VR, Morse AR, Horowitz A, Reinhardt JP. Impact of vision impairment on intensity of occupational therapy utilization and outcomes in subacute rehabilitation. *Am J Occup Ther.* 2012;66:215-223.

37. Scilley K, DeCarlo DK, Wells J, Owsley C. Vision-specific health-related quality of life in age-related maculopathy patients presenting for low vision services. *Ophthalmic Epidemiol.* 2004;11:131-146.

38. Brody BL, Roch-Levecq AC, Gamst AC, Maclean K, Kaplan RM, Brown SI. Self-management of age-related macular degeneration and quality of life: a randomized controlled trial. *Arch Ophthalmol.* 2002;120:1477-1483.

39. Lin MY, Gutierrez PR, Stone KL, et al. Vision impairment and combined vision and hearing impairment predict cognitive and functional decline in older women. *J Am Geriatr Soc.* 2004;52:1996-2002.

40. Travers C, Byrne GJ, Pachana NA, Klein K, Gray L. Validation of the InterRAI cognitive performance scale against independent clinical diagnosis and the mini-mental state examination in older hospitalized patients. *J Nutr Health Aging.* 2013;17:435-439.

41. Haubois G, de Decker L, Annweiler C, et al. Derivation and validation of a short form of the mini-mental state examination for the screening of dementia in older adults with a memory complaint. *Eur J Neurol.* 2013;20:588-590.

42. Cicerone KD, Langenbahn DM, Braden C, et al. Evidence-based cognitive rehabilitation: updated review of the literature from 2003 through 2008. *Arch Phys Med Rehabil.* 2011;92:519-530.

43. Cicerone KD, Dahlberg C, Kalmar K, et al. Evidence-based cognitive rehabilitation: recommendations for clinical practice. *Arch Phys Med Rehabil.* 2000;81:1596-1615.

44. Rovner BW, Casten RJ. Preventing late-life depression in age-related macular degeneration. *Am J Geriatr Psych.* 2008;16:454-459.

45. Cicerone KD, Dahlberg C, Malec JF, et al. Evidence-based cognitive rehabilitation: updated review of the literature from 1998 through 2002. *Arch Phys Med Rehabil.* 2005;86:1681-1692.

46. Hornberger M, Geng J, Hodges JR. Convergent grey and white matter evidence of orbitofrontal cortex changes related to disinhibition in behavioural variant frontotemporal dementia. *Brain J Neurol.* 2011;134:2502-2512.

47. Koedam ELGE, Van der Flier WM, Barkhof F, Koene T, Scheltens P, Pijnenburg YAL. Clinical characteristics of patients with frontotemporal dementia with and without lobar atrophy on MRI. *Alzheimer Dis Associated Disord.* 2010;24:242-247.

48. Kempen GIJM, Ballemans J, Ranchor AV, van Rens GHMB, Zijlstra GAR. The impact of low vision on activities of daily living, symptoms of depression, feelings of anxiety and social support in community-living older adults seeking vision rehabilitation services. *Quality Life Res.* 2012;21:1405-1411.

49. Rees G, Fenwick EK, Keeffe JE, Mellor D, Lamoureux EL. Detection of depression in patients with low vision. *Optom Vis Sci.* 2009;86:1328-1336.

50. Lamoureux EL, Tee HW, Pesudovs K, Pallant JF, Keeffe JE, Rees G. Can clinicians use the PHQ-9 to assess depression in people with vision loss? *Optom Vis Sci.* 2009;86:139-145.

51. Horowitz A, Reinhardt JP, Boerner K. The effect of rehabilitation on depression among visually disabled older adults. *Aging Ment Health.* 2005;9:563-570.

52. Stelmack J. Quality of life of low-vision patients and outcomes of low-vision rehabilitation. *Optom Vis Sci.* 2001;78:335-342.

53. Stelmack J. Quality of life of low-vision patients and outcomes of low-vision rehabilitation. [Review] [58 refs]. *Optom Vis Sci.* 2001;78:335-342.

54. Galaria, II, Casten RJ, Rovner BW. Development of a shorter version of the geriatric depression scale for visually impaired older patients. *Int Psychogeriatr.* 2000;12:435-443.

55. Casten RJ, Rovner BW, Tasman W. Age-related macular degeneration and depression: a review of recent research. *Curr Opin Ophthalmol.* 2004;15:181-183.

56. Horowitz A, Reinhardt JP, Kennedy GJ. Major and subthreshold depression among older adults seeking vision rehabilitation services. *Am J Geriatr Psych.* 2005;13:180-187.

57. Horowitz A. The prevalence and consequences of vision impairment in later life. *Topics Geriatr Rehab.* 2004;20:185-195.

58. Casten R, Rovner B. Depression in age-related macular degeneration. *J Vis Impairment Blindness.* 2008;102:591-599.

59. Williams RA, Brody BL, Thomas RG, et al. The psychological impact of macular degeneration. *Arch Ophthalmol.* 1998;116:514-520.

60. Rovner BW, Zisselman PM, Shmuely-Dulitzki Y. Depression and disability in older people with impaired vision: follow-up study. *J Am Geriatr Soc.* 2000;44:181-184.

61. Brody BL, Gamst AC, Williams RA, et al. Depression, visual acuity, comorbidity, and disability associated with age-related macular degeneration. *Ophthalmology.* 2001;108:1893-1900; discussion 1891-1900.

62. Tolman J, Hill RD, Kleinschmidt JJ, Gregg CH. Psychosocial adaptation to visual impairment and its relationship to depressive affect in older adults with age-related macular degeneration. *Gerontologist.* 2005;45:747-753.

63. Horowitz A, Reinhardt JP. Mental health issues in vision impairment. In: Silverstone B, Lang MA, Rosenthal B, Faye EE, eds. *The Lighthouse Handbook on Vision Impairment and Vision Rehabilitation.* Oxford: Oxford University Press; 2000:1089-1109.

64. Furner SE, Rudberg MA, Cassel CK. Medical conditions differentially affect the development of IADL disability: implications for medical care and research. *Gerontologist.* 1995;35:444-450.

65. National Society for the Prevention of Blindness. Survey '84: attitudes toward blindness prevention. *Sight-Savings.* 1984;53:14-17.

66. Augusto CR, McGraw JM. Humanizing blindness through public education. *J Vis Impairment Blind.* 1990;93:397-400.

67. Davidson K. Declining health and competence: men facing choices about driving cessation. *Generations.* 2008;32:44-47.

68. Corn AL, Sack SZ. The impact of nondriving on adults with visual impairments. *J Vis Impairment Blind.* 1994;88:53-68.

69. Ryan EB, Anas AP, Beamer M, Bajorek S. Coping with age-related vision loss in everyday reading activities. *Educ Gerontol.* 2003;29:37-54.

70. Beck AT, Steer RA, Garbin MG. Psychometric properties of the Beck Depression Inventory: Twenty-five years of evaluation. *Clin Psychol Rev.* 1988;8:77-100.

71. Shiekh J, Yesavage JA. Geriatric Depression Scale: recent findings in development of a shorter version. In: Brink J, ed. *Clinical Gerontology: A Guide to Assessment and Intervention.* New York: Howarth Press; 1986.

72. Davis C, Lovie-Kitchin JE, Thompson B. Life satisfaction with age related vision loss. *Fourth World Congress on Behaviour Therapy.* Gold Coast; 1992:Program and Abstracts 47.

73. Davis C, Lovie-Kitchin J, Thompson B. Psychosocial adjustment to age-related vision loss. *Griffith University Inaugural National Rehabilitation Conference.* Griffith University, Brisbane; 1992.

74. Gould RI, Coulson MC, Howard RJ. Cognitive behavioral therapy for depression in older people: a meta-analysis and meta-regression of randomized controlled trials. *J Am Geriatr Soc.* 2012;60:218-229.

75. Brody BL, Roch-Levecq AC, Thomas RG, Kaplan RM, Brown SI. Self-management of age-related macular degeneration at the 6-month follow-up: a randomized controlled trial. *Arch Ophthalmol.* 2005;123:46-53.

76. Slakter JS, Stur M. Quality of life in patients with age-related macular degeneration: impact of the condition and benefits of treatment. *Surv Ophthalmol.* 2005;50:263-273.

77. D'Zurilla TJ, Nezu AM. Problem-solving therapy. In: Dobson KS, ed. *Handbook of Cognitive Behavioral Therapies.* New York: Guilford Press; 2009.

78. Horowitz A, Brennan M, Reinhardt JP, Macmillan T. The impact of assistive device use on disability and depression among older adults with age-related vision impairments. *J Gerontol.* 2006;61:S274-280.

II

Evaluation

Overview and Review of the Optometric Low Vision Evaluation

Paul B. Freeman, OD, FAAO, FCOVD

OPTOMETRIC LOW VISION EXAMINATION

It is imperative for occupational therapists involved in the low vision rehabilitation process to be familiar with the low vision examination by an optometrist or ophthalmologist. The actual examination will, of course, vary depending on the eye care practitioner. The following is a description of an optometric low vision evaluation (Table 7-1). This evaluation was developed to be performed in a variety of settings, including a professional office, a home, a rehabilitative facility, or a personal care facility. Interpretation of these tests is described in greater detail in Chapter 8.

Case History

The history of a visually impaired patient, as with any other history, is a snapshot of the patient up to the time of questioning. The general areas that this history should cover are listed in Table 7-2. This information may be obtained from a number of sources, including the patient, family, friends, caregivers, therapists, and doctors. From the perspective of the low vision optometrist, among the most common chief visual complaints of visually impaired

patients is the inability to see conventional-size print, the inability to recognize people, difficulty watching television, difficulty seeing medications, difficulty signing any type of document (like a check), and the inability to drive. (To concern yourself about the latter requires, at the very least, know the regulations of the state in which the patient resides.)

It is always important to determine the date and results of the last eye examination. In many cases, individuals who believe they are visually impaired may simply require an eye examination and conventional eyeglasses. This was demonstrated in the Baltimore Eye Survey, which found that "the acuity of about three-fourths of the visually impaired whites and two-thirds of the visually impaired African Americans could have been corrected to better than 20/40 with only eyeglasses."[1]

Once it is established, however, that the patient has a bona fide decrement in visual acuity that cannot be corrected by conventional eyewear, the remaining questions explore the impact of this visual deficit on the patient's ability to visually interact with the environment and the challenges faced. During the case history, the doctor can obtain information about the patient's understanding of the impact of the visual impairment, cognitive level,

Whittaker SG, Scheiman M, Sokol-McKay DA.
Low Vision Rehabilitation: A Practical Guide for Occupational Therapists,
Second Edition (pp 97-105).
© 2016 Taylor & Francis Group.

TABLE 7-1: COMPONENTS OF THE OPTOMETRIC LOW VISION EVALUATION

- Case history
- Distance visual acuities
- Near visual acuities
- Amsler grid testing
- Color vision testing
- Visual/mobility field testing
- Contrast sensitivity testing
- Refraction
- Binocular vision evaluation
- Eye health evaluation
- Magnification evaluation

TABLE 7-2: CASE HISTORY COMPONENTS

- Chief complaint
- Last eye examination
- Visual/ocular history
- Distance visual abilities (present and past)
- Independent travel concerns
- Near visual abilities (present and past)
- Social/emotional review
- General health review
- Environmental challenges (present and past)
- Education and/or vocation and avocation (present and past) needs
- Specific visual goals and desires in prioritized order

TABLE 7-3: FACTORS TO BE CONSIDERED WHEN ASSESSING VISUAL ACUITY

- Lighting
- Contrast
- Specific chart used
- Numbers of targets at each acuity level
- Spacing of the targets
- Difficulty of the targets being identified (ie, letters, numbers, pictures, etc)
- Single letter versus reading acuity
- Type of letters (block, serif, etc)
- Ease with which the targets are identified
- Expressive as well as receptive language skills
- Cognitive functioning
- Eccentric viewing (body positioning, eye/head posture)

motivation, support systems, and previous attempts at vision rehabilitation.

Visual Acuity Information

Visual acuity information is generally communicated as a Snellen fraction, which can be in either feet or metric notation. The numerator signifies the actual or calculated testing distance and the denominator the actual or calibrated target size. For example, 10/200 (3/6M) should be recorded if the physical testing distance was 10 feet (3 meters) and the smallest target size correctly identified was a 200 (60M) size letter. Any of the modifiers listed in Table 7-3 should be included if there is anything unusual or pertinent about the manner with which acuity was measured. These findings are typically obtained for each eye independently, if possible, both with and without the patient's current eyeglass or contact lens prescription. This might also be done with the patient's current low vision devices, if there are any. This last visual acuity measurement will give you an idea of whether the patient is capable of using the device. With low vision examinations, often, the acuity chart is held closer to the person. Instead of testing at the conventional 20 feet (or 6 meters), in the example earlier, testing was at 10 feet (nominally 3 meters). To convert from one distance to another, see Chapter 8.

DISTANCE VISUAL ACUITIES

Distance visual acuities are measured to establish the patient's baseline ability to see at a specific distance, as well as to determine visual disability. Specially designed charts (which allow for better quantification of reduced acuity levels) other than the standard Snellen projected chart can be used, but when doing so, the specific chart used and actual testing distance should be noted (Figure 7-1). Other factors that should be considered that can also affect this measurement when assessing visual acuity at distance, including expressive and receptive language skills and cognitive functioning, are listed in Table 7-3.

There are occasions when a person cannot recognize, identify, or match symbols. In these instances, there are other ways in which the practitioner can establish what a patient can see. In these cases, a more functional approach

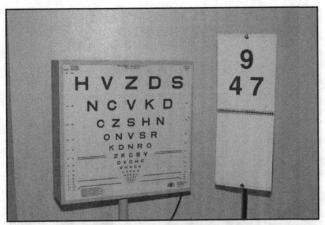

Figure 7-1. Specially designed distance charts for testing visual acuity in visually impaired patients.

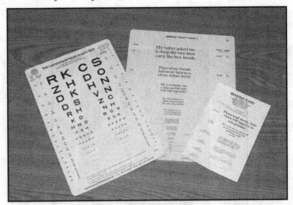

Figure 7-2. Commonly used near visual acuity charts in a low vision assessment.

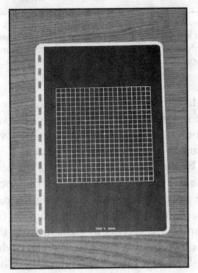

Figure 7-3. Amsler grid.

can be used. For instance, a patient's ability to fixate and follow a light and/or localize a specific sized target (without the actual ability to identify it) at a specific distance can be used to indirectly assess visual acuity.

NEAR VISUAL ACUITIES

The vast majority of activities for which visually impaired patients require assistance revolve around near work. Therefore, a measure of visual acuity should be done at near as well as at distance. This information will not only help the occupational therapist when trying to determine an appropriate sized target to work with, but also helps the optometrist evaluate the consistency between distance and near acuity measurements. As with distance visual acuity measurement, all pertinent information about the test (see Table 7-3) should be made available to anyone reviewing the data. Additionally, knowing whether the target size was

based on identification (discrimination) acuity or actual reading acuity is important, as there can be a difference. The ability to recognize a letter does not always equal the ability to actually read. For this reason, near charts usually require reading. Figure 7-2 illustrates some of the commonly used near visual acuity charts.

Amsler Grid Testing

Using an Amsler grid (Figure 7-3) can help to determine whether a patient is experiencing distortion or has multiple areas of scotoma. A scotoma is defined as "an isolated area of absent vision or depressed sensitivity in the visual field, surrounded by an area of normal vision or of less depressed sensitivity."[2] The Amsler grid measurement can provide information to identify the onset of a pathology, monitor a pathology, or modify the ultimate optical device(s) that might be needed by a patient for a specific task. Functionally, the results can also give guidance as to whether a patient eccentrically views or needs to learn to do so. Figure 7-4 illustrates an example of the distortion of the Amsler grid that can be experienced by a patient with macular degeneration.

COLOR VISION TESTING

Several tests are available for assessing color vision (Figure 7-5). The results of color vision testing can be used to identify the onset of a pathology, monitor a pathology, or alert a therapist to color deficits that might impact a therapeutic regimen for the patient. Color vision deficits are generally not as detrimental to functioning as other losses such as visual acuity, visual field, or contrast sensitivity, but for a visual artist can be very important. Knowing the patient's color vision status can be important in educational, vocational, and social planning or training.

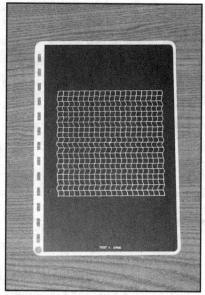

Figure 7-4. Distortion of Amsler grid.

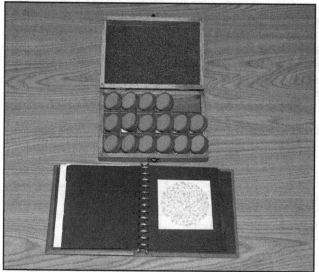

Figure 7-5. Several tests available for color vision testing. The Munsell hue test has a low vision version (top) that is ideal for identifying specific color confusions. The test in the bottom of the figure screens for color deficiency.

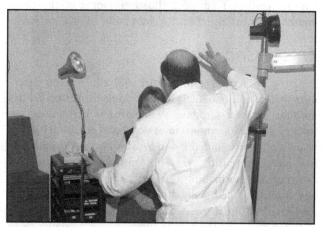

Figure 7-6. Illustration of confrontation field testing.

VISUAL/MOBILITY FIELD TESTING

Perimetry, or visual field testing, is designed to evaluate the depth and breadth of an individual's peripheral vision. Visual field loss can be either absolute or relative, and is described for each eye. An absolute visual field loss is one in which no matter how large and bright the target is, it will not be seen within that blind area. (This is similar to the lack of sight in the "blind" spot created by the optic nerve.) A relative visual field loss, on the other hand, is dependent on the size, brightness, and contrast of the target relative to the environmental background. Most importantly, this translates functionally into variations of visual field awareness consistency based on environmental conditions (the latter is extremely important to remember, as that relationship is what could determine successful rehabilitation). For example, a person with a relative peripheral visual field loss might function better under bright illumination than under dim lighting conditions or at night. Several instruments can formally quantify the extent of the visual field. However, for initial screening, confrontation visual field testing (Figure 7-6) is the method of choice. It is typically carried out by the doctor sitting opposite the patient, each covering the eye on the same side (ie, the doctor's right eye and the patient's left eye), and having the patient then demonstrate awareness of when the doctor's (or a third person's) hand (or object) is brought in from the periphery. As in other testing, notations about environmental conditions should be made (see Table 7-3). This type of testing will uncover gross peripheral visual field deficits, and is useful for determining the presence of a hemianopia (which is absolute) or larger peripheral field defect. This can also be done with both eyes open to determine a bilateral hemianopia. Confrontation visual field testing is not as sensitive for subtle peripheral field loss or for central visual field disturbances.

To more accurately quantify peripheral visual field loss, a formal visual field study must be performed. Typically, a computerized visual field apparatus is used for this purpose (Figure 7-7); this can either be done monocularly or binocularly. However, for purposes of determining visual disability from a medical-legal standpoint, a manual Goldmann visual field test is required.[3] (There are other computations for determining visual disability, but they require calculations based on central vision and amount of side vision loss, and are beyond the scope of this chapter). To test for driving, full visual fields are tested with both eyes open. Most states require 120 degrees of vision along the horizon (a horizontal line through the point of fixation) and that automated or Goldmann perimetry be performed.

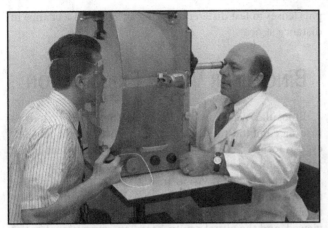

Figure 7-7. Manual visual field apparatus (perimeter).

For central field testing, some clinics have a sophisticated device called a *microperimeter*. This allows a central scotoma to be carefully mapped out in the image of the retina, as well as the retinal position a patient prefers to use during fixation if the fovea is not functioning.

CONTRAST SENSITIVITY TESTING

Contrast sensitivity testing determines the patient's ability to distinguish borders, eg, reading print on different backgrounds, distinguishing between similar-colored medicine tablets, seeing similar-colored steps, distinguishing a gray car against a foggy background, or successfully pouring coffee into a dark cup. It is a method of assessing the qualitative aspects of visual functioning. This is particularly important when following a patient's progress over multiple visits. Patients sometimes report that their sight has changed, but on a standard eye chart (which has a maximum contrast of black and white), there may be no measured difference. These are patients who are noticing real functional difficulties, which vary based on the environment or activity being performed, even though their measured visual acuity has not changed. In these cases, contrast sensitivity testing may demonstrate a qualitative change in vision that confirms the patient's report. This test is also valuable when it is difficult to pinpoint a visual complaint, especially with patients with "good" visual acuities. Proper lighting is integral to this testing. Contrast sensitivity testing and charts are described in Chapter 8.

REFRACTION

Refraction is the term used to describe the evaluation of the optical system of the eye (Figure 7-8). We use the term *refractive error* to describe any deviation from emmetropia. When the optometrist performs the refraction, it can

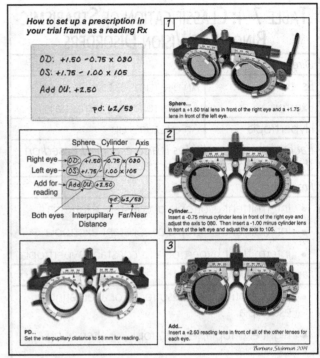

Figure 7-8. Trial frame for checking a refraction for functional activities. (Reprinted with permission from Barbara Steinman.)

be determined whether the eye is emmetropic (absence of refractive error), myopic (nearsighted), hyperopic (farsighted), or astigmatic. The refraction can determine if a patient has a refractive error that needs to be corrected, as well as the exact lens prescription that is appropriate. A phoropter or a trial frame with loose lenses is used to perform the refraction. When a patient is visually impaired, the optometrist must also use information about the refractive error when designing low vision optical devices.

As noted previously, we sometimes encounter patients who appear to be visually impaired or legally blind, but a thorough refraction indicates that the patient simply requires an updated eyeglass prescription to regain "normal" vision. I cannot emphasize enough the importance of performing a careful refraction before initiating any low vision rehabilitation activity. For example, a patient who needs a bifocal correction and is not wearing it may not be able to see clearly through a "simple" stand magnifier. Even if eyeglasses cannot restore normal vision, correction for refractive error will improve vision. A misleading conclusion might be that the patient is unable to cognitively handle the task, when in fact it is simply the omission of the appropriate refractive prescription.

Understanding how a prescription is written can help the occupational therapist appreciate how a prescription might be needed. A simple nearsighted (myopic) prescription is written with a number preceded by a minus sign (ie, –1.00). A simple farsighted (hyperopic) prescription is written with a number preceded by a plus sign (ie, +1.00). An

TABLE 7-4: CLASSIFICATION OF STRABISMIC BINOCULAR VISION DISORDERS

Direction	
Esotropia	An eye turns in toward nose
Exotropia	An eye turns out temporally
Hypertropia	An eye turns up

Each of these conditions is also classified based on the following characteristics:

Frequency

- Intermittent esotropia or constant esotropia
- Intermittent exotropia or constant exotropia
- Intermittent hypertropia or constant hypertropia

Laterality (which eye turns)

- Right esotropia, left esotropia, or alternating esotropia
- Right exotropia, left exotropia, or alternating exotropia
- Right hypertropia, left hypertropia, or alternating hypertropia

Comitancy

- Comitant
- Noncomitant

astigmatic prescription gets a little trickier, as it will have three numbers, which can mix signs (ie, +1.00 −100 × 90), and which can be written with apparently different numbers and signs, but is, in fact, the same (ie, +1.00 −1.00 × 90 is the same as plano +1.00 × 180). Also, depending on the age of the patient, a near lens may be necessary. As a bifocal, this is always written with a plus sign (ie, −1.00 [the distance prescription], and a bifocal of +2.00 [the near prescription]); this is written on the same prescription. Suffice it to say, the prescription is the platform on which the magnification calculation is based. Figure 7-8 illustrates how to make up a trial of a person's prescription using a special "trial frame." The low vision optometrist with whom the therapist works will supply the kit that includes individual lenses and a trial frame. An optometrist may prescribe prism lenses, especially with stronger reading addition. These are placed in the clips just behind the frame so they do not turn when the axis is changed with the flat part of the lens toward the eye. The prescription will indicate the direction of the lens base (thicker part). The occupational therapist need only put the lenses in as directed by the optometrist. The Halberg clip (not illustrated), looks like one side of the trial frame and clips to a person's spectacles and allows the therapist to try different lenses. For example the therapist could put in plus lenses to test different reading addition for a change in distance at near.

BINOCULAR VISION EXAMINATION

Binocular vision is the ability of the visual system to fuse or combine the information from the right and left eyes to form one image. For binocular vision to occur, the information arriving from each eye must be identical, with approximately equal vision in both eyes. To satisfy these requirements, the 2 eyes must be aligned so that at any time both eyes are pointing at the same object that is being viewed, and the visual acuity, based on conventional optics (or refractive error) of the 2 eyes, must be approximately equal. Therefore, it is understandable that many patients with vision impairment do not have normal binocular vision because they lack approximately equal visual acuity in both eyes.

Although binocular problems are frequently encountered if people have a brain injury, it is not uncommon for an older adult with low vision from sensory loss to lose binocular vision as well, which can cause a misalignment of the eyes; this is referred to as strabismus. When strabismus occurs, the eyes may drift in, out, up, or down. Table 7-4 lists some of the common terms associated with binocular vision problems that an occupational therapist may encounter in a low vision examination report.

Clinical Assessment of Binocular Disorders

Some of the common tests used to evaluate binocular vision in patients with low vision include the cover test and tests to assess fusion. Using the cover test procedure, an optometrist can determine many key binocular vision characteristics, including the direction, magnitude, frequency, and comitancy of the strabismus.

Direction of Strabismus

This refers to whether the eyes turn in, out, up, down, or a combination of these directions. Table 7-5 lists the various possibilities, including esotropia (eyes turn in), exotropia (eyes turn out), and hypertropia (one eye turns up).

Magnitude of Strabismus

This refers to the amount of the eye turn. When an eye turn is large, it is quite obvious, even to a nonprofessional. However, it is important to be aware that the magnitude of a strabismus may be moderate or small, and in such cases, the eye turn may be not be visible or detectable without special testing. The magnitude of the strabismus is recorded in prism diopters. For example, you might see the following notation in an optometric report:

TABLE 7-5: COMMONLY USED ABBREVIATIONS IN EYE EXAMINATIONS	
Abbreviation	*Term*
VA	Visual acuity
OD	Right eye (oculus dexter)
OS	Left eye (oculus sinister)
OU	Both eyes (oculus uterque)
XP	Exophoria
EP	Esophoria
XT	Exotropia
ET	Esotropia
AA	Accommodative amplitude
VF	Visual field
PERRL	Pupil equal, round, responds to light
WNL	Within normal limits

25 pd esotropia (or 25Δ)
where pd = prism diopters.

Frequency of Strabismus

Frequency of strabismus refers to the amount of time the eye turns in, out, up, or down (see Table 7-4). For example, it is possible for the eye turn to be present 100% of the time; this would be called a *constant strabismus*. In contrast, the strabismus may occur only part of the time and would be called an *intermittent strabismus*.

For example, you might see the following notation in an optometric report:

25 pd (or 25Δ) intermittent esotropia, or
15 pd (or 15Δ) constant esotropia

Comitancy of Strabismus

The final variable is referred to as comitancy and refers to the uniformity of the size of the strabismus from one position of gaze to another. A strabismus is called *comitant* if it is the same size, regardless of where the patient looks (left, right, up, or down). If there is a significant difference from one position of gaze to another, it is called a *noncomitant strabismus*. For example, if a patient's eyes are aligned when looking straight ahead but deviate when looking to the right, this is a noncomitant strabismus.

Additional tests may be used to evaluate the patient's ability to "fuse" or use information from both eyes in a coordinated way. A popular probe of sensory fusion is stereopsis testing. In this test (Figure 7-9), the patient wears special Polaroid glasses and is asked if any of the figures on the page appear to be floating off the page in 3D. Another commonly used test is called the *Worth 4-dot test*. This test

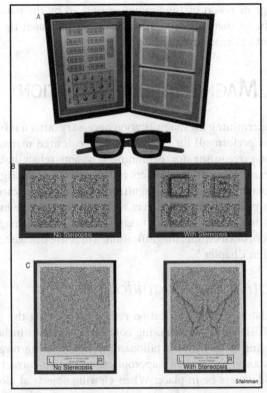

Figure 7-9. Stereopsis test: random-dot stereogram. (Reprinted with permission from Barbara Steinman.)

is very much like the red/green glasses test (see Chapter 8) and is used to determine if the patient has double vision or is suppressing the vision of one eye. The random dot test requires good visual acuity. With impaired acuity a better test has recognizable and large shapes.

The low vision optometrist should provide information about binocular vision to the therapist. This information will help the occupational therapist understand why an optical device was prescribed for just one eye versus both eyes or whether one eye should be occluded when using some handheld optical devices or electronic devices where typically the client uses both eyes.

EYE HEALTH EVALUATION

An eye health evaluation can include, but is not limited to, the following tests: observation of the external structures of the eye and adnexa, intraocular pressure (IOP) measurement, evaluation of the anterior structures of the eye, and evaluation of the internal structures of the eye through a dilated pupil. The goal of the eye health evaluation is to determine the underlying basis for the visual acuity, contrast sensitivity, and/or visual field loss. Many good texts are available for a detailed description of these procedures.[4,5] An ocular health evaluation is indicated prior to beginning any low vision rehabilitation, or if any change in vision or functioning is noticed by the patient, family, or therapist, and periodically as indicated by the patient's primary eye care doctor.

MAGNIFICATION EVALUATION

Determining the magnification necessary (after a refraction is performed) for the patient to see desired materials is the prerequisite for beginning a vision rehabilitation program. Magnification refers to the process of enlarging the image on the retina. Magnification of an object can be accomplished using 4 different methods: relative size magnification, relative distance magnification, angular magnification, or electronic magnification. These are discussed in detail in Chapter 5.

Relative Size Magnification

Relative size magnification refers to enlarging the target. This is similar to taking conventional-size print and enlarging it to fit on a billboard. When viewing targets at distance, the patient's appropriate refractive correction should always be in place. When viewing objects at closer distances, even though enlarged, a compensatory lens for a specific viewing distance must be considered. This concept is reviewed in detail in Chapter 5. Therefore, even when using large print, conventional glasses or bifocals may be needed to see the print clearly, even before other forms of optical magnification are considered.

Relative Distance Magnification

This is accomplished by bringing the object of interest closer. It might be considered similar to "airplane magnification," where at 10,000 feet houses look small, but the closer one gets to the ground, the larger the houses appear. Similarly, a target at 2 inches will give the appearance of being 8 times larger than the same target at 16 inches. Remember that when objects are held at a closer working distance, the patient with "normal" vision must exert additional effort, if possible, to accommodate (focus). This effort, if unable to be done or sustained, can lead to discomfort and eyestrain after short periods of time. Additionally, many older patients are unable to exert this effort due to the decreased flexibility of the natural lens to be able to focus, or due to removal of the natural lens and being replaced by a lens implant, and, along with discomfort, will not see clearly. Thus, an appropriate-powered lens must be used for the target to be seen clearly at that distance. This lens minimizes or eliminates the need for the patient to accommodate (or focus) the eyes for the specific target distance.

Angular Magnification

Angular magnification is the magnification experienced when a person looks through a device like a telescope. This form of magnification is typical of a stand magnifier or a telescope where the relationship between lenses in the system creates an enlarged image. Angular magnification also increases the size of the retinal image, just like relative size and relative distance magnification. The advantage of angular magnification is that it can be used when moving closer to an object or enlarging it is impractical or impossible. Viewing a sporting event is an example of such a situation. If an individual sits far from the action, neither relative distance nor relative size magnification is possible. However, the use of a telescope or binoculars will magnify the object of interest. Telescopic lenses must be focused properly. To see clearly through a telescope, the refractive error must be corrected or compensated for in some manner. This can be done by using glasses or contact lenses, or by adjusting the telescope for the refractive error. However, it should be noted that focusing the telescope for an uncorrected eye may modify the power (or magnification) of the telescope, even though the image will be clear.

Electronic or Projection Magnification

This form of magnification uses electronic equipment viewed at about 40 to 50 cm (16 to 18 inches) and is basically the same as size magnification; practically speaking, it is a combination of relative size and relative distance magnification considerations. Once again, the application of lenses for the near focusing demand must be considered; otherwise, the target may be made large enough to see, but will be out of focus. Big and blurry is not as easy to see as big and clear. In some instances, a clearer image can be recognized with less magnification (ie, smaller on the electronic device), thereby allowing more information to be displayed on the screen at one time.

DETERMINING MAGNIFICATION

When an individual cannot see to perform a task, magnification may be necessary. Simply stated, the magnification required is determined by dividing the patient's actual acuity level by the desired acuity level. For example: An individual has 20/200 distance visual acuity, sees the 20/200 near target at 16 inches (with appropriate glasses), and would like to see 20/50 size print at near. That requires 4× magnification, and can be calculated a number of ways:

1. Using "billboard" magnification (relative size magnification), the target (print size) can be made 4 times larger.

2. Using "airplane" or relative distance magnification, if the 20/200 target is at 16 inches initially, it can be brought 4 times closer to approximately 4 inches, which would require a lens, or accommodation, of approximately +10.00 D. (This gets a little more complex based on whether the patient is myopic or hyperopic).

3. A combination of relative size and relative distance magnification could be provided with electronic equipment like a closed-circuit television (CCTV). For example, the target can be made physically larger on the CCTV monitor, and the patient can sit closer (or farther) than 16 inches, with the appropriate glasses. This formula for equivalent power is used to calculate the overall magnification (see Chapter 5) in terms of diopters.

If this individual needed to see the 20/50 sized target at a 20-foot measured distance, a 4× telescope or electronic equipment that could magnify 4 times at distance could be used. The occupational therapist may help estimate magnification using the actual materials the client might need to see for an activity (see Chapter 8). The limiting physical and optical factors of these, as well as near devices, are the weight, appearance, field of view, and lighting constraints that these systems impose.

These are generalities and should be reviewed with the optometrist who has prescribed the devices in relationship to what the occupational therapist has identified as the visual requirements necessary for the task. However, use of low vision devices for central vision loss is just part of the rehabilitation process. Understanding how these devices are used requires appreciating their optical qualities and practice to get comfortable with their strengths and limitations. Training activities will help make the use of these devices successful.[6]

SUMMARY

This chapter reviewed the low vision examination that an occupational therapist should expect to be performed by the eye care provider. We have also included a sample report from a low vision optometrist, and Table 7-5 provides a list of common abbreviations used in a low vision examination record or report. When receiving such a report, if the occupational therapist has questions about terminology, test results, or any other issues, it is best to contact the referring optometrist.

Trial and error with low vision devices will only further frustrate the often already frustrated patient, and will only serve to convince the patient that "nothing more can be done." A structured approach of assessing the visually impaired patient's needs through a thorough low vision evaluation, and rehabilitation treatment specific to the device(s) is the start of an integrated low vision rehabilitation team approach to the care of these patients. The team effort stressed in this book is one that will ultimately benefit clients with vision impairment who most need the integrated services of both the low vision optometrist and the occupational therapist.

REFERENCES

1. Tielsch JM. Prevalence of visual impairment and blindness in the United States. In: Massof RW, Lidoff L, eds. *Issues in Low Vision Rehabilitation: Service Delivery, Policy, and Funding.* New York: American Foundation for the Blind; 2001:13-26.

2. Cline D, Hofstetter HW, Griffin JR. *Dictionary of Visual Science.* Newton, MA: Butterworth-Heinemann; 1997.

3. United States Social Security Administration. Code of Federal Regulations. 1992.

4. Spalton DJ, Hitchings RA, Hunter PA. *Atlas of Clinical Ophthalmology.* London, England: Gower Medical Publishing; 1984.

5. Harley RD. *Pediatric Ophthalmology.* Vol I and II. Philadelphia, PA: W. B. Saunders Co; 1983.

6. Freeman PB, Jose RT. *The Art and Practice of Low Vision.* 3rd ed. Boston, MA: Butterworth-Heinemann; 1997.

Occupational Therapy Low Vision Rehabilitation Evaluation

8

The *Occupational Therapy Practice Framework* was developed and revised to articulate occupational therapy's unique focus on occupation and daily activities and the application of an intervention process that facilitates engagement in occupation to support participation in life.[1] The framework states that "the evaluation process is focused on finding out what the client wants and needs to do and on identifying those factors that act as barriers to performance."[2] In accordance with this approach, this evaluation takes a "top-down" approach; that is, the evaluation starts by identifying the client's roles, aspirations, and occupations prior to the vision loss and, with the client, develops performance goals. During the interview with a client and others, the evaluation assesses the physical and social environment, or context, prior roles and routines, and "performance patterns." Finally "client factors" are systematically evaluated, not only vision, but also cognitive, motor, and psychological client factors. These must be evaluated with reference to activity demands, such as print size, or fine motor requirements of each specific activity that may be targeted by treatment. The interpretation of these observations and data then leads the practitioner to identify the barriers to performance. The interventions remove these barriers by modifying the client factors and context, and sometimes circumvent the barriers by modifying the

tasks required for an occupation, such as listening to books rather than reading them visually. The evaluation that we present here follows these guidelines. It is also important to remember that under Medicare Part B guidelines, the initial evaluation completed by the occupational therapist is used to determine whether there is medical necessity for low vision rehabilitation.

For example, Ms. Sprout, who presents with a profound loss in vision, was in a caregiving role for an ailing husband and has a performance goal of medication management. Considering activity demand that includes the small print size on the pill containers, the vision evaluation revealed the client would need a high-power magnification to read labels. If low vision were the only barrier to performance, the solution might be a handheld magnifier and maybe an hour of instruction. If the evaluation also revealed other barriers to performance, such as impaired problem solving, low frustration tolerance, and a hand tremor, a more practical solution might be to modify the task and activity demand to avoid teaching the use of such a difficult device; rather, the therapist would recommend a visiting nurse to organize medication into a large weekly dispenser that the client could manage. The best solution depends on much more than vision.

Whittaker SG, Scheiman M, Sokol-McKay DA.
Low Vision Rehabilitation: A Practical Guide for Occupational Therapists,
Second Edition (pp 107-140).
© 2016 Taylor & Francis Group.

In the past, low vision rehabilitation often involved trial and error with devices and interventions. Not only is trial and error incompatible with a success-oriented approach (see Chapter 6), but private and government payers now require an increasingly high degree of cost effectiveness. Unsuccessful trials are costly and discouraging to the client. From the start, an initial evaluation needs to not only accurately predict what devices, environmental modifications, and instruction will enable a client to achieve his or her personal performance goals; the evaluation should lead to the selection of specific devices and use of compensatory strategies that fit into the client's lifestyle and lead to measurable improvements in subjective quality of life. Such predictability is necessary for accurate treatment planning. Payers and consumers now expect this.

For a treatment plan to be accurate, the occupational therapy low vision rehabilitation evaluation first must identify observable and measurable performance goals, including contextual information such as accurately reading a menu in a restaurant, reading a book in a favorite chair at home at a specified rate and duration, or accurately telephoning some close friends and neighbors if help is needed. The evaluation of occupational performance identifies disabled activities of value to the individual that may become a person's goals. Chapter 10, which addresses foundation skills, begins with how to write goals for vision rehabilitation. Information gathered by the occupational therapist, combined with information from the eye care provider, should now identify barriers to performance and what devices, new skills, and changes in the environment are needed for goal achievement, if indeed it is possible to achieve a person's goal. The therapist now should also be able to predict how many sessions are required to achieve specific performance goals. For example, a client who is depressed or somewhat cognitively impaired might require a success-oriented approach (see Chapter 6) and several more sessions than someone whose only impairment is vision.

To accomplish these requirements, the occupational therapy vision rehabilitation evaluation consists of 4 components:

1. Evaluation of occupational performance, disabled activities, and determination of potential performance goals

2. Evaluation of cognitive, psychosocial, context (physical and social), and relevant physical client factors to develop an occupational profile that identifies supports of and barriers to performance

3. A functional vision evaluation to determine visual barriers to performance

4. Determination of specific goals, rehabilitation potential, and cost (of devices, time, and effort) to achieve the goals

This chapter does not provide a comprehensive review of alternative assessment instruments and evaluation techniques; rather, we describe selected instruments that we have used and know will be effective, practical, and affordable based on published research and our own experience. More important than our selection, therefore, is the rationale for our particular selection. The reasons we give for choosing an assessment should guide the reader in the consideration of many acceptable alternative assessment tools.

One important issue for occupational therapists is time management. In almost all clinical settings, the amount of time available for the occupational therapy evaluation is limited to about 1 hour. Important in the selection of assessment tools is administration time. Visual testing, screening for other client factors, and discussion of goals requires about 30 minutes, leaving about 30 minutes for the interview.

OVERVIEW OF THE EVALUATION

In an outpatient setting, the initial evaluation presents a major challenge. One must develop rapport with the client and family, collect a huge amount of information, set goals, and develop a treatment plan in 1 hour. This chapter will follow the sequence of a typical evaluation. The client, who had probably invested hours into arranging for travel and completing forms, must leave this evaluation feeling confident that the proposed treatment plan will be worth the time, effort, and money that will be needed.

Much of the information can be obtained from other professionals before the evaluation session. Low vision care requires teamwork. The eye care professional's role (optometrists, ophthalmologists, neuro-ophthalmologists) is to try and maximize the client's visual function by managing the underlying disease progression, using traditional eyeglasses, and recommending possible low vision visual devices. Selection of optical devices and even use of nonoptical visual devices such as computers, smart phones, and simple handheld magnifiers requires an understanding of refractive error for a given working distance, the underlying visual effects of a disease, and disease progression by an optometrist or ophthalmologist.

Before the evaluation, the performance questionnaires should be sent to the client, but with an indication that sighted assistance will be provided if he or she cannot find someone to help. The client should be asked to bring in all optical devices, eyeglasses, and samples of materials that he or she wishes to read or see, the size of the TV, and viewing distance. Typically, a client is asked to bring in a medication list, prior medical history, and the name and contact information for the eye care providers as well.

To start the evaluation, we suggest that once you have introduced yourself as an occupational therapist and settled into the examination room, it is best to explain to the client that as an occupational therapist, we help people do the things they want to do but no longer can do. One should go on to explain that the purpose of the evaluation is for us to set goals and ask the client "What do you want to do?" Tell the client you will ask him or her lots of questions, do a lot of testing, and at the end will estimate how many sessions, what equipment might be needed, and the likelihood of meeting each goal. Remind the client that he or she will determine the goals.

EVALUATION OF OCCUPATIONAL PERFORMANCE

Occupational performance is defined as the ability to carry out activities of daily life (ADL), including basic and personal ADL, instrumental activities of daily living (IADL), education, work, play, leisure, and social participation.[1] Table 8-1 summarizes activities commonly affected by vision impairment. This list is based on the Low Vision Independence Measure (LVIM)[3] which was developed by focus groups of optometrists, clients, occupational therapists, and other providers of low vision services. The 2008 *Occupational Therapy Practice Framework* provided a basic structure[1] for the development of this list. During the evaluation process, the performance skills and patterns are identified, and other aspects of engaging in occupation, such as client factors, activity demands, and context, are assessed. The occupational performance evaluation should involve objective and subjective measures of performance of an ADL and IADL.

The outcome measures we recommend were inspired by the Canadian Occupational Performance Measure (COPM),[4] where clients are asked to rate the importance of a problem area and then these ratings are used to prioritize the goals. Unfortunately, the COPM uses subjective rather than objective outcome assessments, which are more responsive to the effects of treatment and become the basis for the goals that we need to set. The Melbourne ADL index[5] was developed as an objective outcome measure, but at this writing was no longer being published and is limited to a few areas commonly disabled by performance.

Note that under 2013 Medicare guidelines, outcomes must be converted into measures of percentage disability currently called a *G-code*. There are general strategies for such a conversion. For multistep activities like ADLs and IADLs or the use of assistive devices, the activity can be broken into discrete component tasks, which may or may not require assistance, and are then scored like the Functional Independence Measure (FIM), which indicates what percentage of the steps required assistance. For spot reading or recognizing faces, performance can be measured as a percentage accuracy within a reasonable time limit. If the activity is continual, like fluent reading, then percentage of goal reading speed and endurance can be used. The Pepper Test[6,7] would be appropriate for reading accuracy and speed because it has been validated against passages using meaningful text. Normally, one directly observes performance as part of the initial evaluation, but asking someone to perform an impossible activity is time consuming and discouraging. Inferences about performance can be made from the functional vision evaluation, which involves performance measures. For example, if the reading acuity test reveals that the smallest print someone can read is 2M (16 point), then one can assume 0% accuracy or dependent levels of assistance for everyday reading activities that involve print smaller than 2M (N16) if someone does not have magnification devices.

The location of the evaluation is an important issue to consider, and performance measures should reflect what happens in a person's own environment, not the artificial, idealized settings in the clinic. Ideally, the occupational performance evaluation should take place in the client's home or current living situation. This allows the therapist to explore the various areas of occupation and actually observe the client engaged in these activities in the client's real environment (performance context). This is particularly important because for the low vision client, context issues such as lighting, contrast, glare, home design, appliance setup, and organization are critical to an analysis of occupational performance. In addition, one should observe performance of familiar tasks under somewhat unfamiliar circumstances to evaluate cognitive functions such as problem solving, insight, reasoning, and frustration tolerance. Unfortunately, this is often not practical, but can be approximated by taking video of the activity using a smart phone or based on an interview with a client and caregivers.

This chapter uses published, standardized, current, and validated measures of occupational performance for people with vision disability that list a number of specific activities, such as those activities in Table 8-1 taken from the LVIM,[3] and asks the client to rate the difficulty level of performing each item on a 4-level Likert scale, corresponding to (1) unable, (2) extremely difficult, (3) moderately or slightly difficult, and (4) not difficult. The numbers are then combined into a single number that reflects overall progress that, in turn, can be converted into a G-code.

There are several potential problems with occupational performance measures.

1. Often, a client will wish to focus treatment on just a few activities. Some outcome measures of treatment average performance of relevant activities of interest that were addressed in treatment with a longer list of activities irrelevant to the client that were not addressed in treatment. This will dilute measured improvements in relevant activities with measures of irrelevant activities that did not change so that overall total success is underestimated.

TABLE 8-1: AREAS OF OCCUPATIONAL PERFORMANCE COMMONLY DISABLED BY VISION IMPAIRMENT

SELF-CARE	COMMUNICATION
• Shaving or applying makeup • Identifying toiletries • Brushing teeth/cleaning dentures • Identifying foods when eating • Cutting food on plate • Keeping food on utensil • Managing medication • Identifying clothing	• Requesting assistance • Writing notes/letters/envelopes • Signing your name • Locating/dialing a phone number • Determining the time • Documenting appointments • Using computer/cell phone
HOME MANAGEMENT	**FINANCIAL MANAGEMENT**
• Cleaning floors • Cleaning counters • Washing dishes • Organizing cabinets • Operating washer and dryer • Repairing clothing	• Identifying coins and paper money • Reading bills and receipts • Writing checks • Balancing accounts • Banking online
FOOD PREPARATION	**LEISURE**
• Reading recipes • Pouring liquids • Measuring food • Slicing and peeling food • Seasoning food • Determining food doneness • Using microwave and stove • Identifying foods with similar packaging	• Watching television • Playing games/cards • Reading books/newspapers/magazines • Using technology/iPads/e-books • Doing crafts • Eating out • Participating in community
MOBILITY	**SHOPPING**
• Avoiding obstacles • Wayfinding	• Preparing a shopping list • Locating items • Reading labels or prices • Determining expiration dates • Paying for items

Adapted from items in Theresa Smith's Low Vision Independence Measure (LVIM).[3]

2. Performance measures developed for low vision rehabilitation tend to focus on activities that require vision and are treatable with visual interventions such as magnifiers. Often, effective occupational therapy uses nonvisual options to meet a performance goal, such as recorded books for reading or tactile techniques for ADLs. Ideally, a totally blind person using good adaptive technique and devices should be able to score 0% disability on a low vision functional performance measure.

TABLE 8-2: ADDING OBJECTIVE CRITERIA TO A SUBJECTIVE OCCUPATIONAL PERFORMANCE MEASURE AND CALCULATING TOTAL PERCENTAGE DISABILITY

SUBJECTIVE LEVEL OF DIFFICULTY*	OBJECTIVE MEASURE	SCORE
Unable to perform (impossible)	Requires frequent or intermittent assistance	3
Extremely difficult	Requires occasional assistance and intermittent cues	2
Moderately/slightly difficulty	Requires occasional cues (eg, for problem solving), increased time, or decreased endurance	1
Not difficult	May include use of assistive devices or substitute nonvisual technique	0

*Calculation of percentage disability for G-codes: (1) sum the scores for items of interest, (2) multiply the total number of items of interest by 3, (3) divide #1 by #2 and multiply by 100%.

3. Some tests are too long to administer in the 1 hour allotted to a functional vision evaluation.

4. Performance measures are based on subjective ratings rather than objective measures. We prefer objective measures, which are more responsive in general to interventions and convert directly into the objective goals that are required by payers.

To compromise, we propose for goal writing and evaluation that the instructions to the evaluator link the subjective scale to more objective measures (Table 8-2) that then can be converted into observable and measurable goals. A subjective component is important because an important issue to consider when evaluating the client's performance is how much effort and energy are expended. Warren states that the primary issues to consider regarding performance of ADL are safety and effort.[8] She states that most people with vision loss are technically independent, but expend a great deal of mental and physical effort, with questionable safety and little margin for error. They perform at their maximum capability at all times, leaving them with little energy to enjoy what else life has to offer.[8] This would be reflected in the more subjective measures of performance, such as rated difficulty. In the conversion to objective measures, we leave one level to describe this extra effort. We also propose some changes in the wording of questions to allow nonvisual performance. One should not limit performance goals to those listed on the questionnaires. One should be able to add items and rate them. These changes will invalidate the tests' standardization and use of certain statistical analyses, but are recommended for the practical reasons we describe. Because these tests and the G-codes are currently being developed and may change after this book is published, we have included the latest versions of these tests and a method for converting the results into G-codes (or whatever current outcome measure Medicare requires) in the online appendix (www.routledge.com/9781617116339) in a document entitled "Converting Outcome Measures to G-codes."

We have reviewed several performance measures for this book. One measure in wide use, especially for research, is the NEI VFQ-25,[9] a 25-item Visual Function Questionnaire developed by the US National Eye Institute and used widely in research to evaluate the functional effects of medical interventions. The NEI VFQ-25 is well validated and short, but is *not* recommended for measuring outcomes of low vision interventions because it focuses on a few visually dependent activities and thus will not reflect effective occupational therapy that uses nonvisual interventions, addresses caregiver issues, and restores many spiritual and other user-defined goals and leisure activities. This measure also does not allow for selection of items of interest to the client. Other performance measures include the Veterans Administration measure, the VA LV VFQ-48,[10] and a test of 38 functional outcomes more suited to occupational therapy, the Self-Reported Assessment of Functional Vision Performance (SRAFVP), developed and validated by Velozo et al.[11] The SRAFVP developed by occupational therapists has been widened to include a larger range of ADLs and allow for only relevant activities to be selected. Although these measures allow selection of activates of interest to the client, their measures tend to focus on activities disabled more by visual acuity and central vision loss rather than peripheral field loss, such as hemianopia, which is often encountered by occupational therapists treating in medical rehabilitation settings. Both the SRAFVP and VA LV VFQ-48 have established validity and reliability, and a shorter 20-item version of the VA LV VFQ-48 has been validated as well.[10] The LVIM[3] developed by Theresa Smith includes a broad assessment of ADL and mobility activities that may be initially disabled by vision impairment but can be recovered by visual or nonvisual adaptations. It allows for selection of only activities of interest to the client. Scores from all tests can be converted into G-codes to document the need for rehabilitation and functional improvement (see Table 8-2). The LVIM is recommended because it includes the widest variety of activities, not just those that are usually highly visually dependent, and it potentially can document success with nonvisual techniques. Because it is short, the VA LV VFQ-20 is recommended as a measure of overall progress if an in-clinic assessment is required, but this test needs to be supplemented by any user-defined goals not on the list. Often, a person may focus on just fluent reading. Standardized reading tests like the Pepper Test may be desirable in these cases.

Because of its length, the VA LV VFQ-48, SRAFVP, or LVIM should be administered over the phone or can be sent to the client, who is asked to bring the completed form to the occupational therapy low vision rehabilitation evaluation. The questionnaires will need to be completed with sighted assistance. The occupational therapist can review the questionnaire and elaborate on pertinent issues raised by the client's responses using the low vision rehabilitation evaluation form included in the online appendix. It is important, however, to understand that to sit in front of a client and read off a list of questions is not recommended, but rather to work the questions into a conversation.

The VA LV VFQ-48, VA LV VFQ-24, and LVIM can be found in the online appendix at www.routledge.com/9781617116339

OCCUPATIONAL PROFILE

Early in the evaluation session, the therapist both ascertains occupational performance and develops an occupational profile. Whether vision impairment disables some meaningful activity depends on the context, that is, other client factors and the cognitive, physical, and social environment. For example, one will encounter clients who may no longer be able to perform some chore like cleaning because of vision impairment, but are thrilled that their spouses are finally helping around the house. This change in context and roles would mean the performance limitation is not a disability of interest to this person. The occupational profile, therefore, shapes the evaluation strategy, development of the management plan, and provides the foundation for formulating a rehabilitation prognosis after data about vision and other client factors are gathered. In addition to contributing to better diagnostic and therapeutic decisions, the evaluation process builds the foundation for a good client-therapist relationship.

Building an occupational profile starts with rather general questions (Table 8-3) to help the therapist obtain facts and develop an understanding of the situation from the perspective of the client. Has the client formed performance goals? What is the client's perception of his or her own visual functioning, prognosis and health status, previous eye care, and low vision treatment? What was the client's functional ability before the vision loss? A client's unstructured response to a general question will reveal much about insight, cognitive function, and the psychosocial situation.

TABLE 8-3: SUGGESTED INITIAL QUESTIONS ABOUT VISION LOSS FOR OCCUPATIONAL PROFILE/CASE HISTORY
• What happened and why are you here?
• Do you know the name of the eye disease that has caused your vision loss?
• Can you tell me when this eye disease first became a problem for you?
• What are some things you cannot do now that you did before your vision loss?
• If you could see better, what would be the first things you would do?
• What do you miss the most?
• How long have you experienced trouble seeing?
• Describe your vision?
• What is most difficult to see?
• Do people treat you differently now than before the vision loss?
• Have you ever had a low vision evaluation? When? Where?
• Do you use any magnifiers or special glasses?
• Who gave the magnifiers or special glasses to you?
• Have you had any previous vision rehabilitation services? If so, describe.

Much objective data can be obtained prior to the evaluation from the medical records to verify the client's and family's perceptions. The interview with the client and family is not only necessary to understand the disabilities from the perspective of the client and family, but the therapist also learns what language to use with the client for the most effective communication.

The therapist must first discover the activities that the client perceives as difficult and desirable, which is critical for a treatment plan. These activities then become performance goals and thus require measurement. Questionnaires about performance provide not only a list of common problem areas, but also a means of evaluating performance. Because an ideal outcome measure has not been developed, we will describe current validated performance measures, their limitations, and the rationale for our recommendations.

Interviewing the Client

The rapport established between the occupational therapist and the client will influence the accuracy of the

TABLE 8-4: COURTESIES AND CONSIDERATIONS WHEN DEALING WITH THE ADULT CLIENT WITH LOW VISION

- Announce yourself when entering or leaving the room or when beginning or ending a conversation so the person does not continue to speak after you leave.

- Speak directly to the person, using a normal tone of voice.

- Call the person by name or touch him or her lightly on the arm.

- Always explain what you are going to do before you begin.

- Request permission to touch the person when necessary.

- Be specific in directions. Avoid expressions like "over there" or "right here." Use phrases such as "your magnifier is on the left side of the lamp."

- If in doubt about how to help, just ask the client.

- Do not rearrange the space of a person with a visual impairment.

- Avoid safety hazards. Keep doors fully opened or closed. Push in chairs.

Adapted from Sokol-McKay DA, Michels D. Facing the challenge of macular degeneration: therapeutic interventions for low vision. *OT Practice.* 2005;10:10-15.

information obtained during the interview, as well as the client's confidence in the assessment and his or her response to later recommendations. Therefore, the occupational therapist's attitude should be one of interest, willingness to listen, and empathetic concern. A manner that is friendly and informal will lessen any anxiety associated with the visit. A hurried, indifferent, detached, or unempathetic presence is a barrier to effective communication, which, in turn, may have a deleterious effect on the interview process.[12] Breakdowns in communication frequently result in failure to comply with a professional's recommendations.[13] Because of the client's visual impairment, interaction is different from that typical of a case history with a normally sighted person. Sokol-McKay[14] emphasized the importance of implementing certain courtesies and considerations when evaluating an adult client with low vision. Examples of these courtesies are announcing when entering or leaving the room or when beginning or ending a conversation, speaking directly to the person, using a normal tone of voice, and requesting permission to touch the person when necessary. Table 8-4 provides a list of these suggested courtesies. Typically, one begins the evaluation when first greeting a client and observing his or her navigation walking to the examination area. The therapist should still ask the client if he or she needs assistance. This establishes a concern for the client's safety and deference to the client's choice.

It is best to open an interview with general questions, such as, "Why are you here?" The answer will provide insight into what the client expects, how the client frames the problem, and his or her priorities. An answer such as "I need to read my mail" or "I can't keep up with my reading" or even "To read again" indicates good insight and an ability to quickly focus on performance goals. An answer

such as "For glasses so I can see again" or "To see again" or if an accompanying family member answers for the patient, who, when pressed, only gives general answers, indicates the client needs to better understand the nature of the therapy and will require help identifying performance goals. If a family member answers for a client, observe the interaction between the caregiver and client for a short time to better understand the family and caregiver expectations, but it is important to direct the conversation to the client. With a client who appears cognitively impaired or severely depressed, it is important to have caregivers present, but caregivers and family should sit behind the client and questions directed to the client. The therapist can both acknowledge the others involved with eye contact and can verify client answers by reading the body language of the caregiver while still directing questions to the client. Weaving small talk about interests and family into the early part of the interview will help develop rapport and start the interview on a positive note, but also begin the information-gathering process about where a person lives, how connected the person is socially, and what the client has enjoyed in the past, as well as to evaluate hearing and cognition. A list of areas to cover in these questions is provided in Table 8-5. This casual conversation is a good time to explore prior roles and activities with questions such as, "What did you do last year [before your vision loss]?" As the person reminisces, the therapist can then start picking up on possible goals.

In an interview with clients, especially talkative clients, some therapists might tend to avoid general questions because the client may spend considerable time on an answer. To keep the conversation focused, as the client pauses, the therapist can respond to something a client said,

TABLE 8-5: AREAS OF INTEREST FOR THE OCCUPATIONAL PROFILE

PRIOR AND CURRENT ENVIRONMENT (CONTEXT)

"Where did you live (work)? Did you like it?"

"Where do you live (work)? Do you like it?

- Other household members and relationships
- Working and living physical environment at home and work (photographs)
- Other people at home and work who provided support to you
- Other people, children, or pets who were provided support by you
- Accessibility of places of worship or recreation
- Plans to move and where

PRIOR AND CURRENT LEVEL OF FUNCTION

"What did you do before you had vision problems?"

"What do you do now? Are you satisfied? How difficult is it?"

- Quality of life
- Social roles, routines, and habits
- Specific activities performed and activity demands
- Mobility at home and in the community
- Reading (what specifically did you read, if anything?)
- Use of technology (computer, TV, phones) and tool use
- Shopping and finances
- Homemaking and maintenance
- Leisure and work activities
- Shopping
- Mobility

MEDICAL HISTORY AND CLIENT UNDERSTANDING OF THE CONDITIONS

- Hearing loss
- Hearing aid
- Diabetes
- Dialysis
- Stroke or head injury
- Hypertension
- Cardiac problems or angina
- Arthritis
- Respiratory problems
- Cognitive and emotional health
- Medications

directing the conversation to a more specific question or series of questions to obtain more pertinent information.

Using the previously mentioned occupational performance assessment tools as a basis for exploring particular areas of concern, the occupational therapist can still begin with broad-based questions and move to more focused inquiries. The strategy is to scan potentially important areas and focus in when appropriate, while maintaining sensitivity and flexibility in listening for and pursuing interests.[5]

The key areas to be investigated are listed in Table 8-1 and are included in the low vision rehabilitation evaluation form (see the online appendix at www.routledge.com/9781617116339). These are only suggested starting points. The occupational therapist will need to ask additional questions based on the client's initial responses.

A sample low vision rehabilitation evaluation form can be found in the online appendix at www.routledge.com/9781617116339

Important Areas to Be Addressed in the Occupational Profile

Vision History

It is important to determine the client's understanding of his or her eye disease and vision problem and the level of acceptance. The therapist should ask questions about onset (when did the problem begin), duration (how long has the client been visually impaired), and the date of the last examination, as well as questions to probe the client's understanding of the diagnosis, prognosis, and effects on performance (see Table 8-5). Again, even if a complete report is available from the referring doctor, it is worthwhile to gather this information from the perspective of the client. A client's answers to these questions will indicate stage of coping, expectations, and many aspects of cognitive functioning. One of the critical factors determining the effectiveness of vision rehabilitation is a motivated client who understands the disease process. After discussing onset and duration, ask the client about previous and current treatment and expected prognosis.

We need to know the optical or nonoptical devices that have been prescribed or purchased by the client and the client's efforts at problem solving; always be positive about these efforts and make every effort to incorporate even less desirable solutions by a client and family into the treatment plan. Have there been any previous attempts at vision rehabilitation? If so, who provided these services and were these services helpful? It is also important to determine if the client is aware of support groups and other opportunities in the community to receive help, support, and education about low vision.

Health History

Because the population of clients seen by the occupational therapist will generally be the older adult, many clients will have multiple medical conditions requiring occupational therapy. The health history is an important component of the occupational profile/case history. To save time, much of this information, as well as medications, should be gathered by questionnaire or medical history prior to the evaluation. An understanding of the client's other medical problems, medications, and associated impairments will significantly impact treatment planning. Common examples include peripheral neuropathy secondary to diabetes that limits the use of tactile markings like raised dots on dials, hand tremors that might interfere with the use of optical devices, hearing problems that may preclude the use of assistive devices such as National Library Service (NLS) recorded books, and arthritis that may limit movement and, therefore, the ability to use certain optical devices. Medications might not only have relevant side effects, but may present unique medical management problems, such as with diabetes management.

Premorbid Occupational Performance History

The importance of the occupational history has been summarized in the American Occupational Therapy Association (AOTA) *Occupational Therapy Practice Framework*.[1] A person's expectations about vision rehabilitation are often closely associated with his or her previous level of activity, occupation, habits, routines, and roles. Before establishing that a disabled activity exists, one needs to establish premorbid performance of the activity. Clients typically want vision to be the way it was before the eye disease caused the vision loss. In some cases, improvement in vision may be possible using optical devices with mild vision loss or lighting changes, but treatment often focuses on compensatory strategies and assistive devices that create new and disruptive changes in lifestyle. Current guidelines for a "medically necessary" intervention include sports and sexuality, as well as self-care and homemaking occupations. Vocational rehabilitation and driving are often excluded by medical insurance but are covered by state vocational rehabilitation providers, workers' compensation, and private agencies, with guidelines that vary from region to region.

Client's Needs and Goals

Finally, it is important to let the client tell you what he or she hopes to achieve through vision rehabilitation. As discussed in Chapter 6, it is not unusual to hear some unrealistic expectations from clients. Remember that the prior experience of this client was that new glasses always restored clear vision. Clients often expect the same result even when the vision loss is caused by disease. By the time the client is being examined by the occupational therapist, he or she may have had numerous examinations with an ophthalmologist and perhaps a low vision optometrist. The client has been told that there are no miracle glasses, devices, or drugs that will restore normal vision. Yet, it is not unusual for the client to say, "I want to be able to see well again" or "I am hoping you can prescribe glasses that will help me see well again."[15] They either fail to understand that the vision loss is permanent or are in denial. Denial may be part of the process of adapting to vision loss (see Chapter 6) and is best left alone and not directly contradicted. The best response to such unrealistic statements is to redirect focus from vision to performance, independent of whether an activity is performed visually or nonvisually or how the activity is performed. Once a client enjoys a book by listening to it or finds reading is easier with an electronic magnifier, this initial expectation may change. It is important, however, to revisit client expectations regarding goals and the ongoing treatment plan to check if the original unrealistic expectation had indeed changed. Nothing is more disappointing than, after several sessions working with a device that was found to effectively meet several performance goals, discovering an angry and disappointed client rejecting the device because the initial expectation ("seeing clearly with glasses") was not met.

Once needs and goals have been set, performance of these goal activities must be assessed to justify treatment and modify progress. One problem with all published performance outcome measures for low vision rehabilitation is the focus on visual performance of a task. For example, the VA LV VFQ tests ask a client to rate his or her ability to "read a book or bible with normal size print." If the client had successful rehabilitation outcomes by learning to enjoy recorded books, or by using an e-reader to enlarge print, the answer to this question would not reflect any improvement. One could ask the same questions with a focus on occupational performance rather than visual performance. For example, one should preface the questions about reading by telling the client that reading includes listening or using an electronic device. Unfortunately, to change the wording of a standardized test would invalidate standard error estimates of the score. Such a change, however, would be required to reflect success of nonoptical or nonvisual interventions, and is recommended until improved outcome measures are validated.

Another problem with using the self-rated performance outcome assessments is that a complete evaluation requires that the therapist observe a client's performance, not just depend on the subjective ratings of difficulty. Once the client indicates important activities that are difficult or impossible, then performance should be directly observed. The functional visual evaluation described in this chapter was designed to simultaneously measure performance and vision to save time. For example, for clients with reading goals, visual acuity is measured with reading. If a person cannot read 1M font, then one can assume any ADL reading tasks cannot be performed unless someone has already developed adaptive strategies or uses assistive devices.

Psychosocial and Cognitive Issues

The most emotionally devastating impact of vision loss and psychosocial and cognitive issues related to vision loss are described in detail in Chapter 6. It is critical, therefore, that occupational therapists attend to the emotional impact of the vision loss and the client's ability to cope when providing low vision rehabilitation. Chapter 6 outlined 7 key factors[16] that should be reviewed by the occupational therapist during the occupational profile/case history. These include the type of vision loss, the family's reaction to the vision loss, the client's life stage, significant life events, the client's expectations, the client's self-concept, and the client's personality. In addition, if the occupational therapist is concerned about the client's mental health, we suggest using one of the self-reporting questionnaires described in Chapter 6, such as the Geriatric Depression Scale (GDS). The GDS can be easily administered in a short period of time and is in the public domain (no cost).

Low vision, especially with severe and profound vision loss, creates unique and substantial cognitive demands, especially with spatial perception, which integrates the use and interpretation of other senses. A person with a long-standing visual impairment may have developed an ability to interpret vision differently, such as using a person's hairline and gait to recognize him or her, or using blobs of color to orient in a room. These skills are sometimes informally called *blur interpretation* and may suffice to meet a person's needs.

FUNCTIONAL VISION EVALUATION

The occupational therapist performs a functional vision evaluation to determine visual barriers to performance and to develop a treatment plan to remove or circumvent these barriers. Chapter 1 described and illustrated 5 visual client factors, including visual acuity, contrast sensitivity to larger objects, the central visual field, peripheral visual field, and any eye movement problems. Information about the disease, refractive error, areas of the eye or brain affected, and optical correction for different working distances might corroborate a vision finding or guide an intervention, such as where to hold something to see it most clearly. Depending on the occupational therapist's practice setting, much of this information may be readily available from the referring ophthalmologist or optometrist's records (see Chapter 7). Occupational therapists working in an ophthalmology office, a low vision practice, or any other facility in which an ophthalmologist and/or an optometrist is working will have full access to the client's eye records and the

TABLE 8-6: VISUAL BARRIERS TO PERFORMANCE AND GENERAL INTERVENTIONS

CLIENT FACTOR	ACTIVITY DEMAND	SOLUTIONS
Insufficient visual acuity	Print or object size too small	Improve acuity (eg, lighting), magnify object or print
Insufficient contrast sensitivity	Insufficient object contrast	Improve contrast sensitivity, increase object contrast, decrease glare, optimize light
Central scotoma limits field of view	Larger field of view required for identification	Move eyes to maximize field of view, hold text at a different angle, scroll text or use very high magnification
Peripheral field limitation	Object located in the blind area	Look in the direction of the field loss or use field expansion prism
Oculomotor limitation	Object located out of the range of eye movement, or object position causes double vision or eye strain	Move head, use prism to avoid eye movement, eye movement training (refer to neuro-optometrist)
Perceptual dysfunction due to previously mentioned sensory problems or neurological damage to perceptual processing areas	Visual image distorted	Practice with object identification and localization

required information. Even if the occupational therapist is not working directly with an eye care professional, this information can be requested from the referring doctor. We have included a form in the online appendix that can be used for this purpose. The types of vision loss and recommended tests were reviewed in Chapter 1 and are listed in Table 8-6.

Overview of the Visual Evaluation and Reasoning Process

There is not sufficient time to perform all of the following tests. Before beginning the evaluation, the examiner should consider the diagnosis, as this will indicate the most likely visual barriers to performance and which testing should be performed. For example, a person with low vision from a stroke is most likely to have a peripheral field loss to the right or left and if they have reading problems will need tangent screen testing of the central field. A person with a traumatic brain injury may have scotomas or partial field loss in different areas, as well as eye movement problems. A client with a diagnosis of macular degeneration is more likely to have a central scotoma and will need careful study of reading acuity, contrast sensitivity and lighting, and central field testing. Chapter 3 lists more common visual pathologies that cause low vision and expected visual effects.

The first step in a vision evaluation is nearly always the MNREAD or SKREAD near acuity test because, when properly administered, these reading acuity tests provide considerable information in addition to visual acuity

(Table 8-7) and guide the remainder of the evaluation. The MNREAD quickly estimates the maximum reading rate that could be achieved with magnification alone, as well as the required magnification to barely read and to read at a maximum reading rate (critical print size [CPS]). If fluent reading is achieved with print 3 or 4 lines larger than the acuity threshold, these tests allow one to rule out alexia and literacy problems and to conclude that fluent reading might be achieved by magnification alone. While administering the test, the examiner carefully looks for a pattern of reading errors and hesitations while reading because the pattern may indicate visual field restrictions or eye movement problems. Moreover, this reading task can be quickly and easily adapted to evaluate lighting and colored absorptive lenses (sunlenses).

It is essential that the patient be properly refracted for the test distance, which is usually 40 cm (16 inches), but may be closer if a client has been dispensed stronger reading glasses. For a success-oriented approach, and for proper test interpretation, the examiner should attempt to start with the largest print size that can be read. Many may have not read in years and find that reading again, even with very large letters, to be encouraging. However, nothing is more discouraging to a client than not seeing anything on the chart or during a test. If the interview and initial observations indicate very low vision, then acuity testing should begin with a LEA number booklet. If unfamiliarity with written English, illiteracy, or alexia is suspected, then the examiner should start with a number or symbol chart.

The next test to perform is contrast sensitivity to verify and adjust the range of optimum light and determine if

TABLE 8-7: RECOMMENDED TESTS OF VISUAL FUNCTION

VISUAL FUNCTION	RECOMMENDED TECHNIQUE	ALTERNATIVE TECHNIQUES
Visual acuity at distance	LEA numbers low vision booklet	ETDRS chart
Reading acuity at near	MNREAD test	SKREAD, LEA near vision card, symbols
Peripheral visual field	Confrontation field testing	Confrontation field testing with vision testing wands
Contrast sensitivity	Pediatric near low contrast test booklet	LEA symbol low contrast test 10M
Scotoma assessment	Tangent screen, reading errors	Laser spot on a wall, clock face
Reading assessment/ reading speed	Pepper Test, SKREAD test, paragraph from standardized reading test	Reading material of client's own choosing

absorptive lenses are needed. The contrast sensitivity and acuity tests require a similar task and setup, so the examiner may quickly transition between near acuity and near contrast sensitivity. The examiner may also use the contrast tests to look for partial central field loss and quickly ascertain field of view for reading.

After administering near acuity and contrast sensitivity testing, the examiner has expended about 15 minutes in the visual evaluation, but gained a wealth of information. The examiner has not only estimated prognosis for recovering a fluent reading goal visually and estimated required magnification and lighting for further testing and instruction; the examiner also has some direction for further testing of visual fields and screening for oculomotor problems. Like acuity, confrontation fields are always performed and can be completed quickly. If the diagnosis indicates an expected peripheral field loss, then confrontation field testing will require more time to map out the area of vision loss. If the diagnosis and prior testing indicate central field involvement, then central field testing is indicated. Finally, clients should be screened for eye movement problems.

Tests such as the Pepper Test and SKREAD were designed to be more sensitive to reading errors. Because of administration time, the Pepper Test and the absorptive lens evaluation, and sometimes the tangent screen test for central vision loss, must be conducted during later sessions.

If the visual evaluation of the 5 aspects of visual function does not fully explain disabled performance, then perceptual testing for conditions such as visual/spatial neglect, visual agnosias, or alexia should be pursued. In cases of even mild traumatic brain injury or concussion, people may be left with incipient problems such as headaches and poor reading endurance that require evaluation by a neuro-optometrist. Alexia may require referral to a speech therapist, and balance problems to a physical or occupational therapist specializing in balance problems and vestibular rehabilitation. Orientation and mobility problems ideally should involve a referral to an orientation and mobility specialist and extended home-based treatments;

braille education should be referred to a vision rehabilitation therapist. Cost-effective services require coordination. Since people often must wait for these other services to begin, these referrals should be initiated as soon as possible after the initial evaluation.

The assessments described in this chapter are designed to guide the examiner in developing a treatment plan. One must be careful not to assume the results of formal tests always reflect a person's visual functioning during an activity. Vision often changes during an actual task, especially when field restrictions are involved. Description of the types of errors during reading and visual activities indicates how vision changes during activity. Test interpretations are reviewed in this chapter and are detailed in the chapters that describe the particular treatments in Section III.

An important general concept in determining the visual requirements for an activity is the concept of "functional reserve."[10,17] The visual requirements to perform a task must include a specification of both a client visual factor, such as visual acuity—the smallest print size someone can see—and the activity demand, such as the print size someone must read. Functional reserve indicates the difference or a ratio of the visual property of an object or word during an activity (print size during reading) and at threshold (print size at visual acuity threshold). In reading research, the acuity reserve required for fluent reading is over 2:1; that is, the print size after magnification must be over twice the print size at acuity threshold. Another property, the contrast of print for quickest reading, is nearly 30 times print contrast at threshold. The need for functional reserve is pervasive in rehabilitation. Because clients often resist change and higher magnification is difficult to learn to manage, historically, the tendency in low vision has been to respond to a client's rejection of a strong magnifier with a weaker magnifier because they are easier to use correctly, leaving the client with less functional reserve. The alternative is to use the success-oriented approach (see Chapter 6) and provide the assistance necessary for the client to experience success with higher magnification and then carefully wean a client from the assistance until he or she is reading independently with sufficient functional reserve for acceptable speed and comfort.

Another important part of a visual evaluation strategy is to cross-check visual findings among different tests with the patient's complaints and the diagnosis. If the recommended tests are used and procedures are followed, the results should be internally consistent because the visual evaluation protocol is based on validated tests and well-established principles of optics and visual psychophysics.

Visual Acuity at Distance: The Early Treatment of Diabetic Retinopathy Study Chart

Practice Setting

Recommended for any setting in which the equipment can be set up permanently. If a client presents with very low vision, then start with the LEA number chart.

Equipment Required

- The Early Treatment of Diabetic Retinopathy Study (ETDRS) Chart (Figure 8-1)
- Occluder

Description

This chart, initially developed by Ian Bailey and Jan Lovie,[18] is now the "gold standard" for measuring visual acuity—that is, the ETDRS chart is used to validate other acuity charts.[19] It provides 5 letters per line and standardizes the separation between letters (see Figure 8-1). A unique aspect of this chart is its geometric progression of size differences between lines, referred to as logMAR progression. The letters on each line are 0.1 log unit, or 1.25 times larger than the previous line. This format results in every 3 lines representing a halving or doubling of visual acuity at any given viewing distance. For example, if one starts at 100 and goes down 3 steps (step 1 = 80, step 2 = 80 to 63, and step 3 = 63 to 50), this is one-half of 100. These characteristics allow for consistent and accurate evaluation of visual acuity at different distances. Based on the reliability of these tests, a good general rule of thumb for acuity testing and estimation of magnification is that one line (0.1 log unit) is a significant difference clinically and 2 lines is statistically significant in people with severe vision loss.[19]

The standard test distance is 4 meters, but for low vision evaluations, the test distance is usually halved to 2 meters to ensure a client can read the letters. Testing should be even closer for very low vision. Because of the time involved, distance acuity testing may be skipped during the initial

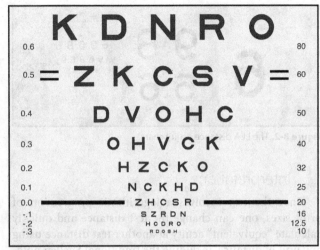

Figure 8-1. The ETDRS chart.

functional vision evaluation unless indicated, although, ideally, it should be performed and is always performed in an optometric evaluation.

Setup and Procedure

1. The client should wear his or her usual glasses. The examiner should be careful to make sure the glasses are clean (clean with cotton cloth and water) and adjusted so the client is looking through the top half of the lens for distance testing.

2. The ETDRS chart is positioned at 4 meters, and the client's left eye is covered with the occluder.

3. The occupational therapist asks the client to call out the letters on the top line.

4. The occupational therapist proceeds until the client can no longer read the letters correctly at 4 meters and records the last level at which the client can read more than 50% of the letters.

5. With all testing, it is appropriate to encourage guessing, eye movements, and eccentric viewing to see the numbers as a means of determining the prognosis for rehabilitation.

6. The occluder is then held before the client's right eye and then both eyes are tested for binocular acuity.

7. If the client is unable to see the largest letters at 4 meters, the chart should be moved to 2 meters and testing should be attempted again.

8. **Time Saver:** Have the client read downward only the first letter of a line until there is some difficulty and then have the client read all of the letters. It also often saves time to have the client read binocularly at first and then cover each eye for a quick check of monocular acuity.

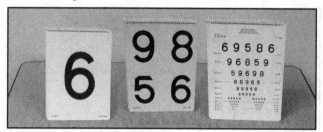

Figure 8-2. The LEA distance acuity chart.

Interpretation

Since the test involves a logarithmic progression of print sizes, one can change the test distance and quickly calculate "equivalent" acuity at another test distance using any unit of distance, including the traditional Snellen notation used widely in the United States. For example, instead of the recommended 4M test distance, low vision testing distances are typically 2 meters. At the 2-meter working distance, the acuity obtained can easily be converted to standard the Snellen 20-ft notation by just adding a zero to the numerator and denominator. For example, a 2/10 acuity measurement becomes 20/100; an acuity of 32M at 2 meters corresponds to a 20-ft equivalent of 20/320. For other distances, one must use a formula. The formula is not only used to convert metric acuity to the traditional Snellen notation; it is also used to estimate equivalent acuity at different distances. This calculation is done frequently by low vision therapists to find equivalent object or print size at distances other than the test distance. There are many ways to perform this calculation. In addition to the shortcut method earlier, a common method is to simply divide the bottom number (denominator) by the top number (numerator) of the original acuity measurement. Then take the quotient of this division and multiply it by the new distance to estimate the threshold letter size at the equivalent distance. Thus, to convert 3/30M to the equivalent Snellen notation (20 feet distance), 20/X, one first divides 30 by 3 (the quotient = 10) and multiplies the top of the equivalent distance (20 feet) number by 10 to estimate the denominator of the Snellen ratio that indicates print size: 200 feet. The acuity equivalent to 3/30 in metric units, thus, is 20/200 in Snellen notation. Using the same formula, we could predict that at near distance, the predicted print size would be 0.4/4M (4M at 40 cm or 4M at 0.4 meters).

However, when determining visual acuity for Medicare documentation and coding, the chart should be placed at 20 feet and the client not permitted eccentric viewing and turning of the head. This will result in lower acuity than the therapist would find if a person uses these adaptive strategies.

Visual Acuity at Distance: LEA Numbers Booklet

Practice Setting

Recommended in any settings. The test has been validated.

Equipment Required

- LEA number booklet (alternatively, the Feinbloom chart may be used)
- Occluder

Description

The LEA chart (Figure 8-2) replaces the Feinbloom chart and is preferred because the measurements agree better with the ETDRS chart measurements, but the differences are small and test-retest reliability is virtually the same.[20] The LEA chart also reports acuity in metric (M) units and changes print sizes in a logarithmic progression, which makes comparison at different distances easier. The LEA chart was calibrated for a 3-meter (10-foot distance). At a 10-foot distance, the acuity range extends from 20/1600 (6/480M) to 20/16 (6/5M), comparable to the Feinbloom chart.

If a client cannot even see the largest letter at 3 meters (about 10 feet), the chart can be moved to 2 meters (about 6 feet) or 1 meter (3 feet). At this distance, the acuity range is extended from 20/1600 to 4800 because decreasing the distance to 1/3 magnifies the letters in the denominator 3×. The same formula described earlier could be used to calculate equivalent Snellen acuity at 20 feet.

Another major advantage of this visual acuity chart is that because of the large visual acuity range that can be assessed, almost all clients with low vision will be able to read at least some letters on the visual acuity chart. This is important from a psychological standpoint. Many clients with low vision have had negative experiences during visual acuity testing if they were unable to even see the large E. Imagine after failing to see the largest letter in a doctor's office, usually the 20/200 or 6/60 letter, the doctor tells you that "you are blind." This can be depressing. The client feels that there is no hope if he or she couldn't see the eye chart at all. With the LEA and Feinbloom charts, however, most clients are able to read quite a few lines, leading to a much more positive experience.[21,22]

Setup and Procedure

1. The client should wear his or her usual glasses. The examiner should be careful to make sure the glasses are clean (clean with cotton cloth and water) and adjusted so the client is looking through the top half of the lens for distance testing.

TABLE 8-8: INTERPRETING THE MNREAD AND SKREAD RESULTS

OBSERVATION	INDICATION
Goal reading rate achieved with larger print	A fluent reading goal could be achieved with magnification alone.
CPS (the smallest print size where maximum reading rate and comfort is achieved)	Optimal near magnification in diopters is estimated as (CPS/GPS)*100/d, where CPS is critical print size, GPS is goal print size, and d is test distance in centimeters.
Fluent reading not achieved within 3 or 4 lines above acuity threshold	Visual barriers other than magnification exist.
Errors on right side of the word being read, pauses at longer words, words spelled out	Right field restriction.
Errors or missed letters or words at the beginning of the word or lines being read, pauses at longer words, skipped lines	Left field restriction, left visual/spatial neglect.
Words and letters are missed, but inconsistently	A central scotoma with unstable fixation.
A narrow range of glare-free light or tinted absorptive lenses required for best visual acuity	Special lighting is required. Lighting evaluation should be repeated with contrast sensitivity testing.

CPS, critical print size; GPS, goal print size.

2. The chart is positioned 3 meters (about 10 feet) away, and the client's left eye is covered with the occluder.

3. The occupational therapist opens the chart to the largest number and asks the client to call it out.

4. The occupational therapist proceeds until the client can no longer read the numbers correctly at 3 meters (10 feet) and records the last level at which the client can read more than 50% of the numbers.

5. It is appropriate to encourage guessing, eye movements, and eccentric viewing to see the numbers[10] as a means of determining the prognosis for rehabilitation, but these observations should be noted, as they indicate other conditions.

6. The occluder is then held before the client's right eye and then neither eye so that binocular visual acuity is tested.

7. If the client is unable to see the largest number at 3 meters (10 feet), the chart should be moved to 2 meters (6 feet) and testing should be attempted again. If the client is still unable to see the largest letter, test at a 1-meter (3-foot) distance. Again, if your performance observations and interview indicate very low vision, then for patient morale, it is better to start closer and move away.

Interpretation

As with all acuity testing, the visual acuity should be recorded as (testing distance)/(last size where numbers were identified). For example, if the testing was performed at 3 meters and the client could identify the 30M size num-

bers, the visual acuity would be reported as 3/30. The same formulae for converting acuity from one distance to another may be used. For easy conversion to equivalent Snellen, a 2-meter test distance may be used with the LEA chart.

Reading Acuity (Visual Acuity at Near With Continuous Text)

Practice Setting

Appropriate for any practice setting.

Equipment Required

Minnesota Low-Vision Reading Test (MNRead Test), stopwatch, task light, and illuminance light meter. The alternative is SKREAD.

Description

Reading is a common goal in low vision rehabilitation. We also know that near visual acuity for single letters (letter acuity) is often different from near visual acuity for reading phrases and sentences (reading acuity). Therefore, to better understand the impact of low vision on reading, it is usually more important to assess reading acuity than letter acuity if time does not permit assessing both. Moreover, the reading tests contain a wealth of information. The interpretation is summarized in Table 8-8.

A popular test for assessing continuous reading acuity is the Minnesota Low-Vision Reading Test (MN Read Test) illustrated in Figure 8-3. An advantage of using this test is that it not only provides an assessment of near visual acuity with continuous text, but the test also can be used

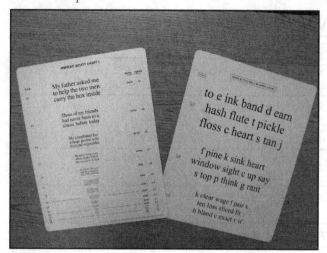

Figure 8-3. MNREAD and SKREAD visual acuity charts.

to estimate magnification required for reading, as well as estimate expected reading speed with magnification. Unlike visual acuity, which is not expected to improve with vision rehabilitation, reading speed is one function that can be improved. Thus, reading speed is one of the areas for which the occupational therapist may be able to document improvements with treatment and justify additional vision rehabilitation in Medicare documentation.

The MNRead acuity chart can be used to provide a sensitive and reliable measure of reading acuity. Each sentence has 60 characters, which correspond to 10 standard-length words, assuming a standard word length of 6 characters (including spaces). The reading or literacy level of each line is controlled at about a third-grade level, so slowed reading is because of vision, not literacy limitations. Each size sentence is presented in 3 single-spaced lines, so line-to-line scanning and the effect of crowding on word recognition within the middle line can be observed. An estimate of reading acuity is given by the smallest print size at which the client can read the entire sentence without making significant errors. (Usually, reading performance deteriorates rapidly as the acuity limit is approached, and it is easy to determine the level where reading becomes impossible.) The examiner uses a stopwatch to record the time required to read each sentence, and this allows a determination of reading speed. The pattern of reading errors and pauses also indicates other visual barriers to performance, like the presence of central vision loss.

The SKREAD resembles the MNREAD except the words and letters in the passages are unrelated. This makes it impossible for a client to infer a word from context; it must be seen. Clients also have difficulty memorizing the passages when testing is repeated. Like the Pepper Test, the SKREAD test was designed so that error patterns indicate how field restrictions affect reading (see Table 8-7). The words are carefully chosen so that if the beginning or end of a word is missed, the word still is recognizable, like the word "manage," which can be recognized by someone with a right field restriction as "man" or left field loss as "age." Although very informative, the SKREAD is at a higher, sixth-grade, literacy level and is generally more frustrating for clients. The SKREAD is a timed test like the MNREAD.

The therapist's goal with this test is to determine the best print size for reading at a given distance. Typically, there are 2 distances at which clients often must read. The most common distance for continuous text reading is 16 inches, or 40 cm. The second common distance is about 32 inches, or about 80 cm (arm's length), the usual distance of stovetop dials and shelf labels.

This test is used for measuring the following:

1. Continuous text reading acuity: This is the smallest print the client can read.

2. Critical print size: The print size just before reading starts to slow—that is, the smallest print that results in maximum reading rate. This is used for estimating magnification.

Setup and Procedure

1. The client should wear his or her usual reading glasses. The examiner should be careful to make sure the glasses are clean (clean with cotton cloth and water) and adjusted so the client is looking through the bottom half of the lenses for near testing, if it is a bifocal, or progressive lens (no-line bifocal) design. A client is usually tested under binocular conditions if he or she typically reads with both eyes, or with the better eye if he or she reads with one eye. Testing might be repeated to determine if occluding one eye improves reading.

2. The usual distance for the MNREAD chart is 40 cm (16 inches) from the eyes. If the patient is reading with stronger reading glasses, the test should be measured at the correct distance for the prescribed glasses. This can be calculated from the reading addition in the report from the eye care provider (see Chapters 5 and 7). This information must be accurate before testing proceeds. Make sure the test distance is maintained throughout the testing.

3. Allow the client to move the card side to side, but be careful to prevent the client from bringing the chart closer as the print size becomes smaller.

4. Adjust the light so it is from the side and there is little or no glare, and set the distance so illumination on the chart is approximately 2000 lux, within the range of optimal lighting for an older adult.[23,24] Ask the client if it is too much light. The client often will accurately indicate if this is the case. Adjust the lighting to a client's preferences to start. (Note this procedure can be modified if a lighting evaluation is concurrently performed to save time; see later.)

5. Instruct the client to begin reading the sentences from the top to bottom of the chart. Note the CPS, the print size just before the line where reading starts to slow. When reading starts to slow, the therapist should ask the client if it is getting hard to see and how. The subjective reports of the clients are valuable.

6. As the client reads smaller print, encourage him or her to keep reading until mistakes are made. The smallest print at which the client can read with no more than one error is continuous text reading acuity.

7. Using a stopwatch, the examiner also records how long it takes to read each 3-line sentence. This information is used to determine the client's reading speed. The MNREAD test comes with a conversion table that allows the examiner to convert the stopwatch measurement of reading time into words per minute (wpm).

8. Now compare eyes by asking the client if he or she can recognize the words at the acuity threshold with each eye covered. If not, then remeasure acuity threshold for the eye with the more impaired acuity. Note because the client can memorize the passages, this testing is based more on subjective impressions.

9. Now repeat testing at CPS under conditions that simulate a typical living room (50 to 100 lux). The client may have memorized the passages, so for an initial lighting evaluation, ask for subjective impressions and increase lighting until optimal reading speed and acuity threshold are achieved; continue to increase illuminance until the client indicates reading becomes more difficult. Measure this range of illuminance with the light meter.

Interpretation

These tests produce considerable information. A summary of test interpretation is provided in Table 8-8. The CPS is the smallest print size read *before* (the line above) the line when reading starts to slow. Print size is recorded using "M" notation and test distance in meters. The client continues reading even if he or she slows down, and the smallest print at which the client can read with no more than one error is continuous text reading acuity, recorded along with distance using metric notation as noted earlier. Typically, CPS is 3 lines above continuous test acuity, indicating a 2:1 acuity reserve. If distance visual acuity indicated that the vision in the left eye was better than the vision in the right eye, the left eye should be tested separately. If the last sentence read before reading starts to slow (CPS) was 1M at a test distance of 40 cm, the result would be recorded as:

Critical print size: 0.4/1M (OS) or "1M at 40 cm"

Acuity: 0.4/ 0.5M (OS) or "0.5M at 40 cm"

Note that acuity, reading performance, and CPS must always include a specification of test distance as well as target size. Because line spacing is logarithmic, if the test distance is changed, then equivalent acuity can be calculated using the formula described above for distance acuity using the ETDRS log chart testing.

One estimates the best near magnification from the MNREAD in units of diopters (see Chapter 5). This is discussed in greater detail in Chapter 14. To estimate, one first must know from the interview what print size a client intends to read—the goal print size (GPS). Then divide the CPS by the GPS. This quotient is then multiplied by 1/d, where d is the test distance in meters, or 100/d if the test distance is in centimeters. If someone is reading at 0.4 meters (40 cm), then 2.5 (1/0.4) diopters of accommodation and spectacle addition is required. To simplify the formula, it is $D = (CPS/GPS)/d$ in meters and $D = (CPS/GPS) * 100/d$ in centimeters. Note that this formula will be used frequently to estimate magnification throughout this book.

Normally people's reading rate does not change as print becomes smaller until CPS is reached. For this reason, it is usually better to err on the side of too much, rather than too little, magnification. If a client reads larger print more slowly, a field restriction or eye movement problem is indicated. In such cases, CPS and estimated magnification should be specified as a range of print sizes that produce maximum reading rate.

The examiner also should carefully observe errors and pauses in reading and to look for patterns that might indicate another visual limitation. These errors contain a wealth of information (see Table 8-7).

Evaluation of Magnification Needs

Practice Setting

May require an electronic viewer; otherwise, appropriate for any practice setting.

Equipment Required

May require an electronic viewer.

Description

For estimation of magnification for purposes other than reading, a direct performance-based approach would have better face-validity. How a person does on an acuity test does not necessarily predict how someone might do watching a TV or seeing his or her knitting. This direct approach estimates magnification by simply magnifying the size of the object or moving it closer until the person identifies some critical detail. For example, a therapist would enlarge a person's sewing on an electronic viewer so an error in stitching can be seen. A limitation of this procedure is that one cannot exactly match the lighting and three-dimensionality for a real task with size enlargement by a picture on an electronic viewer. Another example is to bring a person closer to the object (with optical correction of closer than 50 cm) until it can be seen.

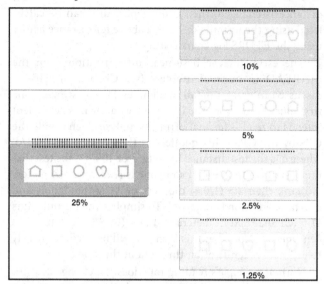

Figure 8-4. LEA Contrast Booklet. (Reprinted with permission from Lea Hyvärinen [www.lea-test.fi].)

Procedure and Interpretation

1. Use optimized lighting (see section on lighting evaluation).

2. For distances less than 1 meter, enlarge a picture of the object(s) being viewed to various sizes. This can be done with a color electronic viewer set to a normal color setting or enlarging color photographs using, for example, a tablet computer, like an iPad.

   a. Present the enlarged images and determine the sizes that would enable performance of the activity at a given test distance. In general, the smaller the magnification, the easier it will be to adapt or use devices.

   b. Select the appropriate enlarged size and divide by the actual size to calculate enlargement ratio (ER). Size can be estimated using any part of the scene as long as it is the same part, such as the size of someone's head, when looking at the same pictures normal and enlarged. One might also put a ruler in the picture.

   c. Divide the ER by distance in meters to calculate equivalent power (EP) of the required magnification device. See Chapter 14 and the occupations sections for selection of appropriate devices of this calculated power.

   d. In a home setting, the therapist might use a hand-held magnifier just to evaluate magnification needs for other devices that are more suitable for the task. One must know for certain the appropriate distance to hold the magnifier (see Chapter 14).

3. For distances greater than 1 meter, bring the person closer to the object (no closer than 1 meter), until the object can be seen. For example, seat a person closer to the TV until he or she reports being able to see the action.

   a. Estimate the equivalent ER or angular magnification (see Chapter 5) by dividing the distance a person wishes to view an object at by the closer distance required for the person to see the object.

   b. The methods in steps 2 and 3 can be combined. One could both enlarge the object directly and move it closer to the client. The combined ER would be calculated by multiplying the enlargement and distance magnification numbers.

4. These methods of estimating magnification may be used for distance devices, like a telescope for viewing a TV, or near devices, such as a magnifier for viewing sewing (see Chapter 14). For example, if a person needs to sit 2 feet away from the TV to see it and would rather sit 4 feet away, then a 2× telescope would give equivalent magnification at 4 feet.

5. Why not just try the optical devices, as is often the current practice? The answer is that an optical device has many characteristics that might affect a person's subjective impression of viewing the object. Devices also significantly restrict a field of view or magnify motion as well as the size of an object. Optical devices can be used, but one must be careful that the devices are perfectly aligned and focused. This is often difficult if a client has a refractive error and cannot use spectacles with the device.

Lighting and Contrast Sensitivity Testing

Practice Setting

Appropriate for any practice setting.

Equipment Required

LEA symbols chart (www.lea-test.fi) (Figure 8-4) or LEA contrast acuity test (Figure 8-5) booklets, stopwatch, task light, and illuminance light meter. The Mars chart has 3 forms with 48 contrast levels and is quite sensitive to small changes in contrast sensitivity. The LEA symbol test has 5 levels of contrast and is considerably less expensive than the acuity chart and MARS chart, but is less versatile.

Description

Contrast sensitivity is the reciprocal of contrast threshold; thus, a decrease in contrast threshold—the lower contrast symbol of a given size that someone can recognize—indicates better contrast sensitivity. For patients with vision impairment, it is important for treatment planning to identify impaired contrast sensitivity because this indicates a need for instruction on glare avoidance, environmental modifications to enhance contrast of steps and tools, an absorptive lens evaluation, and the need to evaluate whether a person can read better with an electronic device that provides higher contrast, white on black letter contrast, or color contrast. Generally, reading performance is the best predictor of the optimum lighting.[25-27] This test is used to validate the lighting findings during reading acuity testing, and it can be quickly performed. Therefore, when performing these tests, it is useful to modify the lighting conditions and determine the effects of these changes. A person must be able to recognize 4M letters or smaller on an acuity chart for these tests to be valid indicators of overall impairment; however, they can be used for a lighting evaluation if acuity is better than 6.3M at the same test distance used for the contrast chart. These tests were chosen because of the relatively quick administration time, portability, and these or similar tests had been validated.[28,29]

Procedure

1. Place the contrast sensitivity test at a distance at which the 4M or smaller letters can be recognized on an acuity chart.

2. Make sure the eyeglasses are clean and appropriate for the test distance.

3. The viewing distance should be selected to ensure that the letters are at least 2 times acuity threshold or more. This is easily done by starting far away and moving the chart closer until the client can barely recognize the darkest symbols. Move the chart half that distance and start testing.

4. Have the client read down the chart until symbols can no longer be recognized. With the Mars chart letter-by-letter scoring may be used. This procedure is described with the instructions that accompany the chart. As with near acuity, this is typically done with binocular viewing, unless a client typically uses one eye only, or if binocular interference is suspected (where binocular contrast sensitivity is worse than the contrast sensitivity of the better eye).

5. Vary the amount of light by varying the distance of the light from the symbol on the chart to determine the range of light levels and type of light that produces the lowest contrast threshold. Note that with light from the side, the symbols closer to the light will have greater illumination. It is best to use a bright enough light source so that it can be positioned far enough away from the chart so that the symbols are uniformly illuminated.

6. Use an illuminometer (digital light meter), which is an inexpensive device that measures light levels in units called *lux*. This allows the therapist to reproduce acceptable light levels accurately under various treatment situations and make appropriate home

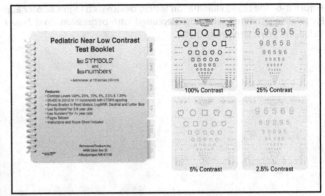

Figure 8-5. LEA contrast acuity test. (Reprinted with permission from Lea Hyvärinen [www.lea-test.fi].)

modifications. If an illuminometer is unavailable, report type of light, luminance, and range of distances that produce the lowest contrast threshold. Because lighting in a home will differ, it is generally better to use a light meter.

7. Although there is little evidence that it makes a difference in performance, one should test lights of different color temperature (warm light, blue light, and natural light) to determine subjective preferences.

8. Once the best type of lighting is determined, the therapist varies the intensity by varying the distance of the light from the material being viewed.

9. Retest with the client wearing light-shaded (about 50% transmittance) yellow-, orange-, gray-, and green-tinted absorptive lenses. Be careful to increase light levels to compensate for reduced light through the absorptive lenses. One can quickly match light level by positioning the lens over the sensor on the light meter and changing light distance until the required illuminance is reached. This will indicate if a tint (spectral filtering) might improve contrast sensitivity.

10. The LuxIQ (Figure 8-6) is a lighting device that is placed over the testing chart. Using 2 sliders and a switch, the practitioner measures the optimum illuminance, color temperature, and hue for contrast sensitivity and high contrast acuity. This can be done in just a few minutes, condensing all of the 9 steps earlier into 3 without any other equipment. With the web app, LightChooser, the clinician can recommend a range of commercially available task lighting options (lamps and bulbs) based directly on the outcome of the LuxIQ's lighting assessment. See www.jasperridge.net for further information. Research is continuing to be performed on the LuxIQ's predictability in real-life situations.

Interpretation

Interpretation of the contrast sensitivity tests is summarized in Table 8-9. In research on reading,[30-32] if text

Figure 8-6. The LuxIQ illumination testing device with LightChooser app for selecting commercial bulbs. (Reprinted with permission from Jasper Ridge. Inc, www.jasperridge.net.)

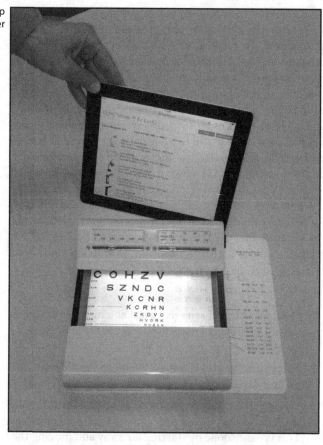

TABLE 8-9: INTERPRETING CONTRAST SENSITIVITY TEST RESULTS

MARS LOG CONTRAST SENSITIVITY SCORE	LEA SYMBOL BOOKLET CONTRAST PER LINE	CONVERSION TO CONTRAST THRESHOLD	INTERPRETATION
0.60 or less	Line 5: 25% contrast	25% or higher: Severe loss in contrast sensitivity	High fluent reading very unlikely even with contrast enhanced and with very careful light control.
0.64 to 1.00	Line 4: 10% contrast	10% to 24%: Moderate/severe loss in contrast sensitivity	Fluent reading unlikely; contrast enhancement and very careful lighting control necessary.
1.04 to 1.28	Line 3: 5% contrast	5% to 9%: Moderate loss in contrast sensitivity	Contrast enhancement (electronic magnification) usually more effective than optical devices. Lighting evaluation indicated.
1.40 to 1.60	Line 2: 2.5% contrast	2.5% to 4%: Mild loss in contrast sensitivity	Increased sensitivity to light intensity level and glare. Contrast enhancement may be more comfortable.
1.64 or greater	Line 1: 1.2% contrast	1.25% to 2.4%: Normal contrast sensitivity	

contrast fell below about 30 times contrast threshold, reading speed dropped, with the most rapid decrease in reading when the letter contrast was less than 10 times contrast threshold. Since objects in the environment vary in contrast from 5% for a carpeted step to about 80% for everyday objects on a contrasting background (see Table 1-3), a conservative estimate of the contrast threshold of 2.5% to 5% or above is generally disabling because even though people can detect most objects in their environment, they do so more slowly, and with some objects or carpeted steps, not at all. This mild level of contrast sensitivity impairment indicates electronic contrast enhancement may be indicated for computers and televisions. If contrast threshold is worse than 5%, one should consider an electronic device that enhances contrast because this will be more effective than optical magnification (see Chapter 15). It also indicates a need for contrast enhancement markings for self-care, homemaking, leisure, and vocational activities. A severe loss (contrast threshold worse than 10%) indicates that fluent reading is unlikely even under optimal visual conditions and the necessity for contrast enhancement and careful lighting control. Use of other senses like tactual techniques and devices for ADLs is indicated as well.

The lighting assessment provides a direct estimate of the optimal range of light intensity and how much changing light will affect visual object recognition. Normally, visual acuity and contrast sensitivity change somewhat up to 1000 lux with the changes in visual function, with low vision being somewhat idiosyncratic.[25-27,33,34] With some who have low vision, optimum vision may only be possible under a much narrower range of light. If a person's vision is relatively stable over a range of about 50 lux (typical room lighting in a house) to 1000 lux (about the brightest indoor lighting one encounters from overhead lights), then a lighting and absorptive lens evaluation is not likely to be necessary unless the client has subjective complaints about lighting. Otherwise, one should dedicate at least one or more sessions to further evaluation and instruction to teach the client how to avoid glare and optimize light (see Chapter 13).

Peripheral Visual Field

Practice Setting

Appropriate for any practice setting.

Equipment Required

The examiner may simply test to see if a client can detect a finger wiggle or count fingers (see Figure 1-12) or use the vision testing wands that turn light-emitting diodes on and off (Figure 8-7) for more precise and reliable measurements (www.guldenophthalmics.com). These are not standardized tests and may be adapted to a setting or client's cognitive status.

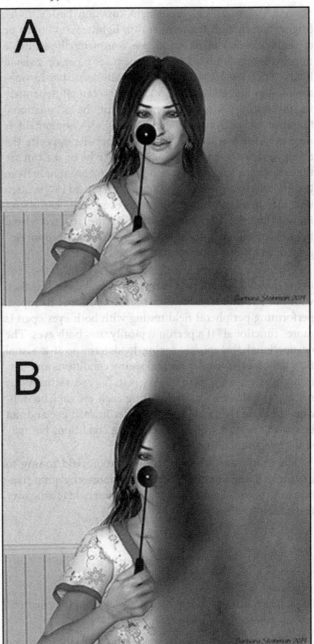

Figure 8-7. (A) Confrontation fields with central sparing. (B) Confrontation fields with a split central field defined with wands. (Reprinted with permission from Barbara Steinman.)

Description

Visual field testing is designed to evaluate an individual's peripheral vision. Visual field loss can be either absolute or relative. An *absolute* field loss has advanced to where a target cannot be seen regardless of target size, contrast, or motion. A *relative* visual field loss, on the other hand, is dependent on the size, brightness, and contrast of the target relative to the environment. This translates functionally into variations of visual field consistency based on environmental conditions. For example, a person with a relative peripheral visual field loss might function better under bright illumination than under dim lighting conditions or at night. Several instruments are commercially available to provide standardized measurements of a person's visual fields. These instruments are generally available in ophthalmology and optometry services, who can bill separately for the testing. A useful alternative for the occupational therapist is confrontation field testing. No equipment is necessary for this testing. The examiner sits opposite the client, and the client has to indicate when he or she can see the examiner's fingers, hands, or any object brought in from the periphery. With acquired brain injury, field loss is often irregular in shape and spotty. Moreover, some can detect motion but not stationary objects in the affected visual field.[35] For this reason, 3 methods are described: count fingers, detect finger motion, and detect a light flash.

When eye doctors assess a client's visual field, the testing is done monocularly, first with the right eye and then with the left eye. However, for the occupational therapist, performing peripheral field testing with both eyes open is more "functional" if a person typically uses both eyes. The occupational therapist is trying to determine if a visual field deficit exists under normal seeing conditions and how it might affect ADL. If the injury is to the eye, retina, optic nerve, or optic chiasm, then testing each eye may be indicated because the field loss may differ in each eye and not be detectable under binocular viewing conditions but may still impact function.

The examiner can adapt confrontation field testing to use more natural testing stimuli and more engaging fixation targets, an advantage of confrontation field testing over instrument testing.

Setup and Procedure

Part 1—Testing for peripheral field loss (field cut)

1. The examiner sits arm's length away from the client, or about 80 cm (32 inches).

2. The examiner's hands should be half the distance between the examiner and the client, or about 40 cm (16 inches).

3. The examiner and the client will see the same thing, except the examiner's right is the client's left.

4. The examiner instructs the client as follows: "Look directly into my eye and tell me if you can see my finger wiggle to the side. Do not look at my fingers, only my eye. Do not look at my hands, only at my eye." The examiner can then observe the patient's compliance with these instructions.

5. Make sure the background is not cluttered. For example, a uniform wall or curtain should be behind the examiner.

6. The examiner positions her or his fingers about 40 cm from the client and then asks the patient to report when he or she sees a finger move. If the patient sees the finger wiggle on both the right and left sides when the fingers are wiggled individually, then wiggle the fingers both at the same time. If, with simultaneous presentation, the client reports seeing only one side even though he or she has vision on both sides, then an inattention or unilateral neglect is indicated. This is called an *extinction procedure.*

7. To screen, the examiner usually tests the client's peripheral vision using 3 positions on the right and 3 positions on the left (ie, presenting the fingers above, at, and below eye level), but often examiners will test more thoroughly on the side of expected vision loss. It is also important to test the client's inferior field, as this area is critical for safe mobility.

8. If the client detects the finger motion, then to test for stationary object detection, present 1, 2, or 3 fingers, then one hand at a time, then both hands until the client counts them reliably. Again, if testing each field reveals intact vision but a person only sees one side when both sides are stimulated, a unilateral inattention or neglect is indicated.

9. If an area of field loss is found, then one reports this finding to the client. Then place the hand in the blind area and move the fingers toward the edge of the blind area until the fingers are first seen. The client will see the arm motion but not the fingers, so attention must be directed to the fingers. Using this dynamic technique, it is important to carefully measure whether the field loss includes central vision. This can be done by moving the fingers toward the face until they are first seen, or asking if facial features on the blind side can be seen. The vision testing wands (see Figure 8-7) were developed to enable an examiner to more accurately measure the extent of the visual field loss and provide a stimulus that is more discrete and can be moved without moving the entire arm for more reliable dynamic testing. The wands also maintain a consistent background to the light.

Interpretation

A visual field loss is indicated if the client is unable to see the target in a particular position on one side. Visual field loss is always described from the point of view of the client and can be drawn using shading and written notes to indicate the area of field loss and stimulus used. Figures 8-7A and 8-7B illustrate what the client sees superimposed on a drawing of the results. If a client is unable to see the target when presented on her or his entire right side, the deficit is called a *right hemianopsia.* The same problem on the left side is called a left hemianopsia. If it is the same for both eyes, it is called a *homonymous hemianopsia.* If the field loss is different from one eye to the other, it is called a *heteronymous hemianopsia*. Using finger testing, the examiner should be able to detect a quadrantopia if a quarter of the visual field is missing. Usually, field loss is smaller than a quarter of the visual field[35] and is difficult to detect using confrontation methods. Likewise, central field involvement significantly affects functions such as reading and object identification because a person does not see part of a word or object. For testing the central field, either the vision testing wands or central field testing methods (discussed later) may be used.

If a person can detect a finger motion or light on one side but the responses are inconsistent, especially when both fields are stimulated at the same time (extinction procedure), then an attention problem or unilateral neglect is indicated (see Chapter 12). When inconsistencies in visual field testing are found, the examiner should be careful that the client is not changing fixation, such as looking toward the expected location of the hand. Also, there may be islands of vision or motion sensitivity.

Assessment of Central Scotoma/ Eccentric Viewing

There are several ways to evaluate central scotoma and eccentric viewing. The complexity, cost of equipment, and accuracy vary dramatically from one technique to another. For example, the most accurate method uses an instrument called the *microperimeter*. Microperimeters allow the examiner to view the patient's retina while testing and the patient is able to see the image of the stimulus when it is presented. The examiner can thus map exactly where scotomas exist and which retinal areas are used for fixation. However, an ophthalmoscopic instrument is expensive and usually only used in large eye clinics. Many private-practice ophthalmologists and optometrists would not have this instrument available. The Amsler grid is inaccurate because people tend to perceptually fill in the area of the scotoma.[36]

Fortunately, less expensive techniques requiring minimal equipment are available. We recommend that the therapist use the clock face technique to start because it is quickly administered and highly informative and then the tangent screen method if someone can maintain steady gaze during a later session.

Clock Face Technique

Practice Setting

Recommended for the home health setting or any setting in which portability is important. Again, the therapist can be creative in adapting this test, using one's face, an object, or chart with discrete symbols, letters, or numbers instead of the clock. The LEA contrast test can be used to detect relative scotomas in which higher contrast targets can be seen but lower contrast targets cannot.

Equipment Required

A clock face is drawn on 8.5-by-11-inch sheet of white/nonglare paper or poster board using a bold-line black marker. Cut a hole in it just above the fixation target so the fixating eye can be viewed at about 40 to 50 cm. This gives you about the same ability to monitor fixation as most microperimeters (1 to 2 degrees accuracy). As mentioned, the clock can be replaced with other stimuli.

Description

As described in Chapter 4, advanced macular degeneration is almost always associated with a macular scotoma or a blind spot in the center of the visual field. This creates a major difficulty for the client when engaged in any ADL requiring vision. Clients with recent loss may tend to look directly at a fixation target, in which case it will disappear. Those who have adapted will use eccentric viewing, looking above, below, or to the side of a fixation target, displacing their central scotoma so the target can be seen using intact peripheral vision.[37-39] See Chapter 11 for further explanation of eccentric viewing. In vision rehabilitation, the therapist will use these tests to teach the client eccentric viewing strategies to improve performance. Therefore, it is important during the evaluation to determine if there is a scotoma and the best position for eccentric viewing.

Setup and Procedure

Wright and Watson[40] describe the following technique used to teach clients how to eccentrically view. We believe that this is also a valuable evaluation tool.

1. Draw a clock (numbers 1 to 12) with a star in the middle on a sheet of paper using a black marker (Figure 8-8[A]). Cut a small peephole in the paper above the star, and view the fixating eye through the peephole.

2. Place the picture of the clock about 40 to 50 cm (16 to 18 inches) away from the client. If you suspect there is a small scotoma, position it farther away.

3. If the client has near eyeglasses, these should be worn for this procedure unless testing is done farther away.

4. Ask the client to look at the clock. If the person has not developed adaptive eccentric viewing, he or she will look directly at the star (centrally fixate) and the scotoma in the center of the visual field obscures the star in the middle of the clock (Figure 8-8[B]). In other words, the star should either be unclear or missing at this point if the person tends to centrally fixate.

5. While the client maintains this position, he or she should see that some of the numbers on the clock are clearer than the star in the middle.

6. Clients who have developed habitual eccentric viewing will tend to move their eye so that the star is most clear. Once the client reports seeing the star, ask if any

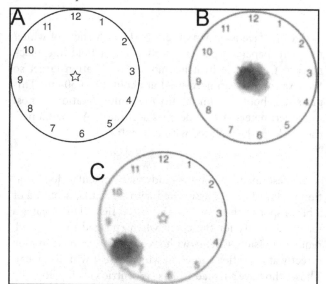

Figure 8-8. (A) Clock face used for evaluation of central scotoma/eccentric viewing. (B) Clock face used for evaluation of central scotoma/eccentric viewing with scotoma covering central star. (C) Clock face used for evaluation of central scotoma/eccentric viewing with central star visible and scotoma down and to left.

numbers disappear. The numbers that disappear indicate the direction of habitual eccentric viewing. If, for example, the 2, 3, and 4 disappear while the star can be seen, then a rightward eccentric viewing is indicated (Figure 8-8[C]). By viewing the eye directly through the peephole, the examiner can see if the client, indeed, is looking to the right. If not, the client might have a paracentral scotoma and intact central vision, a situation not unusual with dry macular degeneration.

7. If it appears the client needs to develop more reliable eccentric viewing or has a maladaptive fixation, then one should try to instruct the client systematically by looking up and toward the right at the number 1 on the clock and continuing clockwise. The difficulty of this step indicates how difficult it may be to teach eccentric viewing if needed.

8. Once an eccentric viewing position is established, if there are still central fixation tendencies, instruct the client to look directly at the star again and notice that it is now blurred or disappears. Then repeat either eye movement as required to regain better clarity.

9. If a patient does not report that the central star or numbers disappear, there might be a relative scotoma or the scotoma might be small or fixation inconsistent. This also is common with atrophic (dry) macular degeneration.

   a. If the patient has unstable fixation, this should be apparent by looking through the peephole.

b. If the patient has a small scotoma, then it should be detected at a longer test distance because of relative distance minification of the target.

c. If the patient has a relative scotoma, it may become more apparent under dim illumination conditions,[41] or lower-contrast numbers could be used.

10. The therapist can adapt this method. Instead of a clock, the examiner could use her or his face and nose as a fixation target and ask if parts of the face are missing or unclear. A chart could be used, and using the first or last letter in a line as a fixation target, ask the client if symbols to the right or left can be seen. If a person has a right eccentric viewing with a relative scotoma, the lower-contrast letters will disappear to the right of the first letter he or she is looking at. This is a good way to check right and left fields of view for reading.

Interpretation

Describe if a scotoma exists, where the client tends to position it relative to the fixation target, and the stability of fixation using direct observation of the eye and reports of what on the clock face disappears.

- If one observes a person consistently looking above a target so the 11, 12, and 1 disappear, then one can conclude that the person already has a central scotoma and uses adaptive eccentric viewing. Eccentric viewing training is not indicated.

- Inconsistent results usually indicate inconsistent fixation and the need for eccentric viewing instruction (see Chapter 11).

- If the star is easily viewed but the 5, 6, or 7 disappears, then the findings indicate a scotoma below fixation can present a safety problem, as clients might miss small obstacles, trip, and fall. Eccentric viewing training is indicated.

- A scotoma to the right of fixation (number 2, 3, or 4 disappears) may impair reading. A scotoma to the left indicates a person might have difficulty finding the next line of text. Further testing should determine if there is a better eccentric viewing position for reading (see Chapter 10), in which case eccentric viewing training is indicated.

- Difficulty following verbal instructions to reposition viewing angle around the clock, for example, indicates more sessions may be needed for eccentric viewing instruction and reliable tangent screen testing.

Tangent Screen

Practice Setting

Recommended for any setting in which the equipment can be set up permanently. In other settings, a laser pointer can be used on a wall with a uniform light color.

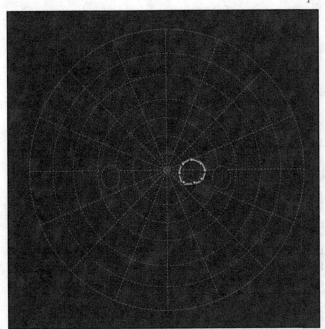

Figure 8-9. Tangent screen (screen only).

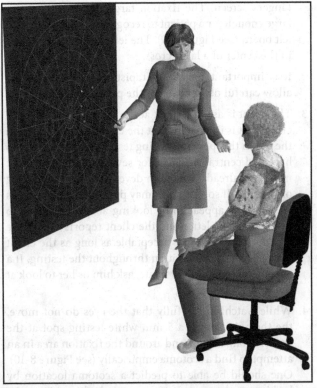

Figure 8-10. Tangent screen showing therapist holding the target, client viewing the screen, and 4 pins showing size of scotoma, which is to the right of fixation. (Reprinted with permission from Barbara Steinman.)

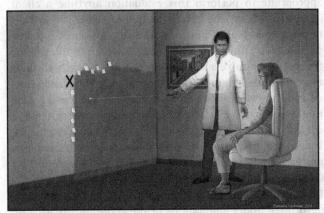

Figure 8-11. Laser on wall with sticky notes used to draw fixation target and to define a quadrantopia with central vision involvement. The client is sitting about 2 meters (6 feet) away from the wall. The blind area is indicated by light gray. The examiner is carefully observing the client's fixation while moving the target from a nonseeing to seeing area. (Reprinted with permission from Barbara Steinman.)

Equipment Required

Tangent screen, laser pointer, and small sticky notes (Figures 8-9, 8-10, and 8-11).

Description

The tangent screen method is less convenient and takes more practice for the therapist to become skilled, but is more sensitive to small scotomas that could be missed with the clock face technique and actually permits the scotoma to be measured.[42] Eye care providers use the tangent screen to evaluate the central visual field of patients. It is a black piece of felt with a white fixation target mounted on a wall (see Figure 8-9). The screen usually has circles of black

thread stitched into it to indicate the degrees from the center of the fixation target (see Figure 8-10). If a wall is used, one can use sticky notes for a fixation target and mark the edge of the scotoma (see Figure 8-11). The size of the scotoma or field loss can be measured and converted to degrees using the inverse tangent function on a calculator to convert scotoma size divided by distance into degrees. This procedure is also used to measure central field involvement or central field sparing in cases of peripheral field loss from stroke or paracentral scotomas from optic nerve damage, encephalopathy and anoxia, or traumatic brain injury. The laser pointer technique has the advantage over the traditional black tangent screen of extending testing well into a person's periphery and can be used in functional activity and natural environments.

In cases of central scotomas, the procedure we suggest combines testing for scotomas with instruction so that scotoma awareness and eccentric viewing training are combined. This procedure is discussed in more detail in Chapter 10. The results of tangent screen testing are useful diagnostically and indicate how to begin eccentric viewing training.

Procedure

1. The tangent screen method involves first positioning the fixation target in the center of a 1-meter-square

tangent screen. The fixation target is usually a letter large enough for a patient to recognize in the center of a felt board (see Figure 8-9). The letter also is positioned in the center of a large cross.

2. It is important for the therapist to be positioned to allow careful observation of the patient's eyes.

3. The client is asked to look at the letter so that it is the clearest. It is important that the client continue to hold the eye in this position during testing. Individuals who have had central field loss for several months or more may have already started to develop eccentric viewing or fixation. If so, the client may position his or her eyes so that they appear to be looking above, below, or to one side of the letter and the client reports seeing the letter. This behavior is acceptable as long as the client maintains this eye position throughout the testing. If a client tends to centrally fixate, ask him or her to look at the center of the cross.

4. While watching carefully that the eyes do not move, the therapist moves a 5-mm white testing spot at the end of a long black wand around the fixation area in an attempt to find a scotoma empirically (see Figure 8-10). One should be able to predict a scotoma location by looking at the eyes. If a person is looking right, the scotoma should be to the right of fixation from the patient's point of view.

5. When the white spot enters the scotoma, the client will report that it disappears. When this occurs, the therapist explains to the client that the scotoma has been found and its size will now be measured.

6. To measure the size of the scotoma, the white target is moved until it is first seen, and the edge of the scotoma is marked with a low-contrast mark or pin (not visible to the client), then quickly moved from a nonseeing area to seeing area and the border of the scotoma is marked several times.

7. Some clients may shift fixation (eg, from looking above to looking below the fixation letter). The therapist can detect these shifts by looking at the eyes and noting inconsistency in where the target is seen. It is important to instruct the client to try not to shift the position of his or her eyes.

8. When the scotoma is mapped, the edges are more clearly marked with white yarn wrapped around the pushpins in the felt board. The patient is instructed to move his or her eyes to see the outlined scotoma.

9. The therapist may instruct the client to look into different positions and with another letter or the wand, demonstrate where the scotoma has moved. This is a training procedure (see Chapter 11).

10. The client may be coaxed with verbal instructions ("look farther to the right"). Sometimes, one needs to give the client a target to look toward, such as waving one's hand above the client's head, to encourage upward eccentric viewing.

11. If one is evaluating central field involvement with a peripheral field defect from a stroke or resulting from brain injury, fixation is usually stable and central. A small target should be used for fixation.

12. If responses are not reliable, watch the eyes carefully for inconsistent fixation and flash the light in various positions in and out of the blind areas, being careful not to be predictable.

Interpretation

The results should be drawn from the point of view of the client, indicating the location of the fixation target. If fixation is not reliable, then results will not be reliable, and eccentric viewing training is indicated.

Absorptive Lens (Sunlens) Evaluation

The lighting and contrast evaluation will indicate the need for a evaluation of absorptive lenses; however, it is appropriate to perform this evaluation anytime a client complains about excessive light (photophobia), regardless of other test results. Someone who is glare sensitive when outside on a sunny or snowy day, driving into the sun, or trying to recognize a familiar person in a brightly lit fluorescent dining hall must try to optimize lighting using tinted sunglasses or sunlenses called "absorptive lenses." One might also use the selected high-transmittance sunlens to cut glare during reading or with an electronic viewer (EV). Indeed, because glare from the table is blocked, sunlenses are preferred to color contrast for EV use. An important component of the occupational therapy evaluation, therefore, involves having the client try on and select sunlenses absorptive under simulations of the conditions that cause problems, although for outdoor use, actually going outdoors is strongly recommended if possible. The general approach to a sunlens evaluation involves trial and error. The "getting started" evaluation equipment for a therapist should include an assortment of wrap-around style sunglasses (Figure 8-12) to demonstrate (see Chapter 16). If absorptive lenses are evaluated as part of the lighting and contrast sensitivity testing, the examiner can predict which tints are likely to be effective. The absorptive lens evaluation is time consuming and will require about 30 minutes in a separate session.

The absorptive lens evaluation involves selecting the style, density (light transmission), and color of the absorptive lens. In general, the best style of absorptive lens wraps tightly above and around the eyes (www.noir-medical.com) to block glare and reflections around the lenses. Relatively inexpensive or more stylish models can be purchased to fit over conventional eyeglasses. With standard commercial sunglasses, this glare can be also blocked with a hat brim or visor, but not as effective.

The density of the absorptive lens describes the amount of light transmitted through the lens, usually described as a light transmittance percentage, where 100% is clear and 0% is completely opaque. Typically, the lightest absorptive lens have transmittance values of 50% to 60%; very dense absorptive lens have transmittance values of approximately 5% to 10%. Absorptive lens also vary in color. Most clients will respond best to yellow or orange absorptive lens that decrease glare or color-neutral lenses (Polarized Gray). Some, however, prefer green hues, and occasionally red and blue. Colored lenses will degrade color vision, but the yellow and light orange hues will improve perceived contrast and decrease glare. Generally, clients will require lighter lenses for indoor use in brightly lit stores like supermarkets or on cloudy days and darker lenses for outdoor use. An indoor site for sunlens evaluation should be about 1000 lux, typical of a brightly lit store or clinic. For an outdoor evaluation, one must wait for a sunny day and evaluate the lens by having the client attempt to identify an object or person next to a glare source, such as reflections off of a car or facing the sun.

Procedure and Interpretation

1. The lenses should be grouped so that those of similar transmittance are together.

2. To save time, the lighting evaluation should reveal the approximate lens density required. The LuxIQ can be used to predict the preferred hue. If a light meter is used, one can hold the meter behind the lens to quickly locate those lenses that will provide the best light levels in a given environment. Use gray absorptive lenses first and then compare colors at the selected transmittance values.

3. The lenses are compared in pairs. The client is asked to look toward a glare source and choose which is better. If the client indicates no preference, then choose gray.

4. In a given setting, one first uses the gray filter and finds the preferred density and allows the client to adapt to the lens for a few minutes, then compares the preferred density with colored lenses of comparable density, using the preferred color for comparison with the next color. Make sure to have the client close his or her eyes while changing lenses so as not to be dazzled by a sudden increase in light.

5. Once a preferred density and color are chosen, the absorptive lenses should be compared to the client's own sunglasses.

Oculomotor Screening

Practice Setting

A screening can be performed in any setting. Because specialized skills and equipment are involved, a functional oculomotor assessment should be performed by an optometrist with appropriate specialization.

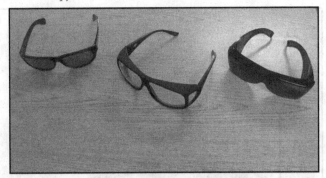

Figure 8-12. Three different shades and styles of fit-over absorptive sunlenses.

Equipment Required

The vision testing wands (see Figure 8-7) or a small LED light in a fixation target, eye occlude, and red/green glasses.

Description

This screening will allow the examiner to see limitations in eye movement and detect strabismus (eye misalignment) with a resulting double vision. Many oculomotor problems are difficult to observe and manifest as subjective complaints of headaches or eye strain that can only be diagnosed by an optometrist with specialization in neurological disorders (and often pediatrics as well). Oculomotor problems can impact treatment and outcomes of clients with "low vision." For example, common age-related changes in oculomotor function include loss in elevation of gaze (the ability to look up) and abduction defects that result in double vision when looking to the side.[43,44] These changes might impact a person's ability to compensate for a central or peripheral field loss with compensatory scanning. Brain injury often results in difficulty maintaining eye alignment in the primary gaze or in certain directions. A person may have normal convergence of the eyes when looking straight ahead or downward to read, but when looking right or left, may have a misalignment of the eyes. In younger clients, optical magnifiers put a strain on accommodation because if a magnifier is slightly out of focus, the client will unconsciously attempt to refocus the eyes rather than adjust the magnifier, with a resulting eye strain. If these complaints persist even if the magnifier is properly positioned (see Chapter 13), then a referral is indicated. The best rule of thumb is to refer patients who complain of discomfort and headaches relating to vision, as well as double vision or obvious convergence problems. Note also that double vision may not be consistent and may come and go. These types of vision problems, brain injury–related vision and perceptual problems, and interventions for occupational therapists are described in the third edition of *Understanding and Managing Vision Deficits* by Mitchell Scheiman.[45]

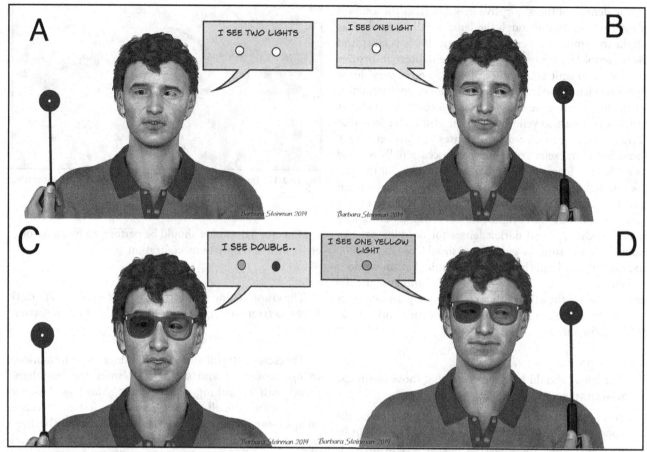

Figure 8-13. Test results with a right lateral rectus paresis. Normal viewing conditions: (A) diplopia response, (B) fusion response. Red-Glass Test: (C) diplopia response, (D) fusion response. (Reprinted with permission from Barbara Steinman.)

Procedure and Interpretation

The red-green glass test can be used to screen for strabismus and other binocular vision disorders (eye misalignment). The oculomotor screening begins without red/green glasses and can be used as a screening for strabismus and convergence. If double vision is present during this part of the test, it will likely be present under natural viewing conditions.

1. Versions (gross assessment of eye alignment)

    a. Hold a small light in front of the client and make sure the client is looking toward a distraction-free, uncluttered background, like a plain wall.

    b. Move the light right and left and then up and down while gently placing the hand on the client's forehead to prevent head movement so the eyes move as far as they can in each direction. Look carefully at both eyes to see if they are moving together and if a nystagmus (eye shaking) is present. A nystagmus often occurs as a result of traumatic brain injury or any brainstem damage. A nystagmus when the eyes are moving as far as possible in one direction

sometimes indicates a limitation in eye movement as well and will generally reduce visual acuity.

2. Convergence screening

    a. To screen for a convergence problem, bring the target toward the client along the midline to the nose. Instruct the client to keep the target single for as long as possible. When the limit of convergence is reached, the client may report double vision and/or you may see one eye drift outward. This is referred to as the "break," and you should record this measurement. If the break occurs at a distance greater than 4 inches (10 cm), this is considered abnormal.[45]

3. Red-green glasses test (Figure 8-13)

    a. While the client wears red-green glasses, hold a penlight in front of the eyes at about 50 cm (18 inches). If the eyes are aligned, the client should report seeing one light; it should appear either yellow or a reddish yellow with some green in it. This indicates fusion—the eyes are working together. One problem is suppression, where the brain shuts down or suppresses one eye; suppression will mimic fusion. If this happens, one light will appear red or green depending on which eye is suppressed. For example, if the left eye with the green filter is suppressed, the light seen by the right eye will appear dark red and will not change if the left eye is covered and uncovered.

b. If the client reports double vision, the eyes are misaligned.

c. Move the light right and left and then up and down while gently placing the hand on the client's forehead to prevent head movement so the eyes move as far as they can in each direction. Ask the client to report if she or he sees double vision in any position of gaze and record this. Also ask if the separation between the 2 lights appears to become greater or smaller as the light is moved from one position to another.

   i. If the separation between the lights varies based on eye position, a cranial nerve palsy is likely to be present.

   ii. Look carefully at both eyes to see if they are moving together and if a nystagmus (eye shaking) is present. (Note on a plot of the visual field from the point of view of the patient where double vision is reported and at what distance.)

d. If double vision is a problem, a first-response intervention is to occlude one eye. In infants, occlusion can cause permanent vision loss, but not in adults. Since occlusion does affect far peripheral field of view, it should be avoided during mobility and used only when the client finds double vision bothersome.

Reading Assessment/Reading Speed

Practice Setting

Appropriate for any practice setting.

Equipment Required

The Pepper Visual Skills for Reading Test (Pepper VSRT) is recommended. Alternatively, the SKREAD test is more quickly administered and informative about reading with different print sizes. The Pepper test has exceptional test-retest reliability and sensitivity to change in performance in clients who have a reading level of ninth grade or higher. Another alternative is the Morgan Low Vision Reading Comprehension Test (LVRCA).[46] These tests have been validated for use with people who have central scotomas and are quite useful for evaluating peripheral field loss with central involvement and reading in people with visual/spatial neglect (see Chapter 12).

Form III

Line		# correct / # item	percent correct
1	x g a j p m u l c d s b r h o	____/15	____%
2	f w z i t b k e n q v y a m r	____/15	____%
3	yes so j pop sat d at c am h in so	____/12	dummy
4	oh of n to am g k in u do of s b	____/13	____%
5	fire side past gold fish own sky help	____/8	____%
6	advice badger slide anyone table mirror	____/6	____%
7	understudy sportsman campground fenders	____/4	____%
8	bad z navy specific g show dog amber	____/8	dummy
9	narrow today penny cream hopped honest	____/6	____%
10	meantime upbringing summertime splendid	____/4	____%
11	quick sand spiteful outlast stops winds	____/6	____%
12	side walk tracking readily overshadow employ	____/6	____%
13	story milk bunny college crayons idea gotten	____/7	dummy

- Total Number Correct (add lines 1-13)= ________
- Mean Percent Correct (sum of percentages/10)= ________ %
- Total Test Time= ______ min ______ sec (Time in Minutes)= ________
- Corrected Reading Rate = Total # Correct/Total Time (in min)= ________

-Error Codes-

Misidentification	substitution written above item	e.g. gust (guest)
Repetition	wavy line placed below item repeated	e.g. red
Spells Word	"sp" placed above word item spelled	e.g. hot (sp)
Omission	circle item omitted	e.g. (to)
Insertion	caret placed where insertion occurs	e.g. f at (of)
Connects Words	line underneath indicating connection	e.g. fear less
Separates Words	slash indicating separation	e.g. eye/sight
Changing Word Order	arrow to where item was read	e.g. p g a
Line Skip	arrow to skipped line →	
Test Termination	1. 10 consecutive errors; 2. skipped line twice	3. fatigue of reader; 4. exceeded time limit

Figure 8-14. Scoring sheet for the Pepper Visual Skills for Reading Test.

Description

The Pepper VSRT is a test in which clients read unrelated words aloud (Figure 8-14). The examiner records reading rate and the occurrence and type of errors. In addition, many compound words are used, so readers may miss either the beginning or end of the words. This would lead to certain error patterns. The examiner can make inferences about the effects of central field loss on reading based on error patterns. For example, a tendency to omit the end of words indicates a scotoma or field loss to the right of fixation in the central field.

The Pepper VSRT engages the client in reading processes that depend either solely or in part on visual sources of information, including word recognition ability, saccade control, return-sweep eye movement control, and scotoma placement while reading.[47] Word recognition ability is required because unrelated letters and words are presented. The absence of contextual information forces clients to rely on vision to identify the items presented. The test becomes increasingly more difficult from top to bottom because line delineation and spacing, word length, and word spacing change as the client reads successive lines. Both saccadic and return-sweep eye movements are also increasingly more difficult because of systematic decreases in either spacing between successive items on a single line or the spacing between successive lines.

The Morgan LVRCA would be particularly valuable as a validated reading comprehension test for treatments of right field loss, which can have a component of alexia (acquired linguistic reading disability). Unfortunately, as of this writing, the test was not commercially available. Another alternative would be the Gray Oral Reading Series (GORT),[48,49] although the reading passages would need to be modified in size for low vision.

Setup and Procedure

1. The examiner should select the appropriate test size based on the reader's acuity. The appropriate VSRT size is at least one size larger print than the reader's acuity. The authors recommend using CPS for best performance.

2. If 4M is not large enough, the reader may use a magnification device. Indeed, this test is usually used to evaluate magnification devices or the effectiveness of a training procedure, which is performed after a magnification device is prescribed. The smaller print sizes are usually used.

3. The client can be encouraged during the test, but feedback about accuracy is not permitted. The examiner must be careful not to provide feedback by tone of voice or types of encouragement. If a reader asks about the correctness of an answer or how she or he is doing on the test, the examiner should give an ambiguous, noncommittal response, such as, "You are doing a fine job, keep going."

4. The reader should be handed the appropriate test, provided the best illumination indicated by the lighting evaluation, and instructed to call out the letters and words aloud. If the reader is using a low vision device, ensure that he or she knows the correct focal distance before administering the VSRT. If necessary, the examiner should point out the beginning of the first line as a localization clue.

5. The test has a coding scheme for recording errors.

6. Readers should be encouraged to guess test items if they are not immediately recognizable.

7. Other details regarding the examination procedure are included with the test.

8. The VSRT should be administered in one sitting. There is a maximum time limit. If the reader is tired or for any other reason unable to finish the test, the examiner should decide whether to readminister the test at another time (because of extenuating circumstances) or score the remainder of the test as errors and count

the administration as the pretest, indicative of the reader's best performance at the time.

9. As soon as the reader pronounces the last word on the test or the test is terminated, the timing of the test is completed.

Interpretation

At the end of the scoring, the examiner should have a profile of the reader's performance that contains the following:

- Accuracy of performance (mean percent correct across lines)
- Reading rate (correctly read words/minute)
- Line mastery for word length or line spacing

A change in reading rate of about 10 words per minute is statistically significant. Four forms of the test are available to enable repeated testing. This test has been used, therefore, to document improvement in performance with therapy or to provide justification for the effectiveness of reading devices using an objective measure of performance.

An evaluation of both the accuracy and rating scores for the reader can provide the clinician with information to make a preliminary categorization of the reader's performance. Typically, low vision readers will be reading as follows:

- Inaccurately and very slowly
- Accurately but slowly
- Accurately with increasing reading rate

The VSRT suggests guidelines that may aid the low vision therapist in making these categorizations. Observations of the VSRT performance of individuals with macular disease suggest that accuracy scores below 75% correct may be indicative of inaccurate performance and rate scores below 20 words/minute may be considered very slow performance.

The VSRT scoring manual also has an extensive discussion of interpretation and analysis of common reading errors, line mastery issues, problems with word length, symbol spacing, omissions, insertions, repetitions, jumping or changing word order, and a variety of other important issues. Although not yet validated by research involving eye movement measurement while people are reading with the test, these errors are likely indicative of maladaptive scanning patterns ("visual skills") during reading.

Putting It All Together

An important part of a visual evaluation strategy is to cross-check visual findings among different tests with the patient complaints and the diagnosis. If the recommended tests are used (Sidebar 8-1) and procedures followed, the results should be internally consistent because the visual evaluation protocol is based on validated tests and well-established principles of optics and visual psychophysics. The examiner should ardently pursue discrepancies in

SIDEBAR 8-1: RESOURCES FOR EQUIPMENT

EQUIPMENT	COMPANY	CONTACT INFORMATION
LEA Charts	Goodlite Richmond Products	www.goodlite.com www.richmondproducts.com
MNREAD Test SKREAD Test	Precision Vision Optelec	www.precision-vision.com www.shoplowvision.com
Tangent screen	Bernell Corporation	800-348-2225 www.bernell.com
Pepper Test	Low Vision Simulators	www.lowvisionsimulators.com
Low Vision Independence Measure (LVIM)	Public domain	www.routledge.com/9781617116339
Veterans Affairs Low-Vision Visual Functioning Questionnaire (VA LV VFQ-48, and VFQ-24)	Public domain	www.routledge.com/9781617116339
Geriatric Depression Scale (GDS)	Public domain	https://web.stanford.edu/~yesavage/GDS.html

findings in search of an explanation. Consistently missed letters at the end of words in the error patterns during reading but not field testing is an example of a discrepancy and might indicate that tangent screen testing missed a small scotoma. If, when near reading acuity is converted to distance-equivalent letter acuity, the actual letter acuity at distance is found to be much better, the explanation might be an incorrect working distance for the near correction during near testing. Differences might also be due to a cognitive problem, such as inattention, alexia, fatigue, frustration, or malingering, all of which are important to consider in the treatment plan. The explanations for these differences are often the most important findings of a functional low vision rehabilitation evaluation. The ability to recognize these discrepancies comes with experience and a thoughtful examination.

ENVIRONMENTAL EVALUATION

Even a well-developed treatment plan will fail unless the therapist considers the location where the client will habitually perform the goal performance in question. For example, a client may successfully perform a task in an office setting using an optical device while sitting at a desk with a task light and a reading stand. However, when the client takes the prescribed device home and sits in his or her favorite chair with inadequate lighting, poor support for materials, and disabling glare, he or she may be unable to perform the identical task. Fortunately, outpatient low vision rehabilitation is a covered service under Medicare B and occupational therapists can provide these services in the client's home. This allows the therapist to evaluate the client's environment.

As individuals age, they often tend to perform tasks in the same place—for example, bill paying is performed on the dining room table. The client knits and reads in the stuffed chair in the living room. Indeed, as people age, the space within which they perform most activities decreases to a favorite chair, referred to as the "personal surveillance zone."[50] This is a sacred place. Individuals resist moving from this place or changing the layout of the space. An environmental assessment, therefore, should focus on the preferred living spaces and seating. This topic is covered in Chapter 13. In general, careful consideration should be given to the following:

- The available lighting and glare sources
- Possible positioning of task lights, reading stands, and tables
- Possible organizational schemes
- Placement and storage of devices
- Ergonomics when performing a task
- Escape and emergency response

ASSESSMENT OF REHABILITATION POTENTIAL

As the therapist performs the evaluation described in this chapter, he or she is not simply gathering bits of unrelated information to be analyzed at the end of the evaluation. Rather, during the evaluation process, the therapist is already thinking about how this information relates to rehabilitation potential and the actual treatment plan.

Experienced clinicians tend to follow a basic clinical reasoning process, which we have outlined here.

To determine rehabilitation potential, the basic reasoning process is as follows:

1. Define the specific performance goal.

2. Look first to evidence-based research and then to clinical experience to ascertain if the visual and nonvisual requirements to perform the goal task are being met.

3. Consider visual performance of the task and ascertain if the visual, movement, and cognitive requirements can be met by available devices or interventions to enhance vision.

4. Consider nonvisual performance of the task and ascertain if other modalities, movement, and cognitive requirements can be met by available devices or interventions. Determine if there is a simpler way to perform the task.

5. Evaluate and document the pre- and postmorbid specific performance deficits or disability.

One must be careful to consider visual and nonvisual options and keep the focus on what the client requires to recover roles, essential function, and quality of life, rather than just visual criteria. For example, arranging for a sighted reader or recorded books for someone who wishes to read again is a successful rehabilitation outcome even if the client is still unable to read fluently and comfortably enough with vision to enjoy a book. Too often, a clinician may be so focused on the visual aspects of the task and visual solutions that he or she ignores a much simpler nonvisual adaptation or solution.

After completing the evaluation, the therapist must make a decision about the client's rehabilitation potential. The information gathered from all 4 components of the evaluation should be used to make this decision. Ultimately, almost any client with low vision has the potential for improving his or her ability to more effectively engage in ADL. To determine rehabilitation potential, however, the therapist must first define the specific performance goal and then follow the other 4 steps listed earlier.

DETERMINING THE PRIMARY DIAGNOSIS

After determining that the client has the potential to benefit from vision rehabilitation, the therapist must determine the primary diagnostic code that will be used for billing Medicare. Medicare considers low vision rehabilitation services reasonable and necessary only for clients with a clear medical need. To establish this need, clients must have a moderate visual impairment of 6/24 (20/80) or worse that is not correctable by conventional eyeglasses and clients

must have a clear potential for significant improvement in function following rehabilitation over a reasonable period of time.

Please note that the primary diagnosis is not the eye disease that caused the vision loss. The occupational therapist does not treat macular degeneration or diabetic retinopathy. Rather, it is the visual disability that is treated. At this writing, coding for low vision was undergoing a substantial change from ICD-9 codes, where vision impairment was coded with a complex system based on visual acuity. These can be found on the Centers for Medicare/Medicaid Services (CMS) website (www.cms.gov). The ICD-10 codes indicated in parentheses and the coding were in proposal form when this book was written.

Four other codes that can be used to relate visual field loss include:

- 368.41 (H53-419)—Visual field defects, scotoma involving the central area

- 368.45 (H53.489)—Visual field defects, generalized contraction or constriction

- 368.46 (H53.469)—Homonymous bilateral field defects

- 368.47—(H53.47) Heteronymous bilateral field defects

The ICD-10 codes for acuity loss simplify coding to 3 categories:

- H540—Total blindness in both eyes

- H5410—Total blindness in one eye, low vision (less than 20/60 acuity) in the other eye

- H542—Low vision in both eyes

Acuity testing used to determine ICD-9 codes can be biased toward lower scores by not allowing adaptive eccentric fixation. Moreover, one letter missed on the 20/60 (6/18) can be considered equivalent to 20/80 acuity, the minimum requirements for reimbursable services. In some cases, visual acuity may still be better than 20/80 equivalent but field loss may be present, and in this case, the field loss codes apply. The secondary code is determined based on information received from either the ophthalmologist or optometrist. In cases where the vision loss is due to acquired brain injury or neurologic disease, the payer will accept a brain injury diagnosis for stroke, multiple sclerosis, or traumatic brain injury, for example. Acceptable rehabilitation codes are frequently updated and posted on www.cms.gov by CMS, which sets the standard for private insurers.

SUMMARY

The objective of the occupational therapy low vision rehabilitation evaluation is to understand the client's functional ability before the vision loss, to define his or her current goals, to evaluate the client's ability to participate in ADL, and to assess his or her social and emotional health.

In this chapter, we described an evaluation consisting of 3 components, including the occupational profile/case history, the evaluation of visual factors, and the evaluation occupational performance.

REFERENCES

1. Amini DA, Kannenberg K, Bodison S, et al. Occupational Therapy Practice Framework: Domain & Process, 3rd Edition. *Am J Occup Ther.* 2014;S1-s48.

2. American Occupational Therapy Association. Occupational Therapy Practice Framework: Domain & Process. *Am J Occup Ther* 2002;56:609-639.

3. Smith TM. Refinement of the Low Vision Independence Measure: a qualitative study. *Phys Occup Ther Geriatr.* 2013;31:182-196.

4. McColl MA, Paterson M, Davies D, Doubt L, Law M. Validity and community utility of the Canadian Occupational Performance Measure. *Can J Occup Ther.* 2000;67:22-30.

5. Haymes SA, Johnston AW, Heyes AD. A weighted version of the Melbourne Low-Vision ADL Index: a measure of disability impact. *Optom Vis Sci.* 2001;78:565-579.

6. Watson GR, Whittaker SG, Steciw M. Pepper Visual Skills for Reading Test (revised). Lilburn, GA: Bear Consultants, Inc; 1995.

7. Watson GR, Baldasare J, Whittaker SG. The validity and clinical uses of the Pepper Visual Skills for Reading Test. *J Vis Impairment Blindness.* 1990;84:119-123.

8. Warren ML, Lampert J. Assessing daily living needs. In: Fletcher DC, ed. *Ophthalmology Monographs: Low Vision Rehabilitation: Caring for the Whole Person.* San Francisco: American Academy of Ophthalmology; 1999:89-125.

9. Stelmack JA, Stelmack TR, Massof RW. Measuring low-vision rehabilitation outcomes with the NEI VFQ-25. *Invest Ophthalmol Vis Sci.* 2002;43:2859-2868.

10. Stelmack JA, Massof RW. Using the VA LV VFQ-48 and LV VFQ-20 in low vision rehabilitation. *Optom Vis Sci.* 2007;84:705-709.

11. Velozo CA, Warren M, Hicks E, Berger KA. Generating clinical outputs for self-reports of visual functioning. *Optom Vis Sci.* 2013;90:765-775.

12. Cotter SA, Scharre JE. Optometric assessment: case history. In: Scheiman M, Rouse M, eds. *Optometric Management of Learning Related Vision Problems.* St. Louis, MO: C.V. Mosby; 1994.

13. Korsch BM, Negrete VF. Doctor-patient communication. *Sci Am.* 1972;227:66-74.

14. Sokol-McKay DA. Facing the challenge of macula degeneration: therapeutic interventions for low vision. *OT Pract.* 2005;10:10-15.

15. Freeman P, Mendelson R. *Believing Is Seeing: Hope for Those Victimized by Macular Degeneration and Other Conditions that Cause Low Vision.* Pittsburgh, PA: Freeman and Mendelson; 1996.

16. Graboyes M. Psychosocial implications of visual impairment. In: Brilliant RL, ed. *Essentials of Low Vision Practice.* Boston, MA: Butterworth-Heinemann; 1999:12-17.

17. Whittaker SG, Lovie-Kitchin JE. Visual requirements for reading. *Optom Vis Sci.* 1993;70:54-65.

18. Bailey IL, Lovie JE. New design principles for visual acuity letter charts. *Am J Optom Physiol Opt.* 1976;53:740-745.

19. Kiser AK, Mladenovich D, Eshraghi F, Bourdeau D, Dagnelie G. Reliability and consistency of visual acuity and contrast sensitivity measures in advanced eye disease. *Optom Vis Sci.* 2005;82:946-954.

20. Hardgrave N, Hatley J, Lewerenz D. Comparing LEA numbers low vision book and Feinbloom visual acuity charts. *Optom Vis Sci.* 2012;89:1611-1618.

21. Freeman PB, Jose RT. *The Art and Practice of Low Vision.* 2nd ed. Boston: Butterworth-Heinemann; 1997.

22. Brilliant R, ed. *Essentials of Low Vision Practice.* Boston: Butterworth Heinemann; 1999:409.

23. Young D. Light the way. Providing effective home modifications for clients with low vision. *OT Pract.* 2012;17:7-12.

24. Hegde AL, Rhodes R. Assessment of lighting in independent living facilities and residents' perceptions. *J Appl Gerontol.* 2010;29:381-390.

25. Fosse P, Valberg A. Lighting needs and lighting comfort during reading with age-related macular degeneration. *J Vis Impairment Blindness.* 2004;98:389-409.

26. Fosse P, Valberg A, Arnljot HM. Retinal illuminance and the dissociation of letter and grating acuity in age-related macular degeneration. *Optom Vis Sci.* 2001;78:162-168.

27. Fosse P, Valberg A. Contrast sensitivity and reading in subjects with age-related macular degeneration. *Vis Impairment Res.* 2001;3:111-124.

28. Mercer ME, Drover JR, Penney KJ, Courage ML, Adams RJ. Comparison of Patti Pics and LEA Symbols optotypes in children and adults. *Optom Vis Sci.* 2013;90:236-241.

29. Ah-Kine Ng Poon Hing D, Vaidhyan JJ, Pathak A, et al. Comparison of visual acuity measured with LEA symbols and LEA numbers at different test distances. *IOVS.* 2007;48:arve.

30. Crossland MD, Rubin GS. Text accessibility by people with reduced contrast sensitivity. *Optom Vis Sci.* 2012;89:1276-1281.

31. Whittaker SG, Lovie-Kitchin JE. The assessment of contrast sensitivity and contrast reserve for reading rehabilitation. In: Kooijman AC, Looijestijn PL, Welling JA, VanDerWildt GJ, eds. *Low Vision: Research and New Development in Rehabilitation.* Amsterdam: IOS Press; 1994:88-92.

32. Whittaker SG, Lovie-Kitchin J. Visual requirements for reading. *Optom Vis Sci.* 1993;70:54-65.

33. Boyce PR, Sanford LJ. Lighting to enhance visual capabilities. In: Silverstone B, Lang MA, Rosenthal BP, Faye EE, eds. *The Lighthouse Handbook on Vision Impairment and Vision Rehabilitation.* Oxford: Oxford University Press; 2000:617-636.

34. Committee on Recommendations for Quality and Quantity of Illumination of the IES (RQQ). Selection of illuminance values for interior lighting design (RQQ report no. 6). *J IES.* 1958;188-190.

35. Trobe JD. *The Neurology of Vision.* Oxford: Oxford University Press; 2001:451.

36. Schuchard RA. Validity and interpretation of Amsler grid reports. *Arch Ophthalmol.* 1993;111:776-780.

37. Fornos AP, Sommerhalder J, Rappaz B, Pelizzone M, Safran AB. Processes involved in oculomotor adaptation to eccentric reading. *Invest Ophthalmol Vis Sci.* 2006;47:1439-1447.

38. Nilsson UL, Frennesson C, Nilsson SEG. Patients with AMD and a large absolute central scotoma can be trained successfully to use eccentric viewing, as demonstrated in a scanning laser ophthalmoscope. *Vis Res.* 2003;43:1777-1787.

39. Whittaker SG, Budd J, Cummings RW. Eccentric fixation with macular scotoma. *Invest Ophthalmol Vis Sci.* 1988;29:268-278.

40. Wright V, Watson GR. *Learn to Use Your Vision for Reading Workbook.* Madison, WI: www.lowvisionsimulators.com; 1995.

41. Lei H, Schuchard RA. Using two preferred retinal loci for different lighting conditions in patients with central scotomas. *Invest Ophthalmol Vis Sci.* 1997;38:1812-1818.

42. Greer R. Evaluation methods and functional implications: children and adults with visual impairments. In: Lueck AH, ed. *Functional Vision: A Practitioner's Guide to Evaluation and Intervention.* New York: American Foundation for the Blind; 2004.

43. Clark RA, Isenberg SJ. The range of ocular movements decreases with aging. *J AAPOS.* 2001;5:26-30.

44. Shechtman D, Shallo-Hoffmann J, Rumsey J, Riordan-Eva P, Hardigan P. Maximum angle of ocular duction during visual fixation as a function of age. *Strabismus.* 2005;13:21-26.

45. Scheiman M. *Understanding and Managing Vision Deficits: A Guide for Occupational Therapists.* 2nd ed. Thorofare, NJ: SLACK, Inc; 2011.

46. Watson GR, Wright V, Long SL. Morgan Low Vision Reading Comprehension Assessment (LUV Reading Series). 1996. (contact www.lowvisionsimulators.com)

47. Watson GR, Baldasare J, Whittaker S. The validity and clinical uses of the Pepper Visual Skills for Reading Test. *J Vis Impairment Blindness.* 1990;84:119-123.

48. Gray WS. *Gray Oral Reading Tests.* New York: Bobbs Merrill; 1967.

49. Greenberg D, Pae HK, Morris RD, Calhoon MB, Nanda AO. Measuring adult literacy students' reading skills using the Gray Oral Reading Test. *Ann Dyslexia.* 2009;59:133-149.

50. Rowles GD. Beyond performance in place as a component of occupational therapy. *Am J Occup Ther.* 1991;45:265-271.

III

Treatment

Overview of Treatment Strategy

MODEL OF CARE FOR LOW VISION REHABILITATION

In Chapter 1, we described our proposed model of care for low vision rehabilitation working in a general rehabilitation or education setting. Because it is often missed and confused with cognitive disability, the first step is to make certain all professionals screen for vision disability. If a vision disability is suspected, then a referral is made to an occupational therapist on staff, who should be able to evaluate and provide the "first-response interventions." These are stopgap interventions that enable a person to participate in therapy, an educational program, and their routines and occupations while waiting for specialized low vision services. A first-response intervention includes assuring that any underlying disease is being managed by an optometrist or ophthalmologist.

With a specialized low vision service, the process usually begins with a referral from a physician with accompanying documentation. In some settings, such as educational settings or in medical rehabilitation settings or outside of the United States, referrals may come from other professionals, but the low vision specialist must find an optometrist or ophthalmologist with whom to collaborate on low vision

rehabilitation. The occupational therapist performs an evaluation (see Chapter 8), where observable and measurable performance goals are set, barriers to performance are identified, and a treatment plan is developed to remove those barriers. In subsequent sessions, the therapist implements the treatment plan. If the course of treatment is lengthy, periodic progress reports are required where progress toward achievement of each goal is measured and reported. Finally, upon discharge, progress toward goal achievement is measured and reported. Note that for occupational therapists, goals and outcomes are measured in terms of performance of an activity, not some visual or physical measure like visual acuity. The treatments involved in low vision rehabilitation are included in Table 9-1. Note that some of the required treatments are beyond the scope of practice of an occupational therapist and require the involvement of other professionals.

Before specialized treatment is started, the occupational therapist should make certain a treatment team is in place for all vision clients so that treatment is being provided for the disorder, impairments, disability, and handicap as defined by the World Health Organization[1] as follows:

- A *disorder* is an anatomical deviation from normal and can be acquired or congenital. Examples of acquired visual disorders causing low vision are diseases such as

Whittaker SG, Scheiman M, Sokol-McKay DA.
*Low Vision Rehabilitation: A Practical Guide for Occupational Therapists,
Second Edition* (pp 143-160).
© 2016 Taylor & Francis Group.

Table 9-1: Treatment for Low Vision: Seven Areas of Treatment

OPTIMIZING CLIENT FACTORS	OPTIMIZING CONTEXT AND TEACHING CLIENT TO MODIFY CONTEXT	TEACHING NON-VISUAL SKILLS	TEACHING USE OF VISUAL SKILLS	SELECTING DEVICES	TEACHING OPTICAL AND ELECTRONIC DEVICE USE	RESOURCES
• Vision • Other senses • Motor function • Cognitive • Psychological • Understanding and adjustment to condition and prognosis	• Lighting and glare control • Contrast • Organization • Orientation • Labeling and markings (visual, tactile, auditory, cognitive) • Relative distance/relative size magnification	• Learn to use NV devices, and techniques (tactile, auditory, smell, and cognitive) • Physical movement and exploration without vision • Orientation • Sensory and concept development and compensation • Optimize social context • Self-regulation • Braille	• Fixation, localization, scanning, and tracking • Eccentric viewing • Visual scanning • Visual skills training without then with a device	• Handheld and headborne • Optical • Non-optical aides • Low vision and non-visual assistive devices • Electronic optical	• Learning to use optical devices • Learning to use electronic devices • Adapting and using computers, e-books telephones, recording devices • Ergonomics/positioning • Implementation into applicable daily activities	• State and other agencies • Assistance purchasing devices • Spiritual • Counseling and psychological • Family and friends • Transportation • Advocacy groups • Medical/rehabilitative management of eye diseases with systemic complications • Reading services (NFB Newsline, radio reading services)

age-related macular degeneration (AMD or ARMD), diabetic retinopathy, and glaucoma. Congenital disorders causing low vision include Stargardt disease, a juvenile form of macular degeneration, and retinitis pigmentosa. Refractive error is also a disorder.

- *Impairment* is a loss or abnormality in function. The impairment can be either physiological or psychological. Visual impairments include decreased visual acuity, reduced contrast sensitivity, central scotomas (blind areas), and constricted visual fields.

- *Disability* refers to a restriction or an inability to perform a task in the normal way. Examples are difficulty reading newspaper print, recognizing faces, and driving a car.

- *Handicap* is a disadvantage that prevents or limits participation in, or the fulfillment of, a role that is normal for the client. Examples are the inability to work or engage in hobbies, and restricted social interactions.

Before the occupational therapist begins an evaluation, an ophthalmologist or optometrist should have evaluated and treated the underlying visual disease, or "disorder," and prescribed corrective lenses if needed. During the evaluation, the occupational therapist might determine the need for other physicians, physical therapists, and psychologists to provide treatments for psychological problems and associated physical disorders. Typically, if the client has usable vision, an optometrist specializing in low vision will be involved to prescribe devices and authorize treatments for visual compensations for the disability and impairment. Other blindness rehabilitation professionals may be required to teach mobility with a long cane or guide dog or braille reading—again, treatment at the level of disability. Because a client must deal with changes in roles as a result of a vision disability, social workers and vocational rehabilitation professionals will often be needed to address an emerging handicap. The participation of these other practitioners is detailed in Chapter 2.

LOW VISION REHABILITATION— GENERAL CONCEPTS

Adult Education Theory and Low Vision Rehabilitation

Malcolm S. Knowles was perhaps the central and most influential figure in the US adult education field in the latter half of the 20th century. His work was a significant factor in reorienting educators teaching adults from "educating people" to "helping people to learn;" facilitating learning rather than teaching. He focused on the notion of "informal education" which emphasized an informal climate (versus formal classroom setting), flexibility of process, use of the experience, enthusiasm and commitment of participants (including teachers). Malcolm Knowles was the first to attempt a comprehensive theory of adult education (through the notion of andragogy).[2a] Adult education theory[2b] (Table 9-2) is based on the science of teaching adults, a very different approach than teaching children—andragogy vs pedagogy. We, as occupational therapists, might find our adult clients unmotivated because we are not teaching them correctly. Adults learn in response to questions they find meaningful and problems that they feel are significant. These and additional adult education principles are identified in Table 9-2 and are contrasted to the process of teaching children.

Optimizing Vision

In low vision rehabilitation, the loss of visual acuity and the visual field is related to a disease process that is usually irreversible. In Table 9-1, one aspect of recovery includes optimizing client factors such as visual acuity or contrast sensitivity. Optometrists improve vision by prescribing corrective lenses; ophthalmologists improve vision by providing surgical interventions such as cataract removal or a vitrectomy to remove blood from the vitreous. Sometimes patients are told that procedures like cataract removal or new eyeglasses will not help when, in fact, some improvement will result even though vision will not be fully restored or the disease cured.[3] The treatment team should encourage clients to consider any intervention that will improve vision, especially if risks are minimal.

One intervention used by occupational therapists that reduces visual impairment is lighting (see Chapter 12). Lighting can profoundly impact visual fields, visual acuity, and contrast sensitivity. The treatments in Table 9-1 provided by occupational therapists and other rehabilitation professionals are considered compensatory interventions, such as using a device that enables the client to reduce disability, that is, perform some activity in spite of impairment. While this essential concept is well known by low vision professionals, clients with low vision may have difficulty understanding and accepting this idea. In the client's previous experiences with blurred vision and other vision disorders, the problems were always solved quite easily with a new set of eyeglasses. It is easy to understand the clients asking, "Why can't the doctor just prescribe stronger lenses?" or "Why can't the doctor just give me a different eye drop?" This difficulty accepting the chronic nature of vision loss is one of the most significant obstacles to successful low vision rehabilitation.

Many clients spend years looking for a miracle that will restore their vision, and valuable time is lost. As discussed below, studies show that vision rehabilitation tends to be more successful when initiated soon after the vision loss and when visual acuity or visual field loss is not too severely

TABLE 9-2: ADULT EDUCATION VERSUS CHILD EDUCATION

ANDRAGOGY	PEDAGOGY
Adult learners help decide what they want to learn; learning is oriented on solving problems and tasks	Child is taught what the teacher/society wants them to know; learning is subject oriented
Adults learn when the need arises, when they need to cope with real-life tasks and problems	Child is taught a particular subject when the teacher/society determines it should be taught
Adults direct and are responsible for their own learning	Teacher is responsible for directing learning
Adult learning is an active process; adults prefer experiential learning—laboratory experiments, discussion, problem-solving cases, simulation exercises, field experience	Child learning should also be an active process, but can be a passive process (lecture and reading)
Adult's desire to learn often is based upon immediate need to know	Child learns for future use
Motivation is internal—self-esteem, self-confidence, and independence	Motivation is often through external pressure or grading
Relationship between adult learner and teacher is a collaborative one; the teacher is a facilitator	The teacher is fully responsible for the learning process; the child is the recipient
Adults bring their significant prior knowledge and experience to the learning situation	Experience is emerging with a child

Adapted from Knowles MS, Holton EF, Swanson RA. *The Adult Learner.* 7th ed. New York: Routledge; 2012.

impaired. There is no doubt that a therapist will encounter the frustration of clients who do not enthusiastically embrace potentially effective attempts at vision rehabilitation because they simply have not yet accepted the fact that the vision loss is permanent. In such situations, the role of the occupational therapist is to provide understanding, acknowledgement, education, and guidance through the stages of coping discussed in Chapter 6. Nonetheless, because of this expectation, clients often respond well to interventions that improve vision or visual devices.[4]

One emerging discovery is that vision can actually be improved somewhat as a result of controlled practice with visual tasks, an improvement that has been attributed to higher-order neuroplasticity following vision loss.[5] This new research supports a traditional clinical dictum that suggests vision might actually improve with use. Although these improvements in visual function are measurable at a higher-order perceptual level, such as word and object recognition, the improvements are not measurable using traditional letter acuity or visual field measurements; rather, they are measured more as improvements in performance, such as reading speed and comprehension. As clients continue to practice and develop skills in using their remaining vision in functional tasks, many areas of visual performance improve considerably. It should be noted, however, that such changes are often subtle or occur slowly and thus may hardly be noticed by the client. Clients often misunderstand that using their vision can damage it. For this reason, clients should always be informed that using

their vision will not make it worse or "use it up," but, in fact, will help it improve.

Compensatory Approaches

Low vision rehabilitation has been successfully practiced for many years with an emphasis on compensatory techniques. Table 9-1 also summarizes compensatory rehabilitation strategies that include the following:

- Modifying the home or work environment, including changes in lighting; organization strategies; and changes in the social environment by educating significant others to reduce caregiver dependence or support resumption of roles and routines at home. Usually, clients must learn to make these modifications themselves (see Chapter 12).

- Teaching nonvisual techniques is now integral in the scope of practice of low vision therapists, and includes feeling for dirt that cannot be seen during cleaning, feeling for stubble during shaving, recognizing the shape and feel of objects by touch, or listening for cars and people during mobility (see Chapter 10).

- Teaching scanning skills such as eccentric viewing, or looking in the direction of a field loss, compensatory scanning, or organizing visual and tactile scanning to not miss important information or objects (see Chapters 10 and 11).

- The selection of optical devices must involve both an optometrist who considers the optical properties of the device and an occupational therapist who considers the task and handling of a magnification device (see Chapter 13). Nonoptical visual devices might include bold-line markers or clocks and calendars with large numbers. Nonvisual devices might include tactile markings or talking clocks. Included are electronic devices and computer software that magnifies, enhances contrast, and reads aloud information displayed on a screen, or a National Library Service (NLS) player for recorded books (see Section IV).

- Teaching people to use the devices must be included in the treatment plan. For many, it may be a few minutes of instruction; for those with cognitive impairment, it might require much longer.

- Providing written instruction and resources in a format accessible to the client is an important part of treatment as well.

These treatments are discussed in detail in Section IV.

Early Intervention Is Critical

One of the key factors in the success of low vision rehabilitation is early intervention. When treatment is initiated earlier in the disease process, visual acuity and visual field loss are generally less severe. With better visual acuity, lower magnification optical aids can be prescribed and it is easier for clients to learn how to use lower-power devices. The working distance of a lower-power device is closer to normal and the field of view is wider. In addition, the use of nonoptical assistive devices is more effective because less magnification is required and a wider variety of appropriate devices is available. Simple rehabilitation strategies such as organization of the environment, enhanced lighting and contrast, and elimination of glare are effective in the early stages of visual loss. Even if the client eventually progresses to more serious vision loss, he or she has already experienced success in low vision rehabilitation and is more likely to be motivated to continue treatment. As a result, early intervention encourages people to begin applying relatively easy compensatory techniques to maintain occupations, routines, and roles.

McIlwaine et al[6] found that there was a relationship between age and success with low vision aids. In their study, there was a significant difference in the use of prescribed aids between clients less than 65 years of age and those greater than age 65. They found that over one-third of clients over the age of 65 never used their low vision aids, compared with only one-sixth of clients under the age of 65 years.[6] Other studies have found that with therapy, the success rates are much higher (see the later section on research). The obstacle to early intervention, however, is that many clients are not emotionally ready for rehabilitation after initially sustaining visual loss.[7] They may still not accept that the vision loss is permanent. Patients often schedule appointments with other doctors for additional options, hoping that there may be a conventional way of restoring vision.

Writing Patient Goals

A person's daily routines could be likened to a wheel moving a person through their roles and toward their aspirations. The spokes of the wheel are the physical, cognitive, sensory, and social requirements to keep going. Disabled performance of some critical activities is like a broken spoke, sometimes weakening and if enough spokes are broken, stopping forward progress. Like repairing spokes of a wheel, achieving performance goals is central to a successful rehabilitation program. Indeed, most payers now require that goals be stated in terms of performance relating to occupation, not impairment. In the evaluation (see Chapter 8), the objectives of the occupational profile/case history are to gather information about the client's prior performance, routines, and roles, identifying what performance areas have been disabled such as grooming, catching up on family news over the Web, reading mail, identifying medications accurately, or cooking for the family on Sunday. Another aspect of the evaluation is identifying what specific impairments present barriers to performance. Impairments might include insufficient visual acuity, visual field loss, frustration tolerance, or lack of knowledge of adaptive skills to perform an activity. Goal definition, however, cannot be written in terms of impairment, but must be written using a performance outcome. The therapist must ask, "What will this client be able to perform once the impairment is reduced?" For example, a defined goal might be to perform a specific reading task, such as reading 8-point type on a medication label; or to identify a lighting problem, correct it, and then read playing cards on a table; or to cook foods to the desired level of doneness and with a safe internal temperature.

The therapist's role is not to define the client's goals, but to guide the client through the process of establishing performance goals. Patients often will require guidance because they may not know what rehabilitation strategies are possible.[8,9] In some of the earliest guides to low vision, Quillman and Goodrich stated that people with recent and severe vision loss may not have been able to think about vision goals.[9] They state that "it is never a good idea for a practitioner to set a goal for a client; it is appropriate to help the client set his or her own goals." This collaborative goal setting is central to adult learning theory and the success-oriented approach (see Chapter 6). According to these approaches, adult clients are self-directed in what they want to learn and how they learn, even in the face of vision loss. The therapist serves as an information resource and guide, enabling the client to delineate and prioritize goals. Goals chosen by the client are relevant to his or her immediate needs, desires, and difficulties faced in personal and work life due to vision loss. Adult clients are problem-oriented. Adults are internally motivated, and it is the therapist's responsibility to discover what factors motivate behavior change. External motivators, such as coaxing and pressuring from outside sources, at best produces short-lived change and often inspires oppositional behavior. Watson suggests using checklists or performance assessment systems to negotiate between felt needs and ascribed needs.[8] In some cases, the client may be depressed and reluctant to establish his or her own goals. In such cases, it is critical for the therapist to acknowledge that a significant loss has occurred, while encouraging the client about proper intervention and motivation.

Introducing a brief high-success, low-cost intervention in an area of stated need at the end of the evaluation can set the stage for ongoing motivation. This is central to the success-oriented approach (see Chapter 6). Some simple examples include teaching the client to identify coins by touch, using a bold-line pen and teaching them to write a grocery list in larger print, or placing a rubber band on the shampoo bottle to help differentiate it from the conditioner. Develop such a list for your own practice. Much can be done to help the client become more independent in activities of daily living (ADL) (see Section IV). Once the goals are established, the treatment plan is organized. Sometimes, if a client is not ready to pursue a goal that the therapist might feel would greatly improve quality of life, the "seed can be planted" by presenting the goal and asking the client to reconsider it later. This "seed" may grow into a goal during the course of treatment, nourished by success achieving other goals.

In Chapter 8 we suggested the Low Vision Independence Measure (LVIM)[10] and the shorter form of the Veterans Affairs Low-Vision Visual Functioning Questionnaire (VA-LV VFQ)[10,11] for in-clinic assessments. These and other lists recognize problem areas and guide the client to consider most areas typically disabled by low vision. Both are in the public domain. Once the goals are defined, in addition to the subjective measures, the therapist must establish corresponding objective performance measures. Guidelines for objective measures are as follows and are based on established standards for goal definition:[13]

The COAST method of goal writing. COAST is an acronym developed by Gateley and Borcherding[13] to ensure all elements of a goal are included:

- **C**lient should be included in the goal
- **O**ccupation should be specified in a directly observable and unambiguous manner
- **A**ssist level
- **S**etting

- **T**imeline (number of sessions may be limited by insurance companies as well)

Examples of goals for ADLs are in Table 9-3. Goals should be set with a specific method of measurement in mind, sometimes simply using an observation of whether a specific task was performed or not. In general, adjectives should be replaced by specific behaviors that indicate if a goal has been achieved or not. If slower progress is anticipated, a measure might be included such as the number of successes out of total attempts or a speed measure like reading rate or time required to perform a task. As occupational therapists, we think in terms of occupational goals. Yet, it is often impossible to describe a general overall goal occupation such as "cooking." A challenge in goal writing is to select a specific, measurable task that is representative of the overall occupational goal. An example might be a representative task, such as "spreading a condiment by obtaining something with a knife during cooking." "The client will independently recognize a person on a television with 5/5 accuracy" would indicate an ability watch and understand what was happening on TV.

The goal should not indicate that it can only be achieved visually unless this is an expectation of the client. For example, instead of "read a medication label accurately," the goal should be "identify a medication accurately." Most people think of identifying products as a visual activity. Indeed, practical spot reading normally requires visual reading, but tactile methods might suffice for someone with low vision. A book or article on the Web can be "read" by listening or using braille, or by using an e-reader so that "reading a novel" usually does not require a specific print size or even vision, but reading speed and endurance can be specified. An example might be, "Client will locate and read a novel, newspaper, or magazine fluently (> 150 wpm) for > 30 minutes and recall principle characters and themes using visual or auditory strategies." In addition, many clients may combine low vision with nonvisual strategies. A specific short-term goal could be "The patient will locate and cut up 2 ingredients and prepare a salad with modified independence." To achieve this goal, a person might locate a cutting board or vegetables visually, but use tactual techniques for safe knife use and cutting consistently sized slices. Limiting performance to visual activity is a problem with most low vision outcome assessment tools.

The following examples include occupational goals. Written under goals that are too general and not observable and measurable are specific task goals that focus on the same occupations, but are written in the required format for reimbursement. Note mod [I] means "modified independence," which implies that the client may use any assistive device or adaptive technique and is considered a level of assistance.

TABLE 9-3: SPECIFIC OCCUPATIONAL PERFORMANCE ITEMS AND EXAMPLE PERFORMANCE GOALS

IN THE HOME, WORK, OR OTHER SPECIFIED SETTING, A CLIENT WILL PERFORM THE FOLLOWING WITH (A LEVEL OF ASSISTANCE OR CUES SPECIFIED) IN (A TIMEFRAME OR NUMBER OF SESSIONS):

- Personal organization activities
  - Access calendar and record appointments w/ 5/5 accuracy

- Self-care
  - Apply makeup resulting in a socially acceptable appearance

- Meal preparation
  - Determine food doneness to personal taste or safety guidelines
  - Open a variety of packages and containers within 30 seconds
  - Prepare cold food item
  - Heat up item
  - Cook single item on stovetop
  - Cook single item in oven
  - Simultaneously prepare >3 food items for a meal
  - Operate small appliances (can opener, toaster oven, microwave, blender, Crock-Pot, indoor grill, wok)

- Housekeeping
  - Locate and retrieve a dropped object within 30 seconds
  - Clean up a spill within 30 seconds
  - Wash dishes until clean
  - Clean flat surfaces thoroughly (counters, floors, tabletops)
  - Make bed; change bed linens with neat results
  - Clean bathroom thoroughly
  - Clean appliances safely and thoroughly
  - Identify toxic chemicals and spoiled food in safe manner
  - Access and operate environmental features (insert plug in outlet, key into key hole, and set thermostat precisely)
  - Perform basic hand mending (sew up a hole or seam, sew on a button, hem a garment) with neat and durable results
  - Thread a sewing machine within 2 minutes
  - Maintain straight, even stitching and consistent accurate seam allowances

- Functional communication
  - Perform mathematical computations with 10/10 accuracy
  - Keyboard with 10/10 accuracy at 20 wpm

- Orientation and mobility
  - Move from a lighted environment to a dark environment and immediately detect low-contrast obstacles greater than 10 cm in size
  - Implement and teach significant others correct human guide (sighted guide) techniques
  - Move within the home avoiding 20/20 obstacles with no bumps or trips as a secondary task
  - Detect an unexpected object within 2 seconds in a cluttered environment with 10/10 accuracy as a secondary task

Based on an ADL checklist developed by Debra A. Sokol-MacKay.

SIDEBAR 9-1: TWO DIFFERENT DEFINITIONS OF INDEPENDENCE

According to the 2014 *Occupational Therapy Practice Framework*: "It is important to acknowledge that clients can be independent in living regardless of the amount of assistance they receive while completing activities. Clients may be considered independent when they perform or direct the actions necessary to participate, regardless of the amount or kind of assistance they require" (p. S6).[2]

Although, the AOTA has defined independence differently, because of conventional use in medical rehabilitation, we recommend in documentation and goal writing that the terms "independence or modified-independence" be used to mean assistance or cues from another person is NOT required.

- Client will read (general occupational goal).
  - Client will read medication labels and package labels that are 1M font with 10/10 word identification accuracy in the home with mod [I].
  - Client will read continuous text in a commercially available book for 15 minutes' endurance at >150 words per minute using vision or text to speech with mod [I].
  - Client will read menus and identify products and prices in printed advertising circulars that are 1M font with 10/10 word and number identification accuracy with mod [I].
- Client will watch TV (general occupational goal).
  - Client will identify different characters and actions on a television with 5/5 accuracy with mod [I].
  - Client will read closed captioning on a TV and correctly answer 3/3 questions on content with mod [I].

Table 9-3 includes properly specified goals for a number of ADL activities. Note that quantitative outcome measures such as the VA-LV VFQ and LVIM are useful for program evaluation, and even documenting overall progress for an individual patient (required by Medicare in addition to specific goals), but the overall score is not acceptable as an individual goal by itself. Rather, the specific tasks from these general outcome tests provide the therapist and client with a suggested list of common problems that can be written as specific performance goals. The overall score might be used to document progress or perform program evaluation, and may be converted into G-codes or other overall performance measures required by Medicare and other insurance companies. Adding a separate overall outcome measure by CMS and medical insurers has been quite burdensome for occupational therapists, as there simply is not time for duplicate assessment. We have adapted these tests so they can be used for both an overall outcome measure and specification of individual performance goals.

In addition to having an observable and measurable specification of performance ("O" in the COAST acronym), a level of assist must be specified ("A" in the COAST acronym). This is best done by indicating how much physical assist or cuing is required. In medical rehabilitation, the words "independent" or "modified independent" indicate another person was not required for cuing and physical assist and this meaning should be assumed in goal writing. The AOTA, however, has a different definition of "independence" that is more relevant to a person's participation (Sidebar 9-1).[2]

Organizing the Individualized Treatment Plan

A treatment plan that includes the areas in Table 9-1 can be organized in many different ways. The purpose of the initial evaluation (see Chapter 8) is to organize an individualized treatment plan, a plan that addresses the unique needs of each client. This model is used in special education and is called an *individualized education plan* (IEP). Defining specific performance goals is central to the reasoning process and not only helps organize a treatment plan, but also provides a framework for the documentation requirements by payers. The summary of the areas of treatment included in Table 9-1 provide the therapist with a list of treatments to consider. Each of these treatments is discussed in depth in subsequent chapters. As mentioned, the evaluation systematically determines which treatments will be needed to attain each goal.

In the current climate of cost-effective health care, the payer and the consumer need to know what health care services are being purchased and for how much. What is being purchased might be described as a treatment plan for the individual performance goals. For the consumer, the cost is not only monetary, but is also in terms of the number and frequency of expected treatments, what equipment will be necessary to achieve those goals, and what other professional treatments will need to be involved. Payers for occupational therapy services need to be assured that the treatments are "skilled," that is, the services require the skill of an occupational therapist and cannot otherwise be performed by a person or family member who is not a licensed occupational therapist.

Payers also usually require the interventions to be "medically necessary." The Centers for Medicare/Medicaid Services (CMS) definition of medical necessity is "[h]ealth care services or supplies needed to prevent, diagnose, or treat an illness, injury, condition, disease or its symptoms and that meet acceptable standards of medicine" (www.medicare.gov/glossery/m.html). For rehabilitation, this includes impairments and disabilities that result from a specific illness, injury, condition, or disease, but what disabilities are treatable is somewhat arbitrarily defined. For example, disabled vocational activities and driving are often excluded by medical insurance payers, but will be covered by state vocational rehabilitation services. In our experience, payment has never been denied for leisure activities and instrumental activities of daily living (IADLs). Historically, a prognosis for improvement has been required, but one recent court ruling in Vermont (*Jimmo v. Sebelius*) suggests that any skilled treatment is reimbursable even if it is only to maintain function after chronic illness. Fortunately, with low vision rehabilitation, the largely compensatory interventions can be shown to quickly improve performance, so progress is rarely an issue.

The occupational therapist summarizes the planned treatments into a "plan of care," which, in most states, requires approval by a physician. In our model of care, an optometrist or ophthalmologist, preferably someone specializing in low vision, should review and approve the plan of care, as well as the referring physician including optometrists. According to CMS, optometrists in all states are now able to sign a low vision treatment plan. The plan of care should be sent to all professionals involved in related treatments and should be revised to coordinate their treatments.

This plan of care can be usually summarized in a page or 2 (this in included in the Initial Evaluation Form provided in the online appendix at www.routledge.com/9781617116339) and quickly and easily transmitted to the participating physicians and professionals. Although it is good practice to review specific performance goals and objectives and perceived/measured progress every session with the client, payers also require periodic progress reports, usually every 10 sessions or every 1 to 2 months, depending on the payer and institution. Ideally, this evaluation and the needed treatments should be developed in an evaluation of about 1 hour. During the subsequent sessions, the plan is reviewed with the client and modified if needed. The plan itself often evolves and will likely need revision within the first few sessions, but the revised plan rarely needs approval unless it deviates significantly from the original. The requirements for a plan of care may differ depending on the requirements of the payer and needs to be verified with the payer before implementation.

Clinical Reasoning Process for Developing a Treatment Plan

Trial and error with devices is no longer an acceptable standard of practice. The key to cost-effective treatment is in the ability of the therapist to predict the outcomes of specific interventions in order to select which interventions and devices to include in the treatment plan. In addition, the therapist must predict how many sessions will be required for the interventions. This section describes the general reasoning process that the therapist will use to select interventions to include in the treatment plan.

First the therapist identifies performance limitations and then, with the client, sets performance goals as described earlier. The next step is to identify what barriers (impairments) prevent a person from goal achievement. To define these barriers or performance-limiting factors, the client must know the "visual and nonvisual requirements" to perform a task. As with any potential barrier to performance, a visual requirement includes not only a client factor such as print size at visual acuity threshold, but also a measure of corresponding environmental factor (print size the client wants to read) and task demand (reading rate and accuracy required).[14] The evaluation also includes other potential barriers and supports in the occupational history, habits, roles and culture context, demand, and finally, the results of current occupational performance assessment.[1] One usually has several goals to address. In the treatment plan, the therapist attempts to use training, devices, and environmental modifications that remove barriers to multiple goals at the same time. For example, one might use the same magnification device for reading mail, reading a mobile phone display, checking fruit for blemishes, and checking knitting for a dropped stitch. As another intervention, the therapist might recommend an assistant come by once a week to set up medications and help with shopping and downloading recorded books on the computer. The treatment plan also includes consideration of a client's morale and need for success, scheduling more easily accomplished, highly valued tasks to be achieved first through the success-oriented approach. If treatment is expected to be lengthy, prioritizing easily attained goals first also enables documentation of progress required by payers.

For example, Ms. Jones, a 72-year-old retired executive, wished to read a novel fluently, make her own meals, and do her own finances. She also had the expected spot reading goals of someone who lived alone, such as reading instructions, correspondence, and medication labels. She had adapted homemaking and meal prep on her own and was quite proud of her accomplishments. At first, she denied problems, but when specifically asked, she admitted problems seeing blemishes on vegetables and fruit, cutting, and measuring. The daughter, who drove her to appointments, reported that she read all her mail for her mother, brought over cooked meals, and did her finances. A quick screen indicated that cognitive and physical barriers were not significant, but Ms. Jones exhibited signs of depression. Her records indicated dry AMD with impaired contrast sensitivity and a moderate reduction in reading acuity. In the functional vision evaluation with the eyeglasses prescribed by the optometrist, the functional vision evaluation predicted the magnification required for reading normal print comfortably was 16 diopters of equivalent power (see Chapter 8). Although Ms. Jones was reassured by her reading with larger print, during testing with the reading acuity chart, she would misread words and numbers. Further testing revealed she required over 2000 lux of illumination and was glare sensitive. The evaluation revealed the following additional nonvisual barriers to performance:

- Low frustration tolerance and mild depression
- Caregiver dependence
- Lack of knowledge about adaptive techniques

Strengths included good problem solving, memory, and insight. Ms. Jones reported her daughter's attempts to help were irritating, but she did not want to hurt her feelings, indicating a desire for increased independence.

Two examples of goals and goal-specific barriers were as follows:

- Identifying blemishes on fruits and vegetables and measuring ingredients for meal preparation with 5/5 accuracy without assistance or cues.
  - Impaired contrast sensitivity and glare sensitivity, high (2000 lux) light levels required
  - Impaired visual acuity
- Spot reading with 10/10 accuracy (see Chapter 15) with modified independence.
  - Impaired contrast sensitivity and glare sensitivity, high light levels required
  - Impaired visual acuity
  - Central scotoma and lack of eccentric viewing skills

Basic food preparation skills and reading directions on food packages were immediate problem areas that Ms. Jones identified in accordance with adult learning theory. Following a mutual discussion of her visual performance barriers and the time, devices, environmental modifications, and instruction estimated to achieve her goals, both the therapist and the client set realistic goals. Ms. Jones and the therapist jointly developed a treatment plan with an estimate of how many sessions and how much practice would be required. The client expressed concern about the need for her daughter to assist her. This issue was first addressed in separate meetings and then together in order to develop a strategy for decreasing caregiver dependence. This included educating her daughter regarding the need for problem-solving therapy and her mother's increased feelings of self-efficacy (see Chapter 6) to avert the development of more severe depression. The caregiver-dependence barrier was thus addressed and reviewed at the beginning of each session. Because of low frustration tolerance and mild depression, the success-oriented approach was used, ameliorating this barrier as well. Because we could predict that the goals could be easily met, her cooking goals were addressed first and easily met with lighting (see Chapter 12) and adaptive cooking strategies (see Chapter 17). The client was given the opportunity to explore the use of color-contrasting and large-print measuring cups on her own with

the therapist's input as needed. She had already proudly reported that she could rely on the nesting feature of measuring cups (one-quarter cup sits in one-third cup, which sits in one-half cup, etc) to determine the size measuring cup she needed, but felt the black measuring cups would meet her needs (see Chapter 17). Because we could predict optimum luminance from the evaluation and used a digital light meter, the first lighting changes tried were effective. We also introduced NLS recorded books to give her an easy alternative for meeting reading goals (see Chapter 15).

Then we turned to other goals that would be more difficult to meet. Because we could predict the optimum magnification for reading devices, the therapist could select and compare devices that were known to have adequate magnification. When a magnifier was first introduced and did not produce the predicted reading fluency, the therapist assumed magnification was correct and quickly narrowed in on lighting as the visual barrier to performance. The therapist tried an alternative device with higher luminance and tried glare-reducing, light-yellow absorptive. Prior to spot reading training, the client was asked to set out several food packages that she would like to read. Within 15 minutes and no trial and error, her spot reading goal was achieved with the therapist providing assistance handling the device. Therapy then focused on teaching device use. Because of her success with reading food packages, she asked to learn how to locate the amount due on her bills. Ms. Jones wanted to read fluently in her favorite chair and had rejected close working distances required of 16-diopter reading glasses, as well as rejected electronic magnifiers such CCTVs. The barriers for device use were basically user preferences. Again, knowing the required magnification, the formula for equivalent power, and lighting and contrast requirements, the therapist quickly narrowed in on the use of a Kindle electronic book reader with white on black contrast and 2.5× print magnification with 6-diopter reading glasses, allowing an acceptable working distance and the needed contrast enhancement and glare reduction for more fluent reading. Under the "standard" model of care (see Chapter 13), the optometrist would recommend alternative devices for magnifying print. Under the advanced model of care (see Chapter 13), the therapist would be able to select the alternative devices and setups. In both cases, the optometrist would prescribe the optical devices used.

TREATMENT APPROACHES

Under the adult learning model, the client is involved in goal setting and treatment planning. Sometimes, a client schedules the initial appointment because of doctor's orders or at the urging of a family member and begins therapy skeptically, needing to be convinced of the value of therapy. The therapist should always begin the rehabilitation program with a careful discussion of performance goals. Fortunately, the evaluation procedure (see Chapter 8) incorporates demonstration that achievement of a performance goal is possible; for example, with the reading acuity test, a person often can read the largest print with relative ease. Often, clients need time for emotional support or to discuss the particular eye disease and the expected course, rather than immediately starting some rehabilitation intervention. The key to acceptance is to encourage the client to focus on the end, a performance goal, rather than on the means. A novel can be enjoyed by listening to it. If someone wishes to read visually, then the therapist demonstrates reading on an electronic viewer and provides maximum assistance and sufficient magnification so reading is relatively easy. The therapist might also show the client how to perform a simple cold food preparation, dial a phone, or find the right cell in her medication dispenser—a task that requires little or no vision to perform. Once the tasks are performed or the book is enjoyed, acceptance may follow and the client might be willing to set more challenging goals. If a client seems reluctant, then under the adult learning model, the goals and treatment plan must be revisited without family present to pressure the client or speak for them.

In cases where a client is reluctant, has a low frustration tolerance, or cognitive impairment, the therapist should use the success-oriented approach (see Chapter 6). This approach is consistent with adult learning theory; it places greater emphasis on demonstration and sequencing interventions to minimize errors and difficulty. Once devices or interventions are demonstrated, the therapist should check in with the client to make sure that he or she is still committed to the goal and treatment plan.

One of the easiest and most economical treatment approaches is the use of environmental modifications (see Chapter 12). It minimizes new learning, and these adaptations can be generalized to other activities. A client can often achieve substantial gains with improved lighting, contrast, and elimination of glare. Therapists will need to evaluate these aspects of the client's environment, educate the client about the importance of optimal lighting and contrast, and then demonstrate possible improvements by making appropriate changes. Clients should be given the opportunity to try different lighting strategies in an effort to discover what works best for them. Other strategies, such as changing the working distance and enlarging target size, are used in this phase of the rehabilitation. If one is providing services in an outpatient setting, at least one home visit early in the treatment is highly recommended, not only for treatment planning, but also because several simple home modifications can be highly effective and easy to implement. One often finds that removing glare and seating a client closer to the TV will easily enable one performance goal to be met.

A large percentage of the clients seen in vision rehabilitation have AMD and, therefore, have a central scotoma. When dealing with a client with a central scotoma, it is best to begin therapy with eccentric viewing techniques. Once the client is comfortable with eccentric viewing, he or she can use these skills throughout the rest of the rehabilitation.[10] Eccentric viewing, scanning, eye movement training, and reading skills training are covered in depth in Chapter 10. Other visual skills that need to be introduced early in treatment might be compensatory scanning training for visual field loss or spatial neglect (see Chapter 12).

Occupational therapists just becoming involved in the field of low vision are sometimes intimidated by the need to develop a knowledge and understanding of optics. New terminology, an understanding of optics, and the impression that there are so many aids available can potentially create an obstacle to getting involved. We feel that it is important to understand that the use of low vision optical devices, although important, is just one aspect of low vision rehabilitation; a collaborating optometrist or ophthalmologist who specializes in low vision rehabilitation will understand optical devices and make recommendations. In many cases, simple environmental modifications and the use of nonoptical assistive devices can be of great benefit to a client. These devices include low vision and nonvisual devices that utilize sensory substitution, such as tactile and auditory assistive devices. Occupational therapists should acquire the various catalogs that are available and become acquainted with a wide variety of available nonoptical assistive devices. These topics, along with information about resources, are covered in Section IV.

Magnification

Up until very recently, electronic and optical magnification were considered separate treatment approaches with different strategies. Today, electronics pervade the lives of even older people who did not grow up with cell phones and computers. The use of optical magnification has been, and still is, of course, critically important in low vision rehabilitation with reduced visual acuity but now they are often used with electronic devices with built-in magnification features. Almost all clients with reduced acuity will be able to perform better with the prescription of appropriate optical aids and, at least, reading glasses are needed in older adults even with electronic magnifiers. These aids will typically be prescribed by the low vision optometrist. In the ideal professional environment, however, the occupational therapist will also be involved in the early phase of selection of optical aids. The occupational therapist can assist in this process by providing critical information about the client's ADL problems and goals. If the client has other physical problems that could interfere with the use of some types of aids, the therapist can make suggestions about optical aids selection based on these needs as well.

Just as computer technology has become important in so many aspects of our lives, it is also gaining importance in the field of low vision rehabilitation. Books, magazines, and correspondence on electronic devices are now becoming as common as paper. The advantage of electronic devices is the ability to change and enhance contrast and color, use text-to-speech, and provide some magnification. For some, computer use is as familiar an activity as cooking. Once a specialty skill, every low vision therapist now needs to understand how to adapt computers for use by people with low vision. Computers themselves have become important assistive devices that enable shopping, leisure, and functional written communication, regardless of the level of vision loss. This generation will want and need to continue using computers and will feel comfortable with computer-assisted technology for low vision rehabilitation. Thus, the use of computer technology has become part of routine low vision rehabilitation.

Nonoptical Assistive Devices and Techniques

Many low vision devices (such as large numbered telephones, color-contrasting cutting boards, and brightly colored stair treads) are common everyday objects that are modified for increased visibility and require little to no explanation for basic use. However, most nonvisual devices (such as talking clocks, knives with a guide, and needle-threading devices) and techniques (determining blade edge of knife or quantity of blush to apply to face) are unique, unfamiliar, and may require instruction. Persons with vision impairment benefit significantly from a multisensory approach to instruction. The client chooses one or more sensory modalities with which to explore an assistive device and uses previous life experience and knowledge to obtain as much information as possible about its setup and use. The client is also taught how to attend to cues. The client directs his or her own learning, requesting feedback from the therapist as needed to become familiar with features of immediate interest.

RESEARCH ON LOW VISION REHABILITATION

One of the most important developments in occupational therapy in the past decade has been a firm commitment to evidence-based practice.[2a] This section will describe and recommend an approach to evaluating research and adopting an evidence-based practice that is particularly well suited for low vision rehabilitation in particular and occupational therapy in general. The second part of this section provides guidelines to help the reader evaluate future research.

In medicine, recent standards for evidence-based practice are based on the Cochrane standard.[15] The Cochrane standard for research provides guidelines for searching for research reports, selecting reports to consider, and summarizing outcomes that ensure objective consideration of all reports, both favorable and unfavorable to specific hypotheses. A more controversial aspect of the Cochrane standard categorizes different research designs into a hierarchy, with the highest level of evidence being the prospective randomized clinical trial (RCT), where, prospectively (before any treatment begins), subjects are randomly assigned to a control (no treatment) and additional treatment groups. Each individual is tested under only one condition. The RCT was chosen as the preferred design because it was less likely to exhibit bias in favor of finding a treatment effect that, in fact, does not exist, known as "type I error."[15] The classification of research designs according to the Cochrane standard, however, was developed for testing medical treatments and has limitations when applied to rehabilitation outcomes. To address these limitations, we consider that for rehabilitation using compensatory interventions (mostly used with low vision), a case-controlled design has more validity than the RCT. In a case-controlled design, each individual who participates in the research undergoes testing under both the control and one or more experimental conditions, such as testing someone's performance reading the mail with and without an assistive device.

When deciding what the best experimental design is, one needs to consider the question being asked that the experiment is designed to answer. With medical interventions or most remediational therapy interventions, the question is whether the intervention is effective or not for the people who meet the selection criteria for the study. With medical interventions, the physiology and anatomy of everyone and a given disease process like wet macular degeneration is assumed to be essentially the same with random variation, so this is a reasonable question that is usually best answered using a randomized trial. Even medical researchers, however, have questioned this assumption for some types of medical research.[16] For compensatory interventions in rehabilitation, especially when devices are involved, a device or intervention strategy is not for everyone. We ask a different question. We ask not "Does it work?" but "For whom does it work?" or "What is the likelihood of effectiveness for people with certain characteristics?" This sort of question is best answered with a case-controlled design. Because the control and treatment conditions have been tested in every individual, we can evaluate on a case-by-case basis whether a treatment was effective or not and evaluate predictors of effectiveness. With an RCT, where each person only experiences one condition, we cannot determine a percentage of success or identify predictors of success.

One problem with repeated measure designs is that a person's performance on some measure, such as reading speed, may be improving or deteriorating because of the natural course of the disease or some learning effect. For example, someone with episodic multiple sclerosis might be tested before some training procedure and then after a training procedure and finds that reading improves. This improvement might result because the underlying condition is improving and may have nothing to do with the treatment. An advantage of the RCT is that this experiment will indicate a treatment effect that cannot be attributed to some "order effect," such as improvements that might be attributed to a person's natural course of recovery from a disease. Each type of experimental design, therefore, has advantages and disadvantages. With devices that only are effective when the device is being used, effects, such as magnification devices or most assistive devices, the effect is reversible. The person may not read small print without the device, but then reads small print with the device and when the device is removed, the small print can no longer be read. In these cases, order effects are easy to control, and the case controlled design is superior to the RCT design.

Because changes in a visual stimulus are reversible, the case-controlled is the most common experimental design in basic research on vision and how visual stimuli affect performance, and represents the empirical backbone of visual science that forms our basic understanding of low vision. In these experiments, individuals are repeatedly tested with variations of some visual stimulus, or the visual property of a device is systematically varied to determine how it affects some visual function or performance such as reading. The purpose of this section is to argue that for much rehabilitation research, a valid case-controlled design should be at the highest level of evidence. This will significantly influence the strength of evidence considered for different low vision interventions.

Levels and Strength of Evidence

In several recent systematic reviews of low vision research,[17-21] the evidence was classified as follows: Level I evidence is based on prospective RCTs. Level II evidence is based on nonrandomized assignment to groups (cohort study). Level III and IV experiments include case-controlled designs that do not have a separate control group. Excluding articles published before 1990, 70 articles were selected from 2356 citations and abstracts. In another comprehensive review, Binns et al[22] classified evidence as (1) very good evidence based on RCT, (2) good evidence based on at least 2 "robust study designs," and (3) evidence based on at least one robust study, including 54 studies from 478 potentially relevant articles.

Practically speaking, the practitioner with assistive devices that have reversible effects, such as different types of optical devices, liquid-level indicator for filing a cup, or a type of light or a line guide for reading. The necessary evidence requires only that the therapist try the device and evaluate performance with and without the device on a case-by-case basis; this is essentially the "repeated-measures" or "case-controlled" design we introduced earlier. If the therapist takes care with the order of testing and uses

TABLE 9-4: LEVELS OF EVIDENCE
• **Practice Standard:** The evidence indicates that an outcome is very likely to be effective for a given set of client and environmental factors and task demand.
• **Practice Guideline:** The evidence indicates that a given outcome is likely, but less certain for a given set of client and environmental factors and task demand. There is a significant number who show no effect. Outcome should be periodically evaluated for each client.
• **Practice Options:** The evidence indicates a given outcome is possible for a given set of client and environmental factors and task demands. Outcome should be frequently evaluated for each client.
Adapted from Cicerone KD, Langenbahn DM, Braden C, et al. Evidence-based cognitive rehabilitation: updated review of the literature from 2003 through 2008. *Arch Phys Med Rehabil.* 2011;92:519-530.

objective outcome measures, then a simple clinical test is more credible evidence for the effectiveness of a device for a particular client than some expensive published RCT. If data are collected from a number of clients on the effectiveness of a device using a proper case-controlled design, then this would offer sufficient evidence for a clinic to stock an item and try it when appropriate. Devices such as electronic magnifiers are expensive to keep in stock and therefore might require a higher level of evidence. The evidence would have to show that such devices would be effective most of the time, or frequently enough to stock them. Lengthy interventions such as instruction to develop compensatory scanning also require evidence that effectiveness would be at least likely or very likely. If an intervention has risk of injury or complications, then the highest level of evidence, near certain success, becomes necessary. Rather than using qualitative terms like "good" or "very good," more meaningful terminology would be a classification that indicates the likelihood for success. For the devices and interventions used in this text, we use terminology similar to the classification of evidence used by Cicerone et al to describe the evidence basis for cognitive rehabilitation interventions.[23,24] Table 9-4 provides levels of evidence that we use to classify an intervention as a practice standard, practice guideline, or practice option.

A practice standard indicates an intervention that is very likely to be effective. Research to establish practice standards ideally should focus on interventions that require a substantial investment of time, funds, or may pose a health risk. For example, to justify lengthy training procedures such as compensatory scanning for spatial neglect, or an inventory of expensive devices such as electronic and optical magnifiers, one should be reasonably certain they will be effective; that is, the level of evidence should be that of a practice standard. Frequent outcome evaluation during the intervention should not be necessary if a practice standard is adopted. Cicerone's group requires the evidence include at least one robust RCT. We accept, indeed require, "robust" case-controlled designs (with control for order effects and other confounding variables but not necessarily a RCT). We expect that to be a practice standard, the effect should be anticipated for nearly every individual who meets the eligibility requirements, not just a group average, which may include people showing a strong effect averaged with people for whom a treatment has little or no effect. Evidence should include a report of not only effect size, but also individual performance or percentages of people who met a performance goal. Since reporting individual data is not customary in RCTs, we accept consistent effects across different experiments and conclusions that are supported by basic science as sufficient for a "practice standard." By including well-controlled, repeated-measures designs,[25] some widely used low vision treatments, such as the use of magnification devices or interventions, can be elevated to a practice standard. The effectiveness of magnification devices that have been classified as having a "questionable evidence base" in a traditional review[13] using the Cochrane standard can be elevated.

A practice guideline indicates an intervention where a positive outcome is likely but less certain. At this time, most instructional protocols, such as eccentric viewing training in low vision rehabilitation, are considered practice guidelines. The clinician can predict successful outcomes, with an expectation of effectiveness, at least *most of the time*. One practice guideline would be that electronic magnifiers, with their contrast enhancement characteristics, are generally more effective than optical devices.[19] This level of evidence, therefore, is sufficient for the success-oriented approach. Because outcomes are less certain, however, the therapist should more frequently evaluate outcomes of specific types of optical devices and training procedures to document effectiveness on a case-by-case basis. Practice guidelines may be advanced to practice standards if clinical eligibility criteria are discovered that indicate for whom an intervention is very likely to be effective and individual data are reported. To elevate the level of evidence from a practice guideline to a practice standard, research should include developing eligibility requirements (client, environmental, and task demand characteristics) that predict a device or intervention will be effective. (This approach has been used in some studies where the effect is compared with people who have visual acuity above and below some criterion, but future work should look at other client, environmental, and task demand characteristics as well.)

Finally, practice options are devices and interventions where evidence exists that an intervention has been shown to be effective *in some cases*. Because evidence does not favor one type of handheld optical device over another, recommendations as to particular optical devices are at the level of a practice option. Most ADL devices like reachers, clothing hooks, and sock donners would fall into this category. The therapist basically uses clinical judgment to predict success and a trial-and-error approach with this level of evidence, depending more on the clinician's prior experience and clinical judgment than on research. For example, if a person cannot see the clock and has sufficient hearing, then the clinician might quickly predict that a talking clock would be appropriate and within a few minutes of testing determine if it would or would not be acceptable. Most assistive devices described in the chapters on ADLs and IADLs would fall into this category, including talking clocks, liquid-level indicators, adapted knives, markings for dials, and so forth. A substantial body of published research evidence is not required for the clinician to try these types of devices and provide their own evidence of effectiveness.

Note that we do not consider expert opinion as evidence at any level (even our own opinions), although specific observations and case reports can be considered evidence at the practice option level. Finally, research is not like bread—it does not go stale and lose credibility after a period of time unless the published work is a literature review or involves technology like electronic magnifiers that has changed in recent years. Omitting research just because it is old is not acceptable. Evidence regarding the effectiveness of optical magnification to enable a person with a given visual acuity to read small print is based on evidence obtained by the Greek philosopher Euclid over 2000 years ago and will never go stale.

Evidence-based practice is not just about reading published research articles; evidence-based practice should be an integral part of every therapist's clinical practice. Indeed, every clinician uses a case-controlled design to evaluate the need for therapy, test progress with specific therapeutic interventions, and assess final outcomes. With proper goal definition, outcome measurement, and attention to confounding variables, every clinician is thus capable of performing evidence-based research and even contributing to a larger body of knowledge. Evidence-based practice is a constantly evolving process. We hope our introduction to low vision rehabilitation in this book not only provides a solid starting point, but will inspire the reader to continue to look to the research literature for better methods. Table 9-5 provides some guidelines for the clinician to evaluate new findings as they occur.

Evaluating the Evidence

Are the Procedures Described Well Enough to Replicate?

Recent reviews indicate that studies of general types of interventions (group vs individualized treatment, occupational therapy vs other treatments) and the professionals involved have produced mixed results,[17,22] but many of the studies reviewed lacked a clear specification of what specific procedures and devices were involved. The credentials of the provider or whether the intervention was provided in a group or with a client alone is probably less important than the specific intervention provided. In general, research on specific, replicable training procedures with performance outcomes had results that more consistently indicated either effectiveness or no effectiveness than did general practice models or general descriptions of types of therapy.[18,19,21,22,26]

Are the Measured Outcomes Subjective or Objective?

One consistent finding that has emerged in the literature on low vision rehabilitation interventions is that observed and measured behavioral outcomes, such as reading speed or performance of an ADL task, has exhibited larger, more consistent effects than self-rated performance or quality-of-life measures.[22] As discussed in Chapter 6, the onset of low vision often has a substantial impact on a person's quality of life, an impact that is not easily or quickly reversed by the ability to perform a few ADLs. Although the primary concern of an occupational therapist should be a client's quality of life and subjective impression of progress, the actual performance of specific tasks is more easily improved by devices and specific interventions than by a person's attitudes and expectations. Both subjective and objective outcomes should be measured and considered when evaluating the effectiveness of an intervention, but an objective measure of performance is most likely to indicate a short-term effect.

Group Designs: Are They Valid?

With a group design, the average performance of 2 or more groups is compared. Sometimes 2 or more treatments are compared. Some designs use a no-treatment control group for comparison. By randomly assigning participants (prospective randomization) to each group, one avoids the possibility of preselecting people who might benefit from an intervention. Use of a placebo treatment for the control group and preventing participants and therapists from knowing who belonged to what group controls for a confounding placebo effect. It has been known since the 1950s that researcher or participant expectations bias research results. "Blinding" (called *masking* in low vision research for obvious reasons) minimizes how much the effect of expectations the researchers or participants might bias results. Thus, the double-masked RCT with a placebo control is considered the highest level of evidence[15] for medical interventions. Threats to the validity of a group design, however, exist. The frequency of dropouts might bias results because people are more likely to withdraw if a treatment is ineffective.[22] Pretesting is essential, and results should be included with the demographics of groups who completed and did not complete the experiment. The major

TABLE 9-5: QUESTIONS TO ANSWER WHEN EVALUATING CLINICAL OUTCOMES RESEARCH

- Are the devices and interventions described well enough to replicate?
- Are the measured outcomes objective or subjective?
  - What is your criterion for a clinically significant change?
  - What type of outcome was measured?
- Group designs: Are they valid?
  - Could groups be biased by selection or dropouts?
  - Does group performance reflect individual performance?
  - What are individual outcomes or outcome distributions of each group?
- Repeated measures and mixed designs: Are they valid?
  - Are order effects measured or controlled?
    - Practice
    - Fatigue
    - Disease progression
    - Lasting effect of a treatment
  - Were predictors of success identified?
- Are the characteristics of the study participants similar to those whom you treat?
- Eligibility criteria: Were participants who might benefit from treatment included or excluded?

threat to the validity of the RCT for rehabilitation outcomes is that the mechanism of disability is unlikely to result in a "normal distribution" of outcomes because many interventions are not expected to have the same effect on everyone. Statistically significant differences in group-average outcomes might reflect that the treatment has a large effect in some, but clinically insignificant or no effect in others. For testing low vision interventions such as training procedures that have lasting effects, a grouped design is necessary. As discussed later, strict eligibility requirements needed to minimize random variability in this design may actually invalidate the experiment by excluding the people who are most likely to benefit from an intervention.

Unfortunately with RCTs, individual results are rarely published, especially the underlying frequency distribution of the experimental and control conditions. Without this information, the reader does not know if the effect is a large effect for a few people with considerable overlap between the control and experimental condition or if there is "normal" underlying distribution.

Repeated Measures and Mixed Designs: Are They Valid?

The case-controlled design is conducted much like a clinician would approach evaluation and treatment—by repeated measurement of a client's performance before, during, and after an intervention. One might test reading rate and accuracy first during a control procedure without a magnification device, then with a magnification device, and, to make sure the person's reading has not improved in general, repeat the control condition again without the device. If a standardized test is used that has confidence intervals, like the Pepper Visual Skills for Reading Test,[26] then statistical significance of a change in performance can be measured on a case-by-case basis and a "practice option" standard of evidence can be established with just a few clients. The statistical power of a case-controlled design, the ability to compensate for individual differences and isolate even small treatment effects or measure mathematical relationships between some visual characteristic and performance, often presents a significant advantage of repeated measures over group designs. Basic research on the visual requirements for reading in people with typical and low vision generally use case-controlled or longitudinal design,[25] providing a substantial body of evidence sufficient to establish as practice standards the use of magnification interventions, contrast enhancement, and interventions that increase field of view.

The general threat to the validity of a case-controlled design is an "order effect," such as a deteriorating physical condition that might result in deteriorating performance that would cancel a treatment effect or recovery from a disease that might be mistaken for a treatment effect. Improvement with practice with the outcome measure is another order effect that might bias results, so that performance might have improved without the treatment condition. With interventions that have persistent effects, the control procedure (no treatment) must only precede the treatment. If the control always precedes the treatment, then the validity of the design is threatened by an order effect. If the person is recovering from some condition such as an exacerbation of symptoms of multiple sclerosis, the client would improve over time, regardless of whether a treatment occurred or not; this is an order effect. Many so-called cures for the common cold reflect an order effect rather than a treatment effect. A person becomes symptomatic, then takes some remedy, and then the symptoms disappear; thus, the person believes the remedy caused the symptoms to disappear. Yet even without any remedy, the symptoms would disappear, as they nearly always do when you get a cold.

If the effect of treatment, such as use of a device, is reversible, then the order effects can be easily controlled by "counterbalancing" the conditions. A participant would be tested first without the device, then with the device, and then finally testing is repeated without the device. This design is adequate for testing the effectiveness of a device clinically with a single case because if it exists, the order effect can be observed and measured by comparing the control condition before and after the device is tested. In a formal research design, half of the participants are randomly assigned the control condition first and last, and the other half are tested with the device first, then the control condition, and then again with the device. Even if an order effect exists, counterbalancing allows order effects to be measured and removed statistically. This is called a *mixed design* and is one of the most powerful and useful designs for rehabilitation research. When treatment effects, like a training procedure, have a lasting effect, a "control-treatment-control" design might be used, but the client is tested at least twice during the first control condition. Any progressive changes within the control condition would indicate any order effects; the repeated measures during a control condition are also called a *baseline*. The control is often repeated later after the treatment to test for the persistence of treatment effects.

The reason a mixed design is so useful for rehabilitation research is because our clients vary so much individually. The case-controlled design can compensate for large individual differences and isolate smaller changes in performance, greatly increasing the power of the test (sensitivity to smaller differences), as well as enable the investigator to retrospectively identify the characteristics that predict who will benefit from a treatment and who will not.

For example, in a case-controlled design with 530 participants, without the magnification device, only 16% could read the small newspaper-sized (8-point) print used to measure the performance outcome. With a magnification device, 94% could read faster than 30 wpm.[28] This experiment involved comparison of performance on a case-by-case basis repeating the same measures of outcome with and without the devices. In this experiment, a retrospective analysis confirmed that visual acuity could be used to predict how much a person might benefit from the devices. Like grouped designs, the repeated-measures designs should have masking and placebo treatments to minimize the effect of expectations of the therapists and participants on the outcomes; this is difficult when testing devices.

When order effects are controlled, a case-controlled design is as valid as an RCT, is more sensitive to treatment effects, and because of the potential of a retrospective analysis to determine predictors of success, a potentially more informative design. Unlike the common cold, most retinal and optic nerve diseases and some neurological diseases that result in low vision are progressive; these impairments are likely to either not change or worsen with time, if anything, reducing a treatment effect. This order effect would actually decrease the likelihood of type I errors (incorrectly reporting a treatment effect). Thus, if participants have a progressive disease, a repeated-measures before-after experimental finding[24] that indicates a treatment improved performance can be considered valid even if order effects are not carefully controlled or measured because, if anything, the order effect would reduce the treatment effect.

Are the Characteristics of the Study Participants Similar to the Clients Whom You Treat?

To reduce the outcome variability and thus increase power (sensitivity to smaller treatment effects), RCT research designs develop inclusion and exclusion criteria that limit the diversity of participants, often eliminating those with multiple disabilities. For example, one widespread and serious flaw in low vision research is a tendency to exclude people with cognitive impairments. Clinically, we have found that people whose only impairment is vision rather quickly learn adaptive strategies and to use many devices; little skilled occupational therapy is needed. Occupational therapy, however, is usually needed for those who have cognitive, motoric, and physical disabilities—the same people who often are excluded from studies of the effectiveness of therapy. The alternative to restrictive criteria would be to have less restrictive criteria and, if a mixed design is used, to perform an analysis of characteristics and attempt to predict who might or might not benefit from an intervention, thus providing important clinical information.

Studies should, and often do, list the average demographic characteristics of the participants in both the treatment and control conditions. Does the study represent people of ages, gender, ethnicity, and with other disabilities that are similar to clients typically treated in your clinic?

Eligibility Criteria: Were the Study Participants Who Might Benefit From the Treatment Included or Excluded?

Usually, studies of magnification devices have an eligible visual acuity criterion that restricts participants to those who could benefit from use of a magnification device. Many studies of instructional interventions, however, often fail to select participants on the basis of a need for an intervention. This serious design flaw is akin to studying the effect of an analgesic on people who are not experiencing pain. For example, the need for skilled training for an electronic magnification device was evaluated in a recent prospective RCT with masked examiners at multiple sites. The study found that longer training by a skilled therapist was not significantly different from the performance after brief training by a salesperson. The authors concluded that "based on these results, outpatient low-vision rehabilitation centers may consider reallocating part of the training resources into other evidence-based rehabilitation programs." This finding was published in a prestigious ophthalmology journal.[29,30] In this study, people with cognitive disability were excluded, as is often the practice for an RCT. The groups were compared. The experimental and control group had comparable diseases, about 75% of which had macular degeneration and comparable visual acuities ranging from about 20/60 equivalent to a little over 20/500 equivalent, with an average of 20/150 equivalent. Because it was a prospective RCT with evidence of unbiased selection of groups, it might be considered the highest level of evidence. In fact, the design was seriously flawed. The problem with this study is that the eligibility requirements did not select people for training who actually needed training. An electronic magnifier is relatively easy to learn to use, especially for someone used to using magnification devices (80% to 90% of the participants had used magnification devices previously). In our experience, instruction on an electronic magnifier may range from about 15 minutes to several sessions, depending on a person's cognitive ability and prior experience with electronic devices and magnification devices. Indeed, the cognitive exclusion criterion in this study actually excluded people who would have benefited from the more intense, skilled instruction used as the experimental treatment. In their review of the effects of low vision services, Binns et al[22] noted that larger effects from low vision rehabilitation services were more likely in studies of people with more severe vision loss, but otherwise, reviews have not paid explicit attention to this design problem, leading many to include that providing therapy beyond the prescription of devices did not improve outcomes.

SUMMARY

This chapter presented an overview of an evidence-based approach to evaluation and treatment that is consistent with what is now required by Medicare, Medicaid, and most payers, as well as critical consumers of health care. Most importantly, by adopting an adult learning approach, therapy becomes client centered and driven by a client's expressed needs. Under this model, a therapist often finds that clients initially reject a recommended device, environmental modification, or intervention. To convince a client to accept devices and interventions, the therapist will find it necessary first to focus on objective goals set by the client, then to consider the reason for an objection and address this concern in a revised treatment plan, and finally, acceptance often results if a therapist can demonstrate performance with and without the intervention to convince the client of its effectiveness. This clinical approach is also called a *case-controlled* research design, which is often more valid for rehabilitation research, especially when assistive devices are being evaluated. Evidence-based practice, therefore, is not just about reading research. Evidence-based practice is an effective method of providing client-centered clinical care.

REFERENCES

1. World Health Organization. *International classification of impairments, disabilities, and handicaps: A manual of classification relating to the consequences of disease.* Twenty-ninth World Health Assembly. Geneva: World Health Organization; 1980.
2a. Amini DA, Kannenberg K, Bodison S, et al. Occupational Therapy Practice Framework: Domain & Process, 3rd Edition. *Am J Occup Ther.* 2014;S1-s48.
2b. Knowles MS, Holton EF, Swanson RA. *The Adult Learner.* 7th ed. New York: Routledge; 2012.
3. Sunness JS, El Annan J. Improvement of visual acuity by refraction in a low-vision population. *Ophthalmology.* 2010;117:1442-1446.
4. Horowitz A, Brennan M, Reinhardt JP, MacMillan T. The impact of assistive device use on disability and depression among older adults with age-related vision impairments. *J Gerontol B Psychol Sci Soc Sci.* 2006;61B:S274-280.
5. Chung STL, Truong SR. Learning to identify crowded letters: does the learning depend on the frequency of training? *Vision Res.* 2013;77:41-50.
6. McIlwaine GG, Bell JA, Dutton GN. Low vision aids—Is our service cost effective? *Eye.* 1991;5:607-611.
7. Graboyes M. Psychosocial implications of visual impairment. In: Brilliant RL, ed. *Essentials of Low Vision Practice.* Boston, MA: Butterworth-Heinemann; 1999:12-17.
8. Watson GR. Older adults with low vision. In: Corn AL, AJ Koenig, eds. *Foundations of Low Vision: Clinical and Functional Perspectives.* New York: American Foundation for the Blind; 2000:363-390.
9. Quillman RD, Goodrich GL. Interventions for adults with visual impairments. In: Lueck AH, ed. *Functional Vision: A Practitioner's Guide to Evaluation and Intervention.* New York: AFB Press; 2004:423-474.
10. Smith TM. Refinement of the low vision independence measure: a qualitative study. *Phys Occup Ther Geriatr.* 2013;31:182-196.
11. Stelmack JA, Rinne S, Mancil RM, et al. Successful outcomes from a structured curriculum used in the veterans affairs low vision intervention trial. *J Vis Impair Blind.* 2008;102:636-648.
12. Stelmack JA, Massof RW. Using the VA LV VFQ-48 and LV VFQ-20 in low vision rehabilitation. *Optom Vis Sci.* 2007;84:705-709.
13. Gateley C, Borcherding S. *Documenting Manual for Occupational Therapy: Writing Soap Notes.* 3rd ed. Thorofare, NJ: SLACK, Inc; 2012.
14. Whittaker SG, Lovie-Kitchin JE. Visual requirements for reading. *Optom Vis Sci.* 1993;70:54-65.
15. Higgins JPT, Green S, eds. *Cochrane Handbook for Systematic Reviews of Interventions Version 5.1.0 [updated March 2011].* www.cochrane-handbook.org: Cochrane Collaboration; 2011.
16. Concato J, Horwitz RI. Beyond randomised versus observational studies. *Lancet.* 2004;363:1660-1661.
17. Arbesman M, Lieberman D, Berlanstein DR. Methodology for the systematic reviews on occupational therapy interventions for older adults with low vision. *Am J Occup Ther.* 2013;67:272-278.
18. Liu C-J, Brost MA, Horton VE, Kenyon SB, Mears KE. Occupational therapy interventions to improve performance of daily activities at home for older adults with low vision: a systematic review. *Am J Occup Ther.* 2013;67:279-287.
19. Smallfield S, Clem K, Myers A. Occupational therapy interventions to improve the reading ability of older adults with low vision: a systematic review. *Am J Occup Ther.* 2013;67:288-295.
20. Justiss MD. Occupational therapy interventions to promote driving and community mobility for older adults with low vision: a systematic review. *Am J Occup Ther.* 2013;67:296-302.
21. Berger S, McAteer J, Schreier K, Kaldenberg J. Occupational therapy interventions to improve leisure and social participation for older adults with low vision: a systematic review. *Am J Occup Ther.* 2013;67:303-311.
22. Binns AM, Bunce C, Dickinson C, et al. How effective is low vision service provision? A systematic review. *Survey Ophthalmol.* 2012;57:34-65.
23. Cicerone KD, Langenbahn DM, Braden C, et al. Evidence-based cognitive rehabilitation: updated review of the literature from 2003 through 2008. *Arch Phys Med Rehabil.* 2011;92:519-530.
24. Cicerone KD, Dahlberg C, Malec JF, et al. Evidence-based cognitive rehabilitation: updated review of the literature from 1998 through 2002. *Arch Phys Med Rehabil.* 2005;86:1681-1692.
25. Legge GE. *Psychophysics of Reading in Normal and Low Vision.* Mahwah, NJ: Lawrence Erlbaum Associates; 2007.
26. Rovner BW, Casten RJ, Hegel MT, et al. Low vision depression prevention trial in age-related macular degeneration: a randomized clinical trial. *Ophthalmology.* 2014; pre publication.
27. Baldasare J, Watson GR, Whittaker SG, Miller-Shaffer H. The development and evaluation of a reading test for low vision individuals with macular loss. *J Vis Impairment Blindness.* 1986;80:785-789.
28. Nguyen NX, Weismann M, Trauzettel-Klosinski S. Improvement of reading speed after providing of low vision aids in patients with age-related macular degeneration. *Acta Ophthalmologica.* 2009;87:849-853.
29. Burggraaff MC, van Nispen RMA, Hoeben FP, Knol DL, van Rens GHMB. Randomized controlled trial on the effects of training in the use of closed-circuit television on reading performance. *Invest Ophthalmol Vis Sci.* 2012;53:2142-2150.
30. Burggraaff MC, van Nispen RMA, Knol DL, Ringens PJ, van Rens GHMB. Randomized controlled trial on the effects of CCTV training on quality of life, depression, and adaptation to vision loss. *Invest Ophthalmol Vis Sci.* 2012;53:3645-3652.

10

Foundation Skills
and Therapeutic Activities

In occupational therapy, occupation is used not only as the goal of treatment, but also as a means for developing necessary foundation skills and abilities that a person might need for many different goals. For example, reading and scanning and playing a card game are engaging activities that help build foundation visual scanning skills for other activities as well. These activities could include teaching the client and caregivers how to recognize and correct problems with lighting, another foundation skill. Treatment for leisure activities like watching TV typically involves using magnification strategies in addition to magnification devices to enable the client to see print and objects and to recognize people. Magnification is an important and widely used foundation intervention for people with impaired visual acuity. Clients with blind spots in the center of their visual field (central scotoma) and peripheral field loss also struggle with reading and spatial localization, and a therapist might use activities valued by a client that require finding and localizing objects in their immediate surroundings and avoiding tripping hazards to provide a foundation for compensatory scanning skills that can be used for other activities as well. Effective reading and scanning of one's environment is closely linked to the

ability to fixate and make accurate, rapid eye movements called *saccades*. One often must relearn saccade control and scanning in order to recover reading and localization of objects in space. Studies demonstrate, however, that in spite of the permanent visual acuity loss and central scotoma, a person can learn to fixate more accurately and make more accurate saccades after vision rehabilitation. Thus, reading and localization of objects in space are foundation skills that have been shown to improve after vision rehabilitation as the client learns to more effectively use remaining vision.

In occupational therapy, the development of meaningful occupation is not only a means but also an end, the ultimate outcome for an occupational therapist. Toward this end, the occupational therapist should consider nonvisual as well as visual solutions to enable someone to enjoy a book or find something in a store. Use of other senses becomes more important in people with more severe vision loss, but is still useful even in cases of milder vision loss. The following chapters elaborate upon the basic therapeutic activities described in this chapter and outline basic principles that form the conceptual foundation for adaptive devices and strategies in the remainder of this book.

Whittaker SG, Scheiman M, Sokol-McKay DA.
Low Vision Rehabilitation: A Practical Guide for Occupational Therapists,
Second Edition (pp 161-179).
© 2016 Taylor & Francis Group.

READING AS A THERAPEUTIC ACTIVITY

Reading is not only a common occupational goal, it is a valuable therapeutic activity to recover visual skills and learn to use assistive devices. Chapter 15 describes how to enable a person to achieve a reading goal using a combination of visual and nonvisual strategies. This section will focus on the use of visual reading as a therapeutic activity. As the first step to recovery of visual reading, the therapist must determine how to meet the visual requirements for reading. The purpose of this section is to enable the therapist to determine the magnification and contrast requirements for reading in order to provide eccentric viewing training and further evaluate lighting and magnification requirements. In our practice, reading provides a framework of treatment. If a client cannot read because of literacy or cognitive impairment, the therapist must be creative in finding alternative methods. Understanding how reading is used as a therapeutic activity will guide the therapist in locating alternative methods for an individual for other activities as well. It is generally advisable to have reading materials available in multiple languages, or one can simply ask the client to bring in reading materials that are short and easy to read.

In using reading as a therapeutic activity, for a success-oriented approach (see Chapter 6), the goal is to have the client succeed at reading, ideally with some personally meaningful or enjoyable material. The reading task must provide the client with immediate feedback if words or numbers are not correctly identified. The Learn to Use Your Vision (LUV) reading series is well designed for this progression.[1,2] For example, from the LUV reading chart, one exercise asks the reader tasks such as "pick out the words that are names of something you find in a grocery store." There are 2 correct responses per line, so the reader knows by the end of the line whether reading was accurate or not.

The occupational therapy evaluation is described in detail in Chapter 8, and how to use the findings to enable a client to reach a particular reading goal is presented in Chapter 15. What follows is a brief review for the purposes of using reading as a therapeutic activity. The therapist must know or measure the reading acuity, letter contrast sensitivity, and visual fields in order to undertake reading rehabilitation (see Chapters 7 and 8).

Visual Acuity and Critical Print Size Assessment

The evaluation and treatment for reading problems related to low vision require an appropriate near reading acuity chart that includes a logarithmic progression of sizes and the same reading level and sentence lengths for different print sizes, such as the MNREAD and SKREAD (see Chapter 8). To quickly review the determination of critical print size, when the therapist evaluates functional reading with a recommended continual text reading test, the client begins reading with the largest print and reads each line as quickly as possible. The smallest print size just before reading slows is the *critical print size*. This is the smallest print size that should be used to begin treatment. Later, as skills advance, the critical print size may decrease. As an additional and significant convenience, charts such as the MNREAD have been designed so that each line is of the same length. The therapist uses a stopwatch to time how long it takes to read each line (reading time) and quickly determines the critical print size as the smallest print size before reading time begins to increase, indicating slower reading rate. As will be discussed later, the pattern of errors may indicate maladaptive fixation and scanning eye movements. For training purposes, we have provided sentences of the same length as the MNREAD sentences. These training sentences have not been standardized for difficulty (see www.routledge.com/9781617116339). Table 10-1 indicates the usual print size for various print media in the more common point scale and the standardized metric (M) scale. Also indicated are the visual requirements for fluent reading for these various types of printed material.

Contrast Threshold Assessment

For reading and lighting evaluation, contrast sensitivity should be measured with a contrast chart (see Chapter 8). The contrast of common print media and contrast threshold requirements are listed in Table 10-2. For functional reading testing, the most relevant results are measured with the test distance chosen so that symbol size is at about 2× to 4× acuity threshold. When using reading as a therapeutic activity, the contrast sensitivity test can be used to assess field of view and detect relative scotomas. Have the subject fixate a single character on the contrast chart and ask if adjacent characters can be seen. Sometimes, a person can see adjacent higher-contrast characters, but with lower-contrast characters, adjacent characters disappear into a "relative" scotoma or area of reduced vision.

Assessment of Field of View

If a client has a reduced field of view, the therapist can estimate and monitor field of view throughout treatment. During an evaluation of central visual fields described earlier, the therapist can assess the characteristics of eccentric viewing and the size and location of the central scotoma. Field of view can be directly measured by having the client attempt to read using words of different lengths while fixating the first letter of the word as described earlier. A therapist can infer field restrictions from actual reading

TABLE 10-1: TYPICAL PRINT SIZES AND ACUITY REQUIREMENTS

TEXT SIZE	SAMPLE		TEXT ACUITY USUALLY REQUIRED
N scale (points)	*M scale*	*Approximate; point size varies with font type*	
3 pt	0.4M	NORMAL acuity threshold at 40 cm	
4 pt	0.5M		
5 pt	0.6M	Ads, bibles	0.3
6 to 8 pt	0.8 M	Telephone book	0.4
8 to 10 pt	1.0 M	Newspaper	0.5
10 to 12 pt	1.25M	Magazines, books, computer	0.6
12 to 14 pt	1.6M	Books, typewriter	0.8
16 to 18 pt	2.0 M	Child and large print	1.0
18 to 20 pt	2.5M	Large print	1.2

TABLE 10-2: TYPICAL PRINT CONTRAST AND CONTRAST THRESHOLD REQUIREMENTS

Contrast Threshold Requirements

TEXT CONTRAST OF READING MATERIAL	USES	SEVERE LOSS *(10:1 contrast reserve) Cannot fully compensate*	MODERATE LOSS *Can usually fully compensate with optimized lighting*
> 95%	Computer and CCTV display with no reflections	Greater than 10% contrast threshold	5% to 10% contrast threshold
85% to 95%	Good quality print	Greater than 8% contrast threshold	4% to 8% contrast threshold
60% to 70%	Newsprint, telephone directory, paperback books	Greater than 5% contrast threshold	2.5% to 5% contrast threshold
50%	Cash register receipts, US paper money	Greater than 2.5% contrast threshold	1.2% to 5% contrast threshold

performance by the error pattern. Clients with restricted fields will tend to spell words, hesitate, omit the end of longer words, or miss the last letters on a line when reading a near visual acuity chart. The SKREAD and Pepper tests described in Chapter 8 were designed to enable users to measure reading speed with different word lengths and to score errors to estimate field restrictions and scanning problems. It is important to attempt to estimate field of view during reading because people with central field loss may use different viewing positions for reading than for other tasks.

A surprising finding in our review of the research on vision and reading is that people can read fluently with a rather narrow 5- to 6-character field of view.[3] This assumes that the client is reading by scrolling text, slowly moving the line of print from right to left while looking straight ahead, rather than scanning left to right with typical eye movement patterns. When someone reads with magnification, he or she typically moves scrolled text from right to left in front of the narrow field of a magnification device or under an electronic viewer, such as a closed-circuit television (CCTV). The major problem created by a restricted field of view is scanning a page for relevant information and losing one's place when reading. Once the line of text is found, however, it can still be read fluently as long as there is sufficient magnification and print contrast.

Central field loss, which generally results from macular degeneration, has a particularly devastating effect on visual reading. Although most people with any level of central field loss can recover visual spot reading sufficient for activities of daily living (ADL) with appropriate magnification, recovery of highly fluent reading cannot be attained with large central scotoma unless nonvisual reading strategies are used.

Assessment of Reading Performance

Performance is evaluated before and during treatment and as part of an ongoing evaluation of intervention strategies. It is useful to have numerous short passages of relatively easy-to-read, engaging material for nonstandardized evaluation during this process. The Pepper Visual Skills for Reading Test[4] is valuable for a standardized reading evaluation (see Chapter 8). This test uses unrelated words that increase in length and line spacing. It has exceptional test-retest reliability, has been validated, and might, therefore, be used to document changes in reading performance as a benchmark test for documenting the efficacy of devices and therapeutic intervention. The test also has diagnostic value in revealing scanning difficulties in people with central field loss. Also designed for adults with low vision, the Morgan Test of Reading Comprehension allows one to document literacy limitations using a validated instrument.[5] Otherwise, one can simply measure word identification accuracy and to calculate reading rate, by counting the number of words a person might read from any reading material that is of interest to the client. Standardized testing becomes important if slower progress in improving reading rate is anticipated and is justified if limits (such as Medicare caps) are reached or exceeded because we must carefully measure and document progress to justify continued treatment. With eccentric viewing instruction, when comparing reading strategies with right field restrictions and, during the treatment of spatial neglect, one needs to measure slower progress (see Chapter 11).

COMPENSATING FOR IMPAIRED VISUAL ACUITY

In low vision rehabilitation, the general approach to treating impaired visual acuity is by magnifying print or an object of interest. In managing impaired acuity, however, one must consider visual acuity as well. Central to the therapeutic reasoning is the concept of "acuity reserve"[3] that was developed from research on reading. Acuity reserve is the difference between print that a client is attempting to recognize and acuity threshold, the smallest target a person is able to recognize. For a person to recognize some text, the letters must be larger than acuity threshold—a positive acuity reserve. For optimal reading, print size must be over 2 to 3 times the acuity threshold for someone with low vision, just like it is for someone with typical vision—a

greater than 2:1 acuity reserve.[3] The 2 general approaches to increasing acuity reserve include magnifying print or improving visual acuity threshold. For example, if a client is trying to read 2M (16-point) print and the acuity threshold is 2M acuity, he or she can barely read typical large print with the zero acuity reserve. To make reading easier, acuity reserve can be increased to twice the acuity threshold by magnifying the print to the equivalent of a 4M (32-point) size. The same 2:1 acuity reserve, however, can also be achieved without changing the 2M (16-point) print size, but rather by improving visual acuity down to a 1M (8-point) threshold with, for example, a refraction. Since large-print books are widely available printed with 2M (16-point) font, improving acuity would enable someone to read without any magnification device. Even though 1M acuity at 40 cm (20/50 equivalent) is not normal, such improvements in acuity can have profound functional impact. This general approach can be applied to any object or target, such as recognizing facial expressions or counting stiches on needlework; for comfortable, efficient performance, the magnified object should be larger than the size where the critical detail is barely recognizable at acuity threshold.

Improving Visual Acuity

Optometrists and ophthalmologists are responsible for remediating and improving acuity loss by performing a careful refraction, clearing the vitreous in the eye, and removing cataracts. Unfortunately, some general eye care practitioners will not perform careful refractions or provide medical interventions such as a vitrectomy or cataract removal if a person will still have impaired acuity after the procedure. Such a doctor might tell the client, "It will not help." Any significant improvement in visual acuity, however, can help by increasing acuity reserve. The therapist should, therefore, ensure that a recent refraction has been done. To determine if it "helps" or not, the low vision therapist can check the refraction using a trial frame to determine if improvements are significant enough to warrant the purchase of new eyeglasses (see Chapter 7). With medical interventions that are risky, acuity potential can be predicted by the treating ophthalmologist using laser interferometer or a Potential Acuity Meter. In such cases, the low vision therapist may speak with the eye care practitioner to determine if the benefit of a surgical or medical intervention is worth the risk.

The therapist may also improve visual acuity by using devices that enhance print contrast and by using lighting strategies that optimize lighting and minimize glare. This determination of glare sensitivity and optimal lighting should be included in the initial evaluation (see Chapter 8). Interventions to optimize lighting are discussed in a following section.

Magnification Strategies

The low vision treatment team generally groups magnification goals into distance goals and near goals because the treatment strategies and optical devices are different. At closer distances (less than about 1 meter), a person's ability to accommodate (focus his or her eyes) and, if a person is using both eyes, to converge his or her eyes greatly impacts performance.

Definition of Magnification

Magnification is a complicated concept due to the varied definitions and different methods for specifying the magnification of different types of devices (see Chapter 5). In low vision rehabilitation, although magnification has a common general definition ("an increase in the apparent size of an object"), the precise mathematical definition varies significantly.

Ultimately, the low vision practitioner is interested in enlarging the size of a retinal image. For example, visual acuity describes the size of the retinal image where the critical detail is just resolvable. Retinal image size is increased either by relative size or relative distance magnification (Figure 10-1). In the scientific literature, retinal image size is reported directly as the retinal image size of the critical detail called *minimum angle of resolution* (MAR). The MAR is one-fifth the size of a letter in minutes of arc. Trigonometry is required to calculate MAR; therefore, it is not practical to use in the clinic. In the low vision clinic, the emerging convention is to describe magnification at a distance greater than about 1M in terms of enlargement ratio (ER). Magnification at closer distances is described using equivalent power (EP) in diopters.[6,7] The functional vision evaluation (see Chapter 8) provides an estimate of the size and the distance of an object or text required by a client to perform a task; required size and distance are compared to the actual size and working distance to estimate the required enlargement or EP in diopters. The magnification of near devices is labeled in terms of diopters. Telescopes are labeled in terms of angular magnification, which is equivalent to enlargement. The therapist then simply selects the predicted device and can further modify overall magnification by changing the size of the object or print being used. For further distances, relative size and relative distance magnification strategies are used. For example, one might achieve size magnification by purchasing a large television screen or clock.

The following concepts of magnification are crucially important for the low vision therapist to understand because if a recommended magnifier is not working, the therapist often must try other magnifiers or change distances and seating, and should be able to set up devices and distances that have a magnification equivalent to the recommended device setup. A few formulas are thus required on the Academy for Certification of Vision Rehabilitation &

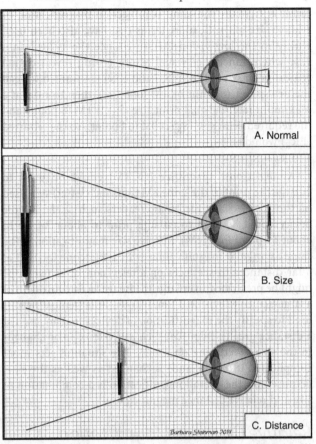

Figure 10-1. Illustration of how the image of a pen on the retina (A) might be magnified by relative size (B) and relative distance (C) magnification. (Reprinted with permission from Barbara Steinman.)

Education Professionals (ACVREP) certification exam for low vision therapists. The best way to become comfortable with these concepts is to practice solving problems. We use metric notation because calculations are much easier, and terms like "diopters" and the M size of print are metric units. We have taken care to reduce the number of formula required to the bare essentials. Five formula have been repeated throughout this book and are listed in Table 13-7.

Relative Size Magnification

Increasing the size of the letter, TV screen, or object (see Figure 10-1) enlarges the size of the image of an object on the retina. The relationship between object size and retinal image size can be approximated as a simple proportion. If you double the size of an object, you double the retinal image size of the object. Enlargement ratio (ER) refers to the ratio of 2 object sizes (S2, S1); thus, ER = S2/S1.[7] Consider an example of a client who wishes to read a goal print size (S_G) of 1M (8 point) newspaper-size font but a required print size (S_R) of 2M print to read fluently based on measured critical print size of 2M. Increasing the size of print from the goal print size (S_G) of 1M (8 point) to S_R = 2M (16 point) at a given distance is an ER of 2×. The definition of ER is virtually the same as projection magnification or relative size magnification, terms that have also been used widely in the low vision literature since the 1970s.[8] In a case where functional visual acuity testing revealed that critical print size was 8M (S_R) and a person wanted to read the newspaper (8 point or 1M font size), then to read at a maximum rate, the goal print size (S_G) is 1M (8 point) and the required print size (S_R) is 8M (64 point), so the required (ER_R) would be 8×.

$$ER_R = S_R / S_G$$

An electronic magnifier (CCTV) could be used to enlarge the print to the same 8M (half-inch letter) size used on the acuity chart. Electronic readers such as the Kindle device could be used to enlarge print to about 2× up to about 16-point font (2M). Relative size magnification is the same as angular magnification with a telescope focused at a far distance. To see faces on a television, a 3× telescope might be prescribed to enlarge the image to an equivalent of a large-screen television 3 times larger. Enlargement ratio is used to specify the magnification of devices that are used at a distance greater than 1M, such as a telescope or changes in the size of lettering on a sign. The situation gets more complicated if the distance is changed as well as the size, because now the overall magnification is a combination of size and relative distance magnification.

Relative Distance Magnification

Since enlarging items of interest is often not practical, the therapist will use relative distance magnification, achieving magnification by moving the client closer to the object of interest, thus enlarging the retinal image (see Figure 10-1). The relationship between object distance and retinal image size is approximated as a negative proportion. If you halve the distance of the object to the eye, you double the size of the retinal image. If you decrease the distance by 25%, you increase the retinal image size by 25%. Achieving relative distance magnification by moving a television screen from 8 feet to 4 feet is equivalent to doubling the size of the television screen.

The therapist seats a client closer to the object of interest—a TV, for example—until she or he quickly and reliably recognizes the object; this is the required test distance (d_R). The customary distance or preferred "goal" distance would be d_G. The required enlargement ratio (ER_R) can be simply calculated by dividing the goal distance by the required distance as follows:

$$ER_R = d_G / d_R$$

So if the client usually sits 3 meters away from the TV (about 9 feet) and must move to a seat 1 meter (3 feet) away to see facial expressions, then the ER required would be 3:1, or 3×. This indicates that if the client wishes to see the TV, he or she will need to enlarge the TV screen, sit closer, or use a telescope (angular magnification), or a combination of size, distance, and angular magnification.

Magnification Strategies at Distance

Very often, a combination of size, relative distance, and angular magnification is required because people find sitting too close to something to be uncomfortable, or higher telescopic magnifications have too narrow a field of view and higher size magnification is not practical.

Overall magnification (M_{OA}) at distances greater than about 1 meter can be calculated by simply multiplying relative distance and relative size magnification as follows:

$$M_{OA} = S_2/S_1 * d_1/d_2$$

where S_1 and d_1 are the original object size and distance and S_2 and d_2 are the new object size and distance.

If, for example, a therapist found in the functional vision evaluation that a client needed to decrease the distance from the television screen from the original distance of 3 meters (9 feet) to the new distance of 1 meter (3 feet) to see the screen, then the previous formula indicates an enlargement (d_1/d_2) of 3×. Now using the formula one can calculate that if the client rejected 1 meter (3 feet) as too close but found 2 meters (6 feet) more acceptable, then the actual magnification would be calculated as the original distance of 3 meters (d_1) divided by the new distance of 2 meters (d_2) equal to 1.5× magnification. Now at the 2-meter distance, a 2× telescope, or doubling the size of the screen from a 20-inch original size to a new 40-inch screen ($S_2/S_1 = 2×$), would result in the same overall magnification as decreasing the distance to 1 meter. Putting these numbers into the previous formula, we find 2 * 3/2 = 3×.

With distances less than about 1M, a client must focus his or her eyes to see clearly and near type devices that focus light must be used that ensure the client can see the object clearly. The amount of focus is specified as "power." The emerging convention is to specify the magnification of near devices in terms of equivalent power (EP).

Magnification Strategies at Near

If someone has refractive error, the eye care provider prescribes corrective lenses (distance correction) to focus objects that are far away on the retina (see Chapter 5). Even with correction for distance, when someone looks at an object up close, the eye must accommodate (focus), and as the lens focuses, it becomes thicker and acquires more power, which is the EP of adding a plus lens in front of the distance correction. This additional need to focus or accommodate for near objects is called *accommodative demand*. As people age, they lose the ability to accommodate and this decreases their ability to focus at near, an aging process called *presbyopia*. Reading glasses or bifocals are plus lenses that are added to a distance correction that allow people with presbyopia to focus at a closer distance. These reading glasses are also called *near vision addition* or *add*. For older individuals, the added plus lenses usually equals accommodative demand. For younger adults who can still accommodate (focus) at near, the required additional plus lens would be less than accommodative demand. The eye care provider estimates a person's ability to accommodate to calculate how much added plus lens is required.

The occupational therapist only needs to understand the power (P) of accommodative demand (expressed as diopters [D], which is calculated directly from the viewing distance). The formula that relates eye-to-object distance (d) in cm to the power (P) required for reading or working on tasks at near is as follows:

P(diopters) = 100/d(cm)

The typical reading distance is 40 cm (16 inches). Using the previous formula, a 2.5 D add is required for objects held at 40 cm. This also is called *accommodative demand*. The accommodative demand is not necessarily the same as the addition prescribed in the glasses, but is a combination of the prescribed addition and the client's accommodation or refractive error.

Equivalent Power Using Size and Distance Magnification

The use of handheld magnifiers, microscopes, telemicroscopes, enlargement, the electronic magnifier (CCTV), or just working at a close distance without glasses are all potential magnification strategies for achieving better performance at near. To compare devices, the therapist must be able to calculate the equivalent magnification for a client to perform a variety of near goal tasks, such as needlepoint, clipping fingernails, bill paying, and reading a book. *Power in diopters* is a universal term that describes the magnification of all near devices. The term *equivalent power* (EP) describes the magnification as "equivalent" to the accommodative demand required for a particular eye-to-object distance. The distance is called *equivalent viewing distance*. For example, a manufacturer might specify the magnification of a handheld magnifier used as "20 D power." This means that the magnifier has magnification equivalent to someone using a 20 D of near add with a lens-to-object distance of 5 cm (even though the actual power of the lenses and distances may differ). This now allows us to use the same term for describing the magnification of another near device. Essentially, the term *equivalent power* describes magnification that is equivalent to the accommodative demand when something is held close enough to see it.

In practice, the formula for EP is different from the formula for accommodative demand. As with distance magnification, estimating overall magnification of the image on the retina requires that we not only consider the distance, but also the enlargement of the object being viewed. As described earlier, the therapist might enlarge print or use larger objects, as well as decrease working distance. Some devices, such as telemicroscopes, enlarge the appearance of objects as well as focus at a closer distance, and the rated magnification is considered the same as size magnification or ER. Equivalent power can be calculated by simply multiplying the accommodative demand (100/d) by the ER. The formula for calculating P is as follows:

P(diopters) = 100/d(cm) * ER

This important formula can be used to approximate the EP of all optical devices or viewing situations at near. For example, if a client requires that regular print be doubled from 1M (8 point) to 2M (16 point) to read comfortably, the ER is 2.0. If he or she is reading at the customary reading distance of 40 cm, the accommodative demand is 100/d(cm), or 2.5 D, and this would be multiplied by an ER of 2 to calculate the EP of 5 equivalent diopters. This would be equivalent to reading the 1M print at 20 cm, a distance at which the actual accommodative demand is 5 D. Note that even when print is simply enlarged or an e-reader or a CCTV is used at a normal reading distance, EP increases even though reading addition or optical devices do not change. The low vision therapist often must change working distance, object size, and the power of magnification to please a client, all while keeping the same overall magnification. If the eye-to-object distance changes, the eye care provider needs to be consulted to prescribe a new reading addition.

One important finding here is that one can estimate required magnification using a reading acuity test for near or relative distance magnification for distance, and one can accurately predict the required magnification of optical devices. With a reading acuity test, the print size can be directly converted into EP by dividing critical print size by the goal print size (usually 1M) and multiplying by accommodative demand (usually 2.4 diopters at a 40-cm test distance). Likewise, bringing the TV or an object closer at distance is easily achieved as well. Because these evaluation procedures are easily performed, one is likely to have an accurate estimate of required magnification for any number of different devices.[9] Trial and error is minimized because it is more likely that the predicted device will work. When one then evaluates a powerful magnifier or a stronger telescope and the device that was predicted using a formula to work does not, then the therapist knows that the problem is not magnification; it is something else, like lighting or improper positioning.

For reading, working in a shop, sewing, or playing cards, the distances are typically 50 cm (20 inches) or less and require near strategies. For adults over 40, some sort of optical device is usually required (see Chapter 13), but the principles of size and relative distance magnification still apply. For example, visual acuity testing with the MNREAD (see Chapter 8) might indicate that the person can fluently read normal 1M print, but only at a distance of 10 cm (4 inches). Strong reading glasses will be required and are often difficult and uncomfortable to use. The therapist might introduce larger print or an e-reader to double the size of the print, allowing the client to now hold the material at a more comfortable 20 cm (8 inches) with reading glasses that are not as strong. A client can read regular-size playing cards when held in the hand at 20 cm, but not if the cards are played on a table 50 to 60 cm away. The therapist might then obtain large-font playing cards with numbers and suits that are 3× normal size, again employing the principles of size and distance magnification. With an older adult, changes in the working distance usually require some optical correction, so an optometrist or ophthalmologist must be consulted. In addition to stronger reading glasses, the therapy team might use handheld magnifiers, telescopes focused at near, stand magnifiers, or electronic devices to enable a person to read or perform a task visually at different distances, all less than about 50 cm. These devices are the focus of discussion in Chapters 13 and 14.

In summary, magnification is usually the method used in low vision rehabilitation to compensate for reduced visual acuity. For working distances less than about 1M, the magnification of any optical device, or just a change in object size, can both be described as EP using equivalent diopters (ED) as the measurement units. At distances greater than about 1 meter, then ER is used to describe required magnification. Five formula are required to apply these important concepts.

LIGHTING AND CONTRAST

Similar to the concept of acuity reserve is "contrast reserve."[10] Contrast reserve is the print contrast (expressed as a percentage) divided by contrast threshold. Print contrast of 100% is the highest possible; 0% is no contrast at all. Contrast reserve can be increased by increasing the contrast of objects or print, or by improving contrast threshold. The contrast of common objects is provided in Table 10-2. Although there is not yet an evidence basis for generalizing the concept, we find it useful for nonreading tasks as well. For example, to detect a carpeted step quickly and reliably, one should make sure the contrast of the step is at least 20 to 30 times the contrast threshold. Contrast threshold is affected by cataracts, blood in the vitreous, retinal edema, or optic atrophy from conditions such as multiple sclerosis and other potentially treatable medical conditions that require the consultation of an eye care provider. Glare and lighting can have significant effects on both object contrast and contrast threshold.

A person who has typical vision can maintain normal visual acuity over a tremendous range of light levels and, as a result, changes in light have little effect on performance. Low vision often greatly narrows the range of optimum light required for performance. Thus, evaluating the effect of light intensity on performance is a critical part of the low vision evaluation because incorrect light levels might result in decreased visual acuity,[11,12] contrast sensitivity, and even increase the size of central scotomas with macular degeneration.[13] Although more light is generally better in older adults, there are significant individual differences in what is optimal lighting[14] that have not been explained or predicted by research. Glare always impairs vision, but people vary in their susceptibility to glare effects. Increasing light inevitably increases glare somewhat. As a result, we have noticed that in highly glare-sensitive individuals, vision might actually decrease with higher light levels.

An individualized lighting evaluation is, therefore, necessary to define the range of optimal light. It becomes essential to measure and optimize light before undertaking a task or performing a therapeutic activity. To avoid time-consuming trial and error, try different lighting with each task; the optimum light levels are measured during the evaluation with a light meter or the LuxIQ (see Chapter 8). The therapist first measures reading acuity or contrast sensitivity with normal room lights, then modifies the lighting (usually increasing illumination) to impress the client that lighting is important and to measure the range of light levels that provide the best acuity and contrast sensitivity. Once this is done, the therapist can use the light meter measurements to simply reproduce the light levels for any given situation or task. One may perform environmental assessment and modification to minimize glare and set these optimal light levels.[12] If a client has the cognitive ability, our preference is to teach the client to evaluate the lighting in a given environment such and to position her or his body, the object of interest, or the light source to minimize glare and optimize light levels. For example, a client might learn that when entering a restaurant, sit with a window to the side for maximum glare-free light. If a person is found to see best over a narrow range of illuminance, the person can learn to use his or her vision to set the correct light intensity; a light meter is not required.

Specific intervention strategies are described in Chapter 12. Some general principles of lighting and contrast enhancement are as follows (see the online appendix for a handout on consumer instructions for lighting). Clients and their families should be educated to manage the clients' lighting requirements. A client usually can use visual benchmarks, like other people's faces or print, to identify poor lighting and apply compensatory strategies.

- Optimizing light levels
  - The low vision therapist is usually interested in measuring illuminance, the amount of light shining onto an object, measured as lux. Luminance may vary from 50 to 100 lux in typical residential settings with shaded table lights, 1000 lux in brightly lit stores, up to over 5000 lux with intense directional task lighting.
  - Light sources like light bulbs are measured in terms of luminance, and the typical measure used commercially is "lumens." Until recently, the luminance of a bulb was described on the packaging as

"wattage," but with newer, energy-efficient lights, wattage is no longer appropriate as a measure of luminance and is being replaced by lumens. Flashlights are usually under 100 lumens, but some are now available over 200 lumens. Halogen spotlights can produce over 1000 lumens.

○ Contrast is usually measured as the illuminance of an object, contour, or letter divided by the sum of illuminance of both the object or contour and the background, varying from 0% contrast (a white letter on a white background) to 100% contrast (a deep flat-black letter on a white background). With electronic devices, "contrast polarity" can be changed from black letters on a white background to white letters on a black background, reducing the glare from the screen.

○ The best method to vary lighting is to vary the distance of a directional light from the object being viewed. Illumination (light falling on an object) increases by an *inverse square law*. As a result, a light that is moved to half the distance might increase the illumination 4 times. This is described in more detail in Chapter 12. Using a directional light on an adjustable arm is usually the ideal choice for lighting because the client can easily position it to minimize glare and the distance adjusted to optimize illuminance on the object or print being viewed. Flashlights are effective and portable light sources.

● Glare avoidance

○ The best position of a light is from the side because there is less reflective glare and contrast is greater. Overhead light tends to reflect off of the lenses of eyeglasses and the page a person is reading, reducing contrast.

○ A hat with a brim is effective in glare control with overhead lighting.

○ A client should be taught to recognize and avoid glare. A glare source is any light or reflection of a light that a person can look at directly.

○ Enhancing the contrast of objects will help those with impaired contrast sensitivity.

○ Wrap-around absorptive lenses (sunlenses) of different colors should be evaluated for bright indoor settings like supermarkets and darker sunlenses for outdoor use. Some colors, especially yellow and light orange tints, or polaroid lenses allow greater light levels by reducing glare.

LEARNING TO COMPENSATE FOR CENTRAL FIELD LOSS

Macular degeneration ranks as the most common cause of low vision in developed countries (see Chapter 4 for details). As the disease progresses to the end stage, it usually restricts damage to the central visual field, the macula, and immediately surrounding area, creating a central scotoma. A *scotoma* is a "blind spot," an island in the visual field with reduced or no vision that is surrounded by better vision. The central portion of our visual field, the macula, comprises the central 15 to 20 degrees of visual angle, an area about twice the width of a fist at arm's length.[1] With macular degeneration, this central region is damaged and creates a central scotoma. Investigators have measured scotoma sizes in people with macular degeneration up to about 30 degrees, an area about the size of 3 fist widths. In addition to macular degeneration, central field loss occurs with untreated diabetic retinopathy and cortical blindness. With these conditions and a severe form of dry macular degeneration called "geographic atrophy," the central field loss might be larger than that associated with macular degeneration.

There are 2 types of macular degeneration. With the *exudative* (wet) type, retinal swelling might distort the shape of objects being viewed, and the person might have multiple scotomas or islands of vision rather than one large central scotoma. With untreated exudative macular degeneration, onset of vision loss occurs suddenly, with more extensive vision loss at first due to hemorrhaging at the retinal level. As blood in the vitreous dissipates, the measured scotoma will stabilize and shrink and contrast sensitivity will improve somewhat. *Atrophic* (dry) macular degeneration usually begins with a *relative scotoma* (ie, an area of reduced visual acuity). This area gradually increases in size and density, allowing the affected individual to adapt to loss of central vision. In some cases, people will experience active hallucinations in the scotoma, referred to as Charles Bonnet syndrome (CBS). Medical treatment for macular degeneration due to retinal pathology may slow the progression of the wet type, but not the dry type. In some instances, there may be some improvement of vision, although typically not enough so that the client no longer has low vision.

Normally when a person looks from one object to another, the eye moves very quickly. This quick eye movement is called a *saccade*, and it results in central fixation of the target—the person positions his or her eyes so that the image of the object projects to the macula, the area of highest acuity on the retina. When a person with a central

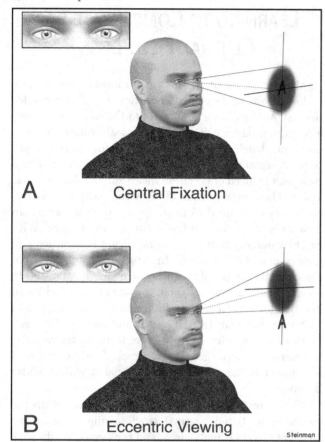

Figure 10-2. (A) Illustration of central viewing. (B) Eccentric viewing with Nilsson technique added. The letter A is the fixation target, and the cross indicates the scotoma center. (Reprinted with permission from Barbara Steinman.)

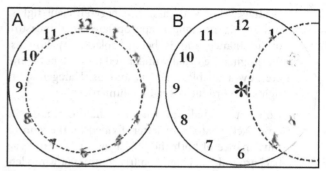

Figure 10-3. Clock face for eccentric viewing instruction. (A) Central fixation with numerals of best acuity indicated to the client's left. (B) Rightward eccentric viewing.

scotoma or blind area looks at an object with a central fixation, the object will suddenly disappear or become less clear because the macular area now has reduced (Figure 10-2). Every study that involves objective measurement of eye movements in people with central field loss found that an overwhelming majority of people with long-standing central field loss adapt by looking above, below, or to the side of the object of interest,[13,15-21] a compensatory scanning strategy now called *eccentric viewing*. From the very first studies,[20,22] it has been found that this eccentric viewing consistently projects the image of a target to one or more retinal areas outside of the macular called a *preferred retinal loci*, or PRL.[23] One study actually measured the development of PRL after loss of central vision in the preferred eye and found that all 25 patients studied had developed at least one PRL after about 6 months. Because of a paucity of randomized clinical trials, recent reviews have questioned whether training people to develop eccentric viewing is really necessary and effective.[24]

We have concluded that as with most instructional protocols, eccentric viewing training is a practice guideline—that is, it is effective in most but not all clients. Howe[15] reviewed 19 experiments, including repeated-measures

designs and case reports, and found the eccentric viewing instruction generally improved reading and ADL performance. As with any instructional protocol, the effectiveness of eccentric viewing instruction depends on whether a person has already developed an adaptive eccentric viewing position. Unfortunately, research has not identified factors that can be used to predict who will benefit from eccentric viewing instruction or not, but we can infer from research when a person might need instruction. With this level of evidence, performance needs to be periodically reevaluated to determine if the eccentric viewing training is affecting some goal activity.

If during the testing described later we find inconsistent fixation, then eccentric viewing training will likely help a person develop a PRL. A goal of eccentric viewing training might be to teach a person who has already developed a maladaptive fixation position a different, more adaptive eccentric viewing position. Rightward eccentric viewing (Figure 10-3) positions the scotoma to the right, reducing the right field of view, and substantial research has found the right field of view to be an important, if not *the* most important, visual factor for reading.[25] We have successfully used eccentric viewing training to teach a person to move the scotoma into a different position, usually upward or downward, to open up the right visual field. Downward eccentric viewing positions the scotoma so it has the same effect as an inferior visual field loss. Inferior visual fields affect safe mobility.[26,27] An upward eccentric viewing position preserves the inferior field of view. This position also preserves the right field of view for reading. For mobility, we often teach people with scotomas to scan laterally to the right and left. Finally, in our experience, eccentric viewing training is a difficult and time-consuming procedure that requires daily practice at home. One must question whether such an arduous procedure is worth the time and effort, given a person's goals and lifestyle.

Although research supports eccentric viewing training as a practice guideline, it does not favor any particular training method.[11,15] As a practice guideline (see Chapter 9), evidence-based practice requires frequent retesting using objective measures as evidence of effectiveness for each

TABLE 10-3: ECCENTRIC VIEWING INSTRUCTIONAL SEQUENCE

1. Perform scotoma awareness training and evaluate scotoma and eccentric viewing skills

2. If no or inconsistent eccentric viewing, train eccentric viewing with central fixation cue

3. Fade out central fixation cue and replace with intermittent to occasional verbal cues

4. If consistent eccentric viewing, attempt to train client to shift eccentric viewing positions with verbal cues

5. Learn to maintain eccentric position for TV watching, fading out central fixation cue

6. Find the best eccentric viewing position for reading

7. Develop habitual PRL for reading using steady eye technique

8. Patient ready for device evaluation and preliminary recommendation by optometrist

9. Reading training with the scrolling technique and introduction to magnification device

10. Final prescription of magnification device—home program with device

11. Tracking with and without a handheld device

12. Scanning without optical devices

individual. In early stages of training, if someone is first learning an eccentric viewing position, outcomes can be measured as the number of correct object or word identifications in a given period of time. For each measure, also describe the cuing, if any. These methods of testing transition into performance speed, such as words read correctly per minute. These data can be collected during training.

In this section we describe procedures developed by Gale Watson[2,5] and personal clinical experience that can be performed without expensive equipment, and includes properties common to all of the training procedures used in research studies that were shown to be effective. We recommend that readers continue to evaluate the research literature for better predictors of who will benefit from training and for more effective instructional methods.

Eccentric Viewing Training

Scotoma Awareness Instruction and Evaluation of Vision and Skills

The steps for eccentric viewing training are summarized in Table 10-3. The first and most important step has 2 objectives. The first is to determine if the client has already developed adaptive eccentric viewing or still has nonadaptive central fixation. The second is to teach the client to become aware of and in some cases visualize the central scotoma. As this instruction is best done by demonstration, the therapist can instruct the client and evaluate eccentric viewing and scotoma size at the same time. The client also requires education regarding the expected prognosis and reassurance that by learning a new way of looking at things, vision will once again become more predictable, although magnification will be required to read and recognize faces and TV again. Learning to eccentrically fixate is

difficult and can be frustrating. Care must be taken to carefully grade activities to ensure early success, to be positive, and to keep training sessions short.

Often, the visual system "fills in" the central scotomas (perceptual completion); the person with a central scotoma cannot see the blind area, but can be instructed to become aware of it. When asked to look at a target "so you can see it clearly," the beginner who has not yet developed eccentric viewing will tend to look directly at the target and it will disappear, but he or she can still see objects to the side. Scotoma awareness training requires demonstration combined with explanation. At the end of scotoma awareness training, the client should be able to describe the shape of the central blind spot and why things appear and disappear. In addition, the client will voluntarily move the blind spot to make isolated targets disappear, as well as position his or her eye to see an object most clearly. The client who has developed eccentric viewing will be able to voluntarily position the eye so that it is looking above, below, or to the side so the target that is straight ahead can be visualized. One case that illustrates this skill involves an attractive young woman who had adapted to a juvenile macular degeneration she acquired at age 16. She described one advantage of macular degeneration: at a party, she could make unattractive guys "go away" just by looking at them, while checking out the cute ones from the "corner of her eye." One might say she had mastered scotoma awareness.

There are several methods to approach scotoma awareness training. We describe 2 useful procedures: the tangent screen and clock face methods. Ideally, instruction should include both techniques. The clock face method is quickly administered; the tangent screen method might require approximately 5 to 10 minutes. A tangent screen is large and cumbersome; we now prefer just using a laser pointer to

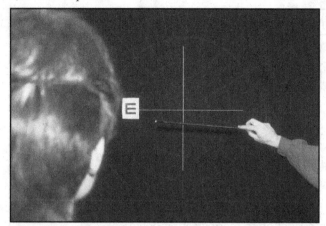

Figure 10-4. Tangent screen method. The E is the eccentric viewing target. The client is looking at the center of the cross, the central fixation cue. The client reports when the dot stimulus at the end of the wand appears and disappears. Often, the cross is eliminated to simplify the task visually.

project a spot stimulus on a light-colored wall. Sticky notes are stuck to the wall to create a fixation target and mark the outline of the scotoma.

The Clock Face Method

Wright et al developed methods available in a workbook that provides excellent worksheets and resources for eccentric viewing instruction.[5] The clock face method involves the use of a picture of a clock (see Figure 10-3) with a star at the center of the clock (we use a letter or a short word). It can be quickly adapted to the size of the scotoma and visual acuity by changing the distance of the clock from the client. The therapist tells the client to "look at the center of the clock so that you can see it." If the client still has central fixation tendencies, the client will report that the center star disappears and that all of the numbers can be seen. If the client cannot see the numerals, the therapist can move the clock closer until they can be seen, or use a larger picture of a clock. If the client has developed eccentric viewing, when asked to describe the shape at the center of the clock, the client will report that a star can be seen but that some of the numbers are missing. The missing numbers will indicate the location of the scotoma and direction of eccentric viewing. For example, if the numbers 2, 3, and 4 are missing, the client is eccentrically fixating to the right (see Figure 10-2). If all of the numbers can be seen and the client reports seeing the star, then 1 of 3 possibilities exists. One is that no scotoma exists. The second, most likely, option is that the client is not steadily fixating; rather, the client is looking around with searching eye movements. The therapist should carefully observe the client's eyes to ensure viewing is stable. This can be done by cutting a peephole above the fixation star so the therapist can look through it at the client's eyes. If the client has steady viewing, the third possibility is that the scotoma might be small or might be a relative scotoma (reduced central vision but enough vision to see shapes). In this case, the therapist moves the clock further away or dims the lights in the room until the client reports that the star fades from view (central fixation) or some numbers disappear (eccentric viewing). During this testing, scotoma awareness training involves explaining to the client about the center "blind spot" and pointing out how it can be moved by looking in different directions.

The Tangent Screen Method

The tangent screen method (see Figure 10-4 and Chapter 8) also can be used to combine central field testing and eccentric viewing evaluation with scotoma awareness training. The viewing target is usually a letter large enough for a client to recognize in the center of the felt board. The tangent screen method involves first positioning the viewing target in the center of the tangent screen. The letter is placed in the center of a large cross. The client is instructed to "look at the letter so that you can see it most clearly." With a large screen, the therapist is able to sit or stand between the client and the screen to carefully observe the client's eyes. The client who has not developed eccentric viewing and is still centrally fixating will fixate the center of the cross and report that the letter disappears. The person with adaptive eccentric viewing will report that he or she sees the letter in the center of the cross, and if the scotoma is large, eccentric viewing should be evident by looking at the eyes. If the client generates random searching movements, gently instruct the client to "look directly at the center of the cross—don't worry about the letter." If the client centrally fixates the cross, the letter will disappear into the scotoma.

If the client has nonadaptive central fixation, while the client continues to fixate and position the scotoma in the center of the cross, move the test spot (on the end of the wand or a laser spot) away from the center until the client sees it (see Figure 10-4). Mark the spot where the wand dot "appears" with a pin, and then start at the center and quickly move to the edge of the scotoma in all directions. The pins should be small or low contrast so they are not visible. Once all of the pins are in place, a thick high-contrast yarn can be placed around the pins to illustrate the size and location of the scotoma. If a wall is used, use light-colored sticky notes instead of pins and dark notes to form a visible diamond shape pattern for fixation and ask the client to look at the center of the grid.

Individuals who have had central field loss for several months or more may have already started to develop eccentric viewing. The client who has already developed stable eccentric viewing will position the eyes to be looking above, below, or to one side of the letter and will report seeing the whole letter. The client may also move the head. The therapist should be able to predict where the scotoma is expected to be located based on where the client's eyes appear to be looking, observing the eyes and not the head, because often the head is moved in the direction opposite to the eyes. Based on this prediction, the therapist moves a white testing spot at the end of a long black wand or the spot from a laser pointer to where the client appears to be looking (see Figure 10-3). It is essential that the therapist carefully watch the client's eyes to be sure that he or she does not move during this procedure. When the test spot enters the scotoma, the client will report that it disappears. Explain to the client that you have found the scotoma and that you will now be measuring how large it is. Move the wand dot until it is first seen and mark the edge of the scotoma with a low-contrast mark or pin (not visible to the client). The key to successful testing is to quickly move from a nonseeing area within the scotoma toward a seeing area and mark the border of the scotoma so that it is mapped in a couple of minutes. The outline of the scotoma should be above, below, or to the side of the letter, indicating the direction of eccentric viewing and the size of the scotoma.

With either the clock face or tangent screen method, if the therapist is not successful in mapping out a scotoma that is known to exist, then the person has not developed a PRL and will need eccentric viewing training.

The Functional Method

The functional method involves error analysis and careful attention to the client's subjective reports. In reading, errors involving the end of words, missed words (especially at the end of a line), and a client's subjective reports of only seeing the first few letters of a word all indicate limitations in the right field of view and a rightward eccentric viewing pattern. Difficulty finding the beginning of the next line or errors toward the beginning of words indicates a leftward eccentric viewing that would restrict the left field of view. People who tend to look downward will skip lines and lose their place, but generally an upward or downward eccentric viewing is ideal for reading. With TV watching or looking at a group of people several feet away, the subjective impressions of the client will indicate the direction of eccentric viewing; the scotoma and habitual viewing position will be indicated by the direction where people or objects tend to be less clear or absent. Note that if a person is scanning to fill in the scotoma, he or she will not report missing objects and people.

Eccentric Training With a Central Fixation Cue

This phase of instruction should be done with clients who have not developed adaptive eccentric viewing and do not give consistent results unless asked to look at the center of the clock or look at the center of the X on the tangent screen. These individuals will fixate more consistently with a cue that will not disappear when they look at it (see Table 10-3). The purpose of this instruction is to eventually have the client eccentrically, not centrally, view; that is, to look in a particular direction above, below, or to the side

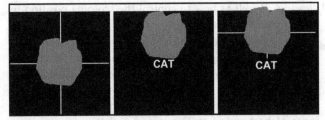

Figure 10-5. (A) Tangent screen with scotoma with central fixation. (B) Upward viewing with word stimulus without a central fixation cue. (C) Upward viewing with a central fixation cue.

of a target—to eccentrically fixate in order to see a target that is positioned at the center of the screen. Note that to avoid confusion we use the term *eccentric viewing target* as the word or shape that the client is trying to see using eccentric viewing. The term *central fixation cue* refers to targets used to encourage the client to look in a particular direction. Central fixation cues are used with beginners who have not yet developed eccentric viewing and still tend to look directly at objects using the macula even though the macula no longer functions. The central fixation cue is used in conjunction with an eccentric viewing target to stimulate the client to position the eyes in a particular direction so that the client might better see the eccentric viewing target. For example, when asked to identify the word "cat" on the screen (Figure 10-5), the beginner will tend to look directly at it and will report that the word disappears (see Figure 10-5[A]). Note that clients who have become well adapted to a central scotoma will automatically eccentrically fixate (see Figure 10-5[B]) even if instructed to look directly at a target. To encourage eccentric viewing, the therapist might ask the client to look at the cross above the word as a central fixation cue (see Figure 10-5[C]). When the client then looks at the cross, the center of the cross disappears, but the word *CAT* now can be visualized and recognized using eccentric viewing. Since the client intends to identify the word *CAT*, it is an eccentric viewing target. The cross is a central fixation cue. Often, the therapist can wave his or her hand to encourage a client to look in a particular direction as a fixation cue instead of a cross.

Clock Face Method

The client is asked to first look at the center of the clock where a star is positioned. If the client tends to centrally fixate, then the client will report that the center star disappears (see Figure 10-3). The clock distance should be positioned so that the shapes of all of the numbers can be seen; bring it closer if the numbers cannot be seen. The therapist then directs the client to look at different clock numerals, which act as central fixation cues. When the client directs central fixation to a numeral, he or she should report that the numeral disappears and the center target appears. Using the disappearing numerals on a clock face for feedback, the client becomes aware of the direction of eccentric viewing, as well as how to control the scotoma position in order to see the central star.

Now ask the client which numerals can be seen most clearly while fixating at the middle of the clock. This report indicates the area of the retina with the best visual acuity. Moving the eye in the direction opposite to the numeral most easily seen (area of best vision) will bring the retinal locus of best vision to the center, and the star or shape in the center of the clock will be seen most clearly (see Figure 10-3). Again, note that the therapist needs to vary the distance of the clock face from the eye depending on the expected size of the central scotoma. For those with better vision and a smaller scotoma, the clock should be held farther away. With the clock method, a copy of the clock can be sent home with the patient with instructions on the correct test distance. The client can practice learning to "move your eyes so you can make each number disappear within 1 second when I ask you to." The goal is to be able to move the eyes to different positions voluntarily.

Tangent Screen Method

Frennesson, Nilsson, and Nilsson[28-30] described a different method that is well suited for a person in the early stages of adaptation with a strong tendency to centrally fixate. This method keeps the eccentric viewing target, a letter, or number stable in the center of the screen and moves the cross above, below, or to the side of the letter on a computer screen. This strategy uses a computer program in the research. A high-contrast cross made out of thin dowels attached to the end of a wand might work as well with a tangent screen. The client is instructed to always direct central fixation and the scotoma to the center of the cross. The cross is then moved until the client reports being able to see the letter. By moving the cross above, below, or to the side of the eccentric viewing target, the therapist encourages the client to redirect the line of gaze eccentrically so that the letter can be seen with side vision. One might think of this technique as enabling the therapist to slowly drag the client's gaze into a desired position. The letters may be replaced with 3- to 4-letter words placed in the center of the screen and different eccentric positions attempted until the eccentric viewing position that produces the best word recognition is found.

Fading Out the Central Fixation Cue and Introducing Natural Eccentric Viewing Targets

This step is quickly performed once clients have demonstrated eccentric viewing during the clock and tangent screen procedures. It should be used to verify that the client can voluntarily adopt different eccentric viewing positions in response to verbal instruction. With cognitively or linguistically impaired individuals, one might just empirically determine the best viewing position and instruct the client to always adopt this one position.

Tangent Screen Method

In this stage of instruction, the tangent screen method is most suitable. The purpose of this step of the instruction sequence (see Table 10-3) is to enable the client to follow verbal instructions to look to each side of the target or above and below the eccentric viewing target without a central fixation cue. Instruction begins with a central fixation cue that is faded out and replaced by verbal cues or no cues. During this instruction, different meaningful eccentric viewing targets are used—3- to 4-letter words for someone who wishes to read, pictures of loved ones, or a TV. Thus, during instruction, the therapist can ascertain the eccentric viewing position that is best for a particular goal task. At first, a central fixation cue is used, such as a cross at the end of a wand or a laser spot to encourage the person to eccentrically view in a particular direction. The central fixation cue is positioned at different points around the eccentric viewing target, encouraging eccentric viewing above, below, and to each side of the target with verbal instruction. The therapist should place a word on the tangent screen and instruct the client to look at the center of the cross (the central fixation cue) until it disappears and determine the position that allows the words to be seen clearly. Then repeat the movement without the wand. As one teaches the client to move their eyes into different positions, one will determine the position most suitable for reading. Occasionally, one finds a client with one PRL with a larger field of view more suitable for reading, and another PRL that allows isolated letters to be seen more clearly. This tangent screen method could be performed on a computer screen or any near card. Variations on the tangent screen can be improvised by using a wall, laser pointer, and a drawn or real-life eccentric viewing target. The eccentric viewing target is centered and a central fixation cue (laser spot) is positioned as needed to the side and eventually faded out so a client can follow directions, such as "look up" and eventually eccentrically fixate a centered target without any cues.

Another therapeutic activity that can be used at this stage of training with either the tangent screen or the clock involves the use of a telescope or small-diameter tube. The client looks through a tube of about 1 cm (0.5 inch). If the person with a central scotoma centrally fixates through the tube, nothing will be seen. If the person eccentrically views, then something will be seen. This exercise may be done with a telescope and provides salient feedback as to whether adaptive eccentric viewing has been achieved or not.

Clock Face Method

Recall that during the initial evaluation, when the client with adaptive eccentric viewing was asked to look at the center star, he or she would report seeing the center star and that some clock numerals would disappear. At this point, the client who has just received completed instruction should also be able to do the same, but much more quickly and on demand. Adopting a different viewing position should become almost automatic, allowing a person to divide attention enough to judge which position provides the best vision for a given task.

Introducing Natural Viewing Conditions

Home exercise or practice also may be performed with pairs of large-print playing cards positioned so that while looking at one card (the fixation cue), the other card (the target) becomes visible. Computer programs that act like flash cards might also help a client practice eccentric viewing by themselves, for example, Magnimaster (Hunstad Magnimaster Reading Improver SMC). The fixation tube, computer program, and clock face may also be sent home for practice as a home exercise program. At this stage of instruction, the client should be able to practice by watching TV, taking care to ensure the TV is close enough to see, sticking a bright orange piece of paper on the edge of the TV as a fixation cue if needed.

During this training, a client may turn the head. This head turn may be in the direction opposite the one to which the client moves the eyes to eccentrically view. There is no evidence that head turning presents a problem except to the therapist trying to observe eye position. Head turning may present ergonomic problems, and clients can be taught to eccentrically view without head turning during advanced instruction. Research needs to be done to better understand the effect of head position. However, eccentric viewing is a difficult skill to learn, and we feel that focusing too much on such technical details as head positioning may be discouraging.

Reading With Scrolled Text

Once the client demonstrates the ability to eccentrically view and identify a single stationary object like playing cards, the client is ready to learn to read while eccentrically viewing. This is an excellent therapeutic activity even in cases where reading is not a primary goal, but if reading is highly unlikely, this difficult step can be avoided. One must be careful to find the best PRL for reading, providing a sufficient field of view for word recognition. Reading is more difficult because the person must move the eyes and scan the text.

The print size used should be at least twice the visual acuity level of the client, or more for early success. The client might also require some magnification device, a microscope (strong reading glasses), a mounted handheld magnifier, a computer, or an electronic viewer (CCTV) for this training period. When practicing with printed text, the client should be sitting at a table in front of a reading stand with the text mounted on a card that slides horizontally on the lip of the stand (Figure 10-6[A]). The client is then directed to eccentrically view the first word. In most cases, looking above the line is best for reading. Once the client can see the word, slowly scroll the text from right to left while he or she tries to keep the eye in the same position.

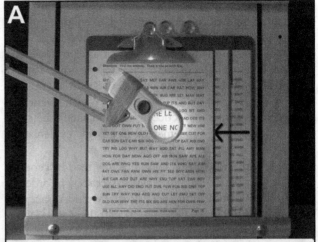

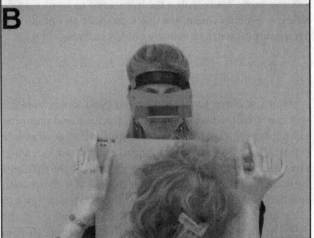

Figure 10-6. (A) Steady eye technique at a reading stand with mounted handheld magnifier. (B) Steady eye technique with the patient using a loupe magnifier while seated with hand-over-hand assistance.

The eye and the head should not move. Watson named this the "steady eye technique." Starting with hand-over-hand assistance, the client holds the text affixed to a clipboard and scrolls the text (Figure 10-6[B]). In addition to reading lines of text, the client needs to learn to return to the beginning of the line. This is accomplished by marking the beginning of the line with a finger and following the line just read back to the beginning and moving down. This is called the *retracing technique*. The therapist gradually withdraws assistance until the client is able to read on his or her own. The client can practice scanning multiple lines and finally more complex activities such as reading bills and bank statements. The key to this technique is that the client slowly moves the material being read from right to left rather than the eyes and head. The MagnaFlyer computer program (SoftOlogy IdeaWorks) was developed for this stage of training. MagnaFlyer is a program developed specifically for eccentric viewing training (www.magnaflyer.net) that uses rapid serial visual presentation (RSVP) to enlarge the print on a computer screen, then successively presents the words on the screen, using existing text, even books. This could be sent home with clients for home-based practice. These different methods have been used to enlarge and display text on a screen and present the text to the client while the client tries to maintain a consistent eccentric viewing position and use a consistent PRL for reading. Similar methods have been shown to be effective without any one method clearly better than another.[31] Which particular method to choose is a practice option and should be carefully evaluated once implemented to provide evidence for effectiveness on a case-by-case basis.

People with more normal visual acuity read by generating rightward quick eye movements (saccades) in order to look from one word to the next. Visually guided saccades are compromised in people without central vision.[32] When using the steady eye technique, a person with central field loss can more easily shift gaze from word to word using a reflexive eye movement, the quick phase of an optokinetic nystagmus rather than visually guided saccades.[33,34]

Tracking and Viewing Through a Handheld Magnifier

After the client has demonstrated good steady viewing and mastered reading scrolled text, tracking and scanning techniques are used along with magnification devices (see Figure 10-6). The procedure begins with steady viewing. The client attempts to identify playing cards as the therapist pulls each card off the top of the deck. Index cards with numbers and short words (4 letters or less) can also be used. Once the client can perform well with steady viewing, the therapist should add movement to the procedure. To do so, the therapist holds the cards while carefully observing the client's eyes. The stack of cards is then slowly moved, and the client should track the cards. Maintaining viewing with a slowly moving target with a predictable motion is relatively easy. Recovering eccentric viewing when viewing is lost presents the greater difficulty, especially if the target disappears into the scotoma. If the client loses visibility of the target during this procedure, the therapist should stop until the client recovers and then continue. At first, the characters should be at least 2 to 3 times the client's visual acuity. Starting from the card position that allows the most consistent eccentric viewing, the therapist slowly moves the cards in various directions (up and to the right, down and to the right, up and to the left, down and to the left), starting with movement away from the scotoma, because movement toward the scotoma will present the most difficulty. Increase task difficulty by increasing the speed of the target movement and then moving the tracking stimulus unpredictably. To further increase the level of difficulty, decrease print size. Note that people will sometimes switch from one eccentric viewing position to another. Let your client know when you observe this happening. Rapid alternation between eccentric viewing positions slows reading and

should be discouraged; this strategy, however, may be adaptable when scanning during mobility.

A practical extension of tracking a large stimulus is to have the client read through a handheld magnifier or stand magnifier held at about 20 to 40 cm (8 to 16 inches) from the eye. Begin with the client seated, and once he or she can master reading in this position, instruct the client to attempt reading through a handheld magnifier or stand magnifier while standing. Recall that the handheld magnifier and the head should rotate together with the lateral movement of the head as the magnifier moves across the page, as if an imaginary rod connects the magnifier through the eye and the head. Scanning with telescopic magnification can also be introduced at this point in the therapy.

Localizing and Scanning

The most advanced task is to have the client scan a room using saccadic eye movements. The goal of scanning training is to enable the client to make an accurate saccade to an object seen peripherally without the object disappearing into the scotoma. Although this is a simple task for a person without a central scotoma, some research suggests that this type of saccadic control is irreversibly compromised with the loss of central vision. A person with a central scotoma requires increased time to make a saccade to an object seen peripherally because these eye movements are inaccurate, and several saccades may be required to scan from one object to the next.[35] To practice scanning, a large, high-contrast eccentric viewing target can be presented in the periphery, such as a waving hand, a person, or a light, in regular, predictable positions at first. Eventually, the targets should be presented in unpredictable positions. A laser light, flashlight, or flash card works well as an eccentric viewing target at this stage.

A more advanced technique for individuals learning to use optical devices is *localization*. With localization, the client scans a room or page of text until fixating a spot where he or she expects to see something of interest. Without breaking eccentric viewing, the client positions a magnification device in front of the eye so that the object of interest is magnified. For example, the client might scan a bill and localize where some numbers are printed that are likely to be the amount due by the layout of the text. The client then positions the magnification device in front of the eye to read the number. Localization will be described in detail in Chapter 13 when discussing optical devices.

As discussed previously, researchers have found that some well-adapted people with central vision loss use different eccentric viewing positions after saccades. This advanced technique can be taught if the evaluation reveals different functional ability for various eccentric viewing positions, such as one PRL that has better acuity and another with a larger horizontal field of view for reading.

Finding the Best Eccentric Viewing Position for Different Tasks

To teach people to use different PRLs, the therapist should select targets that are typically involved in real-life tasks and have the client do free scanning without other cues or targets. Targets should be carefully selected so that a different visual skill is required to best identify the chosen target. For example, one target might be more easily identified with a PRL that works well with longer words, while another target (picture of a face) might be more easily identified with a PRL that has better acuity. Often, different PRLs have different visual acuity ability, requiring a change in required magnification. It is important to understand that for mobility, the use of inferior viewing is dangerous because a scotoma in the lower central field puts people at risk for tripping on objects on the floor.[26] Positioning the scotoma above the text is generally thought to be better for reading.

Equipment for Eccentric Viewing Training and Home Exercise Programs

Ideally, eccentric viewing instruction involves a display for stimuli and a method for the therapist to view the client's eye while he or she is attempting to eccentrically fixate. Rather than a tangent screen, we now use a laser pointer to project a stimulus and stick targets on the wall for early stages of training. The procedures described earlier using playing cards or the clock face can easily be performed at home by the patient without assistance.

The next step, where the client attempts to hold the eye in an eccentric viewing position while presenting the text to the PRL, presents a challenge because considerable practice is usually required, ideally with a home program. When transitioning to more emphasis on home based-practice, the challenge is providing the client with a magnification device sufficient to identify the targets or text used to practice the steady eye technique. Full-field microscopes or loupes can be loaned to the client during the exercise program, while handheld magnifiers that are relatively inexpensive are often prescribed and dispensed for spot reading tasks. The handheld magnifier can be mounted to allow the client to practice the scrolled text. The disadvantage of prescribing and using optical devices before training is that magnification needs might change. A CCTV or a person's computer can be adapted and is preferred because the magnification can be adjusted as the client's skill improves; these might be obtained under loaner programs. A computer can also be used for eccentric viewing training. A final option is to have the client attend office-based treatment sessions and practice before or after the scheduled therapy session in the clinic with a borrowed device.

Finally, once someone has mastered the steady eye technique, he or she is ready to transition to reading continual text. Workbooks are available that provide a sequence of progressively more challenging home exercises for reading,[2] starting with single letters and numbers, then words and single sentences, and eventually to paragraphs and stories. The LUV reading workbook provides this progression of exercises using games and engaging activities. Reading is a valuable therapeutic activity for the development of eccentric viewing because so many tools and materials are available. Even if reading is not the client's primary goal, the skills developed for reading should transfer to other tasks as well. More sophisticated equipment called microperimeters and the predecessor, scanning laser ophthalmoscope[29] allow one to perform training by projecting images of targets directly onto the retina, while at the same time viewing the retina. Although potentially valuable especially for evaluation and research, these devices involve specialized training and are generally too expensive for a low vision practice.

Adaptive Reading Without Eccentric Viewing Training

Many who have lived with macular degeneration for several months or more have developed adaptive eccentric viewing on their own, if they have normal cognition. Many of the early steps required for someone seen soon after a sudden loss can be skipped or completed quickly. If it appears a person has already developed adaptive eccentric viewing, other than teaching them scotoma awareness and to voluntarily move the scotoma using the clock face technique, we often do not attempt more advanced eccentric viewing instruction. Clients often are not willing to spend several weeks of training. In these cases, one can use "supersizing" techniques. Using what is usually an electronic magnifier, one can increase magnification to many times the minimum magnification necessary. If the scotoma is small enough and the text being read very big, then even with maladaptive eccentric viewing, only 1 or 2 letters are obscured and a person can still recognize words, objects, or pictures easily and read with relative ease. This strategy is often used with people with cognitive defects as well.

Eccentric viewing training proceeds much more easily if the client understands complex, multistep instructions; can perform ideational problem solving; and has good semantic as well as procedural memory. If a client is capable of following one-step commands and demonstrates learning with practice, eccentric viewing training may proceed if a helper is present who understands the process and can assist with practice at home that focused on motor learning. One should skip trying to teach this client how to voluntarily shift eccentric viewing positions and use multiple PRLs. Clients with cognitive impairments might have difficulty understanding how to shift eccentric viewing with verbal cues, but might unconsciously have learned one eccentric viewing position with training, and this might be modified with practice using a simple cue with direct feedback. For example, a client with a small central scotoma might have learned to fixate rightward, restricting the field of view to a few letters per fixation. She or he might be cued to "look above the words," opening up the field of view when reading. When she or he does this, reading significantly improves as the client begins seeing words rather than one letter at a time, and this improved reading positively reinforces the behavior. This process of motor learning might effectively teach the client this new habitual position during reading. We do not know why people pick a certain area as a PRL, but suspect it likely is the area of best visual acuity so when someone practices reading, the text must be magnified enough if the new PRL has worse acuity.

LEARNING TO USE NONVISUAL SENSES

Learning to use touch and sound to compensate for vision loss tends to be an approach generally associated with more severe vision loss. We have found, however, that use of other senses often can be combined with low vision to improve the overall experience. For example, even typically sighted people may both look for and try to feel for a blemish on a piece of fruit or some smudge on a table. These strategies would be even more useful if vision was impaired. Using nonvisual techniques typically is the focus of treatment by certified vision rehabilitation therapists (CVRTs), who should be included in the treatment team if nonvisual techniques and braille education are indicated. This chapter will introduce some more basic and widely used nonvisual techniques, as well as methods to evaluate and prepare a person with multiple impairments for more intense treatment by a CVRT, such as the potential to learn braille or a more advanced tactile technique.

Evaluation

To use touch to compensate for vision loss, a person requires not only tactile sensitivity, but also stereognosis (tactile form perception), spatial perception (where things are in space), and working spatial memory to immediately recall the position of objects in peripersonal space, that is, within an arm's length. To quickly evaluate a person's abilities and disabilities to compensate for low vision, we developed a nonstandardized but very informative "coin clock test." Hand a blindfolded person an assortment of 4 or 5 coins and ask them to place a different coin at the 12:00, 3:00, 6:00, and 9:00 positions on the table in front. Observe carefully how accurate the spacing and positioning are. Tell the person you will ask him or her to pick up the coins later. Now perform a different, unrelated task, such as checking hearing or active and passive range of motion, still under

blindfold. Finally, ask the person to put his or her finger on and then pick up a named coin—observe carefully if the person recalls where it is and reaches directly to it. This test will inform the therapist how much grading and instruction will be required for each component. The components tested are as follows:

- Tactile and proprioceptive sensitivity: Can the person feel the ridges on the edge of a coin or size differences?
- Stereognosia: Can the client discriminate types of coins?
- Peripersonal space perception: Does the client place the objects in the correct clock positions on the table?
- Working memory: How accurately does the client follow the instructions, sequence the steps, and recall where the coins were placed?

Instruction

This technique encourages the client to explore the tabletop in a deliberate and methodical manner by first locating the table edge in front. The hands are curled slightly and are moved in a circular pattern away from the edge, locating objects of desire with the fingertips and skirting around others. Another approach involves an up-and-down "patting" type motion that is less likely to knock something over. These approaches are more cautious and deliberate. For fine tactile discrimination, move 2 fingers over a surface together. Movement is important. Therapeutic activities that help a person develop fine discrimination necessary for braille reading, tactile dominoes (www.lss-products.com), and braille flash cards (made using a braille stylus) for numbers are useful exercises. In general, braille should be taught by a CVRT, but while waiting for services, an occupational therapist can introduce some pre-braille skills. Otherwise, the focus should be on the goal activity. For example, if the goal is eating neatly, then the activity should be to apply tactile strategies to practice eating. Specific tactile strategies are discussed under in Section IV.

SUMMARY

Reading is a common goal if someone has low vision and is an activity that builds and solidifies visual skills, including eccentric viewing. The skills can be applied to many activities, and thus reading is a core therapeutic activity. Use of magnification strategies is central to addressing disability that results from impaired visual acuity. For someone with central field loss, development of eccentric viewing and scanning provides foundational skills for reading and finding the face of a loved one in a room, for example. For someone with peripheral field restriction, development of compensatory scanning provides the foundation for orientation and mobility. Compensatory scanning for peripheral field loss is discussed in Chapter 14. Finally, using other senses is not just for people who have profound visual impairment; use of touch, hearing, and smell are important foundation skills for people who have any level of functional low vision because it puts more adaptive tools in the toolbox. We as occupational therapists relish the discovery of therapeutic occupations that continue to teach long after we have formally discharged our client. Yet the occupational therapist must still have the wisdom to appreciate that the ultimate goal of therapy is not just about fixing vision and visual function; it is about using all available resources—touch, smell, and hearing—to help someone find, once again, that flow of living.

REFERENCES

1. Warren M. *Prereading and Writing Exercises for People With Macular Scotomas.* Birmingham, AL: visABILITIES Rehab Services; 1996.
2. Wright V, Watson GR. *Learn to Use Your Vision for Reading (LUV Reading Series).* Lilburn, GA: Bear Consultants; 1996.
3. Whittaker SG, Lovie-Kitchin J. Visual requirements for reading. *Optom Vis Sci.* 1993;70:54-65.
4. Watson GR, Whittaker SG, Steciw M. *Pepper Visual Skills for Reading Test (revised).* Milwaukee, WI: Fork in the Road Vision Rehabilitation Services LLC; 1995.
5. Watson GR, Wright V, Long SL. *Morgan Low Vision Reading Comprehension Assessment (LUV Reading Series).* Lilburn, GA: Bear Consultants; 1996.
6. Bailey IL, Bullimore MA, Greer RX. Low vision magnifiers: their optical parameters and methods for prescribing. *Optom Vis Sci.* 1994;71:689-698.
7. Bailey IL. Equivalent viewing power or magnification? Which is fundamental? *Optician.* 1984;188:14-18.
8. Mehr EM, Freid AN. *Low Vision Care.* Chicago: Professional Press; 1975:107.
9. Cheong AC, Lovie-Kitchin JE, Bowers AR. Determining magnification for reading with low vision. *Clin Exp Optom.* 2002;85:229-237.
10. Whittaker SG, Lovie-Kitchin JE. Visual requirements for reading. *Optom Vis Sci.* 1993;70:54-65.
11. Smallfield S, Clem K, Myers A. Occupational therapy interventions to improve the reading ability of older adults with low vision: a systematic review. *Am J Occup Ther.* 2013;67:288-295.
12. Perlmutter MS, Bhorade A, Gordon M, Hollingsworth H, Engsberg JE, Carolyn Baum M. Home lighting assessment for clients with low vision. *Am J Occup Ther.* 2013;67:674-682.
13. Lei H, Schuchard RA. Using two preferred retinal loci for different lighting conditions in patients with central scotomas. *Invest Ophthalmol Vis Sci.* 1997;38:1812-1818.
14. Fosse P, Valberg A. Lighting needs and lighting comfort during reading with age-related macular degeneration. *J Vis Impairment Blindness.* 2004;98:389-409.
15. Howe J. Eccentric viewing training and its effect on the reading rates of individuals with absolute central scotomas: a meta-analysis. *J Vis Impairment Blindness.* 2012;106:527-542.
16. Whittaker SG, Budd J, Cummings RW. Eccentric fixation with macular scotoma. *Invest Ophthalmol Vis Sci.* 1988;29:268-278.
17. Timberlake GT, Sharma MK, Grose SA, Maino JH. Retinal locus for scanning text. *J Rehab Res Dev.* 2006;43:749-760.
18. Culham LE, Fitske FW, Timberlake GT, Marshall J. Reading performance at different retinal eccentricities using a scanning laser ophthalmoscope. *ARVO Abstracts.* 1991;816.
19. Timberlake GT, Peli E, Assock EA, Augliere RA. Reading with a macular scotoma: II. Retinal locus for scanning text. *Invest Ophthalmol Vis Sci.* 1987;28:1368-1274.
20. Timberlake GT, Mainster MA, Peli E, Augliere RA, Essock E, Arend LE. Reading with a macular scotoma: I. Retinal location of scotoma and fixation area. *Invest Ophthalmol Vis Sci.* 1986;27:1137-1147.
21. Crossland MD, Culham LE, Kabanarou SA, Rubin GS. Preferred retinal locus development in patients with macular disease. *Ophthalmology.* 2005;112:1579-1585.
22. Whittaker SG, Budd JM, Cummings RW. Eccentric fixation with macular scotoma. *Invest Ophthalmol Vis Sci.* 1988;29:268-278.
23. Crossland MD, Engel SA, Legge GE. The preferred retinal locus in macular disease: toward a consensus definition. *Retina.* 2011;31:2109-2114.
24. Kaldenberg J, Smallfield S. *Occupational Therapy Practice Guidelines for Older Adults with Low Vision.* 2nd ed. Bethesda, MD: AOTA Press; 2013:119.
25. Legge GE. *Psychophysics of Reading in Normal and Low Vision.* Mahwah, NJ: Lawrence Erlbaum Associates; 2007.
26. Lovie-Kitchin JE, Mainstone J, Robinson J, Brown B. What areas of the visual field are important for mobility in low vision patients? *Clin Vis Sci.* 1990;4:249-263.
27. Black AA, Wood JM, Lovie-Kitchin JE. Inferior visual field reductions are associated with poorer functional status among older adults with glaucoma. *Ophthalmic Physiol Opt.* 2011;31:283-291.
28. Frennesson C, Nilsson SE. The superior retina performs better than the inferior retina when reading with eccentric viewing: a comparison in normal volunteers. *Acta Ophthalmologica Scandinavica.* 2007;85:868-870.
29. Nilsson UL, Frennesson C, Nilsson SEG. Patients with AMD and a large absolute central scotoma can be trained successfully to use eccentric viewing, as demonstrated in a scanning laser ophthalmoscope. *Vis Res.* 2003;43:1777-1787.
30. Nilsson UL, Frennesson C, Nilsson SEG. Location and stability of a newly established eccentric retinal locus suitable for reading, achieved through training of patients with a dense central scotoma. *Opt Vis Sci.* 1998;75:873-878.
31. Bowers AR, Woods RL, Peli E. Preferred retinal locus and reading rate with four dynamic text presentation formats. *Optom Vis Sci.* 2004;81:205-213.
32. Whittaker SG, Cummings RW. Foveating saccades. *Vis Res.* 1990;30:1363-1366.
33. Cummings RW, Whittaker SG, Swieson LR. Individuals with maculopathies use OKN to scan text during unconstrained reading. *Invest Ophthalmol Vis Sci.* 1989;30:398.
34. Bowers ARMP, Layton CA, Koenig AJ. Eye movements and reading with plus-lens magnifiers. *Optom Vis Sci.* 2000;77:25-33.
35. Whittaker SG, Cummings RW, Swieson LR. Saccade control without a fovea. *Vis Res.* 1991;31:2209-2218.

11

Managing Peripheral
Visual Field Loss and Neglect

OVERVIEW

Clients with acquired brain injury (ABI) often have difficulty with tasks such as reading, recognizing objects or people, and noticing people or things on one or both sides. They often have problems organizing and often lose things. These problems may be the result of peripheral visual field loss, underlying perceptual and attention deficits, or a combination of both. Effective treatment planning requires that the therapist carefully assess and tease sensory deficits apart from the higher-order cognitive or perceptual problems that result from brain injury. Because peripheral vision loss, spatial neglect, and perceptual dysfunctions are all common results of ABI, advanced treatment of these conditions should be part of the basic toolkit of a therapist treating adults with ABI in a medical rehabilitation setting. Field loss and spatial neglect are substantively different impairments that result from damage to different areas of the brain. Even though field loss and spatial neglect have a similar presentation and some treatments are similar as well, the presentation and treatments differ in important ways, and the response to treatment is quite different.

Visual field loss may occur not only from stroke, but also optic nerve diseases such as multiple sclerosis, more widespread systemic conditions like anoxic encephalopathy,

glaucoma, more severe traumatic brain injuries, and brain cancer. Chapter 3 described the common causes of peripheral visual field loss, including diseases and trauma. Damage to the visual pathways beyond the optic chiasm results in homonymous visual field loss (affecting the same areas in the right or left visual field of each eye). Damage to the retina, optic nerve, or optic chiasm usually results in a heteronymous visual field loss (affecting different areas in the right and left visual fields of each eye).

Perceptual problems such as spatial neglect often occur together with a homonymous visual field loss or, because of similar symptomology, can be confused with a visual field loss even though the underlying visual problems are quite different. The treatment sections of this chapter will include diagnosis and treatment of not only visual field loss, but also spatial neglect (also called *visual neglect, unilateral neglect*, or *unilateral inattention*).

Visual-perceptual problems and their etiology are generally described in the neuropsychology, neurology literature,[1-4] and neuro-optometry literature. Optometrists refer to these problems as *information processing disorders*.[5,6] This chapter will describe how to differentiate perceptual dysfunction from visual field loss and review evaluation and treatment of disability associated with some of the more common perceptual disorders encountered by

Whittaker SG, Scheiman M, Sokol-McKay DA.
*Low Vision Rehabilitation: A Practical Guide for Occupational Therapists,
Second Edition* (pp 181-201).
© 2016 Taylor & Francis Group.

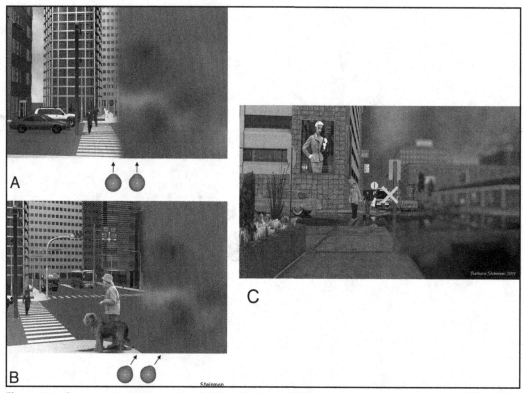

Figure 11-1. Compensatory scanning straight (A) and to the right (B) with homonymous hemianopia. (C) Normally, people cannot visualize the blind area, but tend to perceptually fill it in using visual memory. (Reprinted with permission from Barbara Steinman.)

occupational therapists. Scheiman[5] and Zoltan[7] describe the evaluation and treatment of such perceptual dysfunction in greater detail.

One of the more puzzling features of visual field loss is that the client typically does not see the area of even a large visual field loss as the gray, black, or white area often depicted in simulations (Figures 11-1[A] and 11-1[B]). The brain fills in the blind area, making the individual unaware of the deficit (Figure 11-1[C]). This is referred to as the "perceptual completion." This is puzzling to many of us, who assume that what we see is a faithful reproduction of the actual information being received by our visual system. Visual consciousness, however, has been described as a "reciprocal interweaving of top-down and bottom-up processes that propel and guide movement."[8] At any given moment in time, a person responds to a composition of sensory information (referred to as "bottom-up" processing) and higher-order perceptual and cognitive processing (referred to as *top-down* processing) such as visual attention and short-term visual memory. The result is a person's mental image of the surroundings. Bottom-up damage to the visual pathway, starting at the retina and ending in the primary visual cortex, is considered sensory loss and results in field defects and other sensory impairments, but often leaves these perceptual processing systems largely intact. As a result, with field defects that are total, a person's higher-order perceptual system fills in the missing

area, usually with some reasonably accurate memory of what the person expects to see (visual memory); however, sometimes the blind area is filled with "phantom vision" or visual hallucinations, a condition called *Charles Bonnet syndrome*. The low vision therapist can use the capability of the perceptual system as a treatment strategy to adapt to loss of sensory function by training the higher-order processing to compensate for lack of sensory information and to fill in missing information from memory with object and word recognition tasks. With low vision, where the sensory information has been distorted but higher-order processing is largely intact, the neural processing of the sensory information adapts how the sensory information is processed (called *neural plasticity*) to improve word recognition, for example.[9] The implication of this work is that people who can be taught to actively use their vision will modify visual processing to improve object recognition and spatial estimation. Thus, practice with visual object and word recognition becomes an important part of low vision rehabilitation.

Often, brain injury to areas beyond the occipital cortex affects the perceptual system directly, leaving a person with severe visual impairment even when the sensory system is largely intact. A rather useful starting point in understanding higher-order visual processing is Goodale and Milner's concept of 2 somewhat distinct neurological systems for processing and integrating sensory information: the "what" and "where" systems.[1,10] Starting at the

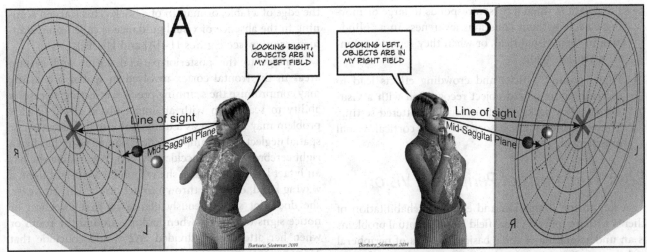

Figure 11-2. Illustration of egocentric (centered on the client's midsagittal plane) and oculocentric (centered at the point of fixation in visual field coordinates) localization. In egocentric coordinates, the dark ball is straight ahead and the lighter ball is to client's left in both (A) and (B). In oculocentric or visual field coordinates, when the client is looking right (A) both balls are in the left visual field and when the client is looking left (B) both objects are in the right visual field. (Reprinted with permission from Barbara Steinman.)

retinal level, the fine-grained parvocellular neurons project through the thalamus and primary occipital cortex into the occipital-temporal ventral stream—the "what" system that processes object recognition, symbol recognition, and what many suggest is conscious perception. The coarse-grained, motion-sensitive magnocellular neurons project to the occipital-parietal dorsal stream—the "where" system that processes spatial information. The dorsal stream organizes and directs action. Damage in the parietal areas involved in the dorsal stream may lead to spatial neglect. Interestingly, part of the magnocellular ("where") system separates into 2 projection systems. One travels along the main projections to the primary visual cortex along with the parvocellular ("what") system. The other projections of the magnocellular or motion system travel through the superior colliculus directly into the dorsal stream in the secondary visual cortex. As a result, sometimes with damage to the primary visual cortex or the optic radiations, a person still may be left with "blind sight," where, with no conscious awareness of vision, the person might still respond to bright lights, motion, and larger objects.[1]

To summarize, visual perceptual disorders associated with visual field loss can be organized as follows:

- Spatial neglect
  - Unilateral spatial neglect, usually unilateral, and on the left side, is associated with right posterior parietal lobe damage and some areas in the right frontal cortex.
    - Usually, spatial neglect is egocentric, to the left of the midsagittal plane of the body, regardless of where someone is looking (Figure 11-2[A]).
    - Left spatial neglect syndrome may be oculocentric (Figure 11-2[B]) or allocentric, resembling a visual field loss in that attention is reduced to the

left of a person's point of fixation, wherever the person looks.
  - Simultagnosia, often associated with Balint syndrome, is essentially a bilateral spatial neglect and is associated with bilateral parietal damage. This presents like an overall visual field loss or "tunnel vision," except it is often egocentric rather than oculocentric and is attention related, so it is possible to see objects in the periphery. In a severe form, a person will see maybe 1 or 2 letters in the center of a word but not the whole word, yet still respond during peripheral field testing.
  - Optic ataxia is a mislocalization of objects in space relative to the body, such as missing an object when trying to pick it up. This also sometimes occurs with spatial neglect and simultagnosia.
  - Clothing apraxia and allocentric spatial defects refer to problems in the organization of parts of a scene or complex object, regardless of where it is relative to the body. Examples include difficulty finding parts of clothes, like the left sleeve, or writing words successively along a single line. We have observed that right-left confusion is associated with neglect syndrome, complicating the process of dressing even further.
  - Anosognosia is unawareness of a deficit,[2,11] which, when combined with emotional volatility,[11] is also associated with left neglect syndrome.
- Charles Bonnet syndrome (visual hallucinations) and other forms of "phantom" vision.
- Alexia is an acquired reading deficit.
- Agnosia is an impaired object recognition.

- Blindsight is when a person responds to large or moving objects without conscious awareness in a "blind" area in their visual field, or when they report no conscious vision at all.

- Figure-ground deficits and crowding effects lead to increasingly impaired object recognition with a visually complex background or visually cluttered setting. These problems are associated with cortical visual impairment.

Basic Functions of Peripheral Vision

A key to the evaluation and effective rehabilitation of clients with peripheral visual field loss perceptual problems is an understanding of the 3 basic functions of peripheral vision: organization of visual scanning, warning, and night vision.

Organize Visual Scanning

The first basic function of peripheral vision is to help an individual organize visual scanning. When someone with normal visual function looks at a larger scene or area such as a room or a restaurant menu, he or she generates a sequence of quick saccades at a rate of 3 to 4 per second. Each saccade ends with a period of viewing on some part of the scene. During this viewing, the visual system samples a different area within the scene. During the approximately one-quarter-second fixation period, the visual system uses the macula with its high resolution and color rendition to collect detail about some patch of the immediate surroundings. Using this sequence of saccades, the visual system rapidly pieces together a detailed and complex 3 dimensional perception of the scene or area into visual working memory. For example, when a person with normal visual function enters an unfamiliar room for the first time, the peripheral vision, with its lower acuity, detects larger, higher-contrast, and moving objects. The person may detect people moving to the left and glance over to see who they are, then check the doors, signs, tables, and chairs seen in the periphery. Within a few seconds, this person has gathered critical information that will allow him or her to interact with the other people, know where the doors are located, and avoid obstacles in the room, as well as read the sign that indicates which doorway to enter. Organization of visual scanning involves not only peripheral vision, but also spatial processing, memory, and other sensory modalities. A person entering a room may use auditory cues to glance over to the left to a radio playing music or to a person talking. The next time this person enters the room, he or she can use memory of the room layout and may know where to look for the faint outline of obstacles or doors even if the lights are out. A person who has lost the visual field will need to become more dependent on memory and auditory cues, as well as develop general nonvisual strategies such as looking toward expected landmarks such as the wall on one side of a room,

the edge of a table, or margin of a book. This learned scanning in the absence of visual guidance is called *compensatory scanning* (see Figures 11-1[A] and 11-1[B]).

Damage to the posterior-parietal cortex and certain areas in the frontal cortex involved in spatial processing may compromise the scanning process, affecting a person's ability to scan even with an intact visual field.[4,12] This problem may manifest as a unilateral visual inattention or spatial neglect. For example, a client named Mary has had a right cerebral vascular accident (CVA). We assume she has an intact left field because she responds to a bright light, a waving hand, or a ball thrown to her on the left. However, she does not spontaneously glance in that direction or notice signs to her left when looking around the room or when her attention is divided. We would conclude that Mary has intact visual fields but a spatial neglect. In some cases, people will have both a spatial neglect and unilateral visual field loss. These individuals cannot see anything on one side and are not aware of the vision loss or that objects exist on the side of the vision loss.

Note that with either unilateral visual field loss or spatial neglect, the pattern of eye movements often will be abnormal, but basic eye movement control, such as saccade control, by itself is not necessarily compromised. With just visual field loss, eye movements often look abnormal because a person loses sight of an object and initiates more corrective saccades in the direction of the field loss to find it.

Therapy for visual field loss should focus on teaching a person to learn to use nonvisual cues or the expected position of objects, visual memory, or organizational scanning patterns. Also, clients are taught habitual scanning to the affected side and to direct the eye movements far enough to the affected side. If the perceptual systems for organizing and directing attention and eye movements to the affected side are intact, people with just a field loss respond quickly to therapy, often with just a few sessions required. With spatial neglect, the abnormal pattern of saccades results from damage to the neurophysiological spatial and temporal processing systems that organize the pattern of saccades required for scanning eye movements and directing attention. The focus of therapy, therefore, should be on attention and initiating and organizing a visual scanning pattern, often by memorizing and overlearning habitual scanning patterns and activities. With left neglect from right frontal or parietal hemisphere damage, a person might learn to pause during an activity to invoke the left hemisphere verbal systems to compensate by using "self-talk" (verbalizing the scanning strategy). Response to therapy is slower, and many sessions are often required.

Use of the Visual Periphery as a Warning System

The second basic function of peripheral vision is as a warning system. This is important for driving, walking in crowds, or mobility in busy areas. Our ability to respond to high-contrast moving objects is a phylogenically ancient system that allows creatures to detect and respond to high-contrast moving objects approaching from the side. That flash of fear we all experience when something unexpected darts rapidly in from the side illustrates this warning system. In humans, this orienting response includes a saccade toward the suspected threat.[13] In our modern era, these threats may be a child running in front of the car, a car suddenly approaching an intersection that we are trying to cross, the unexpected appearance of a rolling ball, or an animal running into our field of view from the side. These events may occur very quickly while we are looking somewhere else. If a client has a peripheral visual field loss and is looking straight ahead, the early warning system associated with the affected side will not alert the client to an unexpected danger unless the person has "blindsight" and may react to larger moving objects like a person approaching. Even with an intact visual field, a person with spatial neglect might be less likely to attend and react when unexpected objects approach on the affected side. Use of a prism that projects an image of the visual scene from the affected blind side to the sighted side serves an alerting function. Therapy focused on learning habitual compensatory scanning—that is, unconsciously looking to the affected side every 1 to 2 seconds while walking—should, if effective, enable a person to compensate for the loss of this warning system as well. With spatial neglect, another compensatory approach involves providing extra stimulation to draw attention to the affected side, such as positioning a person with left spatial neglect so that the right side is to a wall and the left side to a room, or use of electrical stimulation on the affected side.[3,4,12]

Role of Peripheral Vision in Night Vision

The final basic function of peripheral vision is the role it plays in night vision. The peripheral retina has much greater sensitivity to dim light than does the central retina. Loss of peripheral vision, therefore, leads to night blindness, a severe loss of vision when the light levels drop. A person with an overall (bilateral) peripheral vision loss due to advanced glaucoma or retinitis pigmentosa, for example, may report little problems during the day but severe visual disability at night.

Overall Visual Field Loss

The retinal diseases that lead to overall visual field loss or "tunnel vision" usually have a gradual onset, allowing the client to progressively adapt on his or her own using compensatory scanning in all directions. CVA, traumatic brain injury, or cancer that affects both sides of the brain may result in sudden visual field loss or even total blindness that resolves into an overall peripheral visual field loss. Someone who experienced this rapid overall loss in visual fields may report a problem bumping into objects or difficulty finding things and should be taught compensatory scanning (see Figure 11-2). The common challenge in managing people with peripheral loss is addressing the loss of the "warning system." Even when using good scanning technique, a person with an overall peripheral visual field loss will miss an unexpected, quickly moving hazard from the blind side. People with overall peripheral vision loss often experience night blindness as well.

With peripheral visual field loss that has gradually progressed, the client may deny functional problems because the perceptual system fills in the nonseeing area in the periphery while the client still retains high-resolution central vision. People with peripheral visual field loss gradually become accustomed to avoiding particularly disabling situations, such as going out at night. They may not encounter problems because they avoid crowds or new environments, and may be in denial if the prognosis is total blindness. As a result, they may staunchly refuse the best compensation for loss of the warning system: the use of a white cane or guide dog. The denial that occurs with the progressive diseases that cause this kind of impairment lead to total blindness and complicate the introduction of anything associated with what many clients fear most: total blindness (see Chapter 6). As a result, the therapist often must subtly introduce blindness strategies. Even though mobility training should be performed by a certified orientation and mobility specialist (COMS), the low vision rehabilitation therapist could introduce the client to human guide (sighted guide) techniques, use of nonvisual cues, environmental adaptations, and trailing techniques (sliding the back of the hand along a wall while walking), and convince the client to seek training on the use of the white cane (see Chapter 18). Better acceptance might be expected if the therapist introduces a human guide (sighted guide) or the need for a white cane for "walking at night," when the client is less likely to deny the problem. People will gradually become accustomed to the advantages of using these methods at night or when in crowds, and might begin using many of these techniques at all times and if vision further declines.

With more severe field restrictions in people with near-normal visual acuity, sometimes reverse telescopes are prescribed to reduce the size of objects or a scene so the image fits into the smaller visual field. The occupational therapist can evaluate the suitability of this approach by instructing a client to stand further away from something to identify it. If this is successful, an optical solution may be more convenient (see Chapter 14). These are never used while walking or driving a wheelchair.

In our clinical experience, other effective general compensatory treatments of disabilities associated with overall visual field loss incorporate many of the techniques for homonymous visual field loss. Otherwise, the various treatments of overall visual field loss often are task specific and involve tactile methods or devices used for rehabilitation

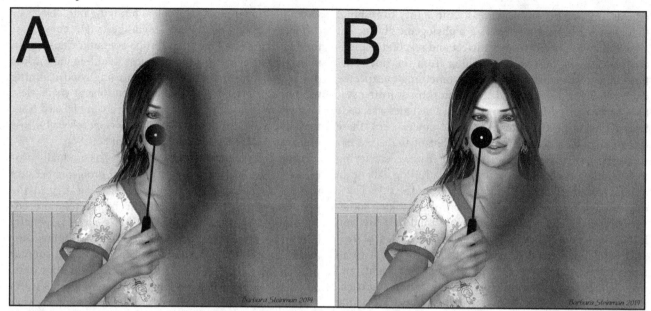

Figure 11-3. Unilateral field loss with and without central sparing during confrontation field testing with wands. The patient detects a light that flashes in the center of the disk. The wands allow stimulus movement without arm movement that might reveal the location of the stimulus. Without the wands, finger movement can be used, but is not as precise. (Reprinted with permission from Barbara Steinman.)

with total blindness. These approaches will be discussed in greater detail in the chapters dealing with specific activities like mobility and homemaking in Section IV.

Unilateral Visual Field Loss

Unilateral visual field loss results from brain injury to the visual pathway after the optic chiasm and is often associated with CVA that has unilateral effects. Damage to the right side of the brain may lead to blindness in the left visual field of both eyes. Damage to the left side of the brain may lead to blindness in the right visual field of both eyes (see Chapter 3). If the blind area comprises nearly half of the visual field starting approximately at the midline of both eyes, the condition is called *homonymous hemianopia* (Figure 11-3). If a quarter of the visual field is affected, the condition is called *homonymous quadrantanopia*.

Unilateral visual field loss usually does not cut the field down the middle, but rather leaves central vision intact, called *central sparing* (see Figure 11-3[A]). Functionally, an individual with a unilateral visual field loss with central sparing will see most of a person's face at about 1 meter (3 feet), but not beyond the face. People with field cuts and central sparing usually have normal acuity and only minor problems with reading (Table 11-1). These individuals will read a single line of text normally, but might lose their place when reading, or may have difficulty scanning a page for information. In some cases, people have a unilateral visual field loss that also bisects the central field (see Figure 11-3[B]). These individuals will report that one half of the examiner's face can be seen during field testing. People with split central fields will only see half of a letter or words they

are trying to identify as well. The resultant loss of basic shape, letter, and face recognition may be confused with higher-order perceptual deficits. People with a right unilateral visual field loss with a split central field will have severe problems with reading.

Functionally, people with unilateral visual field loss will present with a disabled visual scanning and peripheral warning system, often with the functional effects compounded by an overlay of unilateral visual inattention. In addition, a person with recent unilateral visual field loss may present with "wayfinding deficits" and often cannot even retrace his or her steps. A person may have basic problems with wayfinding, primarily due to a unilateral visual field loss rather than a cognitive deficit. For example, if a client with a left visual field loss walks down a hall for the first time, he or she will see one side of the hall to the right. When he or she turns around to retrace his or her steps, the formerly right side of the hall will now be in the blind left visual field. The person doesn't recognize the side of the hall that he or she can now see on the right side because he or she never saw it before. It had been on the blind left side before he or she turned around. In effect, this person has never seen the route he or she is retracing unless he or she uses compensatory scanning. This problem is exacerbated for people who have split central fields and/or unilateral spatial neglect.

Damage to the optic chiasm, which is most often associated with pituitary tumor but sometimes associated with traumatic injury, will cause binasal or bitemporal visual field loss. With binasal deficit, the client cannot see nasally to the fixation objects with each eye and the temporal fields are intact. With bitemporal visual field loss (Figure 11-4),

TABLE 11-1: EXPECTED PROBLEMS BEFORE ADAPTATION

CONDITIONS	MOBILITY ON AFFECTED SIDE		READING				OTHER	
	Detecting people, furniture, traffic	Detecting smaller objects on floor	Finding beginning of each line	Reading text fluently on each line	Reading left half of words	Reading right half of words	Visual acuity	Skimming and visual search
HQ-superior central sparing	Occasional if high obstacles	None	None	None	None	None	None	Occasional
HQ-inferior central sparing	Occasional if unexpected	Occasional if moving	Occasional	None	None	None	None	Occasional
Left HH-central sparing	Intermittent	Occasional if moving	Occasional	Normal	Normal	Normal	Normal	Intermittent
Right HH-central sparing	Intermittent	Occasional if moving	Normal	Mild slowing	Normal	Normal	Normal	Intermittent
Left HH-split central field	Frequent	Frequent	Intermittent	Mild slowing	Intermittent	Normal	Mild loss	Intermittent to severe
Right HH-split central field	Frequent	Frequent	Normal	Frequent	Normal	Frequent with longer words	Mild loss	Severe
HH-motion sensitivity	Less severe than above	Less severe than above	Same as above	Same as above	Same as above	Same as above	Same as above	Same as above

Homonymous hemianopia (HH); homonymous quadrantopia (HQ).

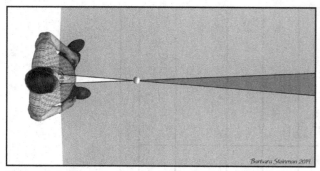

Barbara Steinman 2014

Figure 11-4. An overhead view of distal field loss in someone with bitemporal heteranopia. Objects in the light gray areas are not seen in the temporal field of one eye, but can be seen because it is in the nasal field of the other eye. Objects cannot be seen in the darkened areas directly behind a fixation target where the temporal fields overlap. (Reprinted with permission from Barbara Steinman.)

the client cannot see temporally to the fixation target in each eye and the nasal fields are intact. If one overlaps the visual fields, it appears that the fields are full because one eye will see what the other does not. For example, with binasal defects, the left (temporal) field of the left eye is intact and the right (temporal) field of the right eye is intact. At least in theory, if the 2 eyes look at the same fixation target, the client sees to the right with the right eye and to the left with the left eye and should have a full visual field. There are, however, subtle but disabling problems. A person with binasal deficits will not see some objects closer than the fixation target because closer objects might fall into the nasal field of both eyes. One can demonstrate this by positioning one finger at arm's length and another a few inches from the nose on the midline. Fixate the far finger with both eyes and then close each eye to see how the proximal finger falls into the nasal field of each eye. If a client had a binasal field deficit, he or she would not see the closer object. With bitemporal defects, one will not see some objects further than the fixation target, which can be dangerous. If in addition to the bitemporal defect the central vision is cut in one or both eyes, a client will also have difficulty fixating an object with both eyes at the same time and might have binocular problems as a result.

EVALUATION

Effective treatment starts with an identification of specific potential visual barriers to performance from the functional vision evaluation described in Chapter 8. The evaluation must not only include confrontation visual fields, but also the results of tangent screen fields because central visual field loss significantly affects disability and treatment planning. Ideally, the results of perimetry should be obtained from the optometrist or ophthalmologist involved in treating the client. If this information is not available, and if the client is able to sustain attention for

the approximately 10 minutes required for these tests, the therapist should refer the client for these tests. The most informative tests for rehabilitation treatment planning are the 60-degree or greater visual fields to test far into the periphery (screening is acceptable) and full-threshold fields within the central 10 degrees if central field involvement is suspected.

A visual field loss does not always result in disability. Some people adapt by themselves; others may have been effectively taught adaptive strategies. The disability would be indicated by performance-based tests as follows (see Table 11-1).

Performance-level testing:

- Dynamic functional visual fields. Simply tell the client you are evaluating how well he or she gets around. Do not mention compensatory scanning because the test is to determine if the client will use compensatory strategies without cues. The examiner should closely guard the patient to prevent a fall. First engage the patient in conversation while testing. Have the patient walk down a hallway and around furniture. Have an assistant pretend to walk into the client from the nonseeing side. Place various obstacles on the floor. Ask the client to locate unsafe situations in a kitchen and to look up information in a catalog or on a map. The specific activities should be those that a client would normally perform. If the examiner is required to warn the client or provide any assistance, or if the client makes contact with obstacles, then the examiner documents the need for assistance and/or cues, and this indicates that a disability exists and substantiates the need for treatment. The examiner should note if the client is looking in the direction of the visual field loss to compensate, as this indicates good rehabilitation potential and the absence of spatial neglect. The reason for engaging the patient in conversation is to determine if compensatory scanning is habitual and will occur when attention is divided.

- Laser tag (Figure 11-5). This nonstandardized test provides a quantitative measure of a person's ability to compensate for a visual field loss as a secondary task. The test is conducted in a typical setting with a cluttered visual background on a standard route. In a hospital, it may be a series of hallways. While the client talks about something of interest, the examiner points a laser pointer into the right or left visual field, leaving the spot on until it is detected by the client. The client might hold a laser as well and try to tag the spot when seen or point to it with a finger. If it is detected within 2 seconds, then it is counted as a "hit." Keep a running tally of how many hits and misses occur on the affected side. Randomize the timing and location of the spot so that it is not predictable. Position about half of the spots farther than 45 degrees to the side (but within the

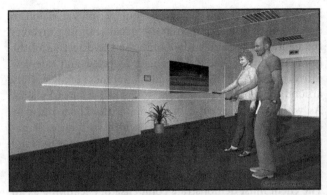

Figure 11-5. Laser tag. The therapist projects a spot on the wall with a laser pointer, keeps it on, and starts timing by silently counting. The client, holding another pointer, has 2 seconds to respond by trying to tag the therapist's spot. Accuracy is not considered, just an obvious response in the direction of the target. (Reprinted with permission from Barbara Steinman.)

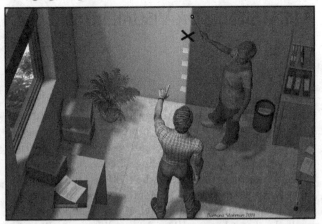

Figure 11-6. Static functional visual fields. The shaded area indicates the nonseeing area. The client maintains straight-ahead fixation (X), and the therapist sneaks up on the affected side or puts objects on the floor to determine when the client sees them. (Reprinted with permission from Barbara Steinman.)

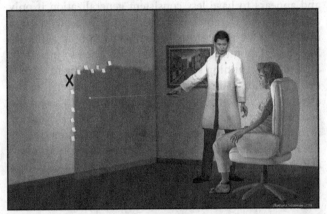

Figure 11-7. Adapted tangent screen fields using a laser pointer target and wall, from the point of view standing in front of the client. Hands of therapist holding a laser pointer to the side projecting a spot on the wall. Fixation X on a sticky note, with several sticky notes along the edge of a superior homonymous quadrantanopia with central involvement). (Reprinted with permission from Barbara Steinman.)

client's field of view). Record how many hits or misses occur out of 10 presentations. Laser tag forms the basis of a training procedure described later.

- The Pepper Visual Skills for Reading Test (see Chapter 8).

- The Bells cancellation task,[14] line bisection, and Catherine Bergego Scale (CBS) will effectively screen for spatial neglect.[12]

Impairment-level testing:

- Static functional visual fields (Figure 11-6). Explain that the test is designed to evaluate side vision and to only look at the fixation target. The client sits or stands looking at an assistant in a large room or hallway, but not anywhere else. The assistant carefully looks for any eye movement, and if these eye movements occur, cues the patient to maintain fixation and avoid looking around. If an assistant is not available, pick a target directly in front of the patient for him or her to fixate. Sneak up on the client on either side and estimate the angle from the midsagittal plane where the person is first detected. Six or more objects, such as bean bags, are scattered on the floor directly in front and the client is instructed to count them, again without looking down. The bean bags can be repositioned and testing repeated to more accurately measure the area of visual field loss.

- Confrontation fields (see Figure 11-3). This was described in Chapter 8.

- Tangent screen fields (Figure 11-7). The client is asked to fixate an X on a sticky note. A laser is used to flash a light around the fixation target at random times and locations to look for an area where the client does not respond to the light—this prevents guessing. Starting in the blind area, move the spot about 12 cm (5 inches) a second until it is seen (dynamic testing). The speed can be varied, but if it is too slow, the client will start looking for it. Use dynamic testing to mark the edge of the blind area with sticky notes, but use static testing—flashing in the seeing area at random times—to prevent the client from anticipating the location. Repeat testing of each point at different times to verify accuracy. The distance from the wall and lighting conditions must be recorded and replicated in future testing (see Chapter 8).

TREATMENT FOR VISUAL FIELD LOSS

Remediation

Some investigators have described a training technique that they claim actually decreases the size of the blind area 5 to 10 degrees in people with a presumably stable visual field loss of 18 months to several years.[15] This instructional technique involved having clients detect flashing lights presented at the edge of the field loss for 1 hour for 3 or more days a week for 3 to 6 months as part of a home program involving specialized training equipment. The results have not been replicated in studies controlling for compensatory scanning eye movements.[16] Therefore, the evidence for this procedure is questionable at this time but it remains a practice option. A variation of this procedure involves repetition of the dynamic tangent screen procedure (see Figure 11-7) described earlier. An assistant slowly moves a laser spot from a nonseeing area in the visual field toward the seeing area and marks the point where the spot is first seen with a sticky note, using these notes to define the edge of the blind area. At home, these markers should be left on the wall, the client should sit in the same place, and the lighting should be similar. The client should practice daily for at least 1 hour. Subsequently, the client can practice alone, moving the laser target him- or herself and noting how far from the edge of the sticky note the spot was first detected. Repetition of this procedure results in repeated stimulation of the edge of a blind area. This allows the client to see if the blind area is changing in size and enhances the client's awareness of the blind area. For this procedure the client must maintain fixation on a central target. It is helpful to have an assistant monitor fixation. A small target at the limit of the client's acuity threshold will help the client self-monitor fixation. This alternative to the commercially available system costs very little, functions to increase awareness of the blind area, and allows clients to determine on their own if the visual field is recovering. The gradual nature of the process allows the client to accept a poor prognosis and to start considering alternatives to driving.

The method that seems to produce the largest and functionally greatest increase in peripheral awareness is called *compensatory visual scanning*. In this technique, the therapist teaches the client to look with quick saccades in the direction of the blind hemifield.[17-19] Although clients often feel like they are recovering visual field, compensatory visual scanning by itself does not actually increase the size of the intact field.

Compensatory Visual Scanning

To compensate for a unilateral visual field loss, the client must change habitual eye movement patterns. Normally we look at an object and depend on our peripheral vision to see on either side. Compensatory visual scanning involves frequently and consistently looking in the direction of the blind area, much like a driver uses rearview and sideview mirrors when driving to maintain awareness of all activity around the car and beyond the range of peripheral vision. As with any therapeutic intervention, the client must be educated about the deficit and provided with an explanation for the compensatory strategy. Understanding and verbalizing the problem or demonstrating improved performance during instructional protocols is not sufficient. The client must demonstrate compensatory scanning as an ingrained habit during real-life activities when attention is on an activity, not the eye movement.

Teaching compensatory visual scanning has not only face validity; there is now ample evidence this intervention is effective when used in the context of everyday activity and appears to have less consistent generalization if only computer-based, more artificial, training protocols are used.[17,20-22] In general, using artificial training activities like cancellation tasks can be effectively used to introduce a client to a scanning strategy, such as scanning to a landmark ("anchor") to cue the client to look far enough to the affected side. The training should then move to a real-life activity in a typical context in which it can be performed in order to maximize generalization of the strategy.[23-26] There is a great deal of room for a creative therapist to adapt activities that are meaningful to the client. The activities should be organized as follows.

Scanning for Expected and Then Unexpected Objects

Recommended materials: Laser pointer, Brain Injury Visual Assessment Battery for Adults (biVABA),[2,27] the *Left Visual Inattention: Workbook*.[28]

We suggest a 3-step sequence for teaching this skill:

1. Looking for expected objects provides direct feedback as to the effectiveness of the scanning effort. The client looks for known objects and knows how many there are. For example, a person is told to look for 10 cards and not stop until all are found, or looks for self-care items that are known to be present.

   a. The first stage in treatment is to engage the client in various search tasks: looking for specified objects in a room, looking for cooking or self-care items, simple puzzles, dominoes, or completing cancellation and drawing tasks from the previously recommended treatment packages. Examples of these treatment strategies have been well described in the occupational therapy literature.[7] This step is quickly mastered by people with intact visual attention, and less easily recovered with clients who have attention deficits and spatial neglect. Easier tasks should be overlearned, including familiar and meaningful

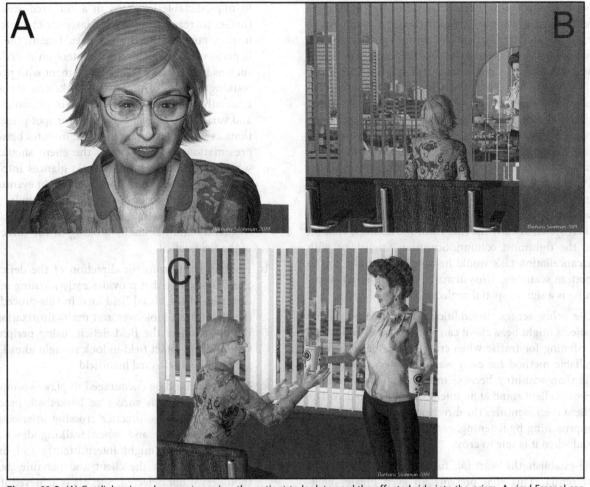

Figure 11-8. (A) Gottlieb prism placement requires the patient to look toward the affected side into the prism. A vinyl Fresnel can be used as an inexpensive, temporary alternative to the Gottlieb prism. (B) The prism can act as a target for compensatory scanning and provides field expansion to the affected side so the image of something or someone in the blind area can be seen as a double image. (C) The client is encouraged to look directly at the target once detected. (Reprinted with permission from Barbara Steinman.)

activities such as brushing one's teeth. Using tasks with expected objects (the brush, toothpaste, and glass) will encourage the client to continue looking until all the components in the visual task are found. These tasks are useful in providing initial instruction on scanning strategies. The difficulty of the task will depend on a client's prior experience; a computer programmer who hates to cook might find locating objects on a computer screen much easier than finding objects in a kitchen.

b. Although people with visual field loss without cognitive or attention deficits quickly learn compensatory scanning,[18,29] direct instruction may be needed to look far enough to the affected side. A classic strategy is to place a brightly colored line and tactile marker down the edge of the page or field being scanned and cueing the client to keep looking until the line is seen; this landmark is sometimes called an *anchor*. A more practical approach is to

have the client use a finger as a landmark on the affected side, or look for a naturally occurring landmark, such as the edge of a book, table, or his or her own shoulder, on the affected side. If a person wears glasses, a vinyl Fresnel prism can be affixed to the edge of the lens on one eye (see later), as this not only provides field expansion, it also acts as an anchor. The client is instructed to look in the direction of the visual field loss until he or she sees the prism (Figure 11-8).

c. Reading provides a person with feedback about the effectiveness of scanning because if words are missed, the meaning is lost. Clients are instructed to reread using appropriate strategies if they lose the meaning of what is being read. Reading, therefore, is an excellent and natural therapeutic activity for visual field loss.

2. Looking for unexpected objects. The previous steps are repeated. Not knowing if an object will be found

becomes challenging because the client does not receive feedback if a scanning strategy does not work. As an example, a client is asked to look for cards or objects, but not told how many. In another example, a person is asked to look in a menu for a dish, but does not know if it is listed or not. When looking for unexpected objects, the client must initiate a systematic scanning strategy to make certain the entire area in question is being scanned. The best search strategy, however, is task dependent. A strategy for looking for coffee cups or a book would be to look for tabletops in a room first. When searching for a food item on a menu organized into columns, the best strategy is to start by scanning section headings vertically from top to bottom and then systematically moving from the leftmost column to the rightmost column. Scanning English or with a cancellation task would involve left to right, top to bottom scanning. Unsystematic, or right to left, scanning is a sign of spatial neglect (discussed later).

3. Use other senses. In addition to anticipating where objects might be, a client can learn to smell and listen. Listening for traffic when crossing a street is a more reliable method for early warning of oncoming traffic than scanning because monitoring is continuous. Have a client stand at an intersection blindfolded. The client then identifies the direction from which cars are approaching by listening, noting traffic light changes and when it is safe to cross.

4. Re-establish the warning function of the peripheral retina. This step presents an even greater challenge because not only is the target unpredictable, but responding to approaching objects from the affected side usually requires habitually scanning to the affected side with divided attention, which is often impaired with brain injury or in older individuals. One approach we have successfully used involves behavior modification of scanning eye movements. The goal is to establish the habit of frequently and quickly looking in the direction of the field defect. Computer programs and equipment have been developed that allow the client to perform this task independently. This author has found any number of computer games where objects fly in unexpectedly from all directions that provide an engaging opportunity for home-based practice as well.

   a. Laser tag (see Figure 11-5) transitions the client to more real-life situations. The therapist and client each hold a laser pointer. The therapist presents the laser spot on a surface such as an uncluttered wall. The client responds by pointing to the light and tagging the spot with his or her laser pointer. At first, the light is flashed at 2 predictable points in the right and left field. The task is graded to become more challenging and more realistic by moving from predictable positions in an uncluttered area

to unpredictable locations in a cluttered area. To further increase difficulty, the laser spot targets can be presented at different distances. Finally, the task is performed when the client's attention is divided, such as in a visually busy environment with people walking around. During this task, the therapist gradually decreases the frequency of presentations and varies the interval between laser spot presentations as well, pausing up to 1 to 2 minutes between presentations. At this point, the client should be walking with frequent automatic glances into the affected hemifield so that when the light eventually appears, she or he detects it within 2 seconds. This instructional sequence should result in the client frequently and habitually looking in the direction of the field deficit.

   b. Holding fixation in the direction of the deficit is another strategy that provides early warning in the direction of the visual field loss. In this procedure, the client must look over and maintain fixation in the direction of the field deficit, using peripheral vision in the intact field to look straight ahead and see into the unaffected hemifield.

   c. The client could be encouraged to play two-on-one ball games such as soccer or basketball, practice walking in crowds, practice crossing intersections with supervision, and when walking down the street, a partner might intermittently and unexpectedly veer into the client and playfully bump shoulders if not detected. Success is achieved if the client automatically maintains most of the fixation between straight ahead and the affected side so as to detect an approaching target within 1 to 2 seconds.

Reading and Object Recognition With a Split Central Field

With a restricted field, the client generally reads better with smaller print, so a recent refraction is necessary to maximize visual acuity. We have found that a small degree of central visual field is spared on both sides of the vertical meridian. Sometimes, visual field loss splits the central field exactly, and the client may need to develop eccentric viewing in the direction of the field deficit and use side vision to expand the field of view, although this reduces reading visual acuity. Since fewer letters are seen in one fixation when larger print is used, the therapist should carefully evaluate reading with print around 1.0 (8 point) to 1.6M (12 point). Therapy focuses on object recognition and reading in addition to the treatment program discussed earlier. This is a practice option level of evidence (see Chapter 9) and thus requires careful outcome evaluation on an ongoing basis.

1. Start with object recognition using objects that require that the client see both sides to identify and orient the object horizontally. Examples of such objects could

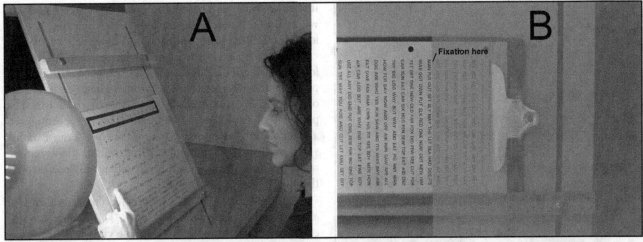

Figure 11-9. (A) A person using fingers and a distinct left landmark to keep place while reading. (B) A person reading vertically oriented text with a right field loss.

be a toothbrush, a hammer, a nut driver, screwdriver, paintbrush, etc. Usually, a client will start by scanning left and right to see the object. To encourage the client to more quickly identify the object by looking toward the affected side rather than scanning back and forth, the therapist gradually slows the duration of the object presentation so the client does not have time to scan back and forth.

2. Reading strategies differ with right and left visual field loss. Pay close attention to the size of the text and distance. Smaller is generally better, but not always, as discussed earlier, so use reading acuity tests to estimate the best size print and what is a comfortable working distance—usually 40 cm (16 inches)—for the client.

   a. Start with single word recognition and number recognition with flash cards. Numbers and compound words (eg, "headlight") are best. Gradually reduce the exposure time so the client can learn to direct fixation toward the affected side. With a right field cut, the client must learn to look toward the end of the words. With left visual field loss, the client must look toward the beginning of words. Start with noncompound words (eg, "caught") so the client will immediately recognize a problem if he or she does not look at the right place. Then move on to numbers and compound words.

   b. Move on to continual text, asking the client to point to the end of words with a sharp pointer at first.

3. With left visual field loss, have the client use a brightly colored ruler or straight-edge to the left of the column of print or a left finger to locate the words at the beginning of the line (Figure 11-9[A]). Most people without visual field loss look to the beginning of words. This becomes less necessary with practice. Another suggestion is to use a strip of Velcro or sandpaper on the left margin so that the client can "feel" the left margin. People can quickly learn to use the tactile sense to drive the saccadic eye movement back to the left margin.

4. With right visual field loss:

   a. Have the client use a pointer and point to the end of each word. Stop and reread when the meaning is lost.

   b. Try turning the text 90 degrees clockwise so it is vertically oriented, requiring the client to look top to bottom, or downhill. With vertically oriented text, the person eccentrically views, using a pointer to direct the gaze to the right of the words so entire words can be seen (Figure 11-9[B]). Pay close attention to head position. It takes several days of practice reading vertically to maximize speed. We have found that people who read vertically usually end up reading downhill or at about a 45-degree angle by a combination of reading and text rotation. Since we have found the results to be inconsistent, be careful to compare vertical and horizontal reading after the practice period. We have also found people with linguistic alexia have considerable difficulty reading vertically. Note that people reading other languages read in different directions, for example, Hebrew is read right to left, and Chinese characters may be vertically aligned.

5. Linguistic alexia is like dyslexia, except it results from a brain injury and results in a loss of reading ability independent of vision. Linguistic alexia occurs with left hemisphere brain injury that might also affect the right visual field. With more severe linguistic alexia, a person cannot even recognize letters or 2-letter words, but can recognize symbols on a LEA symbol acuity chart. A person with a less severe linguistic alexia will

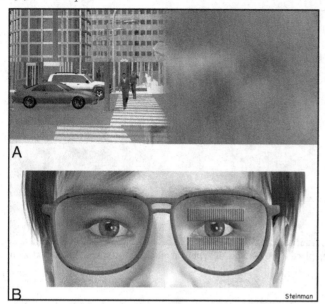

Figure 11-10. The position of the Fresnel prism on spectacles and a simulation of the visual effects. Note that the double image of a potential obstacle approaching from the blind hemifield becomes visible before contact. (Reprinted with permission from Barbara Steinman.)

recognize letters and common words, but has difficulty recognizing less common (harder) words, regardless of the length. It is sometimes difficult to differentiate people with right field loss from linguistic alexia. A person with just a right visual field loss will tend to have difficulty with longer words, regardless of their difficulty, whereas a person with linguistic alexia will find less common words difficult, even if they are short words. People who had marginal literacy or have not read for a long time will exhibit symptoms of linguistic alexia. Because the Pepper Visual Skills for Reading Test[30] contains a mix of easy, uncommon, longer, and compound words, it is ideally suited for this type of testing.

Field Expansion Devices

The use of field expansion mirrors and prisms has been advocated for many years, and some configurations can work as an early warning system, allowing clients to continuously monitor and detect the approach of something on the affected side.[31-34] Fresnel prisms up to 57 diopters (see Figures 11-8 and 11-10) are pressed onto one spectacle lens with the base of the prism in the direction of the visual field loss. The prism displaces an image away from the base toward the point of the prism. (Think of the prism wedge as an arrow that points in the direction in which the person's view will move.) Prisms can be positioned with the base toward the affected side so when a person looks into the prism, images up to about 25 degrees farther into the blind hemifield can now be seen. The prims act like the rearview mirror of a car, allowing someone to quickly glance and see

into the blind area. There is, however, an inherent problem with prisms. When the client looks into the prism on one lens, visual confusion and double vision will be experienced. One image is the normal view as seen by the eye looking through the plain lens. The eye looking through the prism on the other lens will see another image, actually part of a scene displaced from the blind area by the prism. The person will experience 2 different images superimposed and a double of each image somewhere else. Because of this visual confusion and diplopia, we have found clients tend to reject prisms if they are positioned so they will look directly through the prism continually.

Attaching a 20- to 57-diopter prism on the lateral edge of a lens (Gottlieb placement; see Figure 11-8)[31] is not as bothersome because it only creates double vision when the client looks through it, and often the person's nose will block the second image. This prism displaces the image from the blind side toward the unaffected side, but only is effective while the client looks laterally toward the blind side into the prism. This prism placement works well with compensatory scanning training. The prism actually acts as an effective landmark (anchor) when learning to use compensatory scanning because it is available under any situation. These devices are used primarily to detect and avoid larger objects and people. One must be careful, however, because the lateral displacement by the prism can be disorienting. The client should be instructed to locate approaching pedestrians or cars from the affected side by looking through the prism, and then when the object is detected learn to immediately and automatically turn the head toward the affected size until the target is seen directly (outside of the prism). These prisms are available as relatively inexpensive vinyl lenses that stick to the surface of clean spectacles or sunglasses. Better-quality optical devices can be attached to the lens as well (www.hemianopia.net). Evidence that supports the use of the Gottlieb prism is limited to case reports—including our clinical experience—but this prism placement is considered a practice option and thus must be always evaluated for effectiveness before a recommendation is made. Note that effective use of this prism placement requires training in compensatory scanning; it does not allow continual visual monitoring of the periphery.

The Peli prism creates double vision while the patient is looking straight ahead and effectively acts as an early warning system, but is more acceptable because the double vision is peripheral rather than central, where it is most bothersome.[32,33] The prism is attached above and below the pupil so the double vision is in the superior field and inferior field, but the person also has normal single vision in the center of the visual field (see Figure 11-10). When the client is looking straight ahead, he or she might detect some movement, and this will alert the patient to something approaching on the blind side. The client should detect objects in the blind field before the object enters the intact visual field. There are 2 small randomized trials supporting

TABLE 11-2: SYMPTOMS OF LEFT NEGLECT

- Scanning
  - Less scanning to the left side
  - Increased time to "release" fixation
  - Disorganized scanning: starts in the middle and scans right to left
- Attention
  - Detection of stimuli to the left affected by distractions on the right (simultaneous stimulation extinction)
  - Copying picture: leaves out part of the picture on left
  - Reading: skips the first words in a line
- Spatial
  - Inaccurate estimation of distance between objects
  - Copied drawings are spatially distorted on the left
  - Agraphia: writing does not follow a line, or words are not sequenced and spaced properly
  - Left-right confusion
  - Clothing apraxia: difficulty donning and folding clothes
- Apraxia: difficulty learning new complex movements, such as hemiplegic dressing
- Emotional volatility, especially when cued to attend left
- Anosogosia (denial of symptoms) and identifying causal relationships
- Symptoms are significantly more severe and response to treatment is slower if concurrent field loss

effective use in most who try it, a practice guideline level of evidence (see Chapter 9), indicating it should be made available to clients, but should be evaluated as well because some may not find it helpful. Although people with spatial neglect were excluded from the studies that indicated effectiveness of this therapy, we have found Peli prisms to be a useful option if a client with spatial neglect does not learn to use compensatory scanning. Effective use of the prism, however, requires a divided visual attention toward the "ghost image" as well as practice accurately localizing objects when viewed through the prism because the prisms will create an illusory misplacement of objects.

Fortunately, rather inexpensive vinyl Fresnel prisms (www.bernell.com, www.richmondproducts.com) may be trialed by therapists, but an optometrist or ophthalmologist should prescribe the devices and recommend initial placement. Positioning of Peli prisms is difficult, and more advanced training is recommended. Training with the devices is essential and should include compensatory scanning strategies, and may take more than one session. The amount of field expansion in degrees can be approximated by dividing prism diopter by 2, usually between 30 and 57 diopters (about 15 to 25 degrees, respectively).

SPATIAL NEGLECT AND ATTENTION DEFICITS

Spatial neglect is actually a syndrome with a constellation of impairments associated with right hemisphere damage from stroke, traumatic brain injury caused by lateral impact, and brain injuries that affect the parietal and frontal lobes, especially in the right hemisphere. Unilateral inattention is a common impairment associated with this syndrome, leading to the most common term for the syndrome, *spatial neglect*. Other symptoms of spatial neglect syndrome are in Table 11-2. With more extensive brain damage, vision, somatosensory, and motor control are affected, and we find impairments tend to be more severe as more of the brain and sensory systems are involved. Spatial neglect often occurs with visual field loss and can be confused with it. Dementia, encephalopathy, and traumatic brain injury that have a bilateral effect on the frontal and parietal areas result in simultagnosia or Balint syndrome, with what resemble bilateral neglect symptoms. A person with this condition develops what could be described as an "attention tunnel vision"—the person has intact peripheral vision, but when attending to a focal stimulus will tend not to notice stimuli in the periphery. In more extreme forms, a person might see a few letters in the center of a word rather than the whole word and mislocalize objects when reaching for them (optic ataxia).

Evaluation

Validated standardized tests such as the Behavioral Inattention Test (BIT)[35,36] can be time consuming to administer, but might be necessary to justify what is often an extensive course of treatment. Typically, neglect can be detected by looking for the signs and symptoms listed in Table 11-2 within the context of functional activity, where attention tends to be divided or distractions are present. A recent review[12] suggests quickly administered tests that detect spatial neglect, such as (1) clock drawing and picture copying, (2) line bisection, (3) observation donning a T-shirt, (4) extinction of response with bilateral simultaneous stimulation and with more quantifiable tests, including (5) a Bells cancellation test[14] and (6) reading. A highly recommended functional test of visual neglect that is particularly well suited for occupational therapy is the CBS, where an observer rates 10 self-care and functional behaviors on a scale from 0 (no neglect) to 3 (severe neglect). The CBS scale has been well validated[37-40] and measures neglect in personal, peripersonal, and extrapersonal space (allocentric neglect). This test can be found in the *Journal of Neuropsychological Rehabilitation*.[41]

Although validated for use with people with central scotoma, the Pepper Visual Skills for Reading Test is particularly useful in quantifying neglect symptoms as well. Because spatial neglect includes a variety of more specific impairments, a client with spatial neglect may respond differently to these tests. The tests should be used to identify the specific impairments that need to be addressed. For example, problems on the line bisection, writing, and drawing tasks indicate treatment should focus on spatial estimation. Poor performance on one side of the paper with the cancellation task indicates a unilateral attention deficit, whereas missed objects on both sides indicates an overall (bilateral) attention deficit or problems organizing systematic scanning.

Sometimes people who have undergone treatment still have mild neglect symptoms that can be dangerous in a driving situation. These individuals can become "test wise," and their residual neglect can escape detection by the previous tests. We have found that the Trails Test and Useful Field of View Test,[42] which have been used to screen for possible driving disability,[43] are sensitive to mild neglect. Abbreviated versions of these tests are part of a computerized testing program provided by The Automobile Association of America and are available on their website (search for "Roadwise Review"). Note that these are for self-testing by consumers and do not comprise formal clinical testing. People with hemianopic visual field loss or lower quadrant visual field loss are neither safe nor, in most states,

legal to drive.[44] In cases of neglect or visual field loss, a road test by a certified driving instructor is always recommended before driving is resumed.

Treatment for Spatial Neglect

There are both remediational and compensatory interventions for spatial neglect; the intervention best supported by evidence is compensatory scanning. The key for effective treatment of spatial neglect with everyday activities is overlearning. An activity should be automatic and the context kept organized and consistent. It is very important that the nonvisual symptoms of spatial neglect syndrome be addressed because these often are more disabling than the visual symptoms. Pharmacological treatments might ameliorate attention symptoms and emotional volatility—the client should be under the care of a neurologist. The behavioral symptoms of anosognosia, an emotional volatility, create considerable caregiver stress. Normally, it is not unusual in a marriage or family situation for one person to overreact when corrected by another family member. Now add to that a client's heightened emotional response to a cue from anyone and the tendency to deny symptoms resulting from the brain injury. With married couples, it is not unusual to get reports that any cue from a spouse to "look left" quickly escalates into an argument. The argument further distracts the client, and the situation may further deteriorate. Effective treatment also requires highly consistent carryover into the home, often involving the caregiver. As a result, caregiver education must be included in the treatment plan. Generally, a hired caregiver is required, but these situations need to be evaluated individually. Thus, a social worker and a neuropsychologist should be on the treatment team as well. The treatments for spatial neglect are summarized in Tables 11-3 and 11-4.

Remediation With Prism Adaptation

Several studies have shown amelioration of visual and other symptoms of neglect, including compensatory scanning, left side stimulation, mental imagery, and prism adaptation.[3,4,12] Of these, prism adaptation seems to have an effect that persists after the prism has been removed and is thus considered remediation. The treatment protocol is as follows (Figure 11-11):

1. The therapist has a client look through 20- to 40-diopter "yoked" prisms and learn to adapt to optical displacement of a target with the prisms.

2. Both prisms are positioned in front of the client's eyes with the base positioned left for left neglect. The apparent position of a target through the prism is displaced 10 to 20 degrees to the right of where it is actually located so that if a person points to it or throws something at the target, he or she will miss it to the right.

TABLE 11-3: INSTRUCTION ON COMPENSATORY SCANNING WITH AND WITHOUT NEGLECT

COMPENSATORY SCANNING	IF LEFT NEGLECT, ADD THE FOLLOWING
Search tasks for expected objects • Reading • Training using a landmark (anchor) as a target for the initial fixation of a scan that is far enough on the affected side so relevant objects or all words on a line can be seen on the affected side	• Forced fixation on the side of the deficit by shading right • Increased stimulation on the left side, decreased stimulation on the right • Stop and reflect when error is detected or next step of a complex activity begins • Memorize and verbalize strategy for scanning after pause (eg, Lighthouse technique)
Search with unexpected objects by fixating a landmark (anchor) or Gottlieb prism on the affected side	• Reduced stimulation on the right side • Increased stimulation on the left side • Eliminate distractions in general • Memorize and verbalize strategy for scanning and avoiding distraction
Early warning • Behavior modification to develop habitual compensatory scanning of affected side using laser tag • Use Peli prism placement • Holding fixation in the direction of the deficit • Using other senses to detect objects (guarding with extended hand, sound, smell) • Use a long (white) cane	• Slow grading of task complexity and distraction and extended training so scanning is automatic • Avoid distractions; often, divided attention is profoundly impaired

TABLE 11-4: OTHER TREATMENTS FOR SPATIAL NEGLECT

• Prism adaptation therapy

• Mirror therapy

• Focus on familiar activities in familiar context

• Repeat the same movement patterns

• Consider overlearning/errorless learning strategies for dressing and new movement patterns

• Compensatory scanning treatments (see Table 11-3)

• Refer to neurologist, social worker, and neuropsychologist

   ○ Organize home caregiving support for consistent carryover into home

   ○ Address possible caregiver stress

   ○ Carefully coordinate treatment team and use of the same strategies

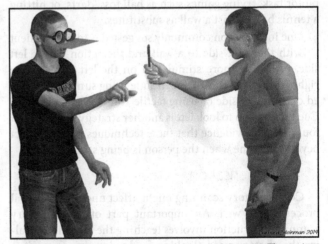

Figure 11-11. The setup for prism adaptation treatment. The patient points to a target. Note that the mask under the eyes prevents the client from seeing the hand or the target until the target is just high enough. The prisms in front of the eye displace the apparent position of the target to the right, so initially the client misses the target to the right until motor learning results in more accurate pointing. (Reprinted with permission from Barbara Steinman.)

3. A mask is positioned so the hand cannot be seen until the object is thrown or the target is reached.

4. With practice, motor learning results in correct localization of the target with pointing or throwing.

5. The prisms are removed after about 100 trials.

6. To test effectiveness, after the prisms are removed, the client should point to or throw an object to the left of where it is actually located, an effect opposite to the error when the prisms were first put on.

7. With one day of treatment, the effect is temporary, lasting only a couple of days. The effect of 10 or more successive daily treatments may last for over 30 days or more.[45,46]

The effectiveness of prism adaptation is not the direct result of any optical intervention because the prisms are removed after training. Although most research supports the effectiveness of this treatment, some good-quality studies do not.[47] Even with randomized clinical trials where there was improved averaged performance, the research is based on grouped data that may have included a mix of people—some were affected and some were not affected by prism adaptation. For this reason, neglect symptoms need to be measured before and after treatments to determine effectiveness on a case-by-case basis. If found effective, the clients are dispensed a kit with the prisms and protocol to be repeated at home on an as-needed basis. Clients often find the task of pointing to a person's finger for 15 minutes a day rather tedious. We suspect that one reason for poor success is noncompliance with the home practice. To improve compliance, we recently tried varying the visuomotor task, trying games such as ball toss, darts, or hitting a tennis ball against a wall as substitutes.

One intervention commonly suggested is to have a client sit with the right side to a wall and the action on the left side, providing more stimulation on the left than on the right. Variants of this theme include using sunglasses shaded on the right side or using tactile stimulators on the left. Cueing a person to look left is another strategy. We have not found strong evidence that these techniques have an effect beyond the time when the person is being stimulated.

Compensation

Compensatory scanning might affect underlying neural processing as well. An important part of compensatory scanning instruction involves teaching the client to verbalize the strategy used (looking for landmarks, pretending to be a lighthouse). This is a metacognitive self-cueing strategy. When a room is first entered, or before starting the next step in a multistep activity such as going from the sauté pan to the cutting board when cooking, the client is taught to stop and think. The client stops and says out loud "look landmark" and then scans the board to make sure no ingredients were missed. The same strategy

is invoked when someone is reading and finds the text no longer makes sense, or if something known to be present is not found. Such an error detection should also prompt the client to stop and think and use the self-cuing strategy. These verbalization strategies could be considered using the left hemisphere's verbal function to substitute for lost right hemisphere function. In our experience, spatial neglect has never been eliminated, and even in someone whose symptoms are not apparent under most circumstances, the left inattention will emerge when attention is divided and the person is fatigued.

In our experience, one compensatory technique to be avoided is using family, friends, and caregivers to cue the client to look left when there is a problem. As discussed earlier, people with left neglect can be more irritable, especially when cued, and conflict can result, particularly if the client is a spouse or relative. Cuing strategies that can be less irritating then telling someone "now remember to look left" might be a tap on the shoulder or a single word or sound. But in general, the compensatory strategy that will increase participation and reduce conflict is to be proactive and structure a person's environment to encourage left attention. If capable of metacognition, the client should be instructed to stop and think and make the following modifications him- or herself before moving into a situation or starting a task:

1. Position him- or herself so that all people and activity are either all on the left or all to the right because if on both sides, the person or activity on the left will be ignored and the client will likely attend to the right.

2. If a person with an egocentric left inattention is reading or using a computer, then the entire screen or page should be positioned to the right of midline.

3. Keeping an organized, decluttered environment where the location of objects does not change will enable a person to function without cues. The client can better predict where an object can be found automatically.

4. Unfortunately, the caregiver might be the person to pick up after the client and keep the environment organized. Cuing or complaining about the messy behavior, especially long after the offending behavior is over, is ineffective and will only lead to conflict.

TREATING PERCEPTUAL DYSFUNCTIONS

When visual temporal areas of the brain are damaged, visual processing might be impaired even though sensory function is largely intact.[1] Examples of perceptual dysfunction include *negative signs*; agnosias, or an inability to recognize and name objects; cortical achromatopsia,

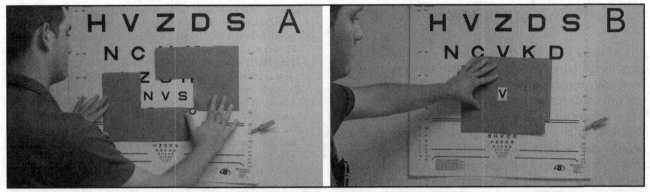

Figure 11-12. How to make a mask for isolating objects and words to eliminate crowding effects. Cut out a gray mask—black creates too much contrast and may cause crowding effects. With a white mask, it is harder for the client to find the target if there is too little contrast. (A) Isolating a line. (B) Isolating a single letter. The clip on the side holds the mask (B) when not in use.

disruptions in color vision; and alexia, an acquired inability to read or recognize letters. *Positive signs* of damage to the retinocortical pathways include various forms of phantom vision; Charles Bonnet syndrome, which includes formed, vivid hallucinations of people and places; and unformed hallucinations, like movement and spots. An assortment of misperceptions of movement (polyopsia) and monocular double vision are associated with brain injury. Palinopsia is where a recently viewed image reemerges later when someone is looking at something else.

Before undertaking treatment for the negative symptoms, one must be careful to rule out sensory involvement. For example, a client who has a homonymous hemianopia with a split central field sees only half of an object when looking at it and may have difficulty recognizing the object. A person with split central fields will also present with reading difficulties that are different from a linguistic alexia.

Although quality evidence is not available, we have found the following strategies to be effective. In treatment of people with both higher-order perceptual problems and low vision, the focus is on functional visual activity and use of multiple-sensory input. For example, Mr. H, a high school principal, had less than a 5-degree central field from a bilateral occipital infarct. He had vivid hallucinations and multiple images, including the vision of teenagers smoking (fortunately, he had a good sense of humor). Treatment first involved blind rehabilitation techniques, such as learning to do activities and recognize objects by touch (see Section IV). He reported that as soon as he touched an object it would appear visually. Mr. H improved in his ability to visualize objects by touch, and with small print that fit into his visual field, could actually read again. He was also encouraged to attempt to identify objects by standing farther away from them, minifying the image of the object so that it would fit into his visual field, and eventually was prescribed a reverse telescope by an optometrist to further reduce the size of an image. With considerable repetition moving around his

house, he recovered his ability to visualize the rooms in his house. During these visual activities, Mr. H reported that the hallucinations were still present but somewhat diminished.

For positive signs like hallucinations and phantom vision, client education is the key to treatment. Carefully ask the client to describe the symptoms and provide reassurance that these symptoms do not indicate underlying psychiatric disorders (as long as the person knows they are not real). The brain must learn how to turn a distorted perception into a recognizable perception. This is accomplished by practice with visual identification followed by tactual or auditory feedback.

It is a standard of practice in treating children with cortical visual impairment to progress visual tasks from visually uncluttered to cluttered settings.[48] A client might see and quickly recognize a cup on a table by itself, but cannot see it when placed among a random assortment of unrelated objects. Visual clutter includes not only other objects, but also patterns on a complex background, such as a patterned tablecloth or reflections, shadows, and glare. Sometimes it is best to evaluate visual clutter by taking a picture of a person's work area because a picture makes the clutter more evident. An example of progressing from uncluttered to cluttered would be reading isolated words, then words in short phrases, then 2 lines double spaced, then 3 lines double spaced, then on to single-spaced lines and eventually paragraphs. Object identification practice should begin on an uncluttered surface, then in a meaningful context. Once again, repetition and progression from uncluttered to cluttered settings appear to be the key to successful treatment. For reading, like measuring acuity, one compensatory technique we have found effective is to view text through a window that isolates words or a line of text (Figure 11-12). Strategies for reading will be discussed in Chapter 15 and blind techniques for other activities are discussed in the other chapters of Section IV.

SUMMARY

Unilateral field loss often presents with similar symptoms as spatial neglect syndrome, but the conditions are completely different in etiology and response to treatment and can occur separately or together. If there are no cognitive deficits or spatial neglect, clients with peripheral visual field loss will naturally develop compensatory scanning because if they cannot see something that they expect to find, they will keep looking around until they see it, just as they did before the brain injury. Instruction on compensatory scanning with just a field loss usually proceeds quickly and effectively within a few sessions. Looking far enough to the affected side and habitual scanning when attention is divided present the greatest challenge. If someone has spatial neglect, then to that person, one side may not even exist in his or her mind and the person does not look in that direction even when he or she hears a person or knows something is present. Spatial neglect thus presents the greatest challenge and significantly prolongs treatment time. Nonetheless, several treatments have been found effective in improving participation in and quality of daily living of people with even severe neglect by using compensatory techniques, sometimes as simple as moving everything of interest to the right side. With mild to moderate neglect, remediational methods and compensatory scanning effectively increase attention to the left. Because evidence is based on group averages rather than individual performance (see Chapter 9), it is important to repeatedly evaluate the effectiveness of interventions on an ongoing basis for every client.

REFERENCES

1. Trobe JD. *The Neurology of Vision*. Oxford: Oxford University Press; 2001:451.
2. Kolb B, Whishaw IQ. *Fundamentals of Human Neuropsychology*. 6th ed. New York: Worth Publishers; 2009.
3. Saevarsson S. Unilateral neglect: a review of causes, anatomical localization, theories and interventions. 2009;95:27-33.
4. Marshall RS. Rehabilitation approaches to hemineglect. *Neurologist*. 2009;15:185-192.
5. Scheiman M. *Understanding and Managing Vision Deficits: A Guide for Occupational Therapists*. 2nd ed. Thorofare, NJ: SLACK, Inc; 2011.
6. Suter PS, Harvey LH. *Vision Rehabilitation: Multidisciplinary Care of the Patient Following Brain Injury*. Boca Raton: CRC Press/Taylor & Francis; 2011:xviii.
7. Zoltan B. *Vision, Perception, and Cognition: A Manual for the Evaluation and Treatment of the Adult With Acquired Brain Injury*. 4th ed. Thorofare, NJ: SLACK, Inc.; 2007.
8. Sanet RB, Press LJ. Spatial vision. In: Suter PS, Harvey LH, eds. *Vision Rehabilitation: Multisensory Care of the Patient Following Brain Injury*. New York: CRC Press; 2011:78-142.
9. Chung STL. The Glenn A. Fry Award Lecture 2012: Plasticity of the visual system following central vision loss. *Optom Vis Sci*. 2013;90:520-529.
10. Milner AD, Goodale MA. Two visual systems re-viewed. *Neuropsychologia*. 2008;46:774-785.
11. Ramachandran VS, Blakeslee S. *Phantoms in the Brain*. New York: Harper Perennial; 1998.
12. Ting DSJ, Pollock A, Dutton GN, et al. Visual neglect following stroke: current concepts and future focus. *Survey Ophthalmol*. 2011;56:114-134.
13. Whittaker SG, Cummings RW. Foveating saccades. *Vis Res*. 1990;30:1363-1366.
14. Gauthier L, Dehaut F, Joanette Y. The Bells test: a quantitative and qualitative test for visual neglect. *Int J Clin Neuropsychol*. 1989;11:49-52.
15. Heikki HA, Julkunen LA. Treatment of visual field deficits after a stroke. *Adv Clin Neurosci Rehabil*. 2004;3:17-18.
16. Reinhard J, Schreiber A, Schiefer U, et al. Does visual restitution training change absolute homonymous visual field defects? A fundus controlled study. *Br J Ophthalmol*. 2005;89:30-35.
17. Pouget MC, Levy-Bencheton D, Prost M, Tilikete C, Husain M, Jacquin-Courtois S. Acquired visual field defects rehabilitation: critical review and perspectives. *Ann Phys Rehabil Med*. 2012;55:53-74.
18. Papageorgiou E, Hardiess G, Mallot HA, Schiefer U. Gaze patterns predicting successful collision avoidance in patients with homonymous visual field defects. *Vis Res*. 2012;65:25-37.
19. Pollock A. Interventions for visual field defects in patients with stroke. *Cochrane Database Systematic Rev*. 2011.
20. Hayes A, Chen CS, Clarke G, Thompson A. Functional improvements following the use of the NVT Vision Rehabilitation program for patients with hemianopia following stroke. *Neurorehabilitation*. 2012;31:19-30.
21. Mennem TA, Warren M, Yuen HK. Preliminary validation of a vision-dependent activities of daily living instrument on adults with homonymous hemianopia. *Am J Occup Ther*. 2012;66:478-482.
22. Pambakian ALM, Mannan SK, Hodgson TL, Kennard C. Saccadic visual search training: a treatment for patients with homonymous hemianopia. *J Neurol Neurosurg Psychiatry*. 2004;75:1443-1448.
23. Cicerone KD, Langenbahn DM, Braden C, et al. Evidence-based cognitive rehabilitation: updated review of the literature from 2003 through 2008. *Arch Phys Med Rehabil*. 2011;92:519-530.
24. Cicerone KD, Mott T, Azulay J, et al. A randomized controlled trial of holistic neuropsychologic rehabilitation after traumatic brain injury. *Arch Phys Med Rehabil*. 2008;89:2239-2249.
25. Cicerone KD, Dahlberg C, Malec JF, et al. Evidence-based cognitive rehabilitation: updated review of the literature from 1998 through 2002. *Arch Phys Med Rehabil*. 2005;86:1681-1692.
26. Ma HI, Trombly CA. A synthesis of the effects of occupational therapy for persons with stroke. Part II: remediation of impairments (structured abstract). *Am J Occup Ther*. 2002;56:260-274.
27. Warren M. *Brain Injury Visual Assessment Battery for Adults: Test Manual*. Birmingham, AL: VisAbility Rehab Services, Inc; 1998.
28. Knauss DS. *Left Visual Inattention: Workbook*. Tucson, AZ: Therapy Skill Builders; 1998.
29. Pambakian AL, Wooding DS, Patel N, Morland AB, Kennard C, Mannan SK. Scanning the visual world: a study of patients with homonymous hemianopia. *J Neurol Neurosurg Psychiatry*. 2000;69:751-759.
30. Watson GR, Whittaker SG, Steciw M. *Pepper Visual Skills for Reading Test (revised)*. Milwaukee, WI: Fork in the Road Vision Rehabilitation Services LLC; 1995.
31. Gottlieb DD, Freeman P, Williams M. Clinical research and statistical analysis of a visual field awareness system. *J Am Optom Assoc*. 1992;63:581-588.
32. Giorgi RG, Woods RL, Peli E. Clinical and laboratory evaluation of peripheral prism glasses for hemianopia. *Optom Vis Sci*. 2009;86:492-502.

33. Peli E. Field expansion for homonymous hemianopia by optically induced peripheral exotropia. *Optom Vis Sci.* 2000;77:453-464.

34. Mehr EM, Freid AN. *Low Vision Care.* Chicago: Professional Press; 1975:107.

35. Wilson B, Cockburn J, Halligan P. Development of a behavioral test of visual-spatial neglect. *Arch Phys Med Rehabil.* 1987;68:98-102.

36. Hartman-Maeir A, Katz N. Validity of the Behavioral Inattention Test (BIT): relationships with functional tasks. *Am J Occup Ther.* 1995;49:507-516.

37. Azouvi P, Bartolomeo P, Beis J-M, Perennou D, Pradat-Diehl P, Rousseaux M. A battery of tests for the quantitative assessment of unilateral neglect. *Restorative Neurol Neurosci.* 2006;24:273-285.

38. Beis JM, Keller C, Morin N, et al. Right spatial neglect after left hemisphere stroke: qualitative and quantitative study. *Neurology.* 2004;63:1600-1605.

39. Azouvi P, Samuel C, Louis-Dreyfus A, et al. Sensitivity of clinical and behavioural tests of spatial neglect after right hemisphere stroke. *J Neurol Neurosurg Psychiatry.* 2002;73:160-166.

40. Bergego C, Azouvi P, Deloche G, et al. Rehabilitation of unilateral neglect: a controlled multiple-baseline-across-subjects trial using computerised training procedures. *J Neuropsychol Rehabil.* 1997;7:279-293.

41. Azouvi P, Marchal F, Samuel C, et al. Functional consequences and awareness of unilateral neglect: study of an evaluation scale. *J Neuropsychol Rehabil.* 1996;6:133-150.

42. Clay O, Wadley VG, Edwards JD, Roth DL, Roenker DL, Ball KK. Cumulative meta-analysis of the relationship between useful field of view and driving performance in older adults: current and future implications. *Optom Vis Sci.* 2005;82:724-731.

43. Classen S, Wang Y, Crizzle AM, Winter SM, Lanford DN. Predicting older driver on-road performance by means of the Useful Field of View and Trail Making Test Part B. *Am J Occup Ther.* 2013;67:574-582.

44. Racette L, Casson E. The impact of visual field loss on driving performance: evidence from on-road driving assessment. *Optom Vis Sci.* 2005;82:668-674.

45. Serino A, Barbiani M, Rinaldesi ML, Ladavas E. Effectiveness of prism adaptation in neglect rehabilitation: a controlled trial study. *Stroke.* 2009;40:1392-1398.

46. Shiraishi H, Yamakawa Y, Itou A, Muraki T, Asada T. Long-term effects of prism adaptation on chronic neglect after stroke. *Neurorehabilitation.* 2008;23:137-151.

47. Turton AJ, O'Leary K, Gabb J, Woodward R, Gilchrist ID. A single blinded randomised controlled pilot trial of prism adaptation for improving self-care in stroke patients with neglect. *J Neuropsychol Rehabil.* 2010;20:180-196.

48. Lueck AH. *Functional Vision: A Practitioner's Guide to Evaluation and Intervention.* New York: AFB Press; 2004.

Environmental Modifications

12

This chapter is designed to present a systematic approach to modifications of the physical environment to maximize the client's function. The suggestions described in this chapter are compensatory. They are designed to improve a client's functional ability despite his or her visual impairment. Duffy et al stress the importance of a careful environmental assessment before attempting to modify the environment. They describe environmental assessment as the process of systematically analyzing the area and surroundings in which individuals with low vision will be living, working, or attending school. To be effective, the environmental evaluation should encompass 2 broad areas: the individual's general environment and surroundings, and the context in which the client performs specific tasks. The assessment provided in *Making Life More Livable* allows the client to take an active role in evaluating and modifying their environment. This provides the client with some ownership of the changes being implemented. It develops their problem-solving skills should future changes be required, and allows them to make decisions regarding cost and ease of maintenance. This approach typifies andragogy or adult learning theory.[1]

EVALUATION

Changing a person's physical environment often must be handled delicately, especially if a person has been living in a given setting for many years or if there are others living in the same space. People with visual impairments depend on consistent organization and placement of objects around them to locate items and navigate. Older people tend to have a favorite chair where they do many activities. Moving the chair or changing the setting around the chair is difficult; asking the person to sit elsewhere to do a task is much more difficult. The first step in organizing environmental modifications, therefore, is to determine if a problem or barrier to performance even exists. Then review the findings from the functional vision evaluation (see Chapter 8), where goals and potential visual and other physical barriers to performance were identified. This can be checked by asking the person to try to perform a goal activity while at home. Be quick to praise and use any modifications a client has discovered on his or her own, even if the modification might not be optimal. Rather than telling a client what to do, help the client discover a solution by setting up a problem so a solution is easily discovered. This encourages a

Whittaker SG, Scheiman M, Sokol-McKay DA.
Low Vision Rehabilitation: A Practical Guide for Occupational Therapists,
Second Edition (pp 203-218).
© 2016 Taylor & Francis Group.

client's problem solving and independence (see Chapter 6). Problem-solving therapy can counteract depression (see Chapter 6) and can continue to be effective long after a "better" idea that a therapist might suggest has become obsolete because of changing vision. Even in cases where a person has cognitive problems and limited problem-solving ability, observation of a failed attempt to perform a task will encourage a client's acceptance of a modification that enables task performance. These observations, therefore, provide a necessary starting point for environmental modifications.

The functional vision evaluation identifies potential visual, physical, and psychosocial barriers that enable the therapist to anticipate potential problems. For example, if we are working with a person with glaucoma who has near normal acuity but is very glare sensitive and the lighting evaluation indicates the need for high light levels, then attention would be paid to lighting but not magnification. If lighting was not found to be critical in the functional evaluation, then this time-consuming aspect of an environmental modification could be skipped. Likewise, the therapist might attend more to tripping hazards if the evaluation revealed impaired balance and a history of falls. Otherwise, if there are no such mobility problems, it is best to avoid asking a person to remove a treasured throw rug.

It is advisable to bring evaluation materials to the environment being assessed, especially acuity charts, contrast charts, strong handheld flashlights, and an illuminometer (light meter) for onsite assessments to check evaluation findings, as well as retest with functional activities. Lighting assessment will be discussed later in this chapter.

INTERVENTIONS

While discussing modification of the environment, Watson states that loss of visual function such as reduced contrast sensitivity or color sensitivity cannot be resolved by prescribing an optical device. She indicates that treatment of these problems requires environmental enhancement and suggests 6 factors that can be manipulated to make the environment more "client friendly." These factors are listed in Table 12-1 and discussed next.[2]

Relative Size Magnification

With relative size magnification or enlargement, the actual size of the object is increased (Figures 12-1 and 12-2). The concept is quite simple (see Chapter 5). If the size of the object is doubled, the size of the retinal image is doubled. To achieve 2× magnification, therefore, we simply enlarge the object twofold. If a client has trouble reading 12-point font, we could print a document on the computer using 24-point font and double the retinal image size. Telephones with large-print number pads, large-print calendars, writing a

TABLE 12-1: FACTORS THAT CAN BE MANIPULATED TO MODIFY THE ENVIRONMENT
1. Size of the object being viewed (relative size magnification)
2. Distance between the object and the client (relative distance magnification)
3. Color
4. Contrast
5. Illumination
6. Figure-ground/visual clutter
Adapted from Watson GR. Functional assessment of low vision for activities of daily living. In: Silverstone B, Lang MA, Rosenthal BP, Faye EE, eds. *The Lighthouse Handbook on Vision Impairment and Vision Rehabilitation.* Oxford: Oxford University Press; 2000:869-884.

grocery list in large print with a bold-line pen, or purchasing a large-screen television are simple and effective applications of size magnification.

This approach is easy, intuitive, and generally well accepted because the client does not require any optical aids and can read at a normal distance. However, as the magnification demands grow and the print size for books and other materials is increased, size and weight become issues. An 18-point large-print version of a document will consist of about 3 pages of large print for every page of 11- to 12-point print.[3] E-books readily increase magnification 2× to 3× and are easy to learn how to use and can enhance print contrast as well. Although size magnification strategies such as large print have been generally considered best suited for clients with mild to moderate loss, this strategy can effectively be combined with optical magnification for those with more severely impaired visual acuity so that magnification devices are easier to use (see Chapter 13).

Examples of the use of relative size magnification are listed in Table 12-2 and illustrated in Figure 12-1.

Relative Distance Magnification

Another simple, intuitive environmental modification that achieves magnification of an object is to move closer to it. As an object is moved closer to the eye, the retinal image of the object increases. If the distance is halved, the retinal image size doubles and 2× magnification is achieved. To achieve 4× magnification, you would decrease the distance to one-fourth of the original distance. If a client is having trouble seeing a 20-inch television at a distance of 12 feet, the therapist can suggest that the client move to 6 feet away. This would double the size of the retinal image of the television and magnify the image twofold (see Chapter 5).

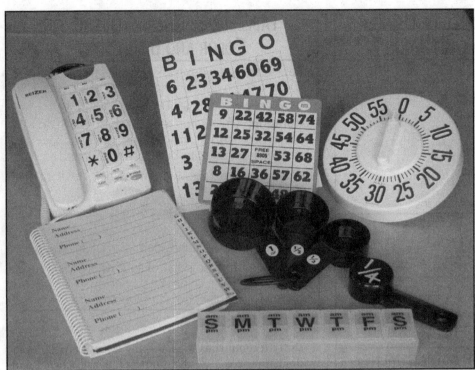

Figure 12-1. Various devices that are examples of relative size magnification.

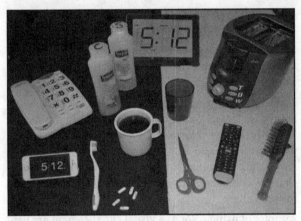

Figure 12-2. Various techniques and devices that illustrate the use of contrast, including iPhone/iPad with clock apps.

If a client is having difficulty reading a newspaper at 40 cm, bringing the newspaper closer to a 10-cm distance would magnify the print 4×. However, moving the newspaper this close creates another problem. The closer an object is brought to the eye, the more eye accommodation is required (the lens must change shape to focus at near). Although decreasing the working distance from 40 to 10 cm achieves 4× magnification, the client would experience blurred vision if he or she is unable to accommodate for that distance. While young children would be able to accommodate even at 10 cm, this would not be possible for an adult, particularly an adult from the age of 40 years and older. To solve this problem in adult clients with limited accommodation, the optometrist prescribes a convex lens

or other optical devices that focus the light on the retina (see Chapter 5).

Lovie-Kitchin and Whittaker compared the effect of relative distance vs relative size magnification on reading rates of adults.[4] They found that the reading rates of the subjects with low vision did not differ significantly with the 2 methods of providing magnification if the magnification provided was adequate. Other common applications of relative distance magnification include getting closer to read a watch or a clock, sitting closer to the stage at a play, and bringing a food package down from the grocery shelf and closer to the eye to read the label. In most cases, if a person cannot see a TV clearly because of impaired visual acuity, bringing the TV closer by moving the chair or TV or both is a quick and effective solution. By purchasing a larger TV, relative distance magnification and size magnification can be combined. For example, if a client can see a TV clearly at 1 meter (3 feet) but can get no closer than 2 meters (6 feet), then buying a TV that is twice as large will achieve the same magnification. The formula for combining relative distance and size magnification is in Chapters 5 and 13.

Color

Color can be used as an effective environmental modification to enhance safety, accessibility, and independent participation in activities of daily living (ADL).[1,5,2] One must perform color vision testing first (see Chapters 7 and 8) because many with visual impairments may have difficulty distinguishing between groups of colors, such as darker colors like navy blue, brown, and black; blue, green,

TABLE 12-2: EXAMPLES OF USING RELATIVE SIZE MAGNIFICATION

KITCHEN/COOKING

- Bold, black, large letters on 3 × 5 index cards to label household supplies
- Bold, black, large letters on spice bottles
- Kitchen timer with large numerals
- Large-print recipes and cookbooks
- Large-print measuring cups/spoons

BATHROOM

- Bold, black, large letters on 3 × 5 inch index cards to label bathroom supplies

COMMUNICATION

- Phone with large-print number pad
- Large-print telephone and address books

MEDICATIONS AND HEALTH MANAGEMENT

- Ask pharmacist to make large-print labels for each medication
- Store medication in pill boxes with large print
- Large-display blood pressure monitor

DRESSING

- Bold, black, large letters on 3 × 5 inch index cards to label clothing

TIME MANAGEMENT

- Large-number watches and clocks
- Large-print calendars

FINANCIAL MANAGEMENT

- Large-print checks and check registers
- Large-print calculator

LEISURE

- Larger TV screen
- Large-print magazines/newspaper (*Reader's Digest, NY Times*)
- Large-print Bingo cards
- Large-print playing cards

TABLE 12-3: CHARACTERISTICS OF COLOR AND BRIGHTNESS

Hue: A color's hue describes which wavelength appears to be most dominant. The terms *red* and *blue*, for example, are primarily describing hue.

Saturation: A fully saturated color is one with no mixture of white. Pink may be thought of as having the same hue as red but being less saturated.

Brightness: Affects how luminous, or full of light, the color appears.

Illuminance: The light falling on a surface expressed as lux.

Luminance: The light radiating from a light source.

Glare: A negative property of light where a light or reflection of a light shines into a person's eyes rather than onto the object being viewed.

Duffy recommends the following general principles for manipulating color in environments to help clients with low vision:[1,5]

- Bright colors are generally the easiest to see because of their ability to reflect light.
- Solid bright colors, such as red, orange, and yellow, are usually more visible than pastels because they are more saturated.
- Lighting can influence the perception of color: dim light can "wash out" some colors; bright light can intensify others. Normally, colors can be best seen using sunlight and full-spectrum or natural-daylight lamps and bulbs that simulate sunlight, but low vision changes color sensitivity, so this needs to be evaluated for each client.

Examples of using color as a visual enhancement are listed in Table 12-4. Often, color saturation needs to be modified to more clearly identify color. For example, televisions often have a setting that changes the saturation of colors. These adjustments may improve the rendition of color for someone with low vision, but be quite unpleasant for others viewing the same TV.

Lighting and the Dilemma of Glare

Before discussing the assessment and modification of lighting, it is important to understand that in people with normal vision, light levels can change considerably from shade to bright sunlight on a snowy day, for example, without significantly affecting visual function. Yet even in older adults without low vision, a difference in illumination between a sunny and a cloudy day can affect their ability to read signs, see detail, and navigate in a building.[6,7] One effect of most eye diseases that cause low vision is that

and purple; and pastels such as pink, yellow, and pale green. The three characteristics of color that must be considered are defined in Table 12-3.

they narrow the range of light over which someone has best vision. Different causes of low vision create different sensitivities to different aspects of lighting. Sometimes people with the same diagnosis respond differently to light, especially macular degeneration and diabetic retinopathy.[8]

Therefore, the appropriate modification of lighting will vary from individual to individual and should involve the client. The lighting evaluation (see Chapter 8) should indicate a range of optimal light levels for each individual, as well as indicate glare sensitivity and a preferred light source. For the therapist who cannot see the effects of lighting on vision, results need to be measured by a digital light meter in order to apply these findings in different environments without time-consuming trial and error. Chapter 10 describes how to instruct clients to manage lighting themselves, as they are the best judge of optimal light levels and glare avoidance.

There are 3 measurements of lighting to consider (see Table 12-3):

1. Luminance, or the amount of light coming from a source such as a light or even a TV screen. Luminance is usually reported commercially as lumens.

2. Illuminance, or the light actually reaching the object being viewed. This is usually the most important measurement. Illuminance changes with not only the luminance of the source, but also the distance of the source from the object being viewed. The distance effect is quite dramatic and usually much more effective than changing the luminance of the source (with a dimmer switch or different light).

3. Glare, which is caused by the light that scatters within the eye, should always be avoided because it interferes with one's ability to see another object, much like light in a room will wash out the image on a screen being viewed. From where a person is sitting and working, a light that the person can see directly or a reflection becomes a glare source. For example, an individual's ability to see the television may be hampered directly by the bright light itself next to the TV or too much indirect light in the room reflecting off the television screen.

Normally, visual acuity, contrast sensitivity, and color discrimination improve as the amount of light increases, but only up to a point. At a certain level, functional improvement plateaus and further increases in the amount of light may be detrimental. Some people with low vision require considerable illuminance for best acuity and contrast sensitivity. Boyce and Sanford report that various diseases that result in low vision affect the significance or benefits from modification of lighting (Table 12-5).[9] These causes include diseases that:

- Reduce transmission of light and require more light to see best (proliferative diabetic retinopathy).

TABLE 12-4: EXAMPLES OF USING COLOR AS A VISUAL ENHANCEMENT

SAFETY

- Use bright colors for light switches, elevator buttons, call buttons, and other critical safety features.
- Mark the leading edge of the first and last steps with bright paint or reflecting tape that contrasts with the background color of the flooring.
- Use solid, brightly colored hallway or stair runners to clearly define traffic flow and walking spaces.
- Use brightly colored duct tape around a pot or pan handle.
- Green grass versus gray sidewalk alerts walker to a surface change.
- Yellow warning markers warn walker of curbs.

IDENTIFICATION

- Use brightly colored index cards to mark clothing on hangers.
- Use brightly colored dots/labels to mark appliances (oven, microwave).
- Upper half of label is red on Campbell's soup can.

VISIBILITY

- Place bright duct tape on magnifier handle.
- Place bright duct tape on memo recorder kept in purse.

COLOR CODING

- Use colored pill boxes to indicate time of day medication is taken (soft morning sun = yellow, intense daytime sun = red, nightfall = blue).
- Green marking on start button on microwave; red marking for stop/clear.

- Cause scatter within the eye or sensitivity to glare (cataract and optic atrophy).
- Have minimal effect on transmission of light, but destroy parts of the retina and neural transmission (glaucoma, retinitis pigmentosa).

Generally, the lighting of the visual environment will always be important in determining how well a client can use his or her remaining vision when the cause of low vision alters the optical characteristics of the eye, such as with cataracts. Finally, in situations where there are combined

TABLE 12-5: LIGHTING REQUIREMENTS AND LIGHT SENSITIVITY FOR CLIENTS WITH COMMON EYE DISEASES

EYE DISEASE	PREFERRED LIGHTING	SENSITIVITY TO LIGHT
Cataract	High	High
Diabetic retinopathy	Moderate	Moderate
Glaucoma	Moderate	Moderate
Macular degeneration	Bright	High
Retinitis pigmentosa	Moderate to bright	High

Adapted from Flom R. Appendix: visual consequences of most common eye conditions associated with visual impairment. In: Lueck AH, ed. *Functional Vision: A Practitioner's Guide to Evaluation and Intervention.* New York: AFB Press; 2004:475-481.

effects, such as macular degeneration, careful attention to lighting has long been recognized.[10] Boyce and Sanford, however, emphasize that this distinction between causes of low vision and the importance of lighting should be used only as a guideline.[9]

In an experiment to determine the effect of lighting on object perception, investigators found that all subjects, regardless of the cause of low vision, showed improvement in ability to recognize objects as illuminance was increased. However, the amount of illuminance at which improvement ceased varied significantly among subjects.[8,11] Another study by Bowers et al (2001)[12] demonstrated the significant effects of lighting in persons with macular degeneration. These effects included ability to read without a magnifier (in cases of mild vision loss), ability to reduce the amount of magnification required (in cases of moderate to severe levels of vision loss), improvement of sentence-reading acuity by 2 times, and increase in reading rate by 40%.

The dilemma of lighting is that increasing the illuminance of an object also increases glare. The challenge is to maximize object illuminance while carefully controlling glare. To create the largest change in illumination of an object, one should change the distance of the light source. To minimize glare, the light source should be shaded and directed from the side or from over a shoulder. Light behind or above usually does not cause glare, but if the light strikes the material from a particular angle, the result might be a reflective glare. Various effects of light positioning on glare and the visibility of lights are illustrated in Figure 12-3. Using a mirror or glossy paper, a person can be instructed how to avoid glare when light is above or behind the head by changing the angle of the paper. Use of visors or brimmed hats and wrap-around absorptive lenses (sunglasses) (Figure 12-4) are effective methods to control glare when it cannot be avoided or light locations cannot be changed (see Chapter 10). Because glare depends on a person's positioning, the client needs to be instructed on how to change positioning and use shades and absorptive lenses to optimize lighting and avoid glare. The best method to optimize lighting is to use a task light with a shaded directional light

source (Figure 12-5). By changing the distance and position of a directional light source, the client can better manage glare and illumination. For this reason, adjustable task lights are nearly always recommended for people who have stringent lighting needs. To test and reinforce understanding of lighting optimization, the client should participate in the environmental evaluation of lighting. It has long been recognized that illumination cannot be standardized and must be tailored to each individual's needs and living situation,[10] and is best left to the client to control and manage using his or her own vision as the "meter" that indicates best lighting. Glare, however, is always deleterious. Glare is usually divided into 2 categories: discomfort glare and disabling glare.

Discomfort Glare

Discomfort glare refers to the sensation one experiences when the overall illumination is too bright, and commonly results from excessive amounts of illumination and/or reflective light off of surfaces that are too bright. Environmental sources of discomfort glare include glossy pages, water, snow, and highly polished surfaces. Discomfort glare is distracting, may cause discomfort and eye fatigue, and may interfere with the ability to see the information being viewed.[13]

Disability Glare

Disability glare refers to glare that interferes with vision by blinding, veiling, or dazzling, and results in reduced visual performance.[14] This type of glare results from aspects of the individual's visual system, including cloudiness in the ocular media, cataracts, and corneal scarring. Corn and Erin note that[13] light passing through the eye is scattered by the ocular media. This scattered light forms a veil of luminance that reduces the contrast and thus the visibility of the target. An example of disability glare would be the familiar experience of being bothered by oncoming headlights while driving at night. One form of disability glare, called

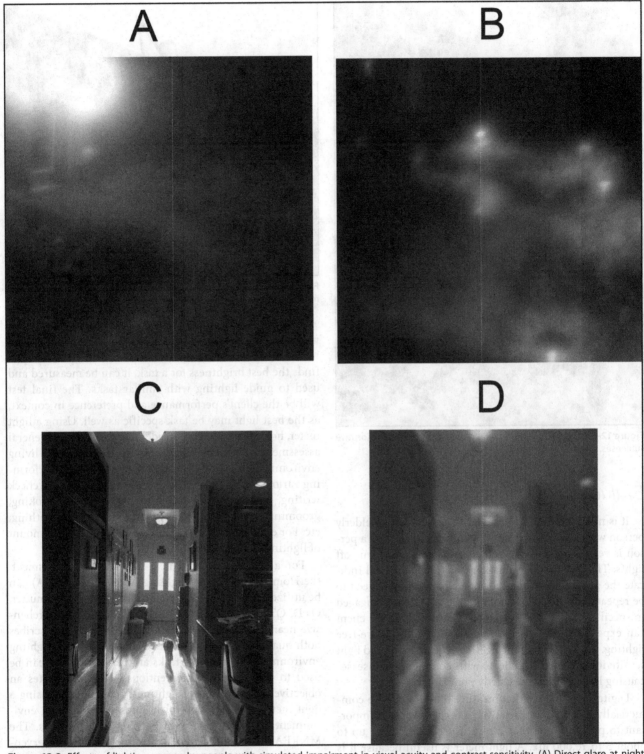

Figure 12-3. Effects of lighting as seen by people with simulated impairment in visual acuity and contrast sensitivity. (A) Direct glare at night with typical entrance lighting. (B) Pathway lighting. (C) Hallway with mostly reflective glare and with a normal view. (D) The same view by visually impaired client. (Where did Sammy the cat go?)

starburst glare, is particularly disabling when someone is viewing white objects against a dark background like white letters on a black background in an electronic magnifier. A light against the dark tends to almost explode like a starburst. Oncoming headlights in the fog at night also simulate

a starburst glare effect. Chapter 11 describes how to teach clients glare avoidance and use glare avoidance devices like absorptive lenses and brimmed hats when they do not have control over the environmental lighting.

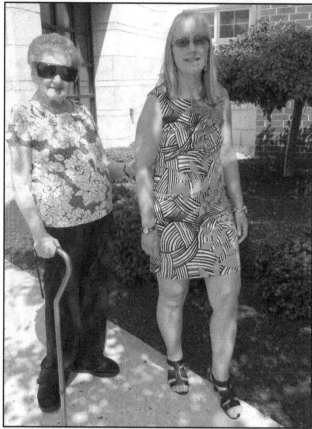

Figure 12-4. Outdoor daylight glare and glare control using absorptive sunlenses.

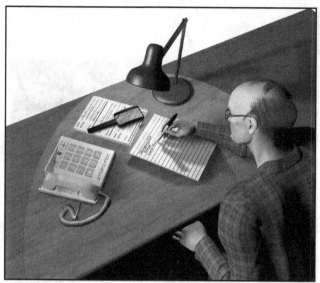

Figure 12-5. Example of a task light setup at desk. (Reprinted with permission from Barbara Steinman.)

Evaluation of Lighting

It is not uncommon to find that the home of an elderly person with low vision is poorly illuminated because a person is very glare sensitive and closes shades and turns off lights. The functional evaluation (see Chapter 8) will indicate the general lighting needs of a client, but may need to be repeated in the client's home while the client is engaged in specific ADL within that environment, where the client can experience the effects of good, directional, glare-free lighting. Table 12-5 lists the lighting requirements and light sensitivity expected for clients with common eye diseases causing low vision in the elderly population.

Digital light meters that measure illuminance are commercially available and relatively inexpensive. It is important to purchase one that can measure illuminance up to about 5 to 10,000 lux. A light meter is useful because it is difficult for a therapist with normal vision to judge absolute illuminance of an object. The therapist can evaluate lighting during the occupational therapy low vision evaluation using contrast sensitivity or visual acuity testing as described in Chapter 8. During testing, the therapist varies lighting by varying the distance of a directional task light from the task and uses a light meter to measure the range of illuminance that produced the best contrast sensitivity or

visual acuity. This same light level can then be reproduced in the clinic or the home. In addition, once the therapist finds the best brightness for a task, it can be measured and used to guide lighting with similar tasks. The final test will be the client's performance and preference in context, as the best light may be task specific as well. Using a light meter, however, will save considerable time. After a general assessment of lighting conditions in the house or living environment, it is important to observe the client performing various ADL. Observe activities such as reading, check writing, reading mail, reading medicine bottles, cooking, grooming, sorting and folding clothing, selecting clothing, etc. For each activity, make observations about the amount of lighting, contrast, and glare.

For a more structured near-task lighting assessment, the Home Environment Lighting Assessment (HELA) can be utilized. This tool was developed by Monica Perlmutter, OTD, OTR/L, SCLV, in 2013 and is the first comprehensive near-task lighting assessment of its type. It describes both quantitative and qualitative aspects of home lighting environments where near tasks are performed and can be used to plan lighting interventions.[15] It incorporates an objective measurement of lighting/illuminance by using a light meter, a description of the presenting lighting environment, and a summary of lighting modifications. The MNREAD is administered at baseline and after intervention to provide a quantitative measure of improvement in reading ability. Clients are also asked to rate the lighting environment pre- and postintervention to provide subjective feedback regarding the benefit of lighting modification.

Recently, a simple, quick, and portable diagnostic system, the LuxIQ, was introduced in the marketplace. The system allows the practitioner to measure and select the right task lighting. It enables the occupational therapist to determine

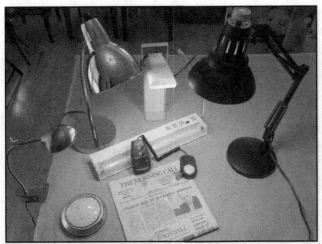

Figure 12-6. Examples of various kinds of commercially available task lights and a light meter.

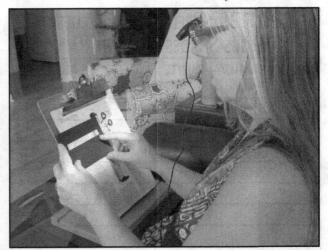

Figure 12-7. Reading with head-mounted VisionEdge and Typoscope. Note lap desk and homemade bookstand that a standard clipboard just slips into.

the amount of light (in lux), as well as the color temperature (in Kelvin), needed by the client at his or her preferred working distance. With the web app LightChooser or Light Bulb Calculator, the clinician can recommend a range of commercially available task lighting options (lamps and bulbs) based directly on the outcome of the LuxIQ's lighting assessment. This is described in Chapter 8.

Lighting Modification

Room vs Task Lighting

Room lighting, also known as ambient lighting, is provided by central ceiling fixtures, wall sconces, torchiere lamps, and the barrel-style table and floor lamps. This type of lighting has a fixed direction. Room lighting should be distributed evenly throughout a room or hallway. Room lighting is used for mobility and detection of large shapes and objects. Task lighting consists of lamps that can be directed to a particular detailed task. Many task lamps have a gooseneck or a swing or hinged arm that will allow one to vary the direction and closeness of the light source. Task lighting can be in the form of a tabletop or floor lamp, a spotlight, a clip-on lamp, book light, flashlight, head-mounted lighting, and lights mounted or built into a spectacle frame (Figures 12-6 and 12-7).

Lighting Enhancement

After assessment, the therapist can modify the lighting conditions by changing the task location, changing the lamp location, altering the type of bulb used, increasing bulb luminance, moving the light source closer, changing the background color so more light is reflected, incorporating supplemental or layered lighting, and reducing glare. Dusting bulbs and cleaning light fixtures regularly will increase luminance from a source. Light bulbs with dying filaments produce less light. An example of changing the

task location would be moving from the kitchen table with overhead lighting to a desk with task lighting to pay the bills. For reading, the lamp should be placed to the side of the better-seeing eye. For writing, placement should be opposite the writing hand to avoid shadows. The lamp shade should be positioned below the eye or over the shoulder.

Light sources have changed considerably in the last 5 years and continue to improve, especially the light-emitting diode (LED) type of lights.[1,16] Table 12-6 lists the different types of light bulbs and their advantages and disadvantages, adapted and updated from Duffy[1] and Kern and Miller.[16] To properly evaluate and modify lighting, the therapist will typically have to evaluate functions with different bulbs so that the types of bulbs and lights can be predicted when the therapist performs a home evaluation. Figures 12-5 and 12-8 illustrate 2 common examples of lighting to enhance a client's ability to participate in ADL. In Figure 12-5, the client is working on finances at his desk, and a gooseneck lamp is placed close to the client's work. In Figure 12-8, a floor lamp with a combination bulb is placed behind the shoulder of the better-seeing eye while the client is reading.

Regardless of the type of lighting used, one of the very important concepts that is routinely used when modifying lighting is the inverse square law. This law suggests that it is more effective to change the distance of a light source than the luminance of the source. If a therapist decreases the distance of a 500-lumens light bulb by one-half, he or she will increase the illuminance of an object 4 times—equivalent to a bulb luminance increase to 2000 lumens. This law is the foundation for the effective environmental modification of moving the light source closer to the client's reading material, rather than increasing the wattage of the bulb.

TABLE 12-6: REFLECTANCE VALUES OF VARIOUS SHADES OF WHITE PAINT	
COLOR FAMILY—WHITE	LIGHT REFLECTANCE VALUE (LRV)
High reflective white	94
Cotton White	87
Extra White	85
Cosmetic Blush	79
Teasing Peach	79
Biscuit	72
Natural Tan	64
Beige	61

Table created using www.sherwin-williams.com/homeowners/color/try-on-colors/color-visualizer.

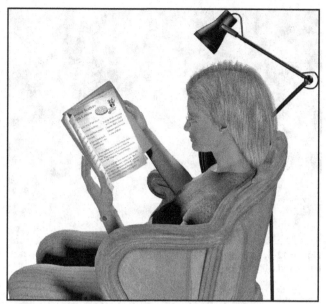

Figure 12-8. Example of lighting/lamp setup while reading. (Reprinted with permission from Barbara Steinman.)

Changing the background color can enhance light reflection. White will reflect more light than yellow and will brighten up an area. This is termed *light reflectance value* (LRV) (see Figure 12-4). The average blackest black has a LRV of 5% and the whitest white 85%. Some yellows can measure up into the 80s or 90s as well. Light reflectance value can be misleading when it comes to yellow. Yellow is one of the most reflective hues in the spectrum and should be avoided if someone is glare sensitive. Table 12-7 provides LRVs for 8 shades of white, underscoring the importance of light source choices in residences. Similarities are noted in all other major color families. Visit www.sherwin-williams.comhomeowners/color/ for the color visualize tool and LRVs of other color families.

Environmental modifications can be implemented that minimize or eliminate glare. Window treatments such as sheers, shades, or blinds can control glare. Antiglare film can be purchased through hardware stores and applied to windows. Removing an environmental surface such as a highly polished floor is generally not practical, but using polish that provides a matte finish or covering the surface is a realistic solution. If an area can be repainted, a shift from high-gloss and semi-gloss paint to eggshell or a matte finish would also be beneficial. Ensuring that a lampshade fully covers the bulb, that all bulbs have shades or fixtures, and using frosted instead of clear bulbs will also minimize glare.

The Illuminating Engineering Society has a website for their lighting education resource portal at www.ies.org/education/index.cfm. The portal has a manual called *Lighting Your Way to Better Vision* (2009) that provides lighting recommendations for the aging eye. There is also a consumer's guide to lighting called *The 5 Ls of Lighting* (2011) that teaches the reader about location, lumens, light bulbs, label and law, and many more resources on lighting. They also have a publication online called *Light in Design—*

An Application Guide that discusses types of lighting and fixtures, proper positioning and location of lighting, and minimal lighting requirements for each room or task.

Contrast

When we discuss contrast, we must consider the sensitivity of a person to lower contrast, such as the first step of carpeted steps. This topic is introduced in Chapter 1 and discussed in detail in Chapter 8. While visual acuity tests measure the smallest high-contrast object that can be recognized, contrast sensitivity measures the lowest contrast where an object or pattern can still be recognized. Contrast and contrast sensitivity are important factors to consider because they are intimately related to performance in ADL and provide information that is not as easily captured by visual acuity measurement. For example, contrast sensitivity is strongly associated with reading performance,[17] mobility,[18,19] face recognition,[20,21] and ADL.[21,22] In vision rehabilitation, occupational therapists can help clients with contrast sensitivity problems by increasing the contrast of objects being viewed. Methods of modifying contrast include environmental modifications and lighting modifications.[23] Generally, increasing the contrast between an object and its background will make the object more visible (see Figure 12-2 for examples). Enhancing contrast between elements of the environment is one of the simplest and most effective modifications to implement in most home, work, and recreational environments.

Visual Clutter

When treating people with perceptual problems due to brain injury, visual clutter emerges as an important factor

TABLE 12-7: COMPARISON OF COMMON LIGHT SOURCES

TYPE OF LIGHT	ADVANTAGES	DISADVANTAGES
Daylight/natural light	• Most natural type of light • Appropriate for most tasks • Provides true color rendition	• Creates glare • Creates shadows • Inconsistent and unpredictable
LED	• Lasts longer • Energy efficient • Portable (as flashlights) • Durable	• Tends to be expensive • Fewer dimmable options • Blue (high color temperature) with more glare
Soft-white CFL	• Readily available in a large variety of wattages • Low cost • Similar to older incandescent light • Yellow (low color temperature) with less glare	• Can create sharper shadows
Bright-white	• Light is concentrated • Better for spot lighting on near tasks • Light does not "flicker" like fluorescent light • Becoming more energy efficient	• Tends to create more glare
Fluorescent (tube style)	• Better for general room lighting • Illuminates a wider area than incandescent light • Does not create shadows	• Tends to create more glare
Daylight CFLs and special lights (OTT light)	• Most natural type of artificial light • Approximates natural light • More accurate color rendition for people with typical vision	• May require the purchase of additional lamps • Specialized lighting fixtures can be expensive
Halogen	• Brighter than incandescent light • Gives more illumination and uses lower wattage • Does not flicker • Ideal for spotlights	• Light is hotter, more focused, and requires a shield • Not recommended for prolonged close work • Bulbs need to be replaced frequently and are more expensive than CFL comparable incandescent lights • May be dangerous for low vision clients because of potential for burns

in a person's ability to recognize and find objects. It is a standard of practice when treating people with cortical visual impairment to progress visual tasks from visually uncluttered to cluttered settings (see Chapter 11).[24] A client might be able to see and quickly recognize a cup on a table by itself, but cannot see it when placed among a random assortment of unrelated objects. Visual clutter includes not only other objects, but also patterns on a complex background, such as a patterned tablecloth or reflections, shadows, and glare. Patterned carpets, wallpaper, and upholstery, or a busy room such as a dining area or restaurant, can visually clutter a background as well. One common source of visual clutter in a clinic is produced by the treatment room itself, if shared by a number of clinicians. A room stuffed with knick-knacks, magazines, and furniture may appear cluttered to a therapist who has never seen the room before, but not to the client who has lived in the room for many years.

Sometimes it is best to evaluate visual clutter by taking a picture of a person's work area because a picture makes clutter more evident. The therapist must be careful in evaluating visual clutter in a person's home environment because one person's clutter may be another's unique organization and collection of treasures. Once a person becomes familiar with a setting and where things are located, the clutter effect can be virtually eliminated.

TYPICAL ENVIRONMENTAL MODIFICATIONS BY ROOM

The following is a list of potential home modifications related to increasing contrast/visibility, reducing glare, enhancing lighting, promoting organization, safety, sensory cues, and increasing access.

General

- Use supplemental lighting such as a touch light or clip-on light in pantries, closets, and other small storage areas. Hang a flashlight in the pantry for ease of access in order to read labels.
- Install automatic lighting in the pantries or closets or encourage use of flashlights.
- A "clap on" lamp is easier to turn on and off.
- Use outlet covers and light switch plates that contrast with the wall, or place color-contrasting tape around its borders.
- Reduce height of, eliminate, or paint door thresholds in contrasting colors.
- Ensure 3-foot-wide clear walking paths through rooms (www.visionaware.com)
- Avoid patterned carpet, flooring (linoleum, tile), bedspreads, tablecloths, and any surface coverings.
- Avoid placement of plants, mobiles, or stained glass decorations in front of windows that block and distort incoming light.
- Use eggshell or flat instead of semi-gloss and high-gloss paint.

- Consider using white paint in closets, pantries, and other small storage areas like cabinets to enhance light reflection.

Kitchen

- Attach lights to the underside of cabinets, use directional task lights on the counter, or replace a diffuse light on the ceiling with track or mounted halogen spotlights that can be directed to work surfaces.
- Keep all cabinet doors and drawers closed at all times. If not, a strip of bright, contrasting tape on the edge of the cabinet door or drawer makes it easier to see when it is left open.
- Replace knobs and handles with color-contrasting or brightly colored models.
- Put color-contrasting tape around the counter edge to increase visibility against the kitchen floor.
- Each workstation should have its own light source, or consider a portable floor lamp on wheels.
- Attach light and dark sheets of contact paper to the wall for measuring liquids near food preparation areas[1,5] or having dark and light cutting mats readily available.
- Use color-contrasting trays to organize kitchen tasks and make products on them more visible.
- Have a dedicated, well-lit countertop workstation for food preparation tasks.
- Mark preferred settings on kitchen appliances—stovetop, oven, dishwasher, toaster oven, and other small appliances (see the section on marking appliances that follows).
- Mount a reading stand that can be swiveled on a counter.
- Consider installing a pegboard or pullout shelves and baskets in cabinets to make contents easier to see.

Dining Room

- The color of the furniture should contrast with the color of the floor and walls, or use a high-contrast table covering and chair back covers (visit www.inmyownstyle.com2013/09/sew-chair-back-covers.html for no-sew chair back covers).
- If the tabletop is dark, use light-colored placemats or dishes.
- Keep chairs pushed under the table.
- Polish table with a matte finish polish, or cover it with a solid-colored, matte-finished tablecloth.
- Avoid glass-fronted cabinets that can produce glare.

- Use frosted instead of clear bulbs in lighting fixtures, or change out the lamp for a covered fixture.
- Use a rechargeable task lamp for a tabletop task light during meals to avoid the need for an outlet and avoid a trailing cord.
- Consider chairs whose legs are straight rather than splayed.

Living Room

- Blinds, shades, or sheers should be used to control direct sunlight.
- Use multiple light fixtures throughout the room to even out lighting.
- Install dimmer switches or use 3-way bulbs to control the amount of light.
- Doors or door frames should contrast with the wall color.
- Space should be provided for the person to move closer to the television.
- A large-screen television should be considered.
- Use a flexible-arm lamp for auxiliary lighting for crafts or reading.
- Remove or cover coffee table with covering that contrasts with carpet or flooring.
- Put a small contrasting rug under coffee table.
- Favor furniture with rounded rather than square corners.
- Consider furniture that contrasts with walls or flooring, or drape a contrasting hanging over chair and sofa backs, or use contrasting pillows.
- Use light-colored lampshades with wide brims at the bottom.
- Move furniture against walls to create a large area of uncluttered space in the center of the room, or consider arranging furniture in small groupings to aid in ease of conversation.
- Use brightly colored accessories such as vases, lamps, and decorations to make furniture easier to locate.

Office

- Place an adjustable lamp on the desk area.
- If desk is shiny, use a matte-finish polish or cover it with a desk pad.
- Keep desk chair pushed under desk.
- In order to take advantage of sunlight, place a reading chair near the window so that the light is projected over the shoulder on the side of the better-seeing eye.

Bedroom

- Ensure the bedspread is a solid color that contrasts with the carpet.
- A nightstand lamp should be operable from the bedside.
- Attach a bed caddy to the side of the bed to hold small items such as eyeglasses, tissues, TV remote, etc.
- Immediately store footwear and dirty clothing to reduce clutter on furniture and the floor.

Hallway

- Use a motion-detector night light.
- Mark or replace thermostat with large/raised print, talking, or interactive model (www.maxiaids.com).

Bathroom

- When choosing a shower curtain, clear plastic (with design) allows more light to be transmitted than an opaque solid color.[25]
- Toothbrushes, cups, and bottles should be brightly colored.
- Purchase towels, washcloths, bathmats, and non-slip rugs in solid colors that contrast with their surroundings.
- Place toiletries such as combs, brushes, and other accessories on a contrasting colored tray.
- Store like items in baskets on shelves in the linen closet (shampoos, conditioners, soaps together; toothpaste, mouthwash, extra toothbrushes, floss, etc).
- Ensure grab bars contrast with walls.
- A towel hung on the wall opposite the bathroom mirror, at the appropriate height, provides a contrasting background for the image of the head and hair. Clients with light hair should use a dark towel; clients with dark hair should use a light towel.[24]
- Install a mirror with long slim lights on each side (www.ies.org/PDF/Education/LightInDesign.pdf).
- Use a small directional flashlight rather than mirror light for makeup and grooming to avoid glare.

Stairs

- Walls and steps should be free of clutter.
- Mark the nosing (the front edge of the stairs) of the top and bottom step to contrast (both visually and tactually) with the treads and risers. Some resources indicate the strip on the nosing should be a minimum of 2 inches in height.[26]

- Paint the stringers (the sloping board beside the treads on each side of the stairs) a color that contrasts with the adjacent risers and treads.[26]

- A contrast nonskid mat at the base of the steps will also alert the individual that he or she is approaching floor level.

- Place a tactile marking under the rail at the second-to-last step ascending and descending to provide individuals with a cue that the last step is next.

- Railings on both sides should extend beyond the top and bottom of the stairs.

- It is best to have light switches at both the bottom and top of the stairs.

- Shine spotlights on the top and bottom steps or use night lights.

Laundry Room

- Ensure the central light in the room has a fixture over the bulb to control the light.

- Mark preferred settings on washer and dryer (see section on marking appliances that immediately follows).

- Mark water controls and fuse box in an accessible manner.

MARKING APPLIANCES AND LABELING

Marking Appliances

Many appliances (stovetop, washer/dryer, thermostat, CD player), as well as other tools with incremental settings (such as measuring cups and timers), often have small and/or poor contrast settings or interval markings. Dials, control panels, buttons, and other surfaces can be marked by visual or tactile markings or a combination of both. A key principle in marking is to avoid overmarking. Before marking, it should be noted whether there are any preexisting tactile or auditory cues or any cognitive approaches that can be taken in lieu of or in addition to marking. For example, it may be observed that a click might be felt and heard as a dial is moved from one setting to the next in a clockwise manner. If the dial represented laundry load size, the dial might start on the left at the first setting "small," one click to the right would be "medium," a second to the right would be "large," and the final click "extra-large." Clock positions or angle of turn may also be used. A stove dial may be turned to a 6 o'clock position or turned 180 degrees to be set on medium.

Marking is an option that provides a unique visual or tactile cue. Table 12-8 provides a listing of both commercially manufactured marking products and alternative materials to make appliances user friendly. Markings come preformed in a variety of shapes, sizes, colors (including transparent), textures, and hardness. Some markings are designed by a thickened liquid paintlike product such as Spot 'n' Line and fabric paint that provides a raised marking once it is fully dry. When markings are first applied, the surface should be cleaned with alcohol to enhance adhesion of the marking. The client should have extra samples of the preferred markings and should know a source for the markings so he or she can instruct a sighted individual how to reapply them (see Table 12-8).

Labeling

Products to be labeled include clothing, medications, frozen and pantry food, financial papers, and CDs, to name the most common. Labeling is similar to marking, in that overlabeling is to be avoided. The kind of label, the extent of information required by the client, the number of garments to be labeled, the ability of the label to withstand extreme temperatures and moisture, and other factors affect the label or labeling system chosen. Labels should be durable, reusable, and easily obtained. Labels are used to aid in product identification. Very basic labels might include a rubber band on a milk carton to differentiate it from a juice carton, or an adhesive label with a bold L to identify the medication Lasix. Fabric paint can be used for labeling, but it needs 1 to 2 hours to dry to touch and longer for sufficient hardness. More complex and comprehensive labeling options might include a recordable label that will not only identify a box of chocolate cake mix, but also give the nutrition label information and the process for preparation, to audible barcode readers and more high-tech "labels" using phone apps that will identify products and their characteristics. Often, an auditory labeling device may have a maximum number of recording hours, which is distributed over the number of labels provided, so in many cases, the label itself does not have a maximum length of recording time (Table 12-9). The phone app readers for people with visual loss have the capability to print personal labels and read commercial labels (Sidebar 12-1).

SUMMARY

A person's personal space is sacred—especially with older clients—and modification should not be considered unless a problem has been identified, is significant, and is persistent. Modifications should only be made with a client's consent and with him or her physically present. Appreciate that one person's clutter may be another's organization, and familiarity tends to make clutter a uniform

TABLE 12-8: COMMERCIAL AND HOMEMADE MARKING

SPECIALIZED	HOMEMADE/GENERAL COMMERCIAL
• Bump dots	• Velcro
• Touch dots	• Sandpaper
• Maxi dots and slashes	• Furniture protectors
• Loc dots	• 3D fabric paint
• Fuzzy dots	• Duct or electrical tape
• Spot 'n' Line	• Adhesive craft foam or fabric paint
• Large-print/high-contrast telephone, microwave, and keyboard overlays	• Elmer's glue
	• Magnetic or wooden letters

TABLE 12-9: COMMERCIAL AND HOMEMADE OBJECT LABELING

HOMEMADE	COMMERCIALLY AVAILABLE
• Rubber bands or hair bands	• Half-inch or 1-inch MagneTachers magnetic labels
• Safety pins, beads,	• Touch-to-See Identifiers
• Index cards and rubber bands	• Magnetic card readers
• Laundry marker	• Pen shaped talking labeling devices
• Freezer tape	• Barcode reader/smartphone apps such as Digit-Eyes
• Self-adhesive numbers and letters	
• Self-adhesive labels	
• Buttons of different shapes	

background. Remember, people do not need vision as much in familiar settings and can often function just fine without optimum visibility.

A variety of techniques and adaptive devices, of both a low vision and nonvisual nature, have been presented, as well as several frameworks from which to expand the interventions available in the area of basic ADL. Much time has been devoted to lighting in this chapter, as we have found that most clients can immediately appreciate changes in lighting. Likewise, adding tactile and other markings are usually appreciated as well. For reference and distribution to clients who are considering moving their place of residence, we recommend Maureen Duffy's work, *Making Life More Livable*,[1] as a well-illustrated and more extensive discussion of effective environmental modifications.

REFERENCES

1. Duffy M. *Making Life More Livable*. New York: AFB Press; 2002.
2. Watson GR. Functional assessment of low vision for activities of daily living. In: Silverstone B, Lang MA, Rosenthal BP, Faye EE, eds. *The Lighthouse Handbook on Vision Impairment and Vision Rehabilitation*. Oxford: Oxford University Press; 2000:869-884.
3. Sutton J. *A Guide to Making Documents Accessible to People Who Are Blind or Visually Impaired*. Washington, DC: American Council of the Blind; 2002.
4. Lovie-Kitchin JE, Whittaker SG. Relative size magnification versus relative distance magnification: effect on the reading performance of adults with normal and low vision. *J Vis Impairment Blindness*. 1998;92:433-446.
5. Duffy MA, Huebner K, Wormsley DP. Activities of daily living and individuals with low vision. In: Scheiman M, ed. *Understanding and Managing Vision Deficits: A Guide for Occupational Therapists*. Thorofare, NJ: SLACK, Inc; 2002:289-304.
6. Elton E, Johnson D, Nicolle C, Clift L. Supporting the development of inclusive products: the effects of everyday ambient illumination levels and contrast on older adults' near visual acuity. *Ergonomics*. 2013;56:803-817.
7. Hegde AL, Rhodes R. Assessment of lighting in independent living facilities and residents' perceptions. *J Appl Gerontol*. 2010;29:381-390.
8. Fosse P, Valberg A. Lighting needs and lighting comfort during reading with age-related macular degeneration. *J Vis Impairment Blindness*. 2004;98:389-409.
9. Boyce PR, Sanford LJ. Lighting to enhance visual capabilities. In: Silverstone B, Lang MA, Rosenthal BP, Faye EE, eds. *The Lighthouse Handbook on Vision Impairment and Vision Rehabilitation*. Oxford: Oxford University Press; 2000:617-636.

SIDEBAR 12-1: DIGIT-EYES: A LABELING APPLICATION

Digit-Eyes is a labeling app for Apple products that will: identify products, instructions for use, ingredients, and nutrition label information by scanning a UPC bar code on a product. A more simplified approach is to use an iPod with internet access versus an iPhone. Digit-Eyes has a database of many millions of products that increase every day as users look for new products. Although Digit-Eyes sells labels, the least costly approach is to make your own labels using Avery products or generic labels. Digit-Eyes clothing labels need to be sewn on or attached to the garment with a safety pin. The clothing labels will tolerate at least 50 standard machine washings/bleachings/dryings, which the Garment Industry reports is the average number of times a piece of clothing will be worn.

This labeling application also has a voice recording to attach your own words to a label—"light blue top goes with the striped blue skirt and the navy blue flowered shorts." Of particular importance is live customer service which will provide individualized training via the phone or Skype. For further information including: extensive tips on scanning; how to create a label; how to find a bar code on a product; audio demonstrations, reviews (by outside evaluators), tutorials on Digit-Eyes; a print manual and much, much more just visit www.digit-eyes.com.

10. Eldred KB. Optimal illumination for reading in patients with age-related maculopathy. *Optom Vis Sci.* 1992;69:46-50.
11. Cornelissen FW, Bootsma A, Kooijman AC. Object perception by visually impaired people at different light levels. *Vis Res.* 1995;35:161-168.
12. Bowers AR, Meek C, Stewart N. Illumination and reading performance in age-related macular degeneration. *Clin Exp Optom.* 2001;84:139-147.
13. Corn AL, Erin JN, American Foundation for the Blind. *Foundations of Low Vision: Clinical and Functional Perspectives.* 2nd ed. New York: AFB Press; 2010:xv.
14. Brilliant R, ed. *Essentials of Low Vision Practice.* Boston: Butterworth Heinemann; 1999:409.
15. Perlmutter MS, Bhorade A, Gordon M, Hollingsworth H, Engsberg JE, Carolyn Baum M. Home lighting assessment for clients with low vision. *Am J Occup Ther.* 2013;67:674-682.
16. Kern T, Miller ND. Occupational therapy and collaborative interventions for adults with low vision. In: Gentile M, ed. *Functional Visual Behavior in Adults: An Occupational Therapy Guide to Evaluation and Treatment Options.* Bethesda: AOTA Press; 2005:127-165.
17. Whittaker SG, Lovie-Kitchin JE. Visual requirements for reading. *Optom Vis Sci.*1993;70:54-65.
18. Marron JA, Bailey IL. Visual factors and orientation: mobility performance. *Am J Optom Physiol Opt.* 1982;59:413-426.
19. Kuyk T, Elliott JL, Fuhr PS. Visual correlates of obstacle avoidance in adults with low vision. *Optom Vis Sci.* 1998;75:174-182.
20. Owsley C, Sloane ME. Contrast sensitivity, acuity, and the perception of 'real-world' targets. *Br J Ophthalmol.* 1987;71:791-796.
21. West SK, Rubin GS, Broman AT, Muñoz B, Bandeen-Roche K, Turano K. How does visual impairment affect performance on tasks of everyday life? The SEE Project. Salisbury Eye Evaluation. *Arch Ophthalmol.* 2002;120:774-780.
22. Rubin GS, Roche KB, Prasada-Rao P, Fried LP. Visual impairment and disability in older adults. *Optom Vis Sci.* 1994;71:750-760.
23. Cummings RW, Muchnick BG, Whittaker SG. Specialized testing in low vision. In: Brilliant RL, ed. *Essentials of Low Vision Practice.* Boston: Butterworth-Heinemann; 1999:47-69.
24. Lueck AH. *Functional Vision: A Practitioner's Guide to Evaluation and Intervention.* New York: AFB Press; 2004:xx.
25. Quillman RD, Goodrich GL. Interventions for adults with visual impairments. In: Lueck AH, ed. *Functional Vision: A Practitioner's Guide to Evaluation and Intervention.* New York: AFB Press; 2004:423-474.
26. Wiener WR, Welsh RL, Blasch BB, eds. *Foundations of Orientation and Mobility: History and Theory.* 3rd ed. New York: American Foundation for the Blind; 2010.

Optical Devices and Magnification Strategies

Reduced visual acuity is the most common visual impairment encountered by the low vision rehabilitation therapist. Optical magnification devices can be used to compensate for visual acuity loss that interferes with a client's ability to perform a particular task. Optical devices compensate by magnifying the retinal image of the target being viewed, allowing the detail to be resolved. People use optical devices for many everyday tasks, such as reading, needlework, bird watching, watching television, enjoying theater or a sports event, repairing appliances, managing medications, and reading package labels.

Recommendation or prescription of any optical device, even a handheld magnifier, requires the collaboration of an optometrist or ophthalmologist with the vision rehabilitation therapist. In Chapter 2, we presented 2 potential collaborative models, which are reviewed here:

1. The standard model involves an eye care provider with advanced skills in low vision rehabilitation working with a therapist who has basic skills. The first section of this chapter provides detailed information required by the occupational therapist working under this standard model. In this model, the low vision optometrist takes the primary responsibility for estimating magnification and prescribing the optical devices. The therapist performs an occupational therapy low vision evaluation (see Chapter 8) and provides information to the low vision optometrist about client goals, such as specific task requirements, and nonvisual impairments, such as a hand tremor or low frustration tolerance. The therapist may also suggest types of devices that seem appropriate. The low vision optometrist recommends devices to try and eventually prescribes the devices. The occupational therapist configures the environment and instructs the client about the use of the recommended device to achieve performance goals. If the client has difficulty performing the required tasks with a recommended device, the therapist consults with the low vision optometrist, who recommends different devices or other solutions.

2. The advanced model requires that the therapist have a more advanced understanding of the principles of magnification and optical devices. In this second collaborative model, the occupational therapist takes a more active role in recommending device magnification, selecting devices, and solving problems relating to magnification and the properties of the devices. The occupational therapist must understand how to estimate the optical device magnification required to perform a task, as well as how optical devices work, and how to identify the limiting visual factor when a device

Whittaker SG, Scheiman M, Sokol-McKay DA.
Low Vision Rehabilitation: A Practical Guide for Occupational Therapists,
Second Edition (pp 219-251).
© 2016 Taylor & Francis Group.

TABLE 13-1: RECOMMENDED "GETTING STARTED" OPTICAL DEVICES

- Illuminated handheld devices with bright white LED-type lights at approximately 2, 5, 6, 8, 10, 12, 16, 20, 25, and 32 D.
- Illuminated stand magnifiers from 10, 12, 16, 25, and 32 equivalent D.
- Open stand magnifier for writing at 5 and 8 D.
- A low power horizontal bar magnifier.
- Hooded visors or loupes at 5, 6, 8, 10, and 12 D that can be worn on the head, with or without eyeglasses.
- Ask the collaborating low vision optometrist to loan half-eye and microscope high near addition.
- Halberg clips with +1, +1.5, +2, +2.5, +3, +4, +5, +8, +10 diopter lenses.
- 1.5×, 2.5×, 3× sports glasses, Eschenbach TV-max (2×), Echenbach Max detail telemicroscope.
- 4×, 6×, and 8× handheld Keplerian telescope.
- One set of 6× and 8× head-mounted telescopes with two 2.5-D caps.
- A metric tape measure, reading stand, and lap tray. Typoscopes, continual text reading card, and directional task light with extension cord. Tape and clipboard to secure the reading material.

does not work as predicted. This level of understanding is required by the Academy for Certification of Vision Rehabilitation & Education Professionals (ACVREP) for certification as a low vision therapist.

This chapter is divided into 3 sections. The first section describes what an occupational therapist needs to understand about optical magnification devices to perform low vision rehabilitation therapy in the standard collaborative model. The second section is advanced and describes additional principles required for the occupational therapist to perform low vision rehabilitation therapy under the advanced model. Finally, some clients with visual impairment also have reduced visual fields. Optical devices have been developed to help compensate for visual field problems. These field expansion devices are discussed in the final section of this chapter.

With mild to moderate loss in visual acuity, optical devices are relatively easy to use and may be sufficient for reading goals. With more severe vision loss, optical devices are difficult to learn to use. With skilled instruction, clients are more likely to accept the higher magnification required for fluent reading. Generally, with higher magnification, electronic devices are easier to use. The success-oriented approach recommends electronic devices be used initially to reintroduce reading to clients who need higher magnification. Indeed, electronic devices as a medium for reading and functional communication are becoming as common as pen and paper. Tablet computers and e-readers enlarge print, enabling lower magnification optical devices to be used. Environmental modifications or nonoptical interventions affect the type of device and magnification of the device required as well.

THE BASIC PRINCIPLES (THE STANDARD MODEL)

Often, low vision optometrists recommend, and some might even prescribe, optical devices for magnification before the therapist has started treatment. When possible, final prescription of optical devices should be discouraged until after instruction has begun and the client has had an opportunity to try the devices. This will increase client satisfaction and decrease the possibility that a device will need to be returned or exchanged. With either model, the occupational therapist should have an assortment of optical devices available that will approximate the devices recommended by the low vision optometrist (Table 13-1). These devices are generally provided by a collaborating optometrist if in the same setting.

Referring physicians and clients also often assume that optical devices are central in the low vision rehabilitation process, leading to an unfortunate expectation by many clients that a device exists that will remediate and restore clear vision. Unlike a pair of eyeglasses designed to correct refractive error and make vision clear and sharp again, optical magnification devices magnify objects to compensate for inadequate acuity. Rather than clear vision, the client experiences an enlarged but still fuzzy view of the object (Figure 13-1).

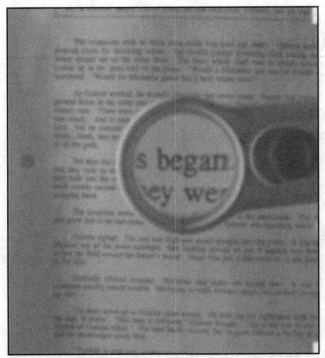

Figure 13-1. Simulated impaired visual acuity of a client as seen with and without an optical magnification device.

The Collaborative Model for Evaluation and Treatment With Optical Devices

The following 7 steps outline our recommended sequence for device selection and implementation (Table 13-2). As described previously, a client should be under the care of an eye care provider and be referred with a diagnosis, prognosis, visual acuity, and a current pair of glasses whose optics are fully described before being evaluated by the occupational therapist. Ideally, as mentioned, the final prescription of a low vision device should occur later in the sequence. The following steps provide an overview of the process of selecting, providing instruction, and evaluating optical devices. The first 4 of the 7 steps have been described in Chapter 8 as part of the occupational therapy evaluation. In the remainder of this section, we describe the basis for selecting devices and instructional procedures.

1. Defining the Goal Tasks and Performance Requirements

The first step in selecting devices is to define the tasks that the client needs to perform, along with observable and measurable performance goals. Performance goals should be specific, as well as whether the task is a brief "spot task," like reading a label, or an "extended task," like reading a newspaper or watching television. The information to be

	TABLE 13-2: WHAT THE THERAPIST CONTRIBUTES TO THE STANDARD COLLABORATIVE MODEL
1.	Define the goal task and performance goal.
2.	Perform an environmental and task analysis.
	2.1. Distance required to see and preferred working distances?
	2.2. Hands-free device required?
	2.3. Illuminated device required?
	2.4. Work surfaces available?
3.	Identify nonvisual impairments.
	3.1. Tremors and impaired fine motor control.
	3.2. Cognitive impairments, impaired problem solving, impaired procedural memory/learning, and impaired frustration tolerance.
4.	Identify visual impairments.
	4.1. Functional reading acuity.
	4.2. Contrast sensitivity and optimum lighting.
	4.3. Field restrictions, central scotoma, and fixation and scanning performance.
	4.4. Complaints of double vision, eye strain, or if vision is better with 1 or 2 eyes.
5.	Recommend type of optical device(s) for all tasks.
6.	In-clinic instruction and device evaluation and final prescription by an optometrist.
7.	Instruction in context.

conveyed to the low vision optometrist is summarized in Table 13-3.

As described in Chapters 6 and 8, goal definition often requires detective work. For example, Ms. Jason, an 86-year-old retired accountant with atrophic macular degeneration, initially denied that she had goals, but she and her husband agreed they had been fighting a lot lately. An examination of her history and interview with her husband revealed medication management errors and frequent arguments about how he manages the bills and checkbook, a job she had been performing for the 43 years of their marriage. She also used to perform cross-stitch. Ms. Jason had not performed this activity for years and did not identify this as a goal because she did not think cross-stitch was possible. She continued to "watch" television, but reported that she could not see the screen very well. Based on this information, 4 goals were identified: 1) improve ability to see television screen, 2) locate amount due and write check for bills and

TABLE 13-3: INFORMATION TO INCLUDE IN REFERRAL TO AN OPTOMETRIST FOR A DEVICE EVALUATION

- Specific goal task and performance requirement.
  - Is the task spotting or sustained?
  - Do high-productivity requirements exist (speed and endurance)?
- Specify exactly what the client is trying to see (size, contrast) and the required working distance if a particular distance is required or strongly preferred.
  - Print size and required distance.
  - Size of the TV and preferred distance.
  - How far a client wishes to sit away from a teacher or player in a sports event to see it.
- Estimate required size and relative distance magnification. If watching a TV, an event, or, with hobbies, indicate the distance at which someone can see the objects or people, or how much the objects must be enlarged to see them.
- Specify if the client reports better vision with both eyes or just the better-seeing eye with good illumination.
- Specify if a task requires both hands.
- Specify tremors, ataxia, or other motor impairments and if a table is available.
- Specify significant cognitive and psychosocial impairments.
- Include visual findings such as continual text acuity, contrast sensitivity, fields, best lighting, and, if field loss, visual scanning performance.
- Recommend types and magnification of devices to consider.

balance a checkbook, 3) read medication labels and identify pills, and 4) perform cross-stitch independently.

2. Perform Environmental and Task Analysis

To be able to recommend magnification, the low vision optometrist needs to know the size and/or distance magnification required to perform a task. Although eye care providers should have continual-text near acuity charts, few eye care providers will have real-life objects like cross-stitch patterns. For reading, the therapist need only specify the required print size and if special working distances are required. For tasks such as hobbies or viewing pictures where the items are portable, the client needs to bring the objects to be viewed to the examination so that the optometrist can estimate magnification requirements. For TV watching or viewing events or activities that cannot be performed in a clinic, the therapist will help determine required magnification.

For distances greater than 1 meter (3 feet), the therapist reports the distance at which the TV or object can be seen and the screen size if a TV. For closer working distances, a tablet computer like an iPad or Kindle can be used to take a picture and enlarge an object to estimate required size enlargement by dividing the enlarged size by the actual size

(Figure 13-2). The therapist can specify this information on the referral form and include this with the performance goal. The therapist needs to consider how the device will be held, if 2 hands are required to perform the task, the demand on fine motor skills, and whether a table is available for support. Hands-free optical magnification devices are available that can be mounted on spectacles or on a table. In the environmental analysis, the therapist needs to consider if lighting can be controlled; if not, an illuminated device might be recommended. A summary of information that should be included on a referral form can be found in Table 13-3. In the case of Ms. Jason, she would be encouraged to bring her cross-stitch to the optometrist, along with samples of bills and medications. The print size required would be specified as "1M preferred, 2M possible" because large-print bills and checks may be obtained.

In the example case report, the environmental evaluation revealed that Ms. Jason preferred to do her cross-stitch and watch television in her favorite easy chair and sort her medication into dispensers and pay bills at the kitchen table. In these settings, reading novels and reading bills can be done at any distance, but cross-stitch and writing in the check register cannot be done closer than about 15 cm (8 to 9 inches). She could use one hand to hold a device for most tasks except cross-stitch. Ms. Jason would require a hands-free device for this task.

3. Evaluate Nonvisual Factors

Clients with tremors and impaired fine motor control require devices with support, such as stand magnifiers, and spectacle-mounted rather than handheld magnifiers. Clients with cognitive impairments such as apraxia, impaired problem solving, impaired procedural memory/learning, and impaired frustration tolerance require simple devices with which they had premorbid familiarity, such as low-power handheld magnifiers. They might require gradual introduction of stronger magnification and are generally poor candidates for handheld telescopes, stand magnifiers, and microscopes. In the case of Ms. Jason, she was cognitively intact and very detail oriented with low frustration tolerance. She had compensated in past years by structuring her routine and environment and avoiding challenging activities. Ms. Jason was resistant to change. For example, she refused to move her chair or television so she could decrease her viewing distance to the television. The therapist summarized all of the information and shared it with the eye care provider who performed the clinical low vision evaluation (see Table 13-3).

4. Evaluate Visual Factors

In the standard model, the eye care provider should perform most of the visual testing (see Chapter 7). The therapist should also perform some or all of the following tests (see Chapter 8):

- Continual text acuity and critical print size. For distance and nonreading tasks, specify how much an object needs to be enlarged and the required distance of the object to see, as well as preferred size and distance.
- Contrast sensitivity and the light levels (using a light meter) that produce the best contrast sensitivity or acuity. In general, if someone has severe contrast sensitivity impairment, electronic magnification devices (see Chapter 14) are preferred because optical devices degrade contrast, while electronic devices increase contrast.
- Visual fields and description of adaptive visual scanning or eccentric fixation if the client has a central or peripheral field loss.
- Determine whether the client performs the task more effectively with both eyes open or by patching one eye.

In the case of Ms. Jason, the therapist might specify (using evaluations from Chapter 8):

- At 40 cm, 4M print acuity (0.4/4M) with her left eye and 0.4M/8 M critical print size to read fluently and comfortably

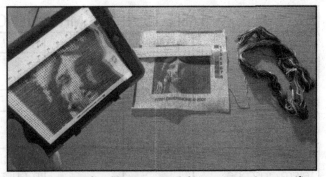

Figure 13-2. Use of a tablet computer (left) to estimate size magnification requirements for a sewing activity. One enlarges the image on the screen until the client resolves necessary detail. To estimate size magnification, measure the size of a 1-cm marking on the ruler in the magnified image, also in centimeters.

- With contrast sensitivity, she has a moderate loss in contrast threshold (7%) with improvement to mild loss (5%) when light levels were increased to greater than 1000 lux. But reported glare sensitivity. She reports less glare if she is viewing only with her left eye.
- Using the tangent screen method, she was found to have stable superior eccentric fixation with a scotoma size of approximately 15 degrees.

5. Recommend Devices

In the referral to the low vision optometrist, the therapist might recommend specific devices based on the occupational therapy evaluation described earlier. A summary of the applications of different types of devices is listed in Table 13-4 and will be explained later in this section. In the case of Ms. Jason, for example, the therapist might recommend consideration of a spectacle-mounted telescope for television watching and an objective lens cap to turn the telescope into a telemicroscope for near work for sewing. The therapist might also recommend an electronic tabletop magnifier (closed-circuit television, CCTV, discussed later and in Chapter 14) for reading and bill paying. The low vision optometrist might then determine the magnification for the telescope and lower-power, full-field reading glasses to use with the electronic magnifier at 30 cm (10 inches) to allow her to use it more easily. The optometrist also might suggest that Ms. Jason use a 10-D illuminated handheld device to write large-print checks and keep a register, and since she is already nearsighted, she could hold it to her eye without her glasses for extra magnification, if needed.

6. Grade the Task: The Success-Oriented Approach

With demonstrations and explanations, most clients will quickly move through the process of selecting devices. Order and manner of presentation are less important. With clients who have cognitive impairments, who are depressed, who are resistant to change, or who have low frustration

TABLE 13-4: MAGNIFIER DEVICES AND TYPICAL APPLICATIONS

Device	Up Close	Far Distance	Arm's Length	Hands-Free	Example
Handheld	Spot	No	Spot	Possible with table and mount	Reading labels, menus, fixing something
Stand	Extended	No	No	No	Reading a letter
Spectacle reading addition	Extended	No	No	Yes	Reading a book or newspaper
Telescope or telemicroscope	Spot	Spot	Extended if mounted	Yes, if mounted on spectacles	Fixing something, reading music, watching TV
Electronic	No	Special camera required	Extended	Yes, if worn on remote camera	Reading book, seeing blackboard, writing

spot: short-duration task; extended: long-duration task.

tolerance, a success-oriented approach is advisable. In the success-oriented approach, evaluation and initial instruction should emphasize successful performance of a goal task (see Chapter 6). Starting with the device most likely to enable successful task performance, have the client try the device in a situation that requires little, if any, learning or skill and with maximum assistance if necessary. This will convince the client that success is possible from the beginning.

The client should experience what it is like to perform the task with a device before facing the challenging task of learning to use it. In the example of Ms. Jason, before trying needlepoint, the therapist might begin by having her watch television with the telescope since this is easier to accomplish and generally successful. Bill paying would be started with the electronic magnifier because success is more likely, and then a handheld device could be attempted later because it is more difficult to use.

If the result with a particular device is unsuccessful, attempt to identify other performance-limiting factors, such as lighting or other visual or physical impairments. Ideally, the eye care provider participates in this problem solving. In the case of Ms. Jason, if her initial attempts to use the telescope were unsuccessful, larger stitches with less magnification and better lighting might be attempted. During this process, the client is often able to decide if he or she wants the device. The therapist should try to find one device that meets several needs. In the case of Ms. Jason, with task modification (using larger stitches), she could use the same telescope to watch television and with a special cap for near work, perform cross-stitch in a favorite easy chair.

7. Instruct in Natural Context: From Ideal to Real

Once a device is selected and successful performance is accomplished in a controlled instructional setting, the therapist provides instruction in the actual setting or a simulation of the actual setting in which a task will be performed. A client who might insist on a particular seating or environment at first may be inspired to change after experiencing how much easier it is to perform a task under the controlled instructional setting. If a device has been prescribed, the client can practice in her or his most comfortable setting and report problems to the therapist during scheduled sessions. At this point, sessions can be scheduled less frequently with more emphasis on a home program. For well-adjusted clients whose only impairment is visual, they will usually be able to quickly learn to use optical devices using adult learning strategies (see Chapter 9) without the requirement of steps 6 and 7. For these clients, the focus can quickly turn to problem solving using the devices where lighting or positioning is difficult.

An Overview of Magnification Strategies and Devices

Relative Size and Distance Magnification

Many devices and strategies can magnify objects to compensate for impaired visual acuity. The term *magnification* has many definitions, but ultimately, magnification refers to changing the size of the image of an object on the retina. The most straightforward magnification method to increase the size of an image on the retina is enlargement, or relative size magnification, and relative distance magnification (Figure 13-3) (see Chapters 5 and 10). Relative size magnification can be accomplished with large-print books, enlarging objects on a copy machine, using larger stitches in a needlepoint task, or using electronic devices such as the electronic magnifier system illustrated in Figure 13-4 (more fully described in Chapter 14). If a device being used does not have sufficient magnification, the therapist can compensate by enlarging the material being viewed.

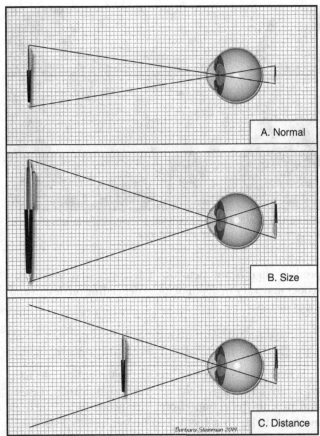

Figure 13-3. Increasing retinal image size with relative size magnification and relative distance magnification. (Reprinted with permission from Barbara Steinman.)

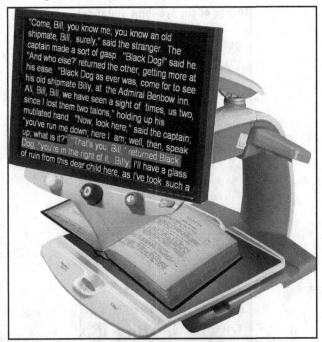

Figure 13-4. A CCTV device magnifies, enhancing contrast by reversing and increasing contrast. (Reprinted with permission from Freedom Scientific, www.freedomscientific.com.)

Another strategy the therapist can use if device magnification is not sufficient is relative distance magnification, which is moving a client closer to the material being viewed. However, one must be careful when using relative distance magnification with near devices; usually, a different device must be used if a person needs to move closer to the object. Handheld magnifiers, spectacles with near reading addition, and stand magnifiers must be used at prescribed distances. Telescopes, however, can be refocused at different distances, so if a telescope is not strong enough, the client can move closer and refocus to achieve increased overall magnification. With some devices like telescopes, magnification depends on how far the device is positioned from the object being viewed—the device-to-object distance.

Magnification and Field of View

Clients ideally want a device that will allow magnification while maintaining a large field of view and a normal working distance. Unfortunately, regardless of the optical device used, there are some universal trade-offs. As magnification increases, field of view necessarily decreases (Figure 13-5). This is easy to understand, because as the image is enlarged, less of it will fit in the person's visual field. Second, the field of view through a device also depends on the eye-to-lens distance.

Positioning a Device

When using devices, the following important distances must be carefully considered (Figure 13-6):

1. Lens-to-object distance is the distance of the lens from the object or page being viewed. The lens-to-object distance determines if the object is in focus or not, and with some devices, magnification is affected by this. The lens-to-object distance should be at or slightly less than the focal distance of the lens, f = 100/D (see Chapter 5), where D is the dioptric power of the magnifier. With a stand magnifier, a stand holds the lens at a fixed distance from the page being viewed to control the lens-to-object distance.

2. Eye-to-lens distance is the distance of the eye from the lens, or in the case of a telescope or multilens system, the distance from the lens closest to the eye (the ocular) and the eye. In general, eye-to-lens distance affects field of view and focus: the closer the lens is to the eye, the larger the field of view. As the lens moves closer to the eye, the effect of eye-to-object distance (working distance) affects focus more than target size.

3. Working or viewing distance refers to how far the eye is from the object being viewed.

Depth of focus describes how much one might change the lens distance and still keep the object in focus. As near optical devices become more powerful, the working

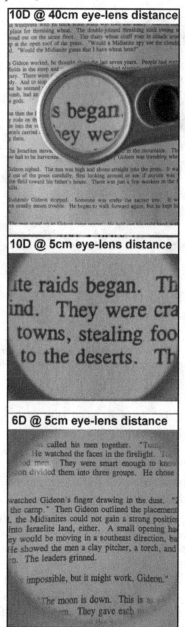

Figure 13-5. Three views through a 10-D handheld magnifier held with a 40-cm eye-to-lens distance (top) and a closer eye-to-lens distance (middle). Lens-to-paper distance did not change. Note magnification does not change, but field of view does change. Eye-to-lens distance in the middle and bottom pictures is the same. Field of view increases only because magnification decreases from the middle lens to the bottom lens.

distance and depth of focus decrease. For example, someone using a 5-D handheld magnifier may vary 20 to 30 mm from the 20-cm lens distance without significant defocus. With a 20-D magnifier, a change of 5 to 7 mm will

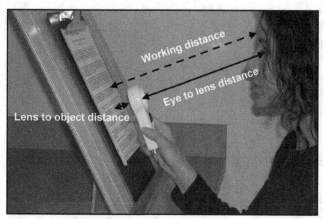

Figure 13-6. An illustration of working distance, eye-to-lens distance, and lens-to-object (page of text) distance.

produce significant defocus. Telescopes and telemicroscopes may vary in depth of focus depending on design and focus distance.

Light Transmittance, Contrast Degradation, and Chromatic Aberration

When a client looks through some optical devices, especially telescopes, light decreases significantly. Lenses also pick up reflections from extraneous lights, such as overhead lights in a room, and poorer quality lenses will scatter light and degrade the contrast of objects being viewed. Antireflective coatings, the use of visors, shielding the lens from light, and positioning light from the side so it does not reflect off the lens will greatly improve lens performance. Very strong, simple lenses act like prisms and turn white light into component colors at the edges and blur the image (Figure 13-7). This is called *chromatic aberration.* Newer, often more expensive, compound lenses have not only become thin and light, but they also have included layers of refraction and defraction-type optics that eliminate chromatic aberration. Clients differ in their sensitivity to chromatic aberration. It is reasonable to suspect that clients who are sensitive to glare and have impaired contrast sensitivity will be more sensitive to reflections off the lenses, defocus, and chromatic aberrations. Newer defraction-type lenses are thinner, lighter, and larger, but more expensive as well (Figure 13-8).

Movement

Devices not only magnify the size of objects being viewed, but also magnify the motion of objects being viewed by the same amount. We all have experienced how difficult it is to hold a pair of powerful binoculars steady, as the motion greatly degrades what is being viewed. Stronger magnifiers require either higher levels of fine motor control and visual motor coordination or external supports and bracing to reduce this movement. Motion sickness can sometimes result from this movement magnification.

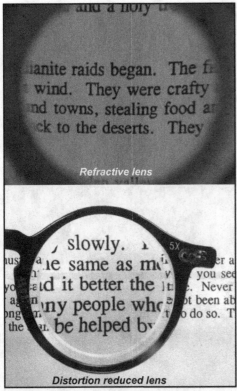

Figure 13-7. Top view through a simple lens. The bottom view is through the Clear Image Lens that is designed to decrease optical aberrations. (Reprinted with permission from Designs for Vision, www.designsforvision.com.)

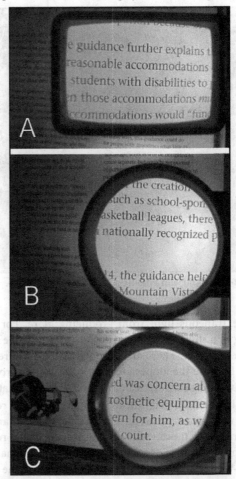

Figure 13-8. Difference in distortion-free field of view through 3 types of 16-diopter lenses (same magnification) in illuminated handheld magnifiers: (A) defractive lens, (B) refractive compound lens, and (C) simple lens.

Properties of Optical Devices

High Near-Addition (Full-Field Microscopes), Half-Eye's, and Loupes

A client young enough to accommodate (focus the eyes) at a close viewing distance might use relative distance magnification, simply moving the eye closer to the text or objects being viewed. An older adult will require microscopes, also called *near vision only* (NVO) reading glasses, to read up close (Figure 13-9). A near add is essentially a plus power lens "added" to a person's distance correction. Near addition lenses that focus at near may take the form of bifocals or variable focus lenses (progressive lenses or no-line bifocals) in the bottom segment of a spectacle lens under about +3.0 D. Stronger near addition that allows one to look above the lens for distance or through the lens for reading, such as reading while watching TV, are called *half-eyes*. Half-eyes are designed to be used binocularly for very close activities and incorporate base-in prisms to improve comfort by decreasing the effort required to converge. A full field high plus lens over one eye is called high-add NVO glasses, or *full-field microscopes* (see Figures 13-7 and 13-9). Full-field microscopes are preferred over bifocals if someone is using only one eye or when high powers (> 10 to 12 D)

are required because the working distance is too close for binocular vision. In addition, NVO glasses enable a broader field of view than bifocals. In some cases, the plus lenses are actually mounted in front of a person's eyes or eyeglasses in the form of loupes or visors (Figure 13-10). For clients working on machinery or doing repair work, crafts, fine furniture, or other tasks in which the client must focus at various distances, flip-up lenses that clip on spectacles can allow a person to quickly change the power of the lens and relative distance magnification. Near addition lenses or bifocals are not recommended for clients at risk for falls when walking because the blur at distance results in tripping hazards.[1]

As mentioned, loupes are plus lenses that clip on to spectacles. Loupes in the form of visors fit on someone's head in front of the eyes or spectacles (see Figure 13-10). Some have multiple lenses, allowing one to change the addition depending on the task. The head visors are a favorite because they easily flip up out of the way, and the shroud

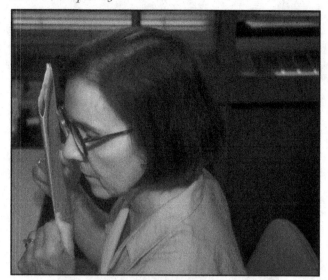

Figure 13-9. Reading with a full-field, high power microscope.

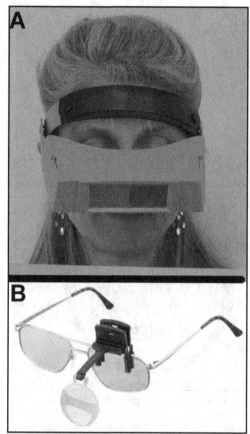

Figure 13-10. (A) A flip-up visor loupe magnifier generally provides some glare control. (B) A spectacle-clip loupe for near magnification. (Reprinted with permission from Eschenbach Optik of America.)

blocks extraneous light from producing glare. For users working in a shop, these devices afford some degree of eye protection as well. These are stronger than typical reading glasses. Because the loupes are positioned farther from the eye, the working distance can be increased somewhat.

Relative distance magnification and microscopes require that the client learn to perform a task at a closer-than-normal working distance. Stronger microscopes also require precise motor control or some external support to maintain the lens-to-object distance and to carefully move the material being read. Because light must be directed between the lens and the object being viewed, lighting becomes difficult with stronger magnification, and illumination built into the magnifier is preferred.

Important Properties of High, Near-Addition, or Microscopes

- Half-eyes with base-in prism enable binocular viewing up to about 10 to 12 D. With more power and a closer working distance, a full-field microscope must be used.

- High reading addition, microscopes, and loupes are often preferred to a handheld magnifier for extended reading, but are not as useful for spot reading because the spotting technique is not possible.

- If the older client is unable to accommodate (focus at near), lens-to-object distance in centimeters is fixed. A person younger than 40 can bring an object closer to achieve additional magnification and still keep it in focus, but this often creates eye strain.

- With higher magnification, working distance is a few inches and the object can go out of focus if not held at the exact distance. External support or good fine motor skills are required. Good ergonomics is critical for success.

- With higher magnification, maintaining good lighting becomes more of a problem.

- Because the lens is close to the eye, the client's visual field through the device is not restricted by optics.

- If a handheld magnifier is held against the reading addition or plus lens put in front of the spectacle lens with a Halberg clip, the power of the lenses will add together.

Handheld Magnifiers

Most clients will be familiar with handheld magnifiers (Figure 13-11), more commonly called *magnifying glasses*. Handheld magnifiers are the least expensive and most versatile of magnification devices. Handheld magnifiers might also be mounted to a table or on a string around the neck to allow a client to use both hands (Figures 13-11 and 13-12). A client can hold the magnifier at any distance from the eye, bringing it closer to increase the field of view. When held close to the eye, the handheld magnifier functions just like a microscope. Like the microscope, the stronger handheld magnifier requires a close lens-to-object distance and good

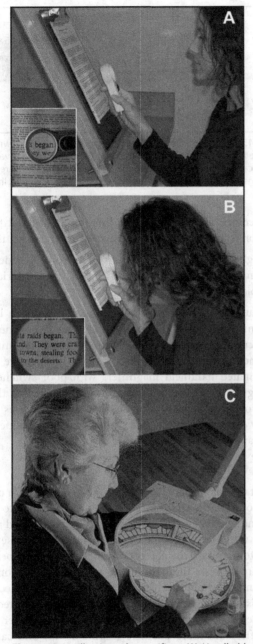

Figure 13-11. Illuminated magnifiers: (A) Handheld at distance (shopping). (B) Handheld at near. (C) Mounted for hands-free use.

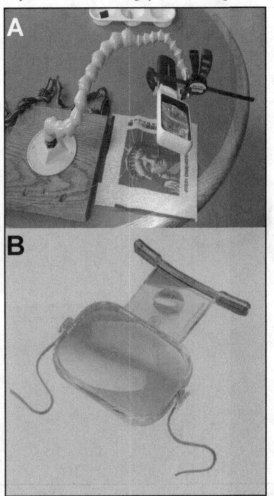

Figure 13-12. Methods for mounting lenses for hands-free use: (A) A holder for a magnifier can be easily manufactured from components available from www.modularhose.com and clamps from a local hardware store. (B) Chest magnifier. (Reprinted with permission from Eschenbach Optik of America.)

fine motor control to maintain this distance and to control the position of the magnifier to avoid losing one's place.

Handheld magnifiers are usually used for short periods. Examples include spot reading, such as reading price tags, bills, and labels; checking medication; checking skin or fingernails; or reading menus. For sustained tasks, the user often quickly fatigues because the magnifier must be held at the precise distance from the objects being viewed. For more sustained work, such as sewing, using loupes stand magnifiers or some hands-free magnifier is preferred.

Important Properties of Handheld Magnifiers

- Handheld magnifiers are usually used for spotting rather than extended use.

- Lens-to-object distance is fixed and can be determined by lifting the lens away from a page until it either focuses the image of a distant light onto the page or maximizes magnification and focus of an object viewed through the lens. If the power of the device is known, lens-to-object distance in centimeters also can be estimated as 100 cm/D, where D is the power in diopters. For example, a handheld magnifier labeled as a 20-D lens would have a lens-to-object distance of 100/20 = 5 cm.

- Decreasing eye-to-lens distance increases the field of view (see Figure 13-15).

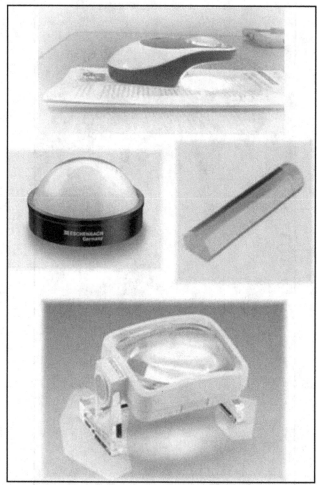

Figure 13-13. An assortment of stand-type magnifiers. Newer-style illuminated stand magnifier (top), bright field and bar magnifier (middle), and magnifier designed for writing. (Reprinted with permission from Eschenbach Optik of America.)

- If the magnifier is held away from the eye, the client looks through the distance (upper) segment of the eyeglasses, or without glasses if he or she does not wear correction for distance. Away from the eye, magnification decreases the closer the magnifier is to the object or paper being viewed.

- The client looks through the bifocal addition or reading addition if the lens is held close to the eye. The combined effect of reading addition and the magnifier will increase overall magnification and maximize field of view.

- A lens with a larger diameter has a lower power. Larger diameter lenses have a larger field of view, mostly because of lower power. Rectangular magnifiers are available to increase horizontal field of view.

- Lower power handheld devices are quite forgiving if not positioned correctly; higher power devices are not forgiving and should not be used for people with

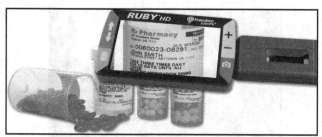

Figure 13-14. An electronic handheld magnifier has a flip-down support like a stand magnifier; can be held in the hand; and has variable magnification, contrast enhancement, and image capture for reading price tags. (Reprinted with permission from Freedom Scientific, Inc.)

tremors, apraxia, or incoordination, or if hand function is limited by problems such as severe arthritis.

- Lighting should ideally be directed from the side and aimed between the magnifier and the material or object being viewed.

- Illuminated handheld magnifiers with built-in light-emitting diode (LED) light sources are generally recommended, especially with stronger magnifiers. Therapists are cautioned to avoid inexpensive illuminated handheld magnifiers with poor switches or regular bulbs and should caution users against them. Broken switches and problems with batteries easily consume considerable clinical time, disable performance, and irritate everyone involved.

Stand Magnifiers

A stand magnifier (Figure 13-13) can be used if a client does not have the endurance or fine motor control to hold the handheld magnifier at the correct distance. Stand magnifiers were developed for extended reading because it is easier to maintain the correct distance for a longer period. One simply rests the base of the stand magnifier on the page and the stand itself maintains the correct object-to-lens distance. Stand magnifiers, however, usually require that the client work on a table or hard surface. Newer style magnifiers are more portable (Figure 13-14) and can be used like a handheld magnifier. Currently, electronic handheld magnifiers are preferred for spot reading and tabletop electronic magnifiers (closed-circuit televisions or CCTVs) are preferred to the more traditional stand magnifiers for extended reading.[2]

Important Properties of Stand Magnifiers

- The client looks through the bottom half of bifocals or reading eyeglasses with the stand magnifier positioned at a prescribed eye-to-lens distance. The prescribing optometrist should provide information about eye-to-lens distance and what reading glasses to use. Estimating these distances is addressed in a later section of this chapter.

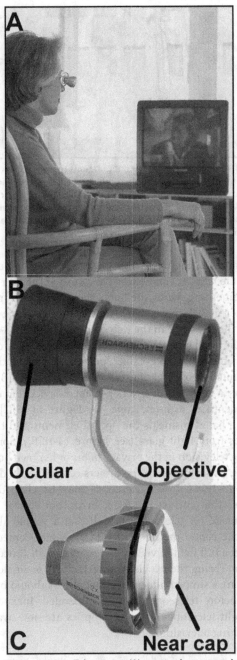

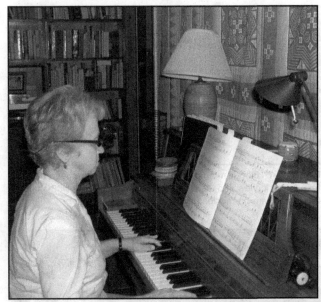

Figure 13-16. Spectacle-mounted telemicroscope (Beecher-Mirage telescope with a near cap) focused at an intermediate distance.

- Higher magnification devices should have built-in illumination. Lower power stand magnifiers (see Figure 13-13) are available as bar readers, or some are adapted for writing as well as reading.

- Portable handheld and desktop electronic magnifiers are often preferred over these devices, especially for reading, because of contrast enhancement and emerging text-to-speech capability.

Telescopes and Telemicroscopes

Devices that are used for seeing sports events, theater performances, the television at distance, or recognizing faces or reading signs are distance devices. Telescopes and binoculars can be handheld or spectacle mounted (Figures 13-15 and 13-16). Spectacle-mounted telescopes may also be mounted on the top of the lens so the client can look through the bottom half of the lenses while moving about, then stop, tip the head downward, and look through the telescope to read a sign or identify someone without touching the device. This is referred to as a *bioptic mount* (Figure 13-17). In many states, people with low vision can legally drive with bioptic-mounted telescopes. Spectacle-mounted telescopes stabilize the device and allow both hands to be free. Spectacle mounting, however, positions the telescope farther from the eye and thus reduces the field of view. Various mounting strategies and devices are available that allow the eye care practitioner to mount the ocular closer to the eye and incorporate correction into the ocular of the telescope. Furthermore, the devices should be mounted to maintain telescopic alignment with the optical axis of the eye. For these reasons, telescopic systems should only be dispensed by an optometrist or ophthalmologist.

Figure 13-15. Telescopes: (A) spectacle mounted, (B) handheld Keplerian telescope, and (C) Galilean telescope (designed for spectacle mount) with near cap in place for close work. (Reprinted with permission from Eschenbach Optik of America.)

- In general, because the lens is closer to the page being viewed, the actual power of a stand magnifier has less magnification than indicated by the power of the lens.[3]

- These devices are generally preferred if someone with impaired motor control needs to use a higher optical magnification.

- These devices are generally preferred over handheld magnifiers for extended reading.

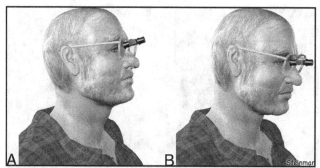

Figure 13-17. Bioptic mount. Someone looking through the carrier lens for a full-field view and the telescope for a magnified view of a target. (Reprinted with permission from Barbara Steinman.)

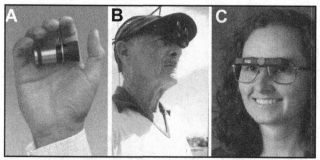

Figure 13-18. Various telescope configurations that are more cosmetically accepted. (A) Handheld; note clip between index and long finger (Reprinted with permission from Eschenbach Optik of America.) (B) Beecher-Mirage using a hat for glare control and to hide the device from others during sailing competition. (C) An Ocutech Keplerian telescope in a bioptic. (Reprinted with permission of Ocutech.)

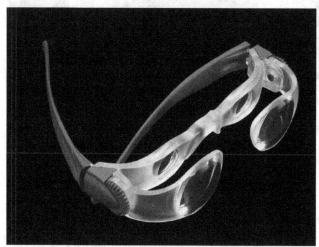

Figure 13-19. Lower-power spectacle telescope ideal for TV watching. A similar-looking, inexpensive, telemicroscope version is focusable at near. (Reprinted with permission from Eschenbach Optik of America.)

Telescopes can be fitted with an extra removable lens (a lens cap) that fits over the lens farthest from the eye (the objective lens) to enable the telescope to focus at arms length (see Figure 13-16) or closer. A telescope that focuses at arms length or closer is called a *telemicroscope*. As anyone who has used binoculars might attest, telescopes and telemicroscopes require good coordination, adaptable visual motor skills, and good fine motor control to focus and use effectively. Spectacle mounting stabilizes the telescope or binocular and makes it much easier to use, but creates cosmetic problems.

Under controlled laboratory circumstances, image motion seems to be the major impediment to the use of telescopes[2]; however, cost and cosmesis are certainly important factors as well. Spectacle-mounted devices may be perceived as odd looking. Imagine a young man or woman with low vision at a party trying to discreetly "check out" someone across the room with a telescope. Imagine an elderly person with low vision watching people out of the front window in her or his neighborhood through a telescope.

Often, telescopes are dispensed to be handheld, as these are cosmetically the most acceptable and are the

least expensive (Figure 13-18). These devices may be worn around the neck or can be worn as a ring. If the user wants to see something, he or she holds the telescope in front of his or her eye. A more stable view is usually achieved by holding the telescope in the web space (see Figure 13-18[A]) so that the hand hides the telescope from the view of others. More cosmetically acceptable spectacle-mounted devices are mounted above the glasses (see Figure 13-18[B]) and hid under a visor, or using a box-shaped device that can be hardly identified as a telescope (see Figure 13-18[C]). The brim of a hat also shields the optical elements and the client's eyes from light glare (see Figure 13-18[B]). Someone watching television in the privacy of his or her own home or watching a sports event often prefers center-mount devices (Figure 13-19). Clip-on telescopes may be clipped onto spectacles that correct refractive error, but special lenses can be made for telescopes. Recall that a simple alternative to the center-mount device that enables someone to maintain a full field of view is to use relative distance magnification (bring the television screen closer or sit closer to the action), a simpler alternative that always should be considered before telescopes are recommended. Inexpensive, lightweight telescopes with good optics are now available for watching television.

Important Properties of Telescopes

- The closer the ocular lens is to the eye, the larger the field of view.

- Viewing through eyeglasses or mounting eyeglasses away from the eye generally results in a smaller field of view than holding the ocular lens to the eye.

- For people with myopia or hyperopia without significant astigmatism, the telescope can be focused to compensate for the refractive error and held against the eye.

- For people with significant astigmatism, the telescope should be viewed through corrective eyeglasses or contact lenses, or special telescopes can be made to correct refractive error.

- For those with tremor, arthritis, or impaired fine motor control, telescopes should be mounted on eyeglasses or a headband.

- Galilean-type telescopes have magnifications up to about 4×, are smaller, are lighter, and have a smaller field of view.

- Keplerian-type telescopes have magnifications greater than 3×, are often larger and heavier, and have a larger field of view.

- Telescopes reduce the amount of light. The larger the objective lens (far lens), the more light is transmitted through the telescope.

- Telescopes can be focused closer for hobbies and sight-reading music. A special cap can be purchased that fits over the objective lens to allow the telescope to focus closer, turning it into a telemicroscope.

Electronic Devices

Electronic versions of several optical magnification devices are emerging in the marketplace. Examples discussed in Chapter 14 include electronic magnifier devices that focus at distance and near, such as telescopes. Handheld electronic devices act much like stand magnifiers, except the magnified image is displayed on a screen (see Figure 13-14). Smart phones can be used as handheld electronic magnifiers. Tablet computers and e-readers can enlarge text to about 2× comfortably, enabling a decrease in the power of a magnifier to half the power needed for regular print. Another advantage of electronic magnifiers is the potential to enhance contrast, as well as magnify the object being viewed and read aloud.

Instruction on Device Use

Evidence indicates that instruction on use of a device is a practice guideline (see Chapter 9); most need instruction, but not everyone. Some earlier research evaluating the use of optical devices simply involved an optometrist prescribing devices without additional instruction. Humphry and Thompson[4] found that 75% of clients never used their devices, but 25% did. In another study of people who were prescribed devices without instruction, 33% never used the devices.[5] With only one session of instruction, the percentage of device use was about 80% 1 year after service.[6] Watson et al found about 85% of veterans continued to use the prescribed device, with generally more severe vision loss after extensive inpatient instruction on device use.[7] An important difference is that in the survey by Watson et al, those who no longer use the prescribed device often had moved on to another device, indicating effective problem-solving strategies.

These and other studies on length of training[8] indicate overall percentage of success, device use, or effect size of improvements increase with greater length of treatment, but one can infer from these studies that many do not require extensive training. A well-adjusted client who has no disabilities other than impaired vision will learn quickly how to use devices of about 16 to 20 D or less working with real-life materials of personal significance to the client, like a medication label, recipe card, or book by a favorite author. For example, in our experience, to teach all of the techniques summarized in Table 13-5 and check for carryover from session to session may require about 1 to 2 sessions—less time if someone has prior experience with optical magnification. Even with experienced users, however, it is important to review the items discussed next to make sure the device is being used properly. The need for instruction, however, can be quickly determined by having the client demonstrate use under challenging conditions with poor lighting and the device out of adjustment to test his or her problem-solving skills with the device. A general training and troubleshooting checklist is provided in Table 13-5. The graded instructions described next are for a more success-oriented approach for a client who might be challenged by multiple disabilities, low frustration tolerance, or depression.

General Strategies for Success-Oriented Instruction

- Complete eccentric fixation training or training on specific compensatory scanning strategies (see Chapter 9) before recommending devices or providing instruction with those devices. Often, a person's functional visual acuity will change as a result of this instruction. In some cases, devices may be used as part of eccentric viewing instruction.

- It is usually advisable to begin instruction at the full magnification that the client will eventually be required to use. Grading the activity by gradually increasing device power requires that working distance, focusing, and lighting strategies be relearned as well. Grade the activity by gradually withdrawing assistance with the manipulation of the device or materials. If the client resists the higher magnification, consider modifying the task to decrease magnification demand—using large print, for example. One might later return to the more demanding task and increased magnification once the skills with a lower power device are mastered.

- Instruction is not complete unless the client is taught not only how to use the device for a goal task, but how to maintain the device, store it for ready access, and solve common problems, such as how to change batteries.

With all devices, the training activities[3] from easier to most difficult are as follows:

- *Focus, fixate, and align.* Have the client adjust the lens to the target distance to keep a single letter or word in focus. The client keeps the device steady while the

TABLE 13-5: SOLUTION CHECKLIST FOR OPTICAL DEVICE USE

POSSIBLE PROBLEM	HIGH NEAR ADDITION	HAND-HELD MAGNIFIER AGAINST EYE	HAND HELD MAGNIFIER AT DISTANCE	STAND-MAGNIFIER	TELESCOPE OR TELEMICROSCOPE
Not aligned	Correct optic axis (line from PRL or fovea through pupil is aligned with center of lens)				
Out of focus	Correct the lens-to-object distance	Correct the lens-to-object distance	Correct the lens-to-object distance	• Place stand firmly against page • Correct the eye-to-lens distance • Look thorough correct near add	• Correct the lens-to-object distance • Correctly focus telescope • Use a lens cap for near
Insufficient magnification	Enlarge print/object Increase power	• Enlarge print/object • Increase power • Use reading correction	• Move lens further from object • Enlarge print/object or increase power • Use distance correction	• Move eye closer to lens and increase reading addition • Increase power	• Move closer to target • Increase magnification
Insufficient lighting	Direct light between lens and object	Use illuminated magnifier	Use illuminated magnifier	Use illuminated device	Increase light on object
Fatigue and eye strain	Correct lens-to-object distance	Correct lens-to-object distance	Rarely a problem	Correct near addition	Adjust focus
Motion sickness	Smooth the motion	• Move magnifier farther from eye • Smooth the motion	Rarely a problem	Use farther from the eye	• Stabilize telescope • Shorten view time through telescope

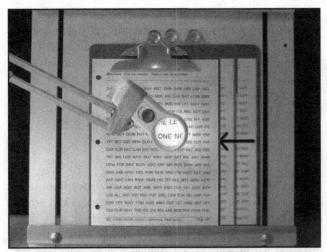

Figure 13-20. Scrolling technique where the reading material is moved from right to left in a smooth, continual motion in front of a stationary optical magnification device such as a mounted magnifier (shown) or full-field microscope (see Figure 13-9).

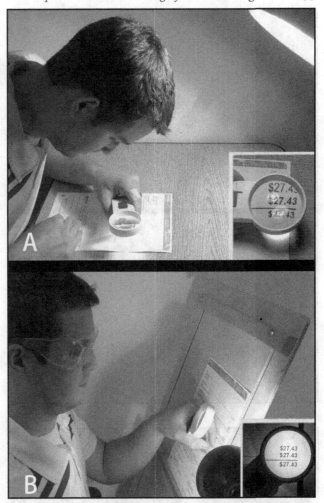

Figure 13-21. Poor (A) and good (B) posture using a handheld magnifier. (A) Working tabletop encourages poor posture and a tilted positioning of the magnifier relative to the eye and object, and exacerbates optical reflections (see Appendix, http://www.routledge.com/ 9781617116339) and shadows from overhead light. (B) Use of a reading stand encourages better posture and correct positioning of the device (perpendicular to the line of sight). The directional light or internal magnifier light is used rather than overhead lights to eliminate lens reflections.

therapist moves the material in front of the magnification device. Move a line of text from right to left in front of the device (Figure 13-20). Then intentionally change the focus of the device until the client self-corrects consistently. With handheld devices, the device needs to be rotated so that a person is looking through the center and the lens is perpendicular to the line of sight. Rotate the device so it is out of alignment and have the client adjust it. Figure 13-21 illustrates correct alignment with a handheld device. With telescopes, alignment is even more critical.

- *Manage lighting.* Lighting should be directed between the lens and target. Instruct the client to adjust lighting to avoid glare and reflections off the optical surfaces (see Figure 13-21). To test the client, create poor and maladaptive lighting for the client to correct.

- *Localization and spotting.* Have the client find an object that is large enough to see unaided with the magnification device. For example, with a telescope, the client carefully fixates the shape of someone standing across the room. While maintaining fixation on the person, the user positions the telescope in front of the eye to see the details (Figure 13-22). With an electric bill, for example, even if she or he cannot read individual words, a client might see from the overall layout of the page where a total would be expected to appear. The client then looks where he or she thinks a total might be located, then without averting gaze, quickly positions a handheld or stand magnifier over the spot to read the total.

- *Tracking.* Slowly move the object being fixated and have the client follow the movement, gradually increasing the speed. Challenge the client's ability to correct focus and device alignment and not lose the target.

- *Scanning and tracing.* Scanning and tracing are methods to skim a space to look for something. With a handheld device or stand magnifier, the client learns to move the magnifier quickly from left to right over a line of text while maintaining gaze at the center of the device, in coordinated head and hand movements. In some cases, the clients skim text by quickly following lines, stopping and reading a couple of words at a time, then skimming over several words until the information they are looking for is found. Scanning and tracing with a telescope require the client to recognize and follow contours, such as following a signpost up to the top where the street sign can be read. This technique is more important for full-field microscopes or center-mount telescopes because the above-localization and

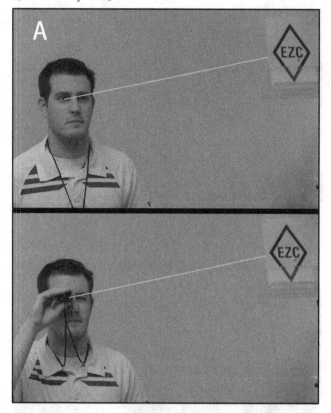

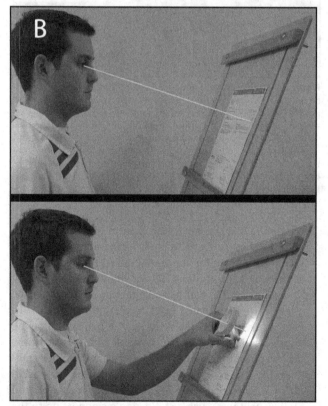

Figure 13-22. Spotting technique with (A) handheld telescope and (B) handheld magnifier.

spotting are not possible. We rarely use scanning and tracing, preferring bioptic mounts for telescopes or using handheld devices. This technique is difficult, time consuming, and tends to produce motion sickness. Clients generally perform much better using localization and spotting strategies.

Specific Strategies for Near Additions, Microscopes, Visors, and Loupes

Ergonomics and Common Applications

Even in well-adjusted clients who may have been users of optical devices, a quick review of ergonomics and proper device use can be instructive.

Ergonomics becomes a significant issue with closer lens distances because at these distances people must lean forward and maintain a precise lens-to-object distance. This is especially true for a client who is somewhat deconditioned or frail because fatigued muscles may become unstable, causing the client to lose precise control of the device. In general, the client should attempt to maintain the hips, knees, and ankles at a 90-90-90 degree posture for maximum stability and minimum muscle strain during reading. If the client reads or works at a table, the use of a reading stand and directional lighting will enable him or her to hold the material steady and sit up straight (see Figure 13-21). If the user leans forward, one hand might be used to support the head with an elbow on the table to relieve neck and back strain. Users often prefer to read with these devices in a favorite easy chair. Lap trays may be used, and other forms of elbow support might help the client steady the material and maintain support for the head and spine as one transitions from the artificial instructional setup to a simulation of the client's home situation.

Optimize lighting by turning off overhead lights. Introduce directional lighting from the side aimed between the lens and paper, being careful to avoid reflections and glare. Use a hat brim or visor to eliminate reflections from the optical surfaces of the glasses from overhead lights.

Overall Instructional Strategy

If the client is expected to have difficulty learning to read with a device, use graded materials in available workbooks, such as the Learn to Use Your Vision (LUV) reading series.[9,10] A typical success-oriented instructional sequence might include the following:

1. Setup and lighting. Start in an artificial work setting most likely to produce successful task performance and allow sufficient control to identify specific impediments. Have the client sit at a table with good posture using a reading stand (see Figure 13-21). Use a typoscope (a black card with a window cut out or contrasting ruler to help the client keep his or her place and reduce glare, see Figure 12-6). Teach the client how to position the light.

2. Grade the activity. Begin with enlarged samples of the materials that the client wishes to read with an uncluttered layout. Start with a reading acuity card and check if the predicted critical print size and acuity are obtained and perform any needed troubleshooting (see later). Use single sentences that are larger (see the online appendix at www.routledge.com/9781617116339), as it is easier for someone to follow a line of text. Menus from restaurants often work well if the print is large enough and the background uncluttered. When reading, use a scrolling or steady-eye technique. The head is kept steady while staring straight ahead. Move a line of text from right to left in front while the client stares straight ahead so the words move to the point on the page where a client is looking. This strategy is most effective if someone with a central scotoma is trying to maintain eccentric viewing (see Figure 13-20). The LUV reading series (www.lowvisionsimulators.com) provides excellent and engaging materials for near.

3. Align, focus, and fixate. Vary the lens-to-object distance and have the client notice the effect with the eye farther and closer to the lens. Then test problem solving by intentionally positioning the lens or paper incorrectly and having the client correct the problem. Finally, just hand the client the magnifier to use.

4. Localization and spotting are possible with half-eyes, a handheld magnifier, or telescope because a client can look over the lens to the target and while still maintaining fixation on the target, tilt the head up or move the magnifier in front of the eyes to look through the device (see Figure 13-22). This cannot be done easily with full-field microscopes or center-mounted telescopes.

5. Scrolling. To instruct the client how to scan, begin with hand-over-hand assistance. Slowly scroll the print from left to right in front of the microscope at the correct distance (see Figures 13-9 and 13-20). To minimize fatigue, the client should move the paper rather than the head. Loose paper should be attached to a clipboard. Gradually withdraw assistance and finally increase task demand by performing tracing/skimming type tasks such as finding the price of items on a menu or an item in a catalog. The pre-reading exercises in the LUV reading series are ideal for this.

6. Writing and nonreading tasks. If the device is to be used with nonreading tasks or writing, these tasks should be introduced after reading instruction, if a person has a reading goal.

7. Natural context. Once good performance has been achieved under controlled circumstances, begin changing the situation to match the home environment. Change seating, external supports, and lighting according to the client's preferred task environment and educate the client regarding the effects of each change. Help the client develop changes in positioning and introduce supports to enable task performance. Consider hats to eliminate reflections on optical surfaces and glare. To decrease light or the effect of uncontrollable glare sources, consider lightly tinted wraparound absorptive lenses. A client resistant to change will be more willing to accept a recommended change in his or her natural context if performance with the recommended situation can be compared to his or her habitual situation.

8. Home program. Once the device has been prescribed, develop a home program with materials graded in size, duration, and task difficulty.

9. Teach the client how to clean, maintain, change batteries in, carry, and store devices.

Common Difficulties and Solutions

The client never sees the object or does not read print as predicted

- Usually, this is because the target is too far from the lens.
- Make sure the client is looking through the center of the lens.
- Using large high-contrast letters or thick lines, check focus by having the client hold the print against the lens and then gradually increase lens-to-object distance until the image appears to clear.
- If the client has a central scotoma, make certain he or she is using an eccentric viewing position (see Chapter 10).
- With high magnification lenses, use a support or a spacer between the lens and paper to help maintain focal distance.
- Turn off overhead lights, adjust lighting, or wear a visor or hat with a brim to eliminate reflections on the lens.
- Recheck near acuity.
- Try larger letters, as the device may have insufficient magnification.

Intermittent object or print recognition

- Check lighting and for reflections on the lenses.
- Check for inconsistent eccentric viewing if there are central scotomas, and provide attritional training with the device if needed.
- Check to make sure the client is viewing through the center of the lens.
- Consider lenses with less distortion.
- With certain conditions such as vitreous floaters, acuity may vary within a session or, with diabetes, from session to session.

Cannot maintain focal distance

- Rest head on hand with elbow on the table using a reading stand to bring the material closer to the lens.

- Start by resting the lens on the object and slowly pulling the lens away.

Inadequate light

- Bring the light source closer and aim the light between the lens and the object.

- Be careful to avoid glare and reflections from the surface of the lenses.

Distortion

- Use better quality optics with less distortion.

- Look through the center of the lens at a closer lens-to-object distance.

- Move it closer to the object being viewed.

Quick fatigue and complaints of headache

- Stop immediately, give the client a rest, and change the task.

- Check to make sure the lens is at the correct distance from the page.

- At close working distances, a change in distance of a few millimeters may significantly change accommodative demand (how much the client must refocus the eyes), and in a younger client who still can focus, this often causes eye strain.

- Rule out inadequate magnification using a reading acuity chart and rechecking.

- Patch the eye with the poorer vision to rule out binocular problems.

- Check posture.

- Task stress may increase blood pressure.

- The client may be developing hypotension, a precursor to motion sickness.

Motion sickness

- If the client starts to perspire, reports a sudden headache, reports feeling cold, or has a measurable drop in blood pressure, stop immediately. These symptoms are precursors to nausea associated with motion sickness.

- Decrease field of view by using a handheld device at distance. Use spotting techniques, not scanning.

- Reduce head motion during reading.

- Reduce irregular image motion, such as a shaky image, by stabilizing the material being viewed on a reading stand.

Loses place when reading

- Use a typoscope, dark ruler, or finger to keep one's place.

Specific Strategies for Handheld Devices

Most clients have prior familiarity with lower power handheld devices, and thus must be carefully instructed if higher power devices are prescribed. Handheld magnifiers are used at about arm's length when spotting, reading a label, or checking skin or nails, or up close to the eye to maximize the field of view for more sustained reading.

Ergonomics and Lighting

Start in an artificial work setting that optimizes vision and ergonomics. Have the client sit at a table with good posture using a reading stand. Provide support for the hand to help maintain working distance. Optimize lighting by turning off overhead lights, and introduce directional lighting from the side. Vary illumination until the best reading speed is achieved. Demonstrate the effects of glare and overhead lights. Reflections on optical surfaces are a common problem with handheld devices. Teach the client to identify offending lights and then position the body or a hat brim to block reflections from overhead lights. If a client is glare sensitive, consider lightly tinted wraparound absorptive lenses and antireflective coatings on optics.

Ancillary Equipment

- A reading stand or lap tray.

- A directional light with a deep shade so it directs light to a specific location under the lens of the magnifier.

- A typoscope, dark ruler, or straight edge.

- Firm pads on which the wrist or an arm might rest.

- Tape or clipboard to secure the reading material.

- A clamp stand or chest stand to hold a handheld magnifier, allowing hands-free use.

Interaction With Corrective Lenses

When reading through the bottom half of bifocals (the near segment of the lens) or reading glasses, bringing a handheld magnifier closer will not only increase field of view; power will increase as well. When the eye-to-lens distance increases, the user should look through the top half of the glasses—the distance segment of the lens. If the user does not wear glasses for distance, then glasses should not be worn when using the handheld magnifier. If the user holds the handheld magnifier farther than about 40 cm from the eye, looking through the lower half of bifocal lenses or reading glasses will actually decrease magnification when compared with looking through the upper distance segment of the lens.

Stand magnifiers are usually designed to be used at an intermediate distance while the client is looking through the reading addition or bottom half of bifocals.

Device Stabilization Strategies

For clients who wish to perform craft or sewing activities, table-mounted magnifiers, usually with light incorporated, are available commercially (see Figure 13-11). Weak (2 to 4 diopters) single-lens devices are readily available in sewing stores and can be hung around the neck to enable hands-free use (see Figure 13-12). Smaller, stronger lenses are often incorporated into the larger lens. Commercially available devices are usually low power (under 5 D).

Mounts for stronger handheld devices are limited only by the creativity of the therapist. The low vision clinic should be equipped with a bin of salvaged table clamps, flexible arms and tubing, and splinting material (see top of Figure 13-12). With a hot glue gun, the therapist can quickly develop a prototype of a lens mount, customized to a client's particular application. Hot glue can be peeled off to modify a design, but is not usually durable enough for permanent use. The final product could use clamps or Velcro to hold the handle of the device to the arm. Magnifiers that come with mounts for craft activities are also sometimes called *stand magnifiers*, but we classify them with handheld magnifiers because the lens-to-object distance is not fixed; one provides instruction and troubleshooting as with a single-lens handheld device. Material for improvising stand magnifiers for any mount or type of device can be found on www.modularhose.com (see Figure 13-12).

Success-Oriented Instruction for Handheld Magnifiers

1. Setup and lighting. Start in an artificial work setting most likely to produce successful task performance and allow sufficient control to identify specific impediments. Have the client sit at a table with good posture using a reading stand. Use a typoscope. Teach the client how to position the light.

2. Grade the task. Begin with enlarged samples of the materials that the client wishes to read and use an uncluttered layout. Initially provide hand-over-hand assistance. Start by laying the lens on the material and providing a slow, controlled increase in lens-to-object distance to well beyond the focal distance and have the client describe the visual effect.

3. Align, focus, and fixate. Instruct the client to control lens distance and align his or her line of sight with the center of the optics. Intentionally position the magnifier incorrectly and have the client correct the problem. Since handheld magnifiers are often used under varied, uncontrolled situations such as shopping, the client should be taught how to solve problems with these devices. Teach the client to hold the device parallel to the line of sight and look through the center of the lens.

4. Device management. Gradually withdraw hand and wrist supports. If such support is necessary, consider

stand magnifiers or head-mounted devices such as loupes or microscopes.

5. Spotting/localizing. Trying to scan a page for information through a magnifier is literally sickening and slow. Instruct the client on how to spot information on a menu, advertising circular, or newspaper without looking through the magnifier. Orient the client to the lines of print or borders of columns and ask him or her to estimate where the information might be by first looking without magnification to where the needed information is expected, then, without averting the gaze, placing the magnifier over that spot (see Figure 13-22).

6. For scanning, start with hand-over-hand assistance. Slowly have the client scan a line of text with a coordinated hand and head movement from left to right. Gradually withdraw assistance, and finally increase task demand by performing tracing/skimming type tasks such as finding items on a menu.

Common Difficulties and Solutions With Handheld Magnifiers

The client never resolved the object or read print as predicted

- Check focus by checking alignment of glasses, and determine whether the client views through the distance segment.
- Check the focus of the handheld device by gradually lifting it from the page to a little less than the focal distance.
- Check for optical distortion, and try better quality optics.
- Turn off overhead lights and adjust lighting.
- Recheck near acuity with and without the magnifier. If larger print is effective, try a stronger magnifier with smaller print.
- With certain conditions, such as vitreous floaters, acuity may vary within a session or, with diabetes, from session to session.

Intermittent object or print recognition

- Check lighting.
- Check for maladaptive central fixation with central scotomas or floaters.
- Check to make sure the client is viewing through the center of the lens.
- Consider a lens with less distortion.
- The client with macular scotoma may require additional eccentric viewing practice.

Inadequate field of view

- Decrease eye-to-lens distance.
- Consider a microscope.

Inadequate light

- Switch to an illuminated magnifier.
- Direct light between the lens and the paper.

Quick fatigue and complaints of headache

- Stop immediately, give the client a rest, and change the task.
- Rule out inadequate magnification by enlarging print and rechecking.
- Check that the lens-to-object distance is at the focal distance.
- Patch the eye with poorer vision to rule out binocular problems.
- Check posture.
- Task stress may increase blood pressure.
- The client may be developing hypotension, a precursor to motion sickness.

Motion sickness

- If the client starts to perspire, reports feeling cold, or has a measurable drop in blood pressure, stop immediately. These symptoms are precursors to nausea associated with motion sickness.
- Decrease field of view by increasing eye-to-lens distance.
- Reduce head motion during reading.
- Reduce irregular image motion, such as a shaky image, by working on a firm surface and using a handheld magnifier.

Loses place when reading

- Use a typoscope, contrasting ruler, or finger to keep one's place

Specific Strategies for Stand Magnifiers

Instruction is identical for the handheld magnifier, except the client does not need to be instructed how to align and position the lens relative to the paper being read. Instead, instruct the client to keep the stand firmly against the page being read.

The client looks through the reading glasses and at a prescribed eye-to-lens distance supplied with the magnifier. Demonstrate the effects of viewing at various distances or without the reading glasses prescribed for the device to determine if the client notices defocus. With stronger magnifiers, these effects will be minimal. Recall that one needs to select stronger stand magnifiers because the indicated power for the lens is higher than the actual power.

Common Difficulties and Solutions With Stand Magnifiers

The client never resolved the object or read print as predicted

- Check focus by checking eye-to-lens distance supplied with the magnifier; try a closer eye-to-lens distance to determine if resolution improves. Make certain the client views through the bifocal or reading glasses.
- Turn off overhead lights and adjust lighting.
- Recheck near acuity, or use a higher power magnifier.
- Enlarge the print. If this works, try a stronger magnifier and contact the prescribing eye care practitioner.

Intermittent object or print recognition

- Check lighting.
- Check for optical distortion, and try better quality optics.
- Check for central scotomas or floaters.
- Check to make sure the client is viewing through the center of lens and maintaining the correct distance.
- Consider a lens with less distortion.
- The client with macular scotoma may require additional eccentric viewing practice.
- With certain conditions, such as vitreous floaters or with central scotomas, acuity may vary within a session or, with diabetes, from session to session.

Inadequate field of view

- Decrease eye-to-lens distance, but with care for a corrected near prescription.
- Consider a half eyes or a full-field microscope.

Inadequate light

- Switch to an illuminated magnifier.
- Direct light between the lens and the paper.

Quick fatigue and complaints of headache

- Stop immediately, give the client a rest, and change the task.
- Check to make sure the client is at the correct distance from a stand magnifier.
- Rule out inadequate magnification by enlarging print and rechecking.
- Patch the eye with poorer vision to rule out binocular problems.
- Check posture. Use a reading stand.
- Task stress may increase blood pressure.
- The client may be developing hypotension, a precursor to motion sickness.

Loses place when reading

- Use a typoscope, contrasting ruler, or finger to keep one's place.

- Slide the device along a straight edge, and secure the page being read.

Specific Strategies for Telescopes
Overall Instructional Strategy

In general, users of telescopes or binoculars, whether handheld or mounted, should be warned to always stop moving before looking through the device. These devices are more stable if someone stops and supports the device or the head. For example, if a client is spotting a street sign, he or she could lean against something while spotting. As an exception to this rule, users may be taught how to use a bioptic during driving or power wheelchair use as a special advanced technique. A person wearing center-mount "sports glasses" to watch television often reduces motion through the telescope if he or she reclines slightly and rests the head on a headrest. Again, ergonomics is critical for near tasks. For example, Ms. Jason would perform her needlework more comfortably if the work were on a raised table so she could sit up straight. The head is more stable if aligned with the spinal column, and she would be more comfortable and the device more stable.

1. Setup. Reassure the client that the task will eventually be adapted to the preferred work environment. Start in an artificial work setting most likely to produce successful task performance and allow sufficient control to identify specific impediments. Have the client sit at a high table with good posture, resting the elbows on the table while holding the telescope in front of the eye. The user should face a large board with lines of sequential numbers that are large enough to be seen through the telescope. Without the telescope, the client should ideally see the numbers as blobs. The poster board should be positioned against a contrasting wall with an uncluttered background at a distance greater than 3M (9 feet) from the user. This allows the user to locate the object if out of focus and identify where the telescope is pointed. If quick learning is anticipated, a television can be substituted for the poster board.

2. Lighting. As telescopes often reduce light, the target should be well lighted. Instruct the client to use a hat brim or visor to shade optical surfaces of the glasses and telescope from overhead lights.

3. Device familiarization. Have the client learn to identify the ocular, objective lens—the focusing ring—and whether it is focused all the way to distance or near without looking through it. If used with glasses, fold the eye cup back so it can be pressed against the lens of the glasses. Have the client describe a strategy for storing and cleaning the device. Have the client set the focus for distance before starting.

4. Align. The user should first master alignment and positioning. The ocular end of the telescope should be held in the web space with the hand resting against the face, not the fingertips, for maximum stability. It should be held as close to the eye as possible to maximize field of view. If properly aligned, the telescope should have a round view, as a crescent view indicates misalignment. With a light shining on the eye, the therapist should be able to look through the objective lens and visualize the user's eye looking back through the telescope—if the telescope is aligned with the eye. Note that a client with macular scotoma may report no view because he or she is not eccentrically viewing properly; with a large central scotoma or if the ocular lens is too far from the eye, central fixation will result in no vision. Mastery of this step requires the client bring the telescope to the eye, quickly align it, and report what he or she is viewing within about 3 seconds.

5. Focus and fixate. Begin with the telescope focused at distance. By changing the distance from a board with high-contrast letters, have the client refocus after he or she has aligned the telescope with the board.

6. Localization/spotting with real-life tasks. Ask the client to look to the spot where he or she would expect to find a particular number on the board without the telescope (see Figure 13-22). The therapist can assist the client by pointing and then having the client bring the telescope in front of the eye without averting gaze and focus the telescope. When the client masters this procedure, the therapist can begin training with real-life goal tasks, such as spotting and recognizing people, a television screen, and a piece of furniture at different distances. Repeat these tasks with the client using hearing to estimate the location of a target.

7. Tracking. Have the client look at someone or something in your hand and continue to follow it as it moves. Then have the client localize and track someone walking in the room.

8. Grading the task. Have the client perform the tasks described earlier while seated and leaning on the elbow of the hand holding the device, then without elbow supports, and finally, while standing. When standing, the client should stabilize the telescope by holding the elbow against the body. The client should lean against something to avoid body sway. If the client cannot stabilize the handheld telescope, consider a spectacle-mounted device. At this point, the device can be dispensed and practice at home can begin.

9. Tracing and scanning. This is rarely performed; localization and spotting (step 6) is a better strategy. Starting in a familiar space, have the client follow contours

such as baseboards, room corners, ceiling edges, door frames, curbs, or signposts to find signs and objects in the room. Have the client do the same to check out other people and discuss discretion. Finally, have the client perform systematic scanning techniques, such as scanning a blackboard for a word, a poster of a group of people for a familiar face, or a room for a particular object such as car keys or a misplaced coffee cup using a left-right or vertical scan pattern. This procedure might induce motion sickness.

10. Moving with bioptics. Now have the client localize and spot objects while walking or moving as a passenger in a car. These spotting maneuvers should be completed in less than a second, like glancing in a rearview mirror of a car, and are appropriate only if a bioptic device is prescribed.

Common Difficulties and Solutions

The client never resolves object detail or reads print as predicted

- Check telescope alignment.
- Make sure it is focused at distance.
- If client has macular scotoma, reassess eccentric viewing, bring the ocular closer to the eye, and realign for eccentric viewing.
- Check for changes in visual acuity.

Intermittent object or print recognition

- Check alignment, lighting, and eccentric viewing.
- Check for central scotomas or floaters.
- Increase field of view (see next).

Inadequate field of view

- Use a Keplerian-type telescope to maximize field of view.
- Bring the ocular closer to the eye.
- If the client wears glasses and has simple spherical refractive error, have the client remove the glasses to bring the ocular cup to the eye and refocus to compensate.
- Refer to eye care provider for special spectacle mount or an ocular lens with refractive correction.
- Consider a lower magnification device and moving closer to the object being viewed.

Loses objects and difficulty tracking

- Practice.
- Increase field of view (described earlier), evaluate visual motor coordination, and consider spectacle mounts.

Cannot focus

- Practice with high-contrast edges.

- Estimate focus by feel (length of telescope) or place tactile or visible marks on focusing apparatus to provide a starting point.
- Consider an auto-focus device.

Inadequate light

- Typically, light cannot be controlled with distance tasks.
- Head visors, hats with brims, or body positioning will decrease disabling glare.
- If light is inadequate with a real-life goal task, consider a telescope with a larger diameter objective lens or lower magnification.

Distortion

- Use better quality optics with less distortion.

Quick fatigue and complaints of headache

- Stop immediately, give the client a rest, and downgrade the task.
- Check focus.

Motion sickness

- If the client starts to perspire, reports a sudden headache, reports feeling cold, or has a measurable drop in blood pressure, stop immediately. These symptoms are precursors to nausea associated with motion sickness.
- Avoid scanning and tracing tasks.
- Stabilize telescope using spectacle mounting.
- Move it farther away to decrease field of view.

Specific Strategies for Telemicroscopes

Telemicroscopes (see Figures 13-4 and 13-5) allow a user to perform tabletop tasks, repairs, sewing, playing cards, or reading music. These devices are widely used by people with more typical vision who need to work with very small objects at near, such as biologists, surgeons, or electronic technicians, and are thus generally available in a binocular mount. Because they have a narrow field of view, telemicroscopes are not as suitable for reading as microscopes, handheld devices, or electronic magnifiers. If carefully fit by an eye care practitioner, the telemicroscope does not require the user to align the device. Telemicroscopes also do not need to be focused. Rather, if the user usually works with a three-dimensional object, then he or she usually compensates if out of focus by moving the head closer or farther from the object being viewed until the correct distance is achieved. Otherwise, the training program is similar to that used for telescopes. Instead of a large poster board with numbers, a smaller paper is used on a table for initial alignment, focus, and practice. Practice localizing, tracking, scanning, and tracing with tabletop activities as well. In general, if clients intend to use the device for a particular task, they should bring in the materials to simulate

SIDEBAR 13-1: SHORTCUT FOR CALCULATING CHANGES IN MAGNIFICATION

If a therapist decides to try a different magnification, how much should the magnification be changed? The answer is that, like acuity, magnification changes in the following logarithmic steps. The size of each step is 1.25%, or five-fourths, larger or smaller than the next step, or one-tenth of a log unit. These steps are psychologically equal. If a person's acuity improves by one step on a log chart, from 1M to 0.8 M, for example, one can reduce magnification one step anywhere on the following scale and the person's performance would be the same. Note that 3 steps equal change by 2×.

Magnification steps in diopters (D):

1.6, 2.0, 2.5, 3.3, 4.0, 5.0, 6.6, 8.0, 10, 12.5, 16, 20, 25, 33,

Note that these numbers are the same as the numbers on most log acuity charts, indicating equal steps in print size:

Print size steps in M:

0.4, 0.5, 0.6, 0.8, 1.0, 1.25, 1.6, 2.0, 2.5, 3.3, 4.0, 5.0, 6.6, 8.0

This progression of magnifiers is what a person should have in stock. Of course, we can estimate. Most manufacturers have 16- and not 15-diopter magnifiers, so the next size up could be a 20 or 21 rather than an 18 D.

These same steps can be used in calculating changes in distance and ER as well. If distance is increased a step (1.25 to 1.5 meters) then ER must be increased by a step (eg, 2.5 to 3.3×).

---

the actual work situation, as many tasks do not require all of the skills required for telescopic use.

ADVANCED CONCEPTS/TECHNIQUES: MAGNIFICATION DEVICES

How therapists and eye care providers collaborate varies considerably from practice to practice. Often, an occupational therapist does not have access to an eye care practitioner who specializes in low vision. General practitioners may be more willing to see low vision patients and prescribe devices if a therapist performs preclinical visual testing and makes specific recommendations regarding devices and magnification. In a busy eye clinic, eye doctors might expect the occupational therapist to recommend initial device selection prior to the formal clinical examination. A therapist will need to problem solve why a recommended device does not work as predicted and find suitable alternatives without consulting the eye care practitioner. In such cases, the therapist must understand some basic principles of optics and magnification and how the devices actually work.

The clinical reasoning remains as illustrated in Table 13-2 except that in step 5, where the therapist recommends optical devices, the therapist would also recommend magnification. To recommend magnification, the therapist must understand the various formal definitions of magnification, strategies for estimating how much magnification is required to perform a task, how to select devices that

have comparable magnification, and how the final amount of magnification depends on interaction with the client's refractive error.

The following list provides a general strategy for determining the magnification of an optical device:

- Make sure the client has had a recent refraction and eyeglasses for distance.

- Estimate the magnification requirements of the task during an evaluation.

- When comparing devices or combining devices with other magnification strategies, make sure the devices have equivalent magnification.

Historically, magnification was estimated on the basis of visual acuity, and the appropriate magnification was determined by trying different devices, often reducing magnification in response to a failure of the device to work as predicted. Trial and error with devices to determine magnification is no longer an acceptable standard of practice. We are now able to use evidence-based evaluation protocols and principles of geometric optics to predict required magnification from the reading acuity chart and select the devices, working distance, and size magnification that will precisely reproduce the predicted magnification requirement. Once this is done, if a given device or situation does not work as predicted, then the therapist's attention can be directed to barriers other than magnification. As a result, the magnification requirements need not be compromised. A shortcut method to calculate changes in magnification without a calculator is in Sidebar 13-1.

Estimating the Magnification Demands of the Task

Definition of Magnification

Magnification is defined and methods for calculating magnification are described in detail in Chapter 10. The important formula and concepts are reviewed here.

Ultimately, the low vision practitioner is interested in enlarging the size of a retinal image. For example, visual acuity describes the size of the retinal image where the critical detail is just resolvable. Retinal image size is increased either by relative size or relative distance magnification (see Figure 13-3). In the low vision clinic, the emerging convention is to describe magnification at a distance greater than about 1 meter in terms of enlargement ratio (ER). Magnification at closer distances is described using equivalent power (EP) in diopters.[3,11] The functional vision evaluation (see Chapter 8) provides an estimate of the ER required to perform a task at a distance preferred by the client. ER is equivalent to angular magnification used to label the magnification of distance devices like a telescope. So, if a client requires an ER of 3× to recognize faces on the TV at 2 meters, then the therapist knows a telescope labeled 3× will have sufficient magnification. Likewise, for near, the functional vision evaluation estimates magnification required to perform a task in terms of diopters of EP. The magnification of near devices like hand-held magnifiers are in diopters. So, if the evaluation indicates 10 diopters of magnification are required to read a utility bill accurately, then the therapist can predict a 10 diopter magnifier will have sufficient magnification. These methods for estimating magnification introduced in Chapter 5 and further developed in Chapters 8 and 10, are briefly reviewed next.

Relative Size Magnification

Increasing the size of the letter or object (see Figures 13-2, 13-3, 13-4) enlarges the size of the image of an object on the retina. The relationship between object size and retinal image size can be approximated as a simple proportion. If you double the size of an object, you double the retinal image size of the object. Enlargement ratio refers to the ratio of 2 object sizes (S1 and S2); thus, ER = S2/S1.[11] Increasing the size of print from 1M (8 point) to 2M (16 point) at a given distance will increase the ER 2 times (2×). The definition of ER is virtually the same as projection magnification or as well as angular magnification, terms that have also been used widely in the low vision literature since the 1970s.[12] As long as working distance does not change, estimating required object or print size for a task is direct and no calculations are required. In the case of the opening scenario, Ms. Jason's functional visual acuity testing revealed that critical print size was 8M, so she required print size be increased from 1M to at least 8M (64 point) to read fluently, which means ER = 8×. An electronic magnifier was used to enlarge the print to the same 8M (half-inch letter) size used on the acuity chart.

Relative Distance Magnification

The retinal image may also be enlarged by relative distance magnification, which is decreasing the distance from the object to the eye (see Figure 13-3). The relationship between object distance and retinal image size is approximated as a negative proportion. If you halve the distance of the object to the eye, you double the size of the retinal image. If you decrease the distance by 25%, you increase the retinal image size by 25%. Achieving relative distance magnification by moving a television screen from 8 feet to 4 feet, for example, is equivalent to doubling the size of the television screen.

Overall magnification (M_{OA}) at distances greater than about 1 meter can be calculated by simply multiplying relative distance and relative size magnification as follows:

$$M_{OA} = S_2/S_1 * d_1/d_2$$

where S_1 and d_1 are the original object size and distance and S_2 and d_2 are the new object size and distance.

Recall from Chapter 10 the example where a therapist found in the functional vision evaluation that a client needed to decrease the distance from the television screen from 8 feet to 2 feet to see it. By dividing the original distance of 8 feet by the required distance of 2 feet, the therapist would estimate a required enlargement of 4×. Now using the previous formula the therapist can calculate that if the client rejected a 2-foot distance as too close, a mounted telescope (see Figure 13-19) that provides a 2× enlargement (S_2/S_1) could be used in combination with decreasing the television distance from 8 feet to a more acceptable 4 feet (d_1/d_2), which would achieve the same overall magnification of 4×.

With distances less than about 1 meter, a client must focus the eyes to see clearly, and near type devices that focus light must be used that ensure the client can see the object clearly. The amount of focus is specified as power. The emerging convention is to specify the magnification of near devices in terms of EP.

Equivalent Power

As with distance, at near the therapist must often trade size magnification against working distance in order to please a client. At near, this process is complicated by the need to make certain the image is focused on the retina by an optical device. Recall from Chapter 10 that, the total focusing power in diopters that is needed for a particular distance is called accommodate demand (see Table 13-6 for the formula). As people age, they develop *presbyopia*. Reading glasses or bifocals are plus lenses that are added to distance correction that allow people with presbyopia to focus at a closer distance. These reading glasses are also called *near vision additions*.

The person's ability to accommodate (focus at near) is added to near vision addition and should equal accommodative demand. For people over 50 near who cannot focus at near, the accommodative demand should equal reading addition. Accommodative demand, reading addition and accommodation are all expressed as diopters. Accommodative demand is a measure of relative distance magnification at near. More diopters indicates more magnification.

For example, the typical reading distance is 40 cm (16 inches). Using the previous formula, a 2.5 D of total focusing power or accommodative demand is required for objects held at 40 cm. At 20 cm (8 inches) the retinal image size will double and the accommodative demand will increase to 5 diopters. An older person who does not require glasses for distance, will need 5 diopters of reading addition to focus an object or text at 20 cm (8 inches). A younger person may be able to accommodate as close as 20 cm (8 inches) without any reading addition.

The use of handheld magnifiers, microscopes, telemicroscopes, enlargement, an electronic magnifier, or just working at a close distance without glasses are all potential magnification strategies for achieving better performance at near. Equivalent power in diopters is a universal term that describes the magnification of all near devices. The term describes the magnification as "equivalent" to accommodative demand (sometimes, called *equivalent viewing distance*). For example, a manufacturer might specify the magnification of a handheld magnifier used as "20D power." This means that the magnifier has magnification "equivalent" to the accommodative demand required to achieve a 5 cm eye-to-object distance. This now allows us to use the same term for describing the magnification of another near device. Essentially, the term *equivalent power* describes magnification that is equivalent to relative distance magnification that resulted from a 5 cm working distance.

In practice, the formula for EP requires that we not only consider the distance, but also the enlargement of the object being viewed. As described earlier, the therapist might enlarge print or use larger objects, as well as decrease working distance. Some devices, such as telemicroscopes, enlarge the appearance of objects as well as focus at a closer distance. Equivalent power can be calculated by simply multiplying the accommodative demand (100/d) by the ER. The formula (see Table 13-6) for calculating P is as follows:

P(diopters) = 100/d(cm) * ER

This important formula can be used to approximate the EP of all optical devices or viewing situations at near. The low vision therapist often must change working distance, object size, and the magnification power to please a client, all while keeping the same overall magnification.

TABLE 13-6: FOUR FORMULAE TO USE TO FIND EQUIVALENT MAGNIFICATION SOLUTIONS

$P \text{ (Diopters)} = \dfrac{100}{d \text{ (cm)}}$	Accommodative Demand
$EP \text{ (Diopters)} = \dfrac{100}{d \text{ (cm)}} * ER$	Equivalent Power (EP)
$\text{Required } ER = \dfrac{d_p}{d_r} * \dfrac{S_b}{S_a}$	Required Enlargement
$\text{Total } ER = \dfrac{d_b}{d_a} * \dfrac{S_a}{S_b}$	Total Enlargement

P = power

ER is $\dfrac{S_a}{S_b}$ where S_a is size after enlargement and

S_b is size before enlargement

d = object-to-eye distance

d_a = object-to-eye distance after, d_b = object-to-eye distance before , d_r = required distance, d_p = preferred distance.

In the case of Ms. Jason, she wished to read and pay bills. Initially, the therapist found with a continual text reading acuity test that she required 8M print to read fluently at 40 cm. To read 1.0M print fluently, she required an ER of 8×. Ms. Jason used her regular reading glasses to view the acuity card at 40 cm (16 inches), an accommodative demand of 2.5 D. Equivalent power would equal 2.5 D multiplied by 8 to calculate a required EP of 20 D. Now one strategy would be to keep the print size at 1M (ER of 1.0) and recommend a 20D reading addition or use a 20D handheld device. Recall Ms. Jason had low frustration tolerance and required a success-oriented approach. In theory, Ms. Jason should be able to read normal 8M print while maintaining a 5-cm (2-inch) lens-to-page distance, but the therapist predicted she would reject this option if presented first because it would be too difficult. This distance also was too close to meet her writing goals. The therapist figured she could double the working distance from 5 to 10 cm, decreasing the accommodative demand (100/10 cm) to 10 D by simply doubling the size of the print from 1M to 2M using standard large-print checks and books. In the previous formula, ER increased from 1× with regular print to 2× with large print. The EP would be 10 D multiplied by 2×, preserving an EP of 20 D.

In summary, for working distances less than about 1 meter, the magnification of any optical device, or just a change in object size, can both be described as EP using equivalent diopters (ED) as the measurement units. Knowing EP allows one to compare several different methods of magnification without changing the overall magnification. Equivalent diopters is calculated using relative size magnification and relative distance magnification. As long as the calculated EP equals that predicted to work by the evaluation, then the therapist knows the magnification of the devices are correct. If the device does not work as predicted, the therapist should search for other barriers and not simply reduce magnification.

Estimating Required Magnification

To estimate the magnification required for a task, the general strategy is to use relative size and relative distance magnification to magnify text or an object until the client is able to perform the task easily. If it is a near task performed at less than about 1 meter (3 feet), one would use the formula for EP to describe the magnification required to perform the task. The therapist must generally perform an evaluation to determine magnification needs at near by changing the size of the object. At distances greater than about 1 meter, the therapist can usually estimate the required enlargement by changing the distance of objects. These strategies are described in detail in Chapter 8 and will be briefly reviewed here.

Estimating Required Magnification at Near

The occupational therapist estimates the required magnification at near by changing the size of the object or text being viewed. In general, an occupational therapist does not have the ability to correct for different working distances at near on older adults because such a change requires a different near reading addition. It is essential that the image be in focus on the retina (ie, that the client is wearing corrective eyeglasses for the specific working distance). For reading, one can maintain near test distance using a continual text reading card, such as the MNRead, where sentences are printed at a progression of print sizes. The client starts reading at the largest print size and reads down the chart until reading starts to slow. The smallest print size before reading slows is *critical print size*. The smallest print that someone can read and still understand is reading acuity threshold. The required magnification depends on the task demands and available print size. If a client wishes to read print fluently, one calculates ER by dividing critical print size by the desired print size. If someone desires only spot reading, then the ER can be somewhat smaller. One then uses the formula for EP and multiplies the ER by accommodative demand of the test distance: 100/d.

For example, assume a client wants to read 1M newsprint fluently and the measured critical print size at 40 cm is 4M. The required EP would be calculated by dividing 4 by 1 and multiplying 4 by 100/40, or 2.5, to estimate a required magnification of 10 D of EP. For spot reading, where speed and endurance are less important, less magnification might be acceptable.

For nonreading tasks, estimating magnification required becomes more of a challenge because it is not easy to enlarge real-life objects. One approach involves using a color electronic magnifier or tablet computer that can magnify virtually anything at a fixed distance using a color view. One would enlarge the image on the screen until the client can identify a critical feature and then calculate the ER by dividing the enlarged size by the actual size. For example, one might display a family snapshot on an electronic magnifier where the heads of the subjects were about 1 cm. The client might recognize the faces when they were enlarged to 5 cm on the screen at 40 cm away. One could then calculate the EP. The ER is 5 cm/1 cm = 5×. The accommodative demand at 40 cm of 100/40 equals 2.5 D. Equivalent power is 5 times 2.5 D, or 12.5 D. Using a 12-D loupe or handheld magnifier should work well to enable this client to see the pictures in this family photo. Another approach is to have photographs or actual samples of different-sized objects.

A still widely used practice is to use a succession of increasingly stronger handheld magnifiers until someone reports being able to see something, but this has the disadvantage that the magnifier must be aligned and positioned at the correct lens-to-object distance. If the client has not yet learned how to use the magnifier, it is difficult to correctly position the magnifier, and the difficulty positioning increases as the power increases. It's much easier to estimate magnification by simply changing the size of an object.

Estimating Required Magnification for Distance

It is an unfortunate tradition to prescribe telescopes to general-criterion visual acuity, such as 20/40 acuity. In general, estimating the required ER should be based on the relative distance magnification required to perform real tasks that are meaningful to the client. At the very least, involving the client in the actual task that he or she wishes to perform will be more engaging than an acuity chart. The visual requirement to perform the tasks, the required ER, can be estimated by first bringing an object of interest (a television, a street sign, or person's face) close enough to the client so that the client can reliably and quickly discern the critical features and note the required distance (d_r). The therapist then estimates the distance that the client prefers (d_p). One then divides the preferred distance (d_p) by required distance (d_r) to estimate the required telescopic ER.

Required ER = d_p/d_r

For example, using an actual street sign, a client can quickly read the sign at 2M (6 ft), but needs to read it just as well across a wide street, about 12M (40 ft). The required ER would be 12/2 = 6×. A similar strategy might be used for face recognition. For example, if a client requires someone be 2M (6 ft) away to reliably discriminate facial expressions, but wants to be able to do this when someone is 3M (9 ft) away, an ER of about 1.3× is required.

In another example, a client wants to watch television and it is determined in the clinic that he or she can see the television at 1M (3 ft). At home, the television is 3M (9 ft) away. In this case, the minimum ER for this task is 9/3 = 3×.

Sometimes an object or picture can be enlarged in addition to being brought closer to a client. A larger TV can be purchased, for example. If it was twice as large, the required ER would decrease in half. The formula for required ER should include this possibility (see Table 13-6).

Selecting Devices

Fortunately, the manufacturers of optical devices specify the magnification in diopters, or in the case of telescopes, as equivalent to ER. The therapist needs only to look up the diopters or power in a specification sheet or read it off the device. How to estimate the magnification of different devices[3] is beyond the scope of this text. With both stand magnifiers the distance of lens from the page is usually less than the focal distance so the diopters (D) specified underestimates actual power. The actual power now depends on the eye to lens distance. Manufacturers will provide tables to make conversions. Likewise, the same principles apply if someone holds a regular hand-held magnifier closer to the page than the focal distance in centimeters, 100/D. Since the convention for magnification can vary, alternative conventions for describing magnifications will be briefly discussed. Some special considerations regarding optical devices are described next.

How Manufacturers Specify Magnification

The emerging convention is to describe the magnification of near devices as equivalent power (EP) in diopters, and distance devices as either angular magnification for telescopes and projection magnification for electronic magnifiers. Angular magnification and projection magnification are virtually the same as enlargement ration (ER), the term we use in this book. For practical purposes these can be considered the same as ER. Power describes the magnification of devices that focus at near, such as near addition or microscopes, handheld magnifiers, and stand magnifiers. Manufacturers, however, have in the past used different and inconsistent conventions for describing the magnification of near devices that persist today.

Describing the magnification property of a device requires reference to the size of one object relative to another. When one reads the magnification of a handheld magnifier as 2×, one must ask "magnification of what compared to what?" For example, when we set the magnification on a copy machine to 2×, this implies the copy will be twice as large as the original. Yet, manufacturers might imprint "2× magnifier" on the handle of a handheld magnifier, leaving the consumer of such a device with no idea what is being magnified compared with what. For example, at 40 cm a client might require print to be enlarged from 1M to 8M to read. This is an enlargement of 8/1 = 8×. If she or he read at 40 cm with reading glasses, the accommodative demand would be 100/40 or 2.5 D. The EP would be 8 times 2.5, or 20 D. One might not know whether an "8×" handheld magnifier should enable Ms. Jason to read the 1-meter fine print on her medicine bottle. Depending on the convention used, "8×" may be equivalent to between 28 to 40 diopters of magnification. On the other hand, if the manufacturer imprinted "20 D" on the device, one would immediately know the exact magnification.

The convention of some manufacturers is to calculate magnification of a handheld magnifier or microscope by dividing the power of the lens by 4; others divide power of the lens by 4 and then add 1, so a 4× from one manufacturer might be equivalent to a 5× from another. These same devices might have different angular magnification, depending on how far they were held from the object being viewed and whether a person was wearing reading glasses while using the device. Rather than attempt to describe the assortment of conventions used by manufacturers, we described how to estimate EP for each near device. If the prescribed device does not fit the task requirements, using the formula for EP, the therapist can select different devices with the same magnification.

Special Considerations: Near Addition, Microscopes, and Loupes

As one common response to inadequate acuity, people will bring whatever they are trying to read or see close to their eyes. A younger person can accommodate or focus at near in response to the accommodative demand of the closer working distance. An older person with presbyopia (who cannot focus at near) will require a near reading addition, which is a plus lens in the form of reading glasses or bifocals. At near, to use 2 eyes, a person at very close distances must converge the eyes more and this can produce eye strain. Try reading this page at a distance of 5 inches—you will likely feel the strain. With stronger reading glasses, a base-in prism must be included in the lens to help someone converge at very close distances. Beyond about 10 diopters of addition—closer than about 10 cm—people usually only use one eye. At these close distances, the therapist must always look for double vision or some sort of interference from the other eye.

A person who is already myopic (nearsighted) will require a weaker near addition lens to achieve a required EP of magnification if the myopia is not corrected (client is not wearing corrective glasses). Uncorrected myopia is equivalent to wearing a plus lens in front of the eye. For example, if a client has 5 D of myopia without distance glasses, he or she needs only an additional 5 D to achieve 10 D of EP. People with high myopia sometimes are able to focus up close by taking off their glasses. If wearing glasses for distance, however, the minus lens acts like a reverse telescope, minifying the image and reducing visual acuity. For these individuals, wearing a contact lens correction for distance will result in better visual acuity than wearing glasses.

A client with uncorrected hyperopia (farsightedness) has insufficient plus in his or her lens and cornea, and extra plus must be added to achieve an EP if the client does not wear spectacle correction. Distance correction in glasses in someone with significant hyperopia will have just the opposite effect as the minus lens in myopia at near. If someone has hyperopia, however, corrective spectacles will act as a weak telescope and provide some distance magnification.

Not surprisingly, when clients use near addition lenses and view binocularly (both eyes open), binocular vision (eye muscle) problems may occur and cause eye strain or double vision that can be relieved by also prescribing base-in prism. If occluding one eye relieves these symptoms, the eye care provider should be informed. The eye care provider may address this issue when prescribing near addition lenses for low vision by adding prism to the lens.

Special Considerations With Handheld Magnifiers

Most clients are familiar with handheld magnifiers or magnifying glasses. Handheld magnifiers are simply plus lenses mounted in a handle. Better magnifiers include thin-lens optics and special compound lenses that reduce chromatic aberration that occurs around the edges of the lens. Many have a built-in light so they can be used to read menus or price tags in a dark store.

Since the therapist often must estimate the power of handheld magnifiers that clients have obtained from a variety of sources, the method for calculating the power of the magnifier will be discussed next.

In theory, if the magnifier is held at the focal distance from the page of text being read or object being viewed, the magnification will not change significantly as the client moves closer to the magnifier (see Figure 13-5). Thus, one need only specify the magnification of the handheld magnifier, such as the spectacle add or microscopes described earlier, in diopters (D).

In general, users often hold handheld magnifiers away from the eye for spotting. Clients should be looking through the distance portion of bifocals when it is held away from the eye. At a greater eye-to-lens distance, the magnification will decrease as the lens is moved closer to the print. Indeed, clients should be taught to start by placing the magnifier flat on the page and then slowly pulling

it away. The image through the lens will enlarge until the focal distance is reached. At the focal distance of the lens, the image becomes distorted, so one actually holds it a bit closer than the focal distance for a distortion-free view with a resulting small reduction in power. When the lens of the magnifier is against the eye or eyeglasses, changing object-to-lens distance changes focus and field of view but not image size. When held against the eyeglasses, looking through the addition will actually increase the magnification by the amount of the addition. The field of view increases dramatically when a handheld magnifier is held close to the eye. Although clients generally do not like to hold a handheld magnifier against the eye, they often will accept an intermediate position of about 20 cm (8 inches), which will improve field of view significantly and reduce distortion.

Special Considerations With Stand and Bar Magnifiers

Unlike handheld magnifiers, stand magnifiers are designed to make it easier for a person to maintain a working distance while reading for a longer period. A stand magnifier is essentially a handheld magnifier set into a stand that rests on the page being read to maintain the lens distance. A bar magnifier (see Figure 13-13) is a low power stand magnifier that magnifies vertically. Some stand magnifiers maintain the lens distance (the distance from the lens to the page) at the focal length of the magnifying lens; like handheld magnifiers, these are used while someone is looking through distance correction. Most stand magnifiers, however, maintain a lens distance that is somewhat shorter than the focal distance of the lens. For a perfectly focused image, one must view the device at a prescribed distance of the eye to the lens and, if presbyopic, through reading glasses prescribed for this particular distance. In some cases, stronger reading glasses will require that the eye-to-lens distance decreases, with an increase in magnification and field of view. This greatly complicates how magnification is specified. Manufacturers have provided the correct eye-to-lens distance, required near addition, and EP, and this information is provided in the online appendix (www.routledge.com/9781617116339).

Unfortunately, one cannot just use the labels on the magnifiers to estimate magnification of stand magnifiers. The dioptric power of the lens that is printed on the device does not indicate magnification because the object is closer than the focal distance of the lens. Tables supplied by manufacturers list the EP for stand magnifiers at a different eye-to-lens distance. A stand magnifier positions the lens closer to the page and has the client look through his or her bifocal at a "virtual" image.[3] As with real objects, a client can increase magnification (increased EP) by moving the lens and virtual image closer. As with real objects, older clients will need stronger near correction as well.

Specific Considerations for Telescopes and Telemicroscopes

When focused at distance, the telescope has no power and, therefore, unlike the other devices and reading situations noted earlier, magnification cannot be specified in terms of EP. Telescopes are described in terms of angular magnification or ER. The convention is that the ER is described by the magnification specification etched on the device, for example, 2×. When focused closer than 1 meter, a telescope technically becomes a telemicroscope, and power can be specified in terms of EP using the general formula for ER and thus directly compared to other near devices (see Figure 13-5).

Two types of telescopes exist: Galilean and Keplerian (see Figure 13-19). Both telescopes have 2 lenses. The lens closest to the eye is called the *ocular lens*, and the lens at the other end is called the *objective lens*. Galilean telescopes are simpler and less expensive. Keplerian systems involve 2 plus lenses spaced farther apart than in Galilean telescopes. In addition to the 2 lenses, a prism or mirror must be incorporated into the telescope to "right" the image. Galilean telescopes have a smaller field of view than Keplerian telescopes of the same magnification. Typically, the smaller and less expensive Galilean telescopes are prescribed for magnification up to 4×.

Since the late 1950s, telescopes have decreased in size and weight, while optical quality has improved. Miniature telescopes can be mounted on spectacles, allowing hands-free, easier use and a decrease in movement.

Normally, just like a set of binoculars or a camera, the user must refocus a telescope when looking at objects at different distances. As with binoculars and cameras, an auto-focus feature is available with some telescopes. Because electronic auto-focus often becomes "confused" and might focus at a different distance than the user intends, it is only recommended if there is a manual override and the user has the ability to "lock" the focus at a given distance. A person can compensate for a smaller, spherical refractive error (myopia or hyperopia) with focus and can thus remove the glasses; however, someone with significant astigmatism may need to wear glasses or have special corrective lenses prescribed and inserted into the telescope.

Although telescopes have become smaller and lighter, the necessary cost of miniaturization is a decrease in the amount of light through the telescope. Light transmission depends on the diameter of the objective lens. The convention is to specify the size of the objective lens after the ER. For example, a 7×50 has an ER of 7× and the size of the objective lens is 50 mm.

Telescopes can also be mounted in the bottom of lenses where the bifocal segment is located (see Figure 13-5). The telemicroscope is focused at near, allowing one to look down to perform a near task with magnification while maintaining a normal working distance. The cost of this greater working distance, however, is a narrower field of view than can be achieved by a simple microscope (near add). Note that most telescopes can be converted to telemicroscopes by purchasing caps that are plus lenses that fit over the objective (far) lens of the telescope. Like near reading add, the value of the cap in diopters is calculated using the formula for accommodative demand (see Table 13-6).

Typically, the power of caps is less than that predicted by the formula because people can add power by focusing the telescope and are in the range of 1.5 to 2 diopters.

Since the working distance used with telemicroscopes is about less than 1 meter, magnification is specified in terms of EP. One uses the general formula for EP to calculate the EP of a microscope. As mentioned, the ER is specified on the telescope. To calculate EP, ER is multiplied by accommodative demand for the particular distance (d) that the telescope is being used using the formula 100/d (cm). If a 4× telescope were used at 40 cm, the EP would be 4 multiplied by 2.5 D, or 10 D. For both distance and near, relative distance magnification and size magnification are often preferred to higher telescopic magnification. Telemicroscopes mounted in the lower segment of the lens as bioptics require the lens be precisely located and angled to match the convergence angle of the eyes. This requires a careful evaluation by an optometrist or ophthalmologist who specializes in low vision. These are also called "surgical microscopes."

Special Considerations
Restricted Visual Fields

Normally with people who have impaired visual acuity, too much magnification will not significantly slow reading. Only if a person has resticted visual fields or requires considerable magnification will too much magnification slow reading because fewer letters can be seen at one time. For example, a client with a visual field restricted to 4 degrees would read text magnified above about 3.6 to 4.0 M at 40 cm more slowly because she or he would see just about 4 letters at a time. In people with normal visual fields, field of view can be limited by the optical device (see Chapter 3), *but the field restriction of optical devices rarely limits reading.* Using a continual text reading acuity test without a magnification device, a clinician can estimate the magnification at which performance is limited by a client's visual field. Normally, reading only slows as the print decreases in size to approach acuity threshold. With significant field restriction, reading also slows as the print is enlarged beyond a given size. One needs to select an optical device magnification based on the print sizes or objects that produce maximum reading rate because too much magnification might impair performance as much as too little magnification.

Clients with field restrictions often have progressive diseases such as retinitis pigmentosa or glaucoma. When these diseases progress to the point that visual acuity is impaired, the residual field of view is often very small. Contrast sensitivity often is impaired as well. In general, these individuals benefit more from electronic devices than from optical devices because electronic devices enhance contrast and optimize lighting, allowing acceptable performance with less magnification. A precise refraction is also needed. Computer systems that provide text to speech, contrast enhancement and controlled lighting, and the future capability to use nonvisual strategies are ideal methods to introduce as alternatives to optical devices with clients who often resist nonvisual strategies.

Central Field Loss

People with central field loss will present with inconsistent reading and visual performance, even with enlarged text rather than an optical device. This condition should be evaluated and the client should be taught compensatory scanning and viewing techniques such as eccentric viewing before optical devices are prescribed. Learning eccentric viewing is difficult and complicates learning new optical devices. As with the introduction of any new technique, learned eccentric viewing strategies may regress with fatigue or frustration. A client who has successfully completed eccentric viewing instruction and is learning to use a telescope for the first time may suddenly complain that nothing can be seen through the telescope because the client has regressed into a maladaptive central fixation or it is not aligned properly. Alignment is difficult because it needs to be off the visual axis of the eye and especially if the pupil is constricted, the margin of the pupil will interfere. Although use of optical devices might be incorporated into the instruction, these devices often are different from the device that will eventually be prescribed. Chapter 9 provides detailed instructions about eccentric viewing strategies.

Poor Contrast Sensitivity

In general, people with impaired contrast sensitivity and impaired acuity will benefit more from electronic magnification where contrast of print may be enhanced and magnified. Avoidance of glare and reflections from lenses becomes essential if someone with impaired contrast sensitivity uses an optical device. Careful control of lighting becomes critical as well; too much light will produce glare. Use of a typoscope (see Figure 12-6), where the client reads through a window cut out of a black card, will decrease glare reflecting off a white page. Matte rather than high-gloss paper will reduce glare as well. Tinted lenses or colored overlays may enhance visual function too.

Cognitive Impairment

Use of optical devices generally requires short-term memory sufficient to learn new materials and the capacity to problem solve. As with any rehabilitation program with someone with impaired memory and problem solving, one must consider the client's premorbid skills and historical roles and activity. A low vision computer system may be complicated to most but relatively easy for someone who worked with computers for 30 years. Clients often have premorbid familiarity with low-powered handheld devices that may enhance learning if similar devices are prescribed, but these people may be in the habit of holding magnifiers farther away from the pages and this complicates learning to use stronger magnifiers, which must be held closer. In general, simple size magnification (for example, using large black marker on a large yellow pad) or relative distance magnification (moving closer to a television, for example) usually are the best solutions. Use of sighted assistance (eg, someone to read a book) provides the client with socialization and is an easy way for 2 people to spend time together.

Impaired Fine Motor Control

People with tremor or incoordination in general respond better to electronic viewers (CCTVs), stand magnifiers, external mounted handheld magnifiers, and spectacle-mounted telescopes. Computer systems with screen magnification and modified keyboard input become excellent alternatives to optical devices for reading and writing tasks.

FIELD-ENHANCEMENT DEVICES

A variety of optical devices have been developed to help people with restricted or narrow fields compensate for a reduced field of view (see Chapter 11). Reverse telescopic arrangements minify a view of the world, but also lead to greater difficulty seeing details.[13-15] For someone who is myopic, a minus lens will reduce the size of objects as well. We have used these devices in people with severe field restrictions (to under 3 to 4 degrees) but who have near-normal acuity. The telescope allows a person to see more of an object and thus recognize it. Use of Fresnel prisms mounted on half of the lens (the affected side) of spectacles has been attempted that moves the view through the prism toward the apex of the prism, which is pointed nasally. These strategies are discussed in detail in Chapter 11. The prism moves the visual scene from the blind field into the sighted field. If the prism includes central vision, then the person experiences double vision. A more comfortable prism placement and double vision is above and below central fixation, so the person can still detect an approaching person.[16,17] Another placement positions the prism on the lateral edge of a lens on the side of the field loss; when the client scans toward the affected side into the prism, the client experiences double vision, but the superimposed prism image allows the person to see about 15 to 20 degrees farther on the blind side without turning the head. By instructing the client to look into the prism, the lateral prism placement also provides a target, or "anchor," for compensatory scanning, ensuring the client looks far enough to the affected side to avoid missing something important.

SUMMARY

Selecting and teaching clients to use optical devices are, and will continue to be, important aspects of low vision rehabilitation. These devices compensate for vision loss and are often necessary for a client to find his or her way back to a valued occupation. The occupational therapist is often the person who must identify why a client is rejecting a device, identify alternative devices or magnification strategies that improve ergonomics, and address cosmetic issues. To do this, the occupational therapist must understand how these devices work and how equivalent magnification can be achieved by changing size, working distance, device position, and the type of device, selecting from among alternative magnification devices and strategies while at the same time not altering the overall magnification. Many "simplifying" assumptions were made to reduce the number of required formula to 4 or 5. The therapist who seeks continuing education on optics to better understand this material will find such knowledge quite useful in solving clinical problems with optical devices.

REFERENCES

1. Lord SR, Smith ST, Menant JC. Vision and falls in older people: risk factors and intervention strategies. *Clin Geriatr Med.* 2010;26:569-581.

2. Goodrich GL, Kirby J. A comparison of patient reading performance and preference: optical devices, handheld CCTV (Innoventions Magni-Cam), or stand-mounted CCTV (Optelec Clearview or TSI Genie). *Optometry.* 2001;72:519-528.

3. Bailey IL, Bullimore MA, Greer RX. Low vision magnifiers: their optical parameters and methods for prescribing. *Optom Vis Sci.* 1994;71:689-698.

4. Humphry RC, Thompson GM. Low vision aids: evaluation in a general eye department. *Trans Ophthalmol Soc UK.* 1986;105:296-303.

5. McIlwaine GG, Bell JA, Dutton GN. Low vision aids: is our service cost effective? *Eye.* 1991;5:607-611.

6. Dougherty BE, Kehler KB, Jamara R, Patterson N, Valenti D, Vera-Diaz FA. Abandonment of low-vision devices in an outpatient population. *Optom Vis Sci.* 2011;88:1283-1287.

7. Watson GR, De l'Aune W, Stelmack J, Maino J, Long S. National survey of the impact of low vision device use among veterans. *Optom Vis Sci.* 1997;74:249-259.

8. Binns AM, Bunce C, Dickinson C, et al. How effective is low vision service provision? A systematic review. *Surv Ophthalmol.* 2012;57:34-65.

9. Wright V, Watson GR. *Learn to Use Your Vision for Reading (LUV Reading Series).* Lilburn, GA: Bear Consultants; 1996.

10. Warren M. *Prereading and Writing Exercises for People With Macular Scotomas.* Birmingham, AL: visABILITIES Rehab Services; 1996.

11. Bailey IL. Equivalent viewing power or magnification? Which is fundamental? *Optician.* 1984;188:14-18.

12. Mehr EM, Freid AN. *Low Vision Care.* Chicago: Professional Press; 1975:107.

13. Bailey IL. Field expanders: choosing the best field expander for increased depth and decreased distortion and loss of acuity. *Optom Monthly.* 1978;130-133.

14. Cohen JM. An overview of enhancement techniques for peripheral field loss. *J Am Optom Assoc.* 1993;64:60-68.

15. Krefman RA. Reversed telescopes on visual efficiency scores in field-restricted patients. *Am J Optom Physiol Opt.* 1981;58:159-162.

16. Giorgi RG, Woods RL, Peli E. Clinical and laboratory evaluation of peripheral prism glasses for hemianopia. *Optom Vis Sci.* 2009;86:492-502.

17. Peli E. Field expansion for homonymous hemianopia by optically induced peripheral exotropia. *Optom Vis Sci.* 2000;77:453-464.

Computer Technology in Low Vision Rehabilitation

OVERVIEW OF TYPES OF ELECTRONIC ASSISTIVE DEVICES AND APPLICATIONS

Case Study 1

The train was late. Dan quickly checked the time and then advanced to the next e-mail on his phone. A flurry of e-mails always seemed to descend from the Internet the day before a critical meeting. Fortunately, like his sighted colleagues, Dan had his e-mails on his smart phone and started reviewing the messages on the train, except he used earphones. Dan could recall just a few years ago when only people with vision disability had personal organizers that read aloud e-mails and messages. Now with the advances in smart phone technology, even sighted people and people with other disabilities have this technology. Dan was a little concerned, however. His coworkers all knew that they should correspond with him by e-mail, messages, or telephone and describe charts and graphs in e-mails so that he could easily process the information, but Dan expected a bundle of printed material from another office. As he entered his office, he gratefully noticed the office secretary

snapping and storing images into his electronic magnifier (EM, formerly called a closed-circuit television, or CCTV) that was also connected to the computer. He now could read the memos that had just been scanned into it.

By habit, Dan arrived 10 minutes before the meeting began. He no longer did so to ensure seating close to the projection screen, because he now had a portable device. He used the extra time to hook the camera up to his notebook computer and point it at the projection screen so that he could also see a magnified view on the screen of his laptop. As an additional advantage, Dan could perform screen captures, allowing him to review more complicated graphics later. When the CEO arrived, she handed him the meeting agenda. Dan flipped the camera attached to his notebook down toward the document on the table, refocused it, and photographed the memo to display and magnify it on his notebook screen with enhanced contrast. When the meeting began, Dan was ready.

Dan could be any young rising executive. Thirty years ago, someone with juvenile macular degeneration and a maximum visual reading rate of 80 to 100 words per minute (wpm) would not have been able to keep up with the paperwork required of someone in Dan's position. Today, with electronic assistive devices, a person with low or no vision can read using text-to-speech technology and process

Whittaker SG, Scheiman M, Sokol-McKay DA.
Low Vision Rehabilitation: A Practical Guide for Occupational Therapists, Second Edition (pp 253-277).
© 2016 Taylor & Francis Group.

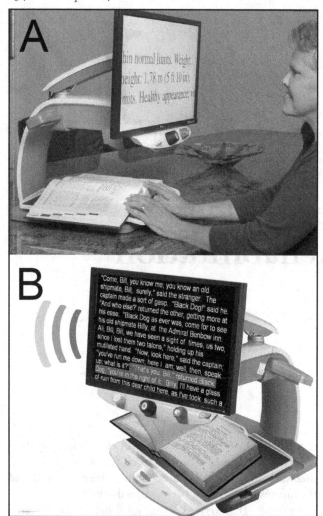

Figure 14-1. Two common desktop electronic magnifiers (CCTVs). (A) A traditional tabletop viewer with natural view and XY table to move the material under the camera. (B) Enhanced black on white for increased contrast and glare reduction that can read aloud using additional document reading software on an attached computer. (Reprinted with permission from Freedom Scientific, Inc.)

numerical information as quickly as someone with more typical vision.[1]

Five years ago, Dan had to purchase special software and hardware to perform these functions. When Apple introduced the iPhone, they set a standard of accessibility for the industry. Using a text-to-speech capability built into the operating system, a totally blind person could access native applications and many commercial applications as well. Currently, with the advent of high-resolution cameras, smart phones, and e-readers; text scanning; easily used magnification gestures; and text-to-speech, the smart phones and tablet computers now are readily accessible, without the need to purchase additional hardware and software. Moreover, a market for automated e-mail readers and other text-to-speech applications have emerged for people to use while they drive. Finger touch is so much

more intuitive than mouse control that this newer technology appears to be more acceptable by older individuals who have not grown up with computers.

Case Study 2

Ms. Wassel refused to move in with her daughter. She loved her house and the morning walk to the coffee shop. She was close to her family in spirit, but they had all moved away and were living in various locations around the world. Ms. Wassel had always loved to write, and even published a short book of poems after she retired. As this 85-year-old woman painstakingly read a handwritten note from her best friend, she momentarily missed the flow and beauty of handwriting. She still added a word or 2 in her own handwriting before signing her printed letters. How she struggled to learn that "darn computer!" Now with the daily e-mails, Ms. Wassel was able to keep in touch with her network of family and friends. This benefit had made the effort worthwhile. Ms. Wassel had macular degeneration, but unlike many with her condition, with the help of a therapist, who had simplified computer access and organized a computer class, Ms. Wassel could once again read and write.

OVERVIEW OF ELECTRONIC ASSISTIVE DEVICES AND PROGRAMS

In general, research indicates that an electronic magnifier (EM) or CCTV (closed circuit TV) (Figure 14-1) is easier and more comfortable to use for extended reading,[2] but the level of evidence is a "practice guideline" (see Chapter 9); that is, an EM is generally better than an optical device for those with more severe acuity loss, suggesting these devices should be available in any low vision service to demonstrate. But any magnification device has to be evaluated on a case-by-case basis. Because the technology changes so rapidly, evaluation of computer based devices has been rarely published, so the devices must be evaluated on a case-by-case basis *before* recommendations are made. Historically, electronic assistive devices for blindness and low vision included CCTV systems and computer-based systems that were generally more complicated for people to learn to use. Now these 2 devices have evolved into several more specialized devices (Table 14-1), many of which are often easier to use than many optical devices. The video-based EMs have evolved so now EMs are all computer-based, and are now more generally called EMs or electronic viewers (EVs), although CCTV is and probably will be a more widely used term. The EM systems can reproduce the image in color (see Figure 14-1[A]) or modify text to make it easier to read (see Figure 14-1[B]). A typical EM (see Figure 14-1) allows the user to vary the image magnification and to increase

TABLE 14-1: TYPES OF ELECTRONIC DEVICES

- EMs, formerly CCTVs
  - Tabletop—camera and display in one unit
  - Component—separate camera and display
  - Optical character recognition (OCR)—images can be processed for more visual enhancement and text-to-speech
  - Split screen—both computer and EM share a single monitor
  - Tablet computer and smartphone apps enable use of the devices for EM
- Software to enable access to personal computers
  - Screen magnifiers—magnify and enhance computer display
  - Screen reader—reads display aloud or converts to refreshable braille
  - Combined screen magnifiers and screen readers
  - Tablet computer and smart phone have magnification and screen reading built in
- Document reader—scans or photographs and reads printed documents aloud
- Personal organizers—portable devices with text-to-speech or braille output, keyboard, or Perkins braille input
- Player for recorded books—reads books aloud using natural speech
- E-reader—allows print to be enlarged and read aloud with a touch of the finger

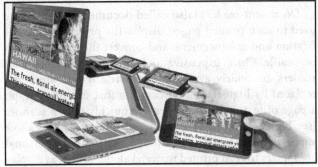

Figure 14-2. A newer EM, the Prodigy, has built-in image capture and optical character recognition that allows customization of fonts, spacing, and other display characteristics, as well as text-to-speech. In this system, the client moves the image on the screen by using a touch pad. (Reprinted with permission from Humanware.)

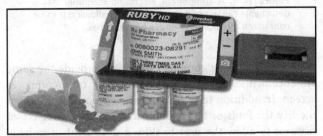

Figure 14-3. A handheld electronic magnifier can use a handle or it can be setup like a stand magnifier stand. (Reprinted with permission from Freedom Scientific, Inc.)

and reverse the image contrast so that the faded black print on a newspaper can be seen as large bright white letters on a dark black page. Since a user must move the material being read under the camera and can easily lose place with a slip of the hand, EMs usually are packaged with special tables that can be moved horizontally and vertically under the camera, enabling the reader to move along a line of text or down a column of numbers with relative ease. Color EMs allow users to see images in natural color and add color contrast enhancements that soften glare, such as using light yellow letters on a dark blue background. Newer systems use touch screen technology (Figure 14-2) to enable a client to move an image on the screen and to capture the image,

identify and read the text aloud, and even automatically move the text on the screen in a scrolling manner, like a marquee.

Once only available as tabletop devices, EMs have become smaller and lighter, the size of a smart phone (Figure 14-3) and can be used to read price tags or perform skin checks by snapping a picture and then bringing it close for viewing. Component systems have cameras that can be pointed at distant objects, such as a blackboard, converting the EM into a telescopic system (Figure 14-4). Component EMs have a detachable camera that can be pointed at a distant object, such as a person or projector screen, and are ideal for nonreading tasks, grooming, or repairing things (see Figure 14-4). Detachable cameras are also available with computers, using the computer display, and with tablet computers (Figure 14-5).

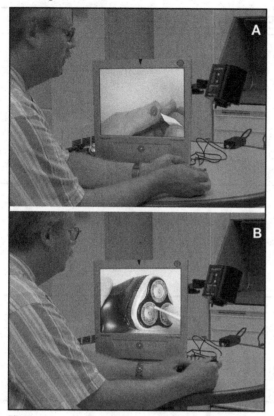

Figure 14-4. A component electronic magnifier has a detachable camera and separate display, allowing it to be configured for vocational and leisure activities.

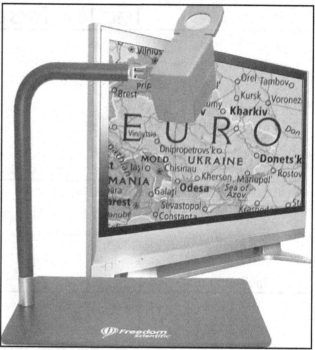

Figure 14-5. A camera connected to a laptop or tablet computer can capture images, allowing distant images to be enlarged. These are popular in classrooms. (Reprinted with permission from Freedom Scientific, Inc.)

Screen magnifier computer programs provide the same enhancements as an EM with the display on a computer screen. In addition to EM features, a screen magnifier can modify the fonts or font spacing and includes a variety of features to allow the user to skim a document or quickly jump from place to place on the screen, such as the lines on a data entry form. A screen reader reads the text displayed on a computer screen aloud or converts the text to a braille display of moveable raised dots. Instead of using a mouse, the blind individual uses key combinations to quickly navigate a screen and read text. Screen magnifiers and screen readers have been combined to allow people with low vision to navigate a page and read with vision enhancement, as well as appreciate the ease and comfort of hearing longer passages read aloud. With these combined systems, people with progressive vision loss can gradually transition from dependence on vision to read, to a screen reader, and gradually learn the more difficult keyboard control required of someone who is totally blind. Currently, free applications are available that allow people with sufficient vision to navigate a computer screen to highlight text and have the computer read it aloud. These systems are ideal for those with hemifield loss and alexia from stroke and other acquired brain injuries (see Chapter 11).

Document readers (also called document scanners) are used to scan printed pages, display the print with magnification and enhancement, and convert the text to speech or braille. Once expensive and cumbersome, document readers are widely available commercially and are being replaced by high-resolution cameras that can photograph a page of text and process it more quickly than a scanner (see Figure 14-1[B]). These "image capture" features allow smart phones, tablet computers, e-readers, and personal computers to read printed material aloud, as well as display the text and figures using screen magnification features. Document readers are also packaged as standalone units that are easy to use. Finally, personal organizers are portable devices that were developed for blind people before they became popular with the general public. The information is presented as computer speech or braille rather than on a visual display. Personal organizers either have keyboards or Perkins braille input. The Perkins braille input is a standard 9-key input used by people to type in braille (Figure 14-6). Personal organizers effectively act as notepads and address books, allowing people with vision impairment to keep personal information, names, and addresses, as well as an appointment book. Smart phones and tablet computers that have built-in text-to-speech capabilities can also be used as personal organizers.

Newer devices enable recorded books to be more easily read. Recordings for the blind (formerly called *books on tape*) are now also computer based. Books are supplied as a single storage device that plugs into a reader. The National Library Service (NLS) (www.loc.gov/nls) now has an online access capability so books can be downloaded as well. Because electronic assistive devices are evolving so rapidly, entire product lines have appeared and disappeared in a few years. In this chapter, we avoid mention of specific products, but rather provide guidance about important features in this technology to guide the reader to making the best selections of equipment.

Before selecting an electronic assistive technology, the therapist must consider the cost and complexity of the devices. For a person with recent vision loss, even simple activities, such as grooming, dressing, cooking, and eating, have become complicated. As a result, such individuals may not welcome the additional complication of a high-technology assistive device. Even the newer EMs with auto-focus features and simpler controls still require relearning complex visual motor coordination, such as moving a book under a camera or moving a finger on a touch pad below the screen while looking straight ahead at the screen. As with optical devices, electronic devices should be introduced in the context of a task that the client deems important. Because people tend to me more intimidated by electronic devices, a success-oriented approach is often necessary (see Chapter 6). Hand-over-hand assistance should be provided to enable the client to quickly achieve success when performing the goal task with the device before confronting more challenging tasks. With repetition and instruction, the assistance can be gradually reduced.

With computer systems, ideally the client should have intact problem-solving skills, but these systems can be used by those with cognitive impairments, especially if they have prior familiarity with computers. Touch screen systems can be used with limited typing or mouse skills. Voice recognition permits these devices to be used by people with good articulation who cannot type, but generally, if someone has writing goals, he or she must have the skills to touch type. Software programs for blind users are available that teach typing/keyboarding, provide an introduction to computer assistive technology, and prepare the client for use of the Web.

Currently, the tablet computer is quickly replacing the personal computer. A typical configuration for an older patient with more severe vision loss is a tabletop EV and a tablet computer and smart phone for browsing the Web, viewing family photographs, and using e-mail. The iPad tablet computer incorporates screen reading, screen magnification, voice recognition, and document scanning capabilities, and is easily accessible if someone has sufficient vision and optical magnification to just read the screen. Other tablet computers have similar capabilities. Because of the small screen size, high spectacle addition and a closer working distance are required. The newer EVs are incorporating this technology as this chapter is being written,

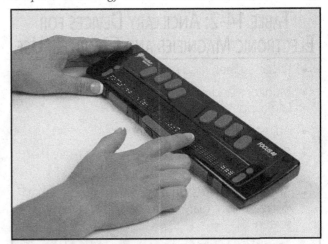

Figure 14-6. A braille display. This is also a keyboard and personal organizer. (Reprinted with permission from Freedom Scientific, Inc.)

and soon, only one device will do it all. One needs only a larger screen and a stand to turn a smart phone into an EV similar to the device in Figure 14-3. The good news is that computer-based accessibility features now open the door so people with both low and typical vision have similar access to the newest technology. The bad news is that the occupational therapist providing even basic levels of care must now keep up with this rapidly evolving technology.

EVALUATION

The Success-Oriented Clinical Reasoning Process for Electronic Devices

The evaluation for electronic devices closely resembles the evaluation for optical devices described in Chapter 13. It is important to anticipate which clients might benefit from electronic devices and present these options concurrently with optical devices. Starting with optical devices and moving on to the more expensive electronic devices, if the optical devices fail, it may discourage a client from considering the EM. With stronger magnification (more than about 10 to 16 equivalent diopters), even if the initial evaluation indicates that an optical magnifier may be as effective as an EM, the therapist should start with a tabletop EM system first because it is easier to use. The client will be encouraged at first just by performing a desired task and developing some basic skills, and will be pleasantly surprised if a less expensive optical device is later found to be sufficient.

Special considerations associated with the low vision evaluation for electronic devices are discussed in the following sections.

TABLE 14-2: ANCILLARY DEVICES FOR ELECTRONIC MAGNIFIER AND COMPUTER USE

- Privacy screen (also reduces glare)
- Monitor stand—variable height, distance, and lateral positioning
- Adjustable office chair on wheels
- Corner desk with swivel chair if using more than one display
- Absorptive lenses (light yellow or orange tint) to decrease light glare from document table and screen
- Special keyboards for screen readers and magnifiers for quick and easy use

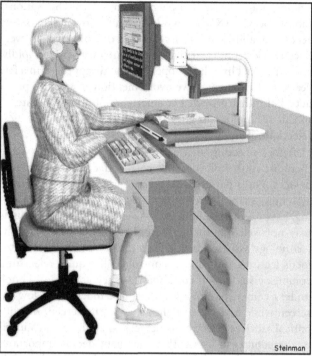

Figure 14-7. Split-screen display where printed material can be presented in real time on the same screen as a computer display. The monitor stand and adjustable computer chair allow for good ergonomic positioning. The computer also includes text-to-speech that can read aloud information from the computer or printed material scanned into the computer. (Reprinted with permission from Barbara Steinman.)

Goals and Performance Requirements

What is the task the client wishes to perform? Examples include correspondence, viewing pictures or graphs, reading short or long passages, and searching for information. What are the performance requirements? Examples include normal fluent reading (for a student or someone working) for longer than 1 hour, skimming, and scanning.

Context, Ergonomics, and Prior Familiarity With Devices

Ideally, devices should be designed around good ergonomics to allow for comfortable performance of a task for long durations without repetitive stress injury and to maximize performance.[3,4] In reality, a person's personal preferences and prior work habits will compromise ergonomics. This includes the range of tolerable working distances for different goal tasks. Are 2 hands required to perform the task, or can the client perform the task holding a device with one hand? Where will the client sit to perform the task? What is the closest possible working distance? Ancillary devices (Table 14-2) such as monitor stands, antiglare privacy screens, adjustable chairs, and specialized adjustable tables should be considered (Figure 14-7). If a person has glare sensitivity issues, then glare-reducing absorptive lenses often will be helpful. Keyboard trays, especially keyboards customized to screen magnifiers and screen readers such as ZoomText and MAGic, are convenient and make learning to use these programs much easier. Figure 14-7 illustrates a work space that has been designed around good ergonomics.

One should carefully consider what computer devices and technology a person has used before, how long ago, and how frequently. People who have been uncomfortable with computers often quickly volunteer this information. Computers have become so ubiquitous in our society, that in a typical clinical setting, expect clients, even those with a cognitive impairment, to readily navigate older versions of Microsoft Windows more easily than they can cook a simple meal.

Optical Devices and Prognosis

If a person's vision is expected to deteriorate, then electronic devices are preferable to optical devices because the magnification and contrast enhancement properties can be adjusted as vision changes. Even when optical devices are not in the treatment plan, eye care providers should be involved. A prescription for a device from a physician will support requests for external funding. Moreover, the client should have proper eyeglasses for the expected working distance from the monitor. In some cases, a special prescription for a closer working distance will enable the user to more easily use the electronic device.

Determination of Display Enhancement Settings

- Start with an estimation of critical print size, which is determined during the functional vision evaluation (see Chapter 8). If impaired contrast sensitivity is found, expect a need for higher contrast. A client who is glare sensitive usually will prefer white letters on a black background, but not always. Those experiencing "starburst"-type glare will reject reverse contrast.

These predictions are important because worse performance indicates other barriers.

- With real objects such a sewing project, one simply magnifies the image with the device until the user is able to easily identify critical features. For picture identification, the most natural color and contrast settings are used. Indeed, this is how one determines the magnification requirements for objects in the initial evaluation (see Chapter 10).

- To compare normal, reverse contrast, and different color contrasts, the therapist should decrease print size until reading speed slows below critical print size, with print size close to visual acuity threshold, where the effects of contrast and color will have the greatest effect. The therapist should then try reverse contrast and different color contrast combinations to determine if reading speed and reported comfort increase. If the print is well above critical print size, these changes will have less of an effect on performance.

- Once the best contrast is ascertained, the therapist should remeasure reading speed using timed reading with different magnifications until an optimum print size is found because critical print size often decreases with other visual enhancements. This testing is most easily performed with different sentences of the same length on the EM. Test sentences are included in the online appendix (www.routledge.com/9781617116339).

- During testing, the therapist should provide hand-over-hand assistance, moving the text to ensure reading speed is only limited visually and not by the client's ability to manipulate the device.

- Just having the client adjust the magnification and contrast to "what looks right" without an objective performance evaluation is not acceptable and often results in the client choosing what is familiar rather than more efficient. After performance is evaluated objectively and the client is informed of the results, client should choose the best configuration.

- With computer systems, several other characteristics of display presentation may be modified as well. Again, some performance measures, such as how quickly someone performs a task, should be combined with subjective preferences in order to decide on the preferred setup.

Selecting Devices

Under the adult learning model (see Chapter 9), if a person's only impairment is visual and he or she has good cognition and is well adjusted, one needs only to describe and quickly demonstrate a device. Give the person time to play with it and experiment. It is better to have the client ask

---

TABLE 14-3: THE SUCCESS-ORIENTED CLINICAL REASONING PROCESS FOR ELECTRONIC DEVICES

1. Define goals and task performance requirements; evaluate with materials specified by the goals.

2. Evaluate and try to approximate prior context, ergonomics, and familiar technology at first.

3. Consider optical and nonoptical ancillary devices with eye care provider.

4. Predict how to setup display from evaluation data NOT trial and error.

5. The therapist performs the setup at first. Use custom keyboards so magnification and other properties can be easily changed with a knob like an EM.

6. Evaluate performance on each device with all necessary assistance to minimize new learning.

7. With alternative devices, respond to a client's concerns about cosmetic, social, financial, and prognosis issues.

8. Teach client to use selected devices starting with goal tasks of high value.

9. On computers, put links to more frequently accessed websites on the Start menu for easy access. Check these sites for accessibility by screen magnifiers and readers.

10. Provide or arrange for support and instruction to teach more advanced use and how to problem solve and change setups at the end.

---

questions then for the therapist to carry on a monologue about each device.

If a client is expected to have difficulties accepting or learning to use devices, use a success-oriented approach (Table 14-3). Begin with the device most likely to be successful. In the success-oriented approach, the first experiences attempting to perform a goal task should be successful. Once success is achieved, then selection of a device requires trying out various options, some of which might be more difficult. Clients will reject a device that could be much more efficient just because it is difficult to use at the time of testing. Learning to use a device often is an expensive and difficult process. Moreover, the client also must obtain the device to practice using it. To avoid the need for instruction and make it easy to use, the therapist should provide as much assistance as necessary to set up and manipulate the device so that all the client needs to do is read or perform the visual task. In this supported setting, the therapist should compare reading speed and comfort using various options, such as less expensive optical solutions, electronic displays, or text-to-speech technology. Performance and rated comfort should be measured during these trials. One must convince the client and any agency funding the program that at the completion of instruction, the client will be able to perform the goal task efficiently.

Objective performance evaluation is essential if the purchase of devices and instructional programs that are more expensive needs to be justified to an agency. Because magnification will affect ease of use, one should use an enlargement ratio (size magnification) and eye-to-screen distance that will produce the same equivalent power (EP) of magnification (see Chapters 8 and 13) for each device evaluated. We recommend that the therapist obtain easy-to-understand paragraphs of the same length and compare reading time with the various options (see online appendix, www.routledge.com/9781617116339). With text-to-speech capabilities, the computer can read the passages aloud at different speeds. Comparison of visual performance with optical devices vs electronic devices can be performed with the Pepper Test, which will be more sensitive to smaller differences. As with optical devices, if performance should be predicted by vision testing, the therapist, in collaboration with the low vision optometrist, should attempt to identify other barriers, such as lighting and other visual impairments.

Cosmetic and Social Considerations

Often, the final selection of a device depends on how it looks or affects a client's social interaction. Does the client require seating away from coworkers? Will the client be working in a public area and be required to deal with stares and questions? These important considerations should follow the performance evaluation because a significant performance enhancement might persuade a client to tolerate these problems.

Instruction

An electronic device should never be recommended unless instructional needs are addressed. Instruction for EM systems or basic word processing can generally be provided by a therapist as an outpatient service in the context of medical rehabilitation for written communication, performing e-mail, and shopping on the Web. Introducing a patient to a keyboard or more complicated screen reading programs that use proprietary software requires considerable instruction that is generally beyond the scope of "medical necessity" and the skill of most therapists. Vocational rehabilitation and college-level educational programs are often available to provide such instruction, although these programs may be expensive and require the client to pay for the instruction. It is the responsibility of the therapist to arrange for such instruction before a device is recommended for such vocational goals.

Affordability

The client ultimately selects a preferred device if he or she is paying for it. If an agency, school system, or insurance pays, the therapist must provide objective performance evaluations and work within the agency requirements.

Some electronic devices are expensive. In the United States, young adults under age 21 who have not yet graduated high school or vocational programs are eligible for what remains the best resource for instruction and equipment—the public school system. If the client is enrolled in a public school system, the school is required by the Individuals with Disabilities Education Act (IDEA) to provide devices necessary for education, including electronic and optical devices. A request for such a device must include clear performance data in support of the recommendation, with data relating the device to the educational objectives as stated in the student's Individualized Education Plan (IEP). The parents should make such a request with the help of the special education teacher who provides low vision services.

By Federal law every state should have blind and vocational rehabilitation services that pay for assistive devices for adults with vocational goals, including primary homemakers and caregivers. In many countries, the government pays for assistive low vision devices as with other medical devices. These agencies, however, have budget limitations. Thus, letters with objective performance data must provide a convincing argument that a device is necessary to perform an essential task for a particular job or to live independently. In the United States, there has been limited success obtaining reimbursement from Medicare, Medicaid, and other medical insurance for assistive devices for low vision and blindness. However, a therapist should at least try to help the patient obtain reimbursement. When documenting the need for devices, it is essential to justify medical necessity. For the EM, for example, the justification might be for medication management, diabetic management, and self-care functions such as skin checks or catheter management.

ELECTRONIC MAGNIFIERS

Electronic magnifiers are composed of 3 basic features: the camera that focuses on the material being read, the display of the enlarged image of the material being read, and the table on which the user rests the material being viewed. Figure 14-1 illustrates a classic tabletop CCTV-type EM system. The display is a commercial monitor/TV screen.

Newer display systems use the lighter and more portable displays with higher resolution that still have critical visual characteristics that are often inferior in some ways to older simpler systems. Newer digital EMs also use digital cameras that may likewise have inferior visual display characteristics when compared to older video cameras. Note that the material being viewed is on an XY table that can be moved horizontally and vertically under a fixed camera. Figure 14-4 illustrates some various uses of a component EM system, where the camera can be detached and positioned for a variety of tasks and the monitor moved as well. The tabletop EM has been used for grooming and small appliance repair too. The detachable camera on a component EM can be set up like the tabletop system, but the component systems are considerably more versatile.

Some component systems allow the camera to be moved manually or electronically to scan and use an XY table accessory. Although this may vary from clinic to clinic, we find the most popular use of the EM is for reading and writing. These activities can easily be performed with the less expensive tabletop EMs. Electronic magnifiers are available that share the display monitor with a computer (see Figure 14-7), allowing the user to quickly switch back and forth from the display of some printed material or information on a screen and the display of a word processor or some other application. These may be used with 2 cameras as well. Split-screen, PC-based EMs still are generally the products of choice in vocational rehabilitation with users in typical white-collar jobs who also use computers, such as Dan in Case Study 1. For home use, tablet computers are replacing the personal computers.

Consider how a person with low vision typically uses an EM. To read, the user will take the page or book and place it on the XY table, center the book, and position it by feel up against a lip so that it is perfectly horizontal on the XY table. When starting, the user must set up and focus the unit. After the setup, the user rarely touches any control except the magnification and a switch between normal view and reading-enhanced view.

- The setup is as follows:
  - For a reading-enhanced view, the user first sets up the color of the display and the contrast. The client might choose high-contrast light yellow text on a black background. Generally, it is better to use tinted absorptive lenses rather than color contrast because they reduce glare from the light that shines on the material being read.
  - Sometimes horizontal or vertical guidelines on the screen are displayed to help the user stay on a line or column.
  - For manual focus, the person increases the magnification to maximum and then adjusts the focus until the letters appear clearest. The EM will then keep the focus throughout the range of magnification as long as the thickness of the reading material does not change. Fortunately, nearly all EMs have auto-focus.
  - Sometimes a clear plastic overlay must be used to hold reading material, like books, flat to stay in focus.
  - The user will adjust the margin stops, place a finger, or move the book so that the table stops at the beginning and end of the lines or column displayed.
  - If possible, adjust the drag of vertical motion so that it is a little easier to move the table horizontally than vertically. This helps a person stay on the line.
- The user adjusts magnification, decreasing to search and find where to start reading, increasing magnification to see.
- The reader then can start reading by moving the book from left to right under the camera of the EM. At the end of the line, the user will quickly move the table back over the line just read and then up slightly until the beginning of the next line is seen.
- For viewing pictures, the client will adjust the EM to use natural color and contrast, switching to contrast enhancement settings like white letters on a black background for reading.
- For writing, the user often will increase the drag on the table so it does not move as easily and angle the entire table and the EM the way someone would angle a paper to write. The table moves while writing.
- For 3-dimensional (3D) objects (eg, trimming fingernails, taking a blood sample, or fixing an appliance), the user must readjust the focus to the correct depth plane. Focusing on lower-contrast objects is difficult. It is often helpful to have high-contrast focusing targets for the client to use. Once the focus is set, it is often easier to lock focus and move the object being viewed closer or farther from the camera to maintain focus than to readjust focus. Most EMs have auto-focus.
- For an experienced user, EM setup can be completed in a few seconds. A beginning user who is more hesitant might find the setup tedious and overwhelming. The success-oriented approach (Table 14-4) starts by having the therapist perform setup and adjustments so the client can have the immediate gratification of reading. Then setups and adjustments can be gradually introduced.

Carrying electronic devices such as EMs and monitors may present a problem for therapists doing home-based or workplace-based low vision practice. For EM evaluation, the therapist may schedule a demonstration by a vendor who will provide the device at the same time a treatment session is scheduled. For instruction, a rental may be arranged. The choice of which devices to demonstrate to clients will depend on the willingness of vendors to provide such support.

TABLE 14-4: IMPORTANT PROPERTIES OF AN ELECTRONIC MAGNIFIER

- Ease of use with controls
  - Levers are better than knobs. Knobs are better than buttons.
  - Magnification control should be quick and easy to access.
  - Easy focus or auto-focus with focus lock for nonreading tasks.
  - One-step switch between natural and contrast-enhanced display.
- Magnification between 1× and 3× enables easier scanning and spotting (High Definition Models).
- High and stable contrast with moving text (low smear and smooth motion).
- Ergonomic flexibility such as an adjustable screen position.
- Easy to move documents and keep one's place with high magnification such as XY tables with adjustable horizontal and vertical resistance, margin stops, and locking capability.
- Handling characteristics if a handheld device.
- Low glare from table illuminator.
- Portability.
- Color.
- Camera stability (component system).
- Product support and integrity of vendor.

Important Properties of Electronic Magnifiers

The following features of EMs have significant functional impact (see Table 14-4). Ideally, several models should be available for the client to try and evaluate, but often the therapist must arrange demonstrations for users by sales representatives. The therapist must, therefore, anticipate which models will be acceptable and suggest 2 or 3 devices for a sales representative to demonstrate, using Table 14-5 as a checklist.

Ease of Use and Controls

Ease of use is not just about positioning the control. It also reflects the intuitive nature of the control—how easy it would be for someone with cognitive impairment to learn.

- In general, levers are better than knobs, and button controls to adjust magnification should be avoided. Digital button controls are the least intuitive for users less familiar with digital technology, but may be easier than knobs for those with motor impairment. Consider hand dominance and manual disability, and rule out devices where controls cannot be reached. If someone has problems with fine motor control then buttons may be easier than knobs.

- The magnification control is most frequently used and should be positioned lower and closer to where the hand must be positioned during the task.

- Focus should be easy and accessible or use auto-focus. Learning to focus the camera and make manual adjustments is difficult. It is easier to read a book that does not lay flat with auto-focus. An auto-focus feature is valuable; however, a focus lock button should be available if the user is using the EM for grooming or examining 3D objects.

- Switching between color and reading modes must be quick and easy. The setting for reading might have contrast enhancement or reversed (white on black) contrast not suitable for viewing pictures or objects. A natural color mode is suitable for viewing pictures and objects, or grooming. Avoid units where switching between these 2 setups is more than one step and is complicated. Some devices require the user to switch through several color combinations in order to find the preferred contrast setting for reading.

Magnification

Often, higher magnification is used as a selling feature. In fact, the ability to achieve lower magnification from 1× to 3× is a most important and useful feature that has become more common with high-definition (HD) systems. To scan and locate information, the client uses lower magnification to view as much of an entire page as possible. The user estimates where critical information might be located by the layout of the page, using a spotting technique similar to that used with optical devices. Once a suspected location is found, the user centers the target and zooms up magnification. People with field restrictions and poor contrast sensitivity appreciate the contrast enhancement features and perform best with lower magnification. Rarely do users set magnification greater than 10X. The visual evaluation should indicate the ideal range of magnification for an individual. With higher magnification, EMs are easier to use if size magnification is combined with relative distance magnification. A user can effectively double the magnification (as measured by equivalent power) by decreasing the working distance from 40 cm (16 inches) to 20 cm (8 inches), enabling a 5× setting on the EM to be used rather than a 10X setting. With tablet computers or EVs with smaller screens, the ability to provide crisp definition

TABLE 14-5: STEPS IN SUCCESS-ORIENTED INSTRUCTION FOR THE ELECTRONIC MAGNIFIER

1. The therapist provides initial setup (sets and controls magnification and contrast, sets margin stops, locates starting position to read).

2. Client learns to use XY table or control to move text horizontally and vertically on the screen.

   a. Use short one-line sentences (see online appendix [www.routledge.com/9781617116339]). Learn to follow a line backward to the beginning.

   b. To find the next line, learn to follow the line just read backward and move down at the beginning of the next line.

   c. Adjust magnification: 1) decrease to find, 2) center on screen, 3) increase to see.

      i. Look at family photos and identify people or look for words on a page.

      ii. Find simple block-formatted text (like a book) of interest to patient or exercises from the LUV reading series (no writing yet), decrease magnification to find starting point, increase to read.

3. Align paper on table or under camera (eg, along guide on table by feel).

4. Review how to adjust magnification and focus (if manual focus). Client will describe the previous strategy.

5. Learn how to find the start of an article or a target.

   a. Start with lowest magnification.

   b. Center it on the screen.

   c. Magnify until it can be read.

   d. Also find food item on a menu, activity on a schedule, person in a photo, passage in a Bible, total on a bill.

6. Learn to switch between natural and enhanced view.

   a. Use catalogues with pictures.

7. Find and follow a newspaper article that is continued or find an announcement in a newsletter or church bulletin.

8. Learn how to adjust brightness in an enhanced-contrast view to maximize contrast.

9. Use the device to read medication bottles and boxes.

10. Write.

    a. Find a finger and then a pen on a screen after placing it on the paper.

    b. Put lines through and then circle and underline targets.

    c. Sign name on a line.

    d. Use LUV reading sentences and fill in the blanks.

    e. Write a passage.

    f. Fill in a form and write a check.

    g. Angle the device for more extended writing.

11. Learn to use the device for grooming, skin inspections, hobbies. This includes learning to focus or to lock an auto-focus at a given distance.

12. Learn how to move the device (if portable) and set up the device, how to set margin stops, maintenance instructions, advanced features like line guides and color contrast.

of letters and 1.5× to 3× magnification becomes important because optical magnification often must be used as well.

High definition is becoming common with EMs. Although the now crisp image on the screen can be appreciated by people with low vision, the major advantage is that with HD, magnification can be reduced so that an entire page can be seen on the screen without losing critical definition.

High and Stable Contrast With Image Motion (Low Smear)

A major advantage of an EM over optical systems is the ability to increase print contrast. This advantage can be negated by smear or ghosting. To evaluate smear on a given device, set an EM to reverse contrast and decrease the magnification, and then move the page under the camera quickly. Note that the letters will fade when the page is moved. With some EMs, especially those with HD or that use computer processing, smear appears quite significant and the image motion is not smooth. Smear becomes functionally important in people with poor contrast sensitivity who are reading with lower magnification, such as someone with diabetic retinopathy, advanced glaucoma, or retinitis pigmentosa. With more magnification, smear is less of a problem. In general, users appreciate the highest contrast possible. If illumination creates glare (eg, from a bright white letter on a black background), consider one or more of the following additional EM features:

- Turn down monitor brightness (or have the user wear lightly tinted polarized or yellow absorptive lenses) (see Figure 14-1[B]).
- Use a color unit with different color contrasts (the most popular is light yellow on a black background).
- Use normal black-on-white contrast with a curtain feature that darkens all but the line being used, like a typoscope.
- Wear light shaded (indoor) absorptive lenses while using the device. Avoid polarized lenses that interact with LCD displays.

Ergonomic Flexibility

A moveable monitor provides the most ergonomic flexibility. For example, a detachable monitor can be set up and positioned at any distance or height and angled with commercially available 3D monitor stands. Newer product lines have display monitors that can be adjusted as well. This is an important feature for those requiring higher magnification, where relative distance magnification is used in combination with relative size magnification on the screen. With a closer working distance, one often must bring the monitor closer and raise it to enable an upright posture. With a separate monitor, the user can put the monitor on an adjustable stand and change the elevation and working distance to achieve a comfortable posture (see Figure 14-7). With older people of short stature, the ability to move the monitor as close as possible to the table becomes important. The center of the monitor should be slightly below the eyes, even lower if a person is viewing though a bifocal.

Table Characteristics and Handling Characteristics

The table is where the client positions the page to be magnified. In general, tabletop EVs should have a movable XY table. An XY table moves both horizontally and vertically so the user can smoothly and easily slide material under the camera of the magnifier. The magnifier magnifies any movement, however, so jerky and irregular movements can induce motion sickness. For someone with motor impairment, low frustration tolerance, and/or incoordination, table characteristics become the most important features of an EM.

- A table should at least have a lip against which the material can be rested to ensure it is positioned horizontally.
- The table should have greater resistance to movement vertically than horizontally to help the user stay on the same line.
- The table should have tab stops to stop movement when the beginning or end of a line is reached.
- The table should have a locking mechanism or mechanism for increasing drag if someone plans to use the EM for viewing and working on objects or writing. Electronic magnifiers that have separate cameras (see Figure 14-4) often do not have XY tables, so a person must drag reading material over the surface. In such cases, separate XY tables can be purchased from the vendor. Newer systems scan in pages and provide alternative methods to move the page on the screen, such as a touch screen, touch pad, or, with a personal computer, a mouse.

Handheld devices require the client move the camera over the page being read. These devices should have stands like a stand magnifier so the client can rest the magnifier on the page. Some devices have handles so they have the look and feel of a handheld magnifier, but the stand makes extended reading on a flat surface easier. Because books and magazines often do not lie flat, in general, handheld devices are better for spotting (see Figure 14-3). Tabletop devices are better for extended reading (see Figure 14-1).

Glare From Table Illumination

Since the EM is often most useful for people with impaired contrast sensitivity, glare from the light illuminating the material being read becomes a significant problem. Directional lights from the side of the page produce the least amount of glare. Newer machines require less light and produce less glare. If glare is a problem, the client might use wraparound light-colored yellow or orange absorptive lenses to reduce glare from the table top. Avoid polarized lenses.

Portability and Screen Size

There is a trade-off between screen size and portability; the screen size now limits how small a device can be, rather than the other electronic components of the system. Electronic magnifier systems in general have become smaller and lighter, but typically have smaller screens. Tablet computers, e-readers, and smart phones all have magnification capability, but the screen size limits the field of view with higher magnification, so those who need higher magnification generally need either a tabletop EV or some way to hook up a larger screen to the device. The solution to this problem is found with spectacle-mounted displays. With spectacle-mounted displays, one needs to carefully measure the contrast, smear, brightness, and how large the virtual image actually is. Spectacle mounted displays have been tried but as of 2015 have not yet been commercially successful.

Color

Color features used to add cost and complexity to a CCTV, but now are standard. However, color only enhances reading if the user appreciates color contrast features, such as yellow letters on a black background, to decrease glare. A person does not need color vision to appreciate these features. Otherwise, color becomes useful for those using the EM to enjoy pictures or read tables, graphs, maps, and color illustrations.

Camera Stability and Rotational Camera Adjustment

With component EM systems (see Figures 14-4 and 14-6), the camera often attaches to an arm, which might easily bounce and magnify any movement of the table on which it rests. Likewise, when a camera is pointed at a target from an oblique angle, the object will be viewed as rotated on the screen. Some units allow one to rotate the camera to compensate. For those using the EM for skin inspections or to work in a shop, one also should consider how the camera might be mounted. A camera with a conventional camera screw mount is an advantage, as one might be able to use the assortment of relatively inexpensive camera mounting systems, including table and tube clamp mounts and tripods, available in a photography store.

Product Support/Integrity of Vendor

Unlike optical devices that only can be prescribed by an eye care provider, EM devices can be sold and dispensed without any special qualifications. Moreover, most low vision services cannot afford to stock and maintain the plethora of expensive and ever-changing product lines. A good relationship between a vendor of such products and a therapist becomes essential for effective delivery of low vision rehabilitation services. The therapist can provide the vendor with valuable advice as to what products will sell and provide a vendor with an opportunity to sell his or her products. If a vendor is frequently demonstrating and selling products at a site, the vendor is often willing to provide demonstration units at no charge for the therapist to demonstrate and use for training. Outpatient therapists may depend on vendors to correctly configure a device in a client's home and provide some home-based instruction. Vendors can keep therapists abreast of new technological developments and train therapists in how to use new equipment. If a vendor is unwilling to support his or her product, oversells expensive features, and fails to respond to queries from consumers, the therapist often must provide the additional support a client requires. The therapist has a responsibility to carefully document complaints by consumers and address them with and report unethical behavior, first to the distributors and manufacturers of the product, and then possibly to regulatory agencies. Fortunately, manufacturers and distributors of electronic devices are keenly aware of maintaining a good reputation among a group where word of mouth can make or break these businesses.

Instructional Strategies With Electronic Magnifiers

For someone with intact cognitive function and who is comfortable with technology, an EM might take 10 to 15 minutes of instruction to master. For those with cognitive problems, who are resistant to technology, or have depression, a graded success-oriented approach may be needed (see Table 14-5). Generally with an EM, one begins instruction with use of the XY table, setup of the device, reading, writing, and finally other special applications suited to an individual client's interest. To motivate an ambivalent or resistant client, or someone who is expected to find learning the EM difficult, the therapist should begin with an activity that directly addresses a client's interest or individual goal, teaching actual use of the device after it has been demonstrated. We have presented an order of instruction used for a client with recent vision loss who is resistant to change and is expected to find learning an electronic device difficult. If setup is taught later, however, the client cannot practice at home or independently until demonstrating competency with setup and basic trial-and-error problem solving. The therapist might try to instruct a helper on setup if someone is available. Indeed, for the reluctant client, the therapist should not recommend purchase of the device until competency with task performance has been demonstrated or a helper can set up the device and solve problems. For younger, vocationally-aged clients and students, or more adventuresome tech-savvy older people, the strategy may be completely different. One might start by showing the client all of the features of the device and setup. Indeed, in these cases instruction can often be completed in less than one session.

One challenge in providing EM instruction is gaining access to these expensive devices. A well-equipped clinic will have at least one EM system, with most extras that can be set up to simulate a less expensive system. All of the instructions described later, except for the setup, will rather easily transfer to another EM as long as the design of the XY table is similar. In the case of the reluctant client, to avoid transfer of learning issues, the therapist should recommend the device be available for instruction in the clinic.

Tips for Success: Getting Started.

In the success-oriented approach (see Table 14-5), the first activity a client performs with a difficult device should be of interest and part of a stated goal. Reading is the most common goal, but if the client had hoped for the day when he or she could perform cross-stitch again, then the demonstration material should be a photograph of cross-stitch, and the task might be "looking for missed stitches." The well-equipped service will have life-size photographs of a variety of nonreading activities for such clients as a starting point. Photographs will be much easier to manipulate at first than 3D objects. If a client has central field loss, the following instruction can be incorporated into eccentric viewing training (see Chapter 9) as the "steady eye technique" once development of eccentric viewing of isolated targets has been mastered.

For someone with cognitive impairments or low frustration tolerance, the change in the visual motor demands of reading or any task presents the greatest challenge with the EM. Typically, people are accustomed to directly looking at whatever they wish to see. For this reason, optical devices and tablet computers with touch screens are more natural to use. With an EM, the user must look at a display positioned above or to the side of the object being viewed. When someone tries to locate something under an EM, the beginning user will often first try to look directly at the book or material on the XY table, rather than at the display.

- For someone who wishes to read, the best starting point is to set up the EM (CCTV) with optimum equivalent power magnification predicted by the evaluation or pictures of tasks or family photos. Determine the required display enhancements (Chapter 8).

- Any text of interest will do, but keep the passages short and use greater-than-normal spacing between the lines. The therapist sets up the device and simply has the client look at the screen.

- The client places her or his hands on the table, but the therapist moves the table.

- Gradually the therapist withdraws assistance until the client is moving the table without any assistance both horizontally and vertically. Keep distracting verbal instructions to a minimum; this is a motor learning process. Continue until the client reads several lines without any assistance or cues.

- Now teach the client how to change magnification, locate a different spot on the page, center it on the screen, and increase magnification. This can be best done with family photographs. Once the client actually performs the tasks, verbalize the strategy.

- Introduce other controls, such as switching between a natural picture view and text-enhanced view.

- Teach setup and maintenance last.

- Then teach additional features, such as how to adjust brightness to enhance lower-contrast materials.

With electronic devices and the resistant client, the therapist should attempt to make the task as easy as possible. To upgrade the activity and teach problem solving, position the paper incorrectly so that the lines are on a diagonal and challenge the client to identify and correct the problem. Move the table so that a few words are skipped or a line is skipped, and have the user find the beginning of the line once again.

Reading and Writing

Reading instruction continues from scanning sequential numbers and letters to simple sentences, isolated short words, and more complicated sentences, as described in Chapter 9. At first, the exercises should only involve reading successive horizontal lines across a full page (see the online appendix at www.routledge.com/9781617116339). Wright and Watson's Learn to Use Your Vision (LUV) reading series (www.lowvisionsimulators.com) provides an excellent source of graded engaging exercises for reading rehabilitation.[5] Initially, material should be selected that involves sentences or sequenced words or numbers to provide immediate feedback if the user skips a line or some words. Activities involving random words and numbers can be presented once skipping errors are minimal. As this practice can be somewhat tedious, the exercises should involve games such as counting words that describe people or finding numbers that add up to 10. Writing can be incorporated into the reading exercises in a graded manner. First, the client might simply draw a line through selected words or numbers, then draw a line under the word, then a circle around, and finally a square around selected words or numbers. These graded activities are built into the sequence of exercises in the LUV reading series.

If the client is having difficulty writing at the magnification level used for reading, then writing practice should occur separately at first. With an EM, the setup for writing should involve a dark-flow pen (ballpoint pens and pencils are not recommended) on regular lined paper. Normally, a person writes with a dark felt-tip pen with thick lined paper. To grade the task for those with severe acuity loss, a felt-tip pen on dark lined paper can be used with lower magnification.

To begin, the client must learn to find the pen under the EM camera and become accustomed to a different visual motor orientation using the following steps:

- The client points to a high-contrast target on the XY table at a random location and then moves his or her hand on the table until the target and tip of the finger are displayed on the screen, and finally the use of a pen is added.

- This task is first performed at minimum magnification and graded to increased difficulty with higher magnification.

  ○ Start with putting lines through targets, then circling or underlining targets. These activities are in the LUV reading series beginning lessons. Practice with this task should enable the client to adapt visual motor coordination with the EM so that positioning objects for a better view feels more natural.

  ○ Have the client practice his or her signature and then write single words and phrases.

  ○ Then have the client complete fill-in-the-blank exercises.

- Once the client feels comfortable writing enlarged print at a lower EM magnification setting, grade up the difficulty of the task by using the contrast/color settings used for reading, then progressively increase EM magnification with paper or forms with smaller, more typical lines.

- Turn the whole machine to a slant for writing rather than the page on the table. Then the table can be moved left to right while writing with increased resistance and the person can maintain a natural posture. A swivel screen is ideal for this activity, but a fixed screen usually can be viewed as well.

Once the user is competent reading lines of text, the difficulty of the task might be increased by presenting reading material in columns and then interspersed with figures, tables, and ads, as is typical of a newspaper or magazine.

Localization

A more difficult but functionally important task with an EM is localization. This involves spotting strategies where first the material is viewed with lower magnification and the approximate location of the critical information is estimated from the layout of the material as seen with lower magnification. The user centers the suspected location of the critical information on the screen and increases magnification to read. If in the wrong place, the user uses the material just read to better estimate the location of the critical information. The user decreases magnification somewhat to enlarge the field of view and moves the

material and increases the magnification to read when the target is expected.

Functional reading, such as reading medicine labels, finding the total on a bill, finding information in a printed advertisement, reading a recipe or instructions, and finding and identifying faces in a photograph, involves localization strategies. Localization practice proceeds first with having the client locate sequential numbers in the corner of a blank page, then to the middle of a page. Then the client might practice finding and naming the first word in successive paragraphs, locating the byline or headline, and reading a picture caption. This phase of instruction can be completed using bills, medicine labels, instructions, and recipes. Note that the user is frequently changing magnification. Users require convenient access to the magnification control for such advanced skills.

Grooming/Diabetic Management/ Reading Labels

To begin this step in instruction, the client should demonstrate competency with EM setup and problem solving, especially with focusing (if no auto-focus). Tabletop EMs can be used to inspect hands and trim nails visually. The client should be competent with visual motor coordination with an EM, such as writing tasks.

To start, a target is applied to a finger or picked up and viewed after focus is adjusted. The therapist instructs the user to inspect his or her hand and find the target. The goal is for the client to be able to move an object and position it so that it is in focus. Subsequent practice tasks might include fastening buttons, adjusting zippers, simple sewing activities like separating seams, cutting, and painting 3D objects. These activities may require that the EM be refocused but it is generally better to lock the table and focus and learn to move the objects to focus and center them on the screen. Subsequent activities can be varied according to the client's interests and needs.

To read a medicine label or syringe, or to blot a bead of blood onto a test strip, the hand or object being viewed should rest in the center of the XY table so the distance from the camera does not change. In most cases, the table should be locked or friction increased for stability. A medicine bottle or syringe might be rotated while resting on a firm surface. To facilitate this activity for someone with impaired motor control, the therapist might easily fabricate stands and holders from scraps of splinting material or dispense some firm theraputty to a client to stabilize objects.

Working With Crafts and 3D Objects, Grooming, and Skin Inspections

These activities are more easily performed with component EM systems (see Figure 14-4). With a detachable or adjustable camera, the objects are often viewed at odd angles so the image on the display appears rotated. If the camera does not have a rotational adjustment, the user should position the camera with direct horizontal or vertical alignment with the object rather than direct the camera at an oblique angle. For example, if setting a camera to magnify a screen at the end of a rectangular table, the user should position the camera directly in front of the screen, at the other end of the table, rather than from the side. If a component EM is used as a mirror substitute for grooming, the camera might be directed at a mirror so the view is reversed like a real mirror. Otherwise, the user may need to readapt because the view will appear reversed from working in front of a mirror, although component systems usually can be switched to mirror view. If the camera can be handheld, component EMs can be used for skin inspections. Component systems may also allow the camera to be mounted for self-catheterization. The challenge with all of these tasks is learning to approximate the correct camera positioning by feel or with the use of visible markers or tactile cues. Tablet computers and hand-held EMs can now be used to take pictures for skin inspections.

Skimming, Scanning, and Text-to-Speech Features

Skimming and scanning is the most advanced reading task and presents a challenge when done visually. In some cases, the user cannot use localization strategies because the layout of the page in an unmagnified view does not indicate where critical information is located. The client must now magnify the text until it can be read and perform systematic left-right vertical scanning to look for some text. The task might be to search text for particular words or numbers. In most cases, a combination of scanning and localization can be used. For example, when looking up a passage in the Bible or some reference book, the reader can view the headings on the top of the page under magnified view to find the correct page and then once within the page, read a few words under magnified view, reduce the size to whole-page view, reorient to where the information is located, and magnify to read again.

Skimming, scanning, and, for some clients, even reading can be done more quickly and comfortably on a computer. Now that EM and computer technology are merging, newer features include the ability to transfer images to a computer and search the document, or even a whole book, by typing in words to match, or have the device read the text aloud. To perform these functions, the EM must convert the image of a page to a file format where letters can be recognized by computer programs, called *optical character recognition* (OCR), is necessary for more advanced computer features discussed later. Once images are digitized by OCR, the EM becomes a computer system. At this time, some newer EMs have HD cameras that are sufficient enough to not only reduce the size of a page so the whole page can be seen on a screen without losing detail, but OCR can be performed too.

Computer Systems

The increasing popularity of the personal computer in the early 1980s was a breakthrough for people who were blind. The first operating systems (eg, MS DOS) displayed text one line at a time in a form that could be easily transmitted to text-to-speech conversion hardware. People who had difficulty reading visually now could read and write as quickly and efficiently as a typically sighted user. The advent of the now-standard graphical user interface (eg, Microsoft Windows, Apple Macintosh) and dependence on the mouse then presented the blind user with a major obstacle to full access to the world of computing. Since the advent of the graphic interface, software developers and computer engineers, many of whom were blind, fought back with innovation and advocacy that encouraged manufacturers of operating system software to make their interface systems accessible. This was true not only for people with visual impairment, but also for those with a variety of other impairments. When tablet computers and smart phones were introduced, Apple built screen magnification and text-to-speech capabilities into their iPad and iPhone. The screen magnification features are limited by the small screen. The text-to-speech feature, called *voiceover* on Apple products, is usually the accessibility feature of choice, even by people with low vision. Because a finger touch is needed to select objects and voice recognition can be used, the new Apple products are more intuitive and do not require touch-typing skills for basic operation. Other tablet computers, e-readers, and smart phone devices have followed, but may not be as fully accessible and should be fully evaluated before recommendations are made. Likewise, apps are not always fully accessible even for the iPad and iPhone.

The personal computer and tablet computer remain the potentially most powerful assistive device to enable a user with any level of vision loss to easily access print and numerical information and to recover inclusive functional written communication. People can read by listening as quickly, comfortably, and efficiently as a typically sighted person. Not only can a user with low vision access e-mail and other information on the Web, but with document readers that are now reasonably inexpensive, the computer user can scan and read printed information with magnification and visual enhancement with screen magnifiers or with speech or braille using a screen reader.

Getting Started

Now that computer systems are so widespread, the therapist must be proficient in adapting these systems for vision impairment. To provide clients with access to these powerful tools, the therapist must learn how to adapt computer systems and operate common assistive equipment, but he or she does not need to become a computer expert. This chapter provides a "getting started guide" to computer assistive systems. The information changes so rapidly that specific instructions and product recommendations would become quickly outdated (we do mention products that have been available for more than 10 years). We will direct the reader to resources where this information can be found and provide recommendations about what to look for when evaluating equipment and software. This chapter will also provide the reader with an overall strategy on how to narrow in on specific equipment, skills, and procedures for using computer-based assistive technology. For the clinic that cannot afford to stock and maintain the expertise to teach all competing products, selection of 1 or 2 preferred systems often is sufficient. Therapists can obtain free demonstration software for evaluation and introductory instruction. Extended instruction on use of the equipment typically is beyond the scope of a low vision service and can be provided by vendors or separate agencies.

Although the vendors of such equipment and instructors have special expertise with computers and the specialized programs and applications, these individuals often do not have special training in low vision rehabilitation and require a collaborating therapist with such training. These instructional and equipment providers require a therapist to set up the equipment and workplace so that the client with low vision can easily read the display. To share the equipment, the collaborating therapist providing vocational rehabilitation might consider working in the same facility with computer instructors and vendors.

Required Equipment and Skills

In typical outpatient, home-based, or workplace-based low vision rehabilitation settings, the therapist needs to be prepared to perform basic evaluation and introductory instruction with affordable equipment and basic skills. The hardware, software, skills, and resources required are listed in Table 14-6. A therapist can avoid the necessity of owning and learning many devices by having just 1 or 2 available. Most clients will depend on the therapist for specific product recommendations. Using the guidelines in this chapter, the therapist should evaluate the different devices available at least once a year and select 1 or 2 of the best products for demonstration and instruction.

As mentioned, carrying electronic devices such as computer monitors presents a problem for therapists providing home-based or workplace-based low vision services. Clients interested in computers usually already own a computer. It is recommended that the therapist have all of the necessary software on his or her own (portable) computer and use that computer for evaluation and demonstration rather than the client's computer. Computer programs for the visually impaired often conflict with other programs and may require special hardware. Loading the software on a client's computer often results in many technical problems.

The therapist, however, usually can easily connect his or her own computer to the client's monitor and keyboard without such problems. If a client wishes to use a program for instruction and home practice, these programs will need to be loaded on the client's own computer. At this stage, the compatibility of the software with the client's computer will be important to consider in evaluating this device. The therapist is advised to refer the client to a vendor who can address installation and compatibility issues.

Minimally necessary equipment and skills include the following (see Table 14-6):

1. An approximately 21- to 26-inch monitor on a stand where height and distance can be adjusted (see Figure 14-7).

2. A laptop computer with headphone jacks, speakers, and scanner.

3. A tablet computer and smart phone (eg, iPad and iPhone).

4. Learn how to use screen enlargement and the basic gestures for the text-to-speech system (eg, VoiceOver). Have a quick reference guide for common gestures for the clients and your own use.

5. Summaries in large print and audio format should be written and saved when a client's computer is adapted describing modifications to common operating systems (versions of Windows, tablet operating system), common web browsers, word processors, and e-mail programs, as well as recommended computer programs. These modifications can be made to a client's computer or a shared computer and saved under a user login name to be automatically recalled later when the user signs onto the computer. These instructions should indicate how to:

   a. Change display font and background colors.

   b. Enlarge icons and print.

   c. Enlarge and change the contrast of print.

   d. Turn text-to-speech systems on and off.

   e. Use other magnification features under accessibility options.

6. Demonstration screen magnifiers (eg, MAGic by Freedom Scientific or Zoom Text by AI Squared). These programs enlarge and enhance text displays much like an EM enlarges printed material. Select a screen magnifier that can be combined with a screen reader or that incorporates screen reading features. Selection depends on availability of product sales and support.

7. Demonstration screen readers (eg, JAWS). These programs read aloud text or numbers displayed on a screen or display the text on a braille display. Many will indicate the position of graphics and even descriptions of

TABLE 14-6: BASIC EQUIPMENT AND SKILLS FOR EVALUATION AND INSTRUCTION WITH PERSONAL COMPUTERS

EQUIPMENT

- An approximately 20- to 26-inch monitor.
- A height- and distance-adjustable monitor stand.
- A laptop computer with speakers, scanner, regular keyboard, popular operating system, Web browser, word processor, and e-mail program.
- A tablet computer with built-in zoom and screen reader.
- Demonstration screen magnification programs.
- Demonstration screen reader programs.
- Demonstration document reader programs.
- Special keyboard that works with the program.

THERAPIST SKILLS

- How to set up operating system with simplified menus and presentation.
- How to set user profiles (names used to log on to an operating system).
- Set accessibility display features of an available operating system, word processor, Web browser, and e-mail system, including:
  - Enlarged icons and text
  - Different and enhanced color contrast
  - Change print spacing if possible
  - Turn on/off text-to-speech features if available
  - Enlarge and enhance the mouse pointer
- Use other magnification features under accessibility options.
- Know how to use the demonstration magnification, screen reader, and document reader program.
- Know how to teach a client to use the basic features of a simplified word processor, e-mail system, text messaging, photo display, and favorite web pages, and to change templates so these programs automatically start with required user settings.

RESOURCES

- A relationship with local vendors and agencies that provide instruction.
- A commitment to continuing education on technology for the visually impaired.

graphics in some cases. Currently, free screen readers are available for those with reading disability that allow a reader with partial vision to highlight text to be read aloud. Windows has recently included a screen reader/magnifier as an accessory to Microsoft Office, available at no additional charge.

8. Demonstration document reader (eg, Kurzweil) software. This includes OCR software and a display enhancement.

9. On the demonstration personal computer that supports different users, create a new user, "Mr. Easy," under the operating system, then remove all icons and features from the operating system except those minimally necessary to operate just the applications a client needs: a word processor, the typing teaching program, the operating system e-mail program, and a simplified Web page. If possible, disable all specialized key combinations that can initiate features unexpectedly if a user strikes the wrong keys. The goal here is to create a close equivalent to a typewriter.

10. Necessary computer skills. The therapist needs to develop the skills and a summary of instructions to introduce a client to a word processor, 1 or 2 demonstration Web pages, and e-mail using the demonstration screen magnifier and screen readers. Focus on one common e-mail program, such as Microsoft Outlook. Avoid Web-based mail systems, as websites are often incompatible with screen readers. Choose sample Web pages with good compatibility and generally high interest value, such as the website for a news source. Web pages for demonstration and instruction can often be duplicated on the hard drive of the therapist's computer so the therapist can avoid problems with Internet access.

11. A template for a written report. The therapist should have a document template that can be completed to describe all of the steps required to set up a system so that a user can see what is on a screen, including necessary optical devices, magnification, screen enhancements, working distance, and ancillary devices such as an adjustable monitor stand. The summaries describing changes to software described earlier can be added to this document. This report is provided to consumers and all instructors working with consumers who depend on the vision therapist to communicate the optimal visual settings.

12. A relationship with a local vendor or agency that provides instruction on use of computer assistive equipment.

13. A commitment to attending continuing education on assistive technology and constantly looking for new products.

Resources

Access World, one of best sources of objective information about assistive technology by and for consumers of these products, is published by the American Foundation for the Blind and available online for no cost (www.afb.org/aw/main.asp). The publication provides product reviews and unbiased information on what's new in computer technology. The following websites are also good sources of information for updated product information:

www.afb.org
www.nfb.org
www.resna.org
www.csun.edu
www.disabilityresources.org

Maintaining updated versions of the software can be costly unless one has demonstration versions that are free. Demonstration software usually is fully operational, but with time limits. There are 2 basic strategies for limiting time. First, the therapist may limit the time a person can access the software to about 30 minutes each time the computer is turned on. This limitation is usually sufficient for evaluation and initial instruction. The second strategy is for the software to run normally for a fixed number of days and then stop functioning. This, of course, is not satisfactory. Therapists are encouraged to contact vendors and manufacturers to provide demonstration versions that can be used by practitioners for evaluation and instruction for more than a limited number of days.

Prerequisite Client Skills and Abilities

Computer assistive devices for the PC continue to be difficult to use, but can be simplified for users. Tablet computer and smart phone screen readers are intuitive to use, but the gestures are complicated and difficult to learn for someone with an apraxia or motor impairment; however, there are accessibility features that allow for customized gestures to be programmed. The key to enabling easy access to computers is to reduce the clutter and limit the options at first to those that most interest the client. Once the client can perform some basic functions comfortably, more options can be added.

Although the tablet and smart phone computers and newer software for the PCs now have excellent speech recognition, touch typing is still needed for efficient use of a computer to write. A potential user with even moderate vision loss must learn to touch type before he or she can use a computer with efficiency. Close working distances in order to see the screen or the keys generally render the "hunt and peck" method impossible. Fortunately, programs like Talking Typing Teacher (MarvelSoft Enterprises, Inc) or Talking Typer (www.aph.org) have been developed that teach people who are blind to type on a computer. Simplified talking word processors are also available. To locate typing programs for the blind, search the Web using the key terms *typing instruction blind* and *word processor blind*. In general, if a person is physically able, typing is preferred to speech recognition software. Detecting and correcting errors that inevitably result from speech recognition is still slower than typing it correctly the first time. These typing programs are actually an excellent way to reintroduce a client to the computer.

As with other devices, the success-oriented approach for the tentative user puts setup at the end of the instructional sequence after basic operation has been mastered. The therapist or a helper should set up the computer at first. Once the PC is set up with assistive software, the setups can be recalled and implemented automatically every time the user logs on to the computer.[6] If the user shares the computer, then a user account must be set up and the client instructed how to sign in. The following steps will enable a client to more easily access a tablet computer or PC:

- The therapist should set up assistive software and save the settings so they are implemented automatically on startup.

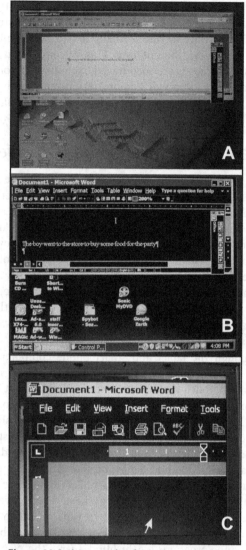

Figure 14-8. An example of a screen magnification program for Windows. Newer tablet computers or operating systems designed for touch screens allow users to use pinch and expand gestures to quickly minify and magnify text, but these have been less reliable in working with all applications.

- Enlarge text and enhance contrast (up to about 2.5× magnification).

- Drag all applications from the desktop and put them in folders, except the applications that a client will use frequently. On versions of Windows with a Start menu, simplify the menu as well.

- Eliminate background pictures—just have a single color to eliminate visual clutter.

- Set up text-to-speech capability to "verbose" where it reads everything if it is available.

- For smart phones and tablets that have shortcuts, teach the client to turn the text-to-speech feature on and off. For example, if using an iPad, it can be

set up so 3 quick presses of the Home key will turn on VoiceOver. A person can use vision and normal gestures to locate text on the screen with minimum magnification and strong reading glasses and then turn on VoiceOver to have it read aloud without learning more complicated gestures.

- Teach the client only gestures or actions needed to perform preferred basic operations.

Screen Magnification Options

Display Enhancement: Mild/Moderate Vision Loss

For those with approximately 20/80 to 20/100 acuity or better who can read 2M print or smaller print fluently at 40 cm (16 inches) (required magnification of less than 10 diopters [D] EP), use of optical devices with a standard operating system is usually sufficient. The user requires an adjustable monitor stand and an ability to touch type. Icons, text, and mouse pointers can be easily enlarged 2× (5 D EP) using standard operating systems (Figure 14-8). These modifications do not change the essential layout of the operating system and are thus easiest to learn. The setup steps are as follows:

- The mouse setup features allow enlarged mouse pointers to be used. An "inverted" feature should be selected so that the pointer automatically changes color on a background to reverse contrast.

- By finding the Accessibility or Ease of Access options in the setup software (in Control Panel in Windows) the operating system can be set to double the size of all text displayed. The accessibility setting also allows various reverse and color contrast settings. The setup features for the display also can be adjusted to provide white on black or any required color contrast. Icons can be enlarged using the display control as well.

- Once set in the operating system, the screen enhancements should automatically apply to the menus of common word processors, spreadsheets, database programs, and Web browsers. If one needs to enlarge the text displayed within the particular program (the text the user is typing in a word processor, for example), the "normal" template must be modified so the view or zoom setting is set to an appropriate magnification. In the View menu, Web browsers can be set to enlarge the print of pages and change contrast of Web pages as well.

- Despite all of these changes, Windows accessibility features are inconsistent—for example, sometimes messages will appear in an unmagnified view. For this reason, the user should always have additional alternative optical magnification devices available that allow seeing normal displays.

- Both Macintosh and Windows operating systems now have separate magnification programs that enlarge everything on the screen to sizes greater than 2×. These may be more convenient to use than changing display characteristics. The primary advantage of changing display characteristics is that the whole screen is visible. Magnification programs like EMs only display part of the screen.

Clients can magnify the screen up to 5 diopters (D) EP or 2× enlargement, but sometimes up to 10 D (4×) will be tolerated. The use of a full-field microscope prescribed by an eye care provider, along with an adjustable monitor stand, will enable the user to sit up straight and bring the monitor closer to the eyes (see Figure 14-7). Because the hands are now obscured by the monitor, touch typing is required. By combining relative distance magnification and operating system enhancements, one can achieve up to 4× to 6× enlargement (10 to 20 EP magnification). Additional screen reader features are available that allow the user to highlight text and have the computer read the text aloud. This same strategy can be used with tablet computers, which are easier to position and handle.

We do not recommend Fresnel magnifiers (magnifiers that adhere to the screen) or optical magnifiers that are positioned in front of the screen. One can achieve the same magnification more easily and inexpensively with a clearer image of the screen with relative distance magnification with a correction for near prescribed by an optometrist.

If a client must use a number of different computers (eg, he or she is a computer support person), the client should have optical devices available that are sufficient to access computers on a regular basis. Examples of such devices are full-field microscopes with hand magnifiers for additional magnification and a telemicroscope if the client is instructing someone or needs to provide hardware repairs.

Display Enhancement: Moderate to Severe Vision Loss

For those requiring more than 2× to 4× enlargement, consider a screen magnification program supplied with the operating system or a separate screen magnifier program like MAGic or ZoomText. The screen magnifier has more additional features than an EM (Table 14-7) but is similar in concept. Beyond 2× magnification, the text is too large to fit on the screen, so just as an EM enlarges a portion of the printed page, screen magnifiers enlarge a portion of the screen (see Figure 14-8). Figure 14-8[A] illustrates a normal view of a Windows desktop, a [B] view with reversed and enhanced contrast and about 2 to 3× magnification, and [C] a view of a magnified and contrast-enhanced portion of the desktop with higher magnification. Note most of the desktop is off the screen. The user uses the mouse to move the desktop much like he or she would move a page under the camera of an electronic magnifier to view the magnified portion. The user must now learn scanning skills, often

---

TABLE 14-7: IMPORTANT PROPERTIES OF SCREEN MAGNIFIERS

- Reliability (most important): the computer does not stop working properly while program is running.
- Ease of use for simple applications such as e-mail and word processing and the programs used by the client.
- Magnification down to 1× and up to 10X.
- Quick and easy magnification adjustment.
- Use with screen reader.
- Quick and easy change from contrast that is best for reading and normal view.
- Script files can be written so setups can be customized for applications.
- Targeting feature: the view can be preset to jump to targets frequently accessed with a keystroke.
- Font modifiability.
- Scroll features.

---

using the mouse or a gesture on a tablet computer to scan the entire screen. As with an EM, scanning can be a time-consuming and difficult skill to master. Screen magnifier programs, unlike EMs, have features that allow one to automatically jump to areas of interest on a screen. For example, with a word processor, one might use a mouse to scan and read a document being typed, but as soon as a letter key is pressed, the screen magnifier will jump to the place in the text where the text is being typed. If a message box appears on the screen, the screen magnifier can be set to automatically jump to the text displayed in the box and then back to where the user was previously reading once the box is closed.

With software that a client uses often, such as database programs, screen magnifiers can be preprogrammed using script programs. When the software is started, the script file will change magnification and display characteristics for that particular software. For example, the script program will assign special control keys so that the user can, with a key press, jump to a particular area on the screen for data entry rather than searching the screen to find it. This is called a *targeting feature*. These are used primarily by clients with vocational goals and require advanced instruction and support beyond the scope of a general low vision service.

Screen magnifier programs have features that can modify text characteristics, such as font type and spacing, to allow the user to more easily read without changing the font of the document being read or written. For example, ZoomText will display the text in a long document in a marquee fashion, scrolling the text from left to right at a preset speed. The reader no longer needs to hunt for the beginning of lines, but can use the steady eye technique to more easily read without moving his or her head or gaze position. This feature can be set up and used for training steady eye technique for people with central field loss (see Chapter 9). Most importantly, several screen magnifiers can be combined with screen readers, allowing users to read and listen to text at the same time. These combined systems are the software of choice for most people with low vision—even moderate vision loss. Table 14-7 lists the important properties of screen magnifiers.

The most important property is reliability and that the program does not stop working unexpectedly. For someone with normal vision, software malfunctions are frustrating but generally obvious. For someone with low vision, it is often difficult to distinguish a software malfunction from a user error.

Text-to-Speech/Braille Software

Once used only by people with profound vision loss or total blindness, the screen reader allows a blind individual to navigate a computer screen, but is now used by people with any level of vision loss or even reading disability. The screen reader reads text and numbers displayed on a screen using computer speech or braille displays. Screen readers might also read entire documents, lines, sentences, or paragraphs at a time at a preset speed so that a user can read a document of several pages. Braille displays are pads that are about twice the length of a spacebar with moveable pins that are usually positioned just under the spacebar. The device in Figure 14-6 can be used as a braille display. The pins, representing braille characters, are raised and correspond to the text displayed on a line on the screen. Special translation software converts text to braille.

Most screen readers work with a mouse, reading whatever text or numbers are displayed where the mouse pointer stops. On touch screen displays, any icon or text someone touches can be read aloud. In general, someone with low vision will use a computer much more efficiently with only keyboard controls, avoiding the mouse as much as possible. Using the keyboard, the user must, therefore, memorize dozens of key combinations that direct the cursor to scan a page horizontally or vertically; jump through text a word, sentence, or paragraph at a time; start reading; read faster or slower; or jump to preset locations in a particular application.

Using only the keyboard, a user can control all of the features and position the cursor on all major operating systems, word processors, spreadsheets, database programs, and Web browsers. The screen reader still reads what is being displayed at the location of the cursor. One needs to

TABLE 14-8: IMPORTANT PROPERTIES OF SCREEN READERS
• Reliability.
• Ease of use for simple, common applications and the applications used by the user.
• The screen reader used with magnifier uses the same controls as a screen reader used alone.
• Quick speed adjustments, repeat reading a line aloud or sentence with a single keystroke.
• Script files and targeting features.
• Web compatibility.
• Compatibility with software applications required by the client, including DOS.
• Full compatibility with common applications such as Outlook, Word, Excel, Internet Explorer, and Access.
• Adobe PDF file compatibility.
• Users do not need to see to set up or use.

search the website for the software manufacturer for this information (a common search phrase is "shortcut keys"). In general, a convention has developed where the control features are listed in text format at the top left of the screen with all programs, starting with "File." One can press the alt key and the underlined or first letter on this menu for keyboard access. For example, holding the alt key down and pressing f followed by a p will open the File menu to the Print screen. The script file and targeting features described earlier for screen magnifiers actually are available from major commercially available screen readers to allow the user to jump the cursor to preset locations with key combinations.

Graphics, graphical icons, and unusual formats in Web pages, documents, and software present a continual challenge to the operation of screen readers. At the very least, screen readers normally announce to the user that it has encountered a graphic or a graphic control. All major programming languages, operating systems, and Web designs now have this feature. Some, unfortunately, have not used it so when a blind user encounters a picture all they hear is "image" rather than a description of the picture. One useful service a therapist might provide is to identify software and websites that are fully accessible by a blind user using a screen reader and put shortcuts to these sites on the desktop. Software is available that checks sites for accessibility. These programs can be found by searching "accessible web sites blind" on the Internet. Of the many features that are most important for the beginning user (Table 14-8), stability remains the most important. Screen readers tend to have the most problems with stability, especially with the Web.

Print Reading Systems

This author recalls in 1975 the first document or print reader (the Kurzweil machine) that could read normal print and cost about $40,000 in 1970s dollars. Developed by a collaboration between Ray Kurzweil and people who were blind, the reader was effective, but slow. Scanners and software are now available for a few hundred dollars, and apps for tablet computers and smart phones have features that convert printed text into speech relatively quickly and for a few dollars. Although the sophisticated visually impaired client can use the inexpensive systems, commercial scanners were not developed with blind users in mind and thus are often difficult to access with screen readers. Several manufacturers currently sell programs that work on standard PCs. Document readers are also sold as standalone products that are specifically designed for users with low or no vision and are easier to use than computer-based systems. Inevitably, document readers make mistakes and sometimes do not read print in the correct sequence when textbooks or documents have multiple columns. The systems designed for the blind user allow errors to be avoided or more easily corrected. Standalone systems are more expensive, but are easier to use and more stable than systems designed to work with conventional computers. Most recently, EMs include document readers or remote cameras that connect to computers and have sufficient resolution for OCR. The features that are most important for successful use by the beginner are summarized in Table 14-9.

Recordings for the Blind and Sighted Readers

The NLS, formerly the National Library for the Blind and Physically Handicapped, is a federally funded agency that provides recordings or braille transcriptions of current novels and magazines to users who cannot read because of visual, physical, or cognitive disability. Reading Ally (formerly known as Recordings for the Blind, or RFB) is a private agency that provides a similar service for little or no fee. Reading Ally more often provides textbooks and teaching materials (www.readingally.org). Many countries have these services.

The technology involved in presenting recordings of books and magazines is rapidly changing. In 2005, recordings were generally available on audiotape cassettes that were specially formatted to store twice as much as conventional cassettes. Special players are required; these are generally available for free from NLS. Now NLS record the books digitally. These players use a single cassette that stores the entire book digitally and are easy to use and have excellent sound quality. The books can be ordered by mail or downloaded. The players have features that allow the

TABLE 14-9: IMPORTANT PROPERTIES OF DOCUMENT READERS
• Reliability.
• Ease of use for the reluctant client.
• Low error frequency even with poor-quality print and unpredictable formats (evaluation with a newspaper is recommended).
• Low error frequency if original is not aligned properly.
• Fast image processing, with scanners that automatically feed multiple pages, is very helpful.
• For low vision users, items can be read aloud while documents, charts, and figures are simultaneously viewed with screen magnification.

user to skip to specific chapters and to place and jump to bookmarks as well. The NLS provides a player and books to rehabilitation providers who can then authorize access to this service and demonstrate and teach clients how to use these devices and order books. Normally, one needs to only quickly show a user features in a few minutes. People reading the Bible, magazines, or books for research appreciate the advanced player that has controls to place and return to bookmarks and advance one chapter or article at a time. Cognitively impaired clients should use the simpler player without these controls. Teaching a cognitively impaired user to use the player involves the following steps:

1. Start with operation of the power on and play buttons.

2. Teach the sleep button that turns off after a time (the default is 15 minutes) so the playing will stop if someone falls asleep. Then teach holding down the rewind button, rewinding 15 minutes.

3. Teach use of the Fast-forward tabs.

Digital talking books, available from RFB and commercial sources and other private suppliers, use CDs or flash drives to store both a recording by a reader (as opposed to computer speech) and a digital transcription of the material. With digital talking books, the user can much more easily scan the recording for specific phrases or terms. The user must acquire special CD players or software that can be installed on any PC to use this technology. iPhones, iPods, and other MP3 players are able to store music, audio books, podcasts, and radio broadcasts that can be downloaded from the Web to play on demand.

Personal Organizers and Other Devices

As mentioned, blind users used personal organizers before they became widely used by those with typical vision. These devices essentially are keyboards. Instead of a display, the device uses text-to-speech features played through standard earphones. Some models have special keyboards and displays for braille users as well. Talking cell phones, talking global positioning devices, and echolocation devices that use sound to indicate obstacles are available as well (see Figure 14-6).

EVALUATION

Computer systems should be considered assistive devices as well as adaptations for those who aspire to use computers as a performance goal. As a general rule, clients for whom an EM would be seriously considered for a reading or writing goal might benefit from adapted computer systems as well. For those with reading and writing goals that do not necessarily involve computers, evaluation of clients for use of assistive computer systems is virtually identical to the evaluation performed for the EM, except one tends to avoid computer systems if users have lower frustration tolerance or decreased problem-solving ability because of inherent unreliability. Many just dislike this technology and wish to avoid it.

Computers should be considered for clients who must engage in writing more than is required for activities of daily living. Word processing is often easier than handwriting for those with moderate vision loss, especially if they already can touch type or have incoordination impairment or arthritis. People with vocational goals involving extensive reading and writing, data processing, searching for information, and virtually anyone working at a desk will benefit from assistive computer systems. In addition, therapists should perform an evaluation of people with mild vision loss who have included computer use in their performance goals.

Computer systems are similar to EMs in the following ways:

- Evaluate reading performance with text-to-speech capability vs reading vs both.
- Evaluation of other physical requirements relevant to ergonomics.
- Evaluation of cognitive capability. The client requires good frustration tolerance and some level of trial-and-error problem solving. Don't rule out computers for people with cognitive disability. Computer systems are routinely used successfully for many with developmental disabilities and can be adapted for cognitive impairment as well.

Instructional Strategies

In general, instruction with computer systems depends on the specific configuration provided and is beyond the scope of this text. Some general strategies for the more reluctant user are as follows:

- Choose systems primarily on the basis of stability. Nothing is more frustrating to a beginning user than when a computer stops working and the user cannot tell if he or she made a mistake or if it is a "system error."
- The first skills to learn are how to start and restart a computer. The user should be taught "escape strategies"—how to return to a comfortable, familiar place in the computer, such as the Start menu, if the computer starts doing the unexpected.
- Do not begin with instructions on setup. Often setup can be automated so that when the client signs onto the computer as a user, the assistive programs start and configure automatically, and the desktop will appear in a familiar format. Once the therapist determines the optimum setup, this information can be stored and transferred to another computer with the help of a computer-savvy assistant.
- Begin with a typing instruction program (Talking Typing Teacher or Talking Typer) if necessary, then a simplified word processor, and then to e-mail.
- Use optical devices and modifications in operating system software if possible with clients with milder vision loss, rather than special screen magnifiers or screen readers.
- Remove all icons from the desktop. Place applications frequently used on the top of the Start menu. See the Help menu for the operating system for instructions on how to do this.
- Have available a simplified computer for demonstration using a different name (Mr. Easy) for evaluation and initial instruction.

ACCESSORIES AND ERGONOMICS

A visually impaired student, worker, or leisure participant using a computer system or EM will be moving the head a lot more than a typically sighted user and is thus at risk for repetitive strain injury. When recommending electronic systems, the therapist must use a variety of methods to enable good ergonomics (see Table 14-7). The use of a monitor stand is the most important. The workspace should be set up so that the user can switch quickly among all of the devices that must be used. For example, a user providing customer service by telephone needs to easily access the telephone, so a headset is essential. Someone using an optical device to read documents requires a task light and workspace for visual reading. Someone typing from print might require the magnified view of the original positioned to be read with good posture with a reading stand or EM. The corner of a corner desk with a swivel chair allows one to avoid lateral back movement. Split-screen EMs also have a feature where the user can switch between the EM and computer display with a foot switch, allowing one to copy without moving the head (see Figure 14-7).

Another configuration involves having the computer read the typed material aloud while the client is reading visually. This is an excellent strategy for the beginning typist. Glare is often a problem in a large office area. A privacy screen positioned in front of the monitor allows only the person directly in front of the monitor to see what is displayed without decreasing the light from the display. This is the best method to eliminate glare and allows for privacy for someone who is displaying a magnified image on the screen.

SUMMARY AND VIEW OF THE FUTURE

The tablet computer and smart phone are revolutionizing assistive technology for those with vision impairments. What were once expensive and difficult add-ons are now being built into the basic operation of this technology. The demand for multitasking and using devices while driving encourages the development of voice-control and text-to-speech capabilities for everyone, not just people with disabilities. Moreover, the cost of these devices is starting to decrease to where EMs are replacing optical devices. Another trend is for EMs (CCTVs) to merge with computers, so in a few years EMs will have all of the capability of a personal computer. Once familiarity with assistive technology was a specialized practice for providers of low vision and blindness rehabilitation services; today, all low vision therapists need to be familiar with this technology at a basic level. The challenge faced by the provider of low vision services is to keep abreast of this technology. Optical devices should always be considered with assistive technology. The client should have a near-vision-only (not bifocal) correction for the eye to screen distance with good ergonomics. Secondly, the client should have backup magnification when the computer system is not working properly.

Finally, one unfortunate consequence of emerging technology has been an apparent decline in human-to-human contact that for all of us is most important. For the older, often lonely, client who has recently lost vision, a friend reading the newspaper or helping read mail provides so much more than the achievement of efficient reading performance.

REFERENCES

1. Hensil J, Whittaker SG. Comparing visual reading versus auditory reading by sighted persons and persons with low vision. *J Vis Impairment Blindness*. 2000;94:762-770.
2. Smallfield S, Clem K, Myers A. Occupational therapy interventions to improve the reading ability of older adults with low vision: a systematic review. *Am J Occup Ther*. 2013;67:288-295.
3. Watson GR, Ramsey V, De L'Aune W, Elk A. Ergonomic enhancement for older readers with low vision. *J Vis Impairment Blindness*. 2004;98:228-240.
4. Lund R, Watson GR. *The CCTV Book: Habilitation and Rehabilitation With Closed Circuit Television Systems*. Froland, Norway: Synsforum ans.; 1997.
5. Wright V, Watson GR. *Learn to Use Your Vision for Reading (LUV Reading Series)*. Lilburn, GA: Bear Consultants; 1996.
6. Whittaker SG, Young T, Toth-Cohen S. Universal tailored access: automating setup of public and classroom computers. *J Vis Impairment Blindness*. 2002;96:448-451.

IV

Occupational Performance

15

Reading and Writing

READING

Ms. Tuttle, a 94-year-old, loved to read sitting in her recliner by the window, starting with the newspaper in the morning, then the mail, her prayer book, and then a novel later in the afternoon. This had been a routine for over 10 years, that is, until she could no longer see the print because of atrophic macular degeneration. Ms. Tuttle claimed she could still read, but it was just too hard.

Jerry, a first-year college student, was diagnosed with a progressive juvenile macular degeneration at age 16. As his vision slowly declined, Jerry compensated by bringing the print closer to his eyes. He had figured out how to adapt his iPad tablet computer, his iPhone, and his Windows PC, but found himself sitting closer and closer to the screen and reading slower. His vision teacher in high school had recommended various devices, which he had rejected because he was concerned about appearances, but now in college Jerry was falling further and further behind in his assignments. He had always been a straight-A student and was quite distressed. He wanted to go to law school.

People with low vision often present upon initial evaluation with performance goals that involve reading. The visual requirements and performance demands of a reading activity vary considerably depending on the particular task.

Reading a medicine bottle, finding the total on a credit card invoice, finding the departure time on a bus schedule, meditating on a familiar passage in the Koran alone during morning prayer, reading the Torah in Hebrew in front of synagogue, locating a sign on the street corner, and enjoying the latest Tom Clancy novel involve substantially different assistive devices, motor skills, and visual demands. School systems, state offices of vocational rehabilitation, and medical insurance companies recognize literacy as medically, vocationally, and educationally necessary. Not surprisingly, reading has become the cornerstone therapeutic activity in a treatment plan for a variety of visual impairments and performance goals. Reading is so often the focus of treatment because the skills transfer to other tasks as well.

Although reading is almost universally identified as a visual task, successful rehabilitation requires the therapist to move beyond the process of typical reading to appreciate the meaning of reading as an "occupation" to each individual. Ms. Tuttle and Jerry both wish to read books and had similar levels of vision impairment, but will require very different interventions because of context, task demand, roles, expectations, and a willingness to try new things. The act of reading might be viewed as purely functional, the process of transmitting information from

Whittaker SG, Scheiman M, Sokol-McKay DA.
Low Vision Rehabilitation: A Practical Guide for Occupational Therapists,
Second Edition (pp 281-300).
© 2016 Taylor & Francis Group.

the printed page into the brain. From this functional perspective, whether the reader uses vision, hearing, or touch to "read" becomes less significant. A person can acquire the information printed in a newspaper visually with an optical device, tactilely using a braille transcription, listening to someone read, or as auditory reading using a computer equipped with a screen reader that reads Web pages aloud. For students like Jerry and those employed with productivity demands, people who want to read quickly, the most efficient solution often is text-to-speech. For others like Ms. Tuttle, however, the performance goal might focus on the process. How one reads a spiritual text often becomes a focus in religious ritual, as with unison recitations in a church or synagogue, the reading by a young man during his bar mitzvah, or the recitation of the Divine Office by a priest. Productivity might be less important than the process, or *how* we read. In this case, treatment planning should consider the process as well as speed and efficiency of information acquisition.

First-Response Interventions

Tailoring goals and treatment to a client's long-term needs and occupations usually requires a thorough evaluation and a thoughtful treatment plan involving optical devices, electronic devices, and environmental modifications. A therapist who does not specialize in low vision rehabilitation will rarely encounter "low vision" as a primary diagnosis. More often, the therapist will identify low vision in a person with multiple disabilities, or an older individual being treated for medical or orthopedic problems. A person with typical age-related vision loss may be disabled by glare or poor lighting often typical in a home environment. For example, some years previously a home therapist working with Ms. Tuttle after a hip replacement first identified that the client was struggling with reading based on a visual screening. The therapist also performed the initial evaluation and first-response intervention, which basically involved improved lighting that enabled her to read her home exercise program as well as her other reading materials. This therapist made certain Ms. Tuttle's optometrist was aware of the problem, and the doctor prescribed slightly stronger reading glasses as well.

Chapter 1 provides the therapist with the tools to screen for and initially evaluate vision disability. For most, a sudden loss of the ability to read presents immediate problems that need to be quickly solved. The therapist might suddenly find that a client cannot read written instructions or engage in a variety of therapeutic activities because of a vision disability. A person who loves to read will be cut off from his or her favorite leisure activity, often in a hospital setting when there is not much else to do except watch TV. The person may be cut off from use of a telephone or e-mail and messaging on his or her cell phone. The first-response evaluation in Chapter 1 is designed to provide quick

solutions while a client waits for advanced low vision rehabilitation. The first-response evaluation, however, includes the basic elements of the more advanced evaluation and treatment by the eye care provider and low vision therapist. A client who requires first-response interventions should be referred for advanced treatment that typically involves optical and electronic devices as well as specialized training procedures.

- **Impaired reading acuity.** The first-response intervention is to enlarge the text and optimize the lighting to enable reading.

  - If, with optimal light and glare reduction, a person can read 2M or smaller fluently on the reading acuity chart, then using large-print books and materials is an easy solution. Recall that we multiply 2M by 8 to convert this number to 16 *point*, which is a term used by printers and word processors to describe font size. Large-print books are published at 16- to 18-point fonts. These print sizes can be easily achieved with e-readers and tablet computers, and setting larger fonts on a PC as well. In younger individuals like Jerry who can focus their eyes at close distances, holding something closer can improve vision, although this might cause eye strain. Younger people should be referred for a vision evaluation even though they can apparently read without difficulty.

  - If a person can read print smaller than about 8M (64 point), the therapist can use larger fonts or a dark bold line marking pen for written instructions, but normally sized written material generally will need to be read aloud. If a person is still struggling or requires greater than 2M font, then National Library Service (NLS) or Learning Ally, formerly Recordings for the Blind and Dyslexic (RFB&D) should be ordered for leisure reading, or someone should read aloud to the client.

  - For marking and labeling, large lettering or color coding can be used even with acuities worse than 8M. Telephone dialing or use of a call system can be done by feel or marking the buttons.

  - Newer smart phone and tablet computers have built-in features that read everything displayed aloud. Optical devices, even handheld magnifiers, require a prescription from an eye care practitioner (Chapter 14).

- **Impaired contrast sensitivity, glare sensitivity, and lighting needs.**

  - A dark, bold print for marking items such as medication bottles will enhance contrast.

  - If contrast sensitivity and reading acuity improve when glare is eliminated by carefully positioning a light source to the client's side during testing, and teaching a client how to avoid glare by positioning their body or using a hat with a brim.

- ○ If adjusting lighting by changing the distance of the light significantly affects contrast sensitivity and reading acuity, then instruction on controlling light levels is indicated. Most strategies described in Chapter 12 to modify lighting can be used as first-response interventions and are especially effective in older individuals with mild age-related vision loss.

- **Field loss.**

  - ○ A recent central field loss usually severely impacts reading until a person learns eccentric viewing (looking above or below the text being viewed) (see Chapter 10). If it is a barrier to reading, then a client will miss words or letters even when the print is enlarged. Using text-to-speech on electronic devices, using recorded books, and a friend reading aloud provide the most immediate chance of success. For written instructions, "supersizing" the print often will enable visual reading, as the print will outsize the smaller central blind spot (scotoma).

  - ○ Peripheral field loss from stroke, especially field loss that includes the central visual field, is well within the scope of practice of a general occupational therapist. Since reading is an important therapeutic activity, the occupational therapist is advised to learn advanced treatment strategies in Chapter 11 about field loss, which provides detailed strategies for the recovery of visual reading. Otherwise, extended reading on tablet computers or personal computers can be immediately achieved using text-to-speech applications. For the PC, inexpensive or free applications allow a person to navigate visually, a valuable therapeutic activity, and then highlight text to be read aloud.

- **Oculomotor impairment.** Often people with vision problems from concussion and traumatic brain injury also have developed impaired oculomotor control. While waiting for an evaluation and treatment recommendations by a neuro-optometrist or neuro-ophthalmologist, the occupational therapists might try occluding one eye during reading to eliminate double vision, or if there are limitations in the range of eye movement, have the client hold the reading material in front of the eye and then scroll the text from right to left in front of the eye. Most people will naturally position their heads to optimize vision, resulting in an abnormal head position. By repositioning the target or reading material, the therapist might be able to get the head into a more ergonomically appropriate position. If any of these strategies are effective, the findings should be sent to the consulting eye care providers.

TABLE 15-1: STEPS FOR READING REHABILITATION

EVALUATION

- Determine reading context (lighting, glare, seating, ergonomics).
- Determine font characteristics and availability of alternative media (braille and recordings).
- Ascertain reading task demand (duration, rate, comprehension requirements).
- Consider and present available nonvisual options to client.
- Evaluate visual requirements for reading: identify performance-limiting factors to address in treatment.
- Evaluate reading performance.

TREATMENT (IF VISUAL REQUIREMENTS CAN BE MET)

- Address performance-limiting factors:
  - ○ Inadequate acuity reserve—use assistive devices.
  - ○ Inadequate contrast reserve—use assistive devices.
  - ○ Central field loss and compensatory scanning strategies.
  - ○ Provide initial instruction under idealized settings.
  - ○ Transition to natural context and perform necessary environmental modifications.

Advanced Reading Evaluation

Overview

Since reading is the most common goal addressed in low vision rehabilitation, we will elaborate on the theoretical basis for the treatment strategies to equip the therapist with the skills for creative problem solving for his or her clients. The steps for evaluation and treatment for reading rehabilitation are summarized Table 15-1. The evaluation begins with consideration of the context in which the reading will occur, and the instruction ends in this natural context. If one does not consider context, a successful demonstration of good reading performance in the "ideal" clinic will not carry over into the home or workplace. The evaluation of context begins with the physical and social settings. Then one considers the font characteristics of the reading material and availability in other media. Is the material available in large print or as an audio recording? Next one considers

TABLE 15-2: TYPICAL PRINT SIZES AND ACUITY REQUIREMENTS[6]				
TEXT SIZE ONLY M SCALE IS STANDARDIZED			**SAMPLE**	**TEXT ACUITY USUALLY REQUIRED**
N scale (points)	*Jaeger (J)*	*M scale*	*Approximate; point size varies with font type*	
3 pt	J1	0.4M	NORMAL acuity threshold at 40 cm	
4 pt	J2	0.5M		
5 pt	J3	0.6M	Ads, bibles	0.3
6 to 8 pt	J5	0.8 M	Telephone book	0.4
8 to 10 pt	J7	1.0 M	Newspaper	0.5
10 to 12 pt	J9	1.25M	Magazines, books, computer	0.6
12 to 14 pt	J11	1.6M	Books, typewriter	0.8
16 to 18 pt	J13	2.0 M	Child and large print	1.0
18 to 20 pt	J14	2.5M	Large print	1.2

the task demand. Does the client need to read a few words on a label, or can he or she read more slowly while relaxing and enjoying a novel? Does a lawyer or a student like Jerry need to scan and read hundreds of pages all day long? The therapist performs a functional vision evaluation and, with the help of a consulting low vision optometrist, decides if the visual requirements for reading can be met and, if so, what options are most appropriate. The evaluation identifies the nonvisual and visual barriers. Then the various options are discussed with the client, who participates in the treatment plan.

In a case like Ms. Tuttle, where a client might not fully understand the options and outcomes, the success-oriented approach is used to demonstrate first and discuss and choose later, starting with the options that are most likely to enable goal performance. It is usually advisable to start with the nonvisual options first, as text-to-speech options often are the easiest to implement. The use of sighted assistants or NLS can quickly enable the goal task while the more difficult rehabilitation of visual reading is undertaken. Ms. Tuttle ordered a free Bible in digital format to play on her NLS digital talking book player (visit www.audiobibles-fortheblind.org for alternative formats and languages). The evaluation should predict the devices, magnification, lighting, and adaptive techniques that are most likely to succeed. Instruction begins out of context, in a setting where ergonomics and visual conditions can be carefully controlled to more easily remove these barriers so the client can experience successful performance, then moved to the person's preferred context like a favorite chair.

Context

The therapist should first determine where each goal reading task will be performed, such as reading price tags in a grocery store, reading a novel in a favorite chair in

the living room, or managing medications at a table in the kitchen. Instruction should begin on a table that encourages good posture and support for the upper body that is required for finely controlled movement of text, optical devices, and the head. The use of a table also allows for easy repositioning of a directional task light. During this phase, the therapist must reassure the client that the task will eventually be adapted to his or her preferred habitual context. As the therapist transitions from the ideal setting to the habitual setting, the client will become aware of the effects environmental changes have on reading ability. For example, a client might be reluctant to move the chair so that it does not face a window when initially suggested. However, once the client has experienced more comfortable reading in the clinic with appropriate directional lighting from the side, she or he may be more open to repositioning the chair at home. Evaluation of context should include attention to lighting and potential glare sources, the potential for mounting reading stands or assistive positioning devices, and ergonomics. Often, optical devices for reading are more easily used if the client stabilizes the material being read and the upper body on a table. In the case of students like Jerry, or for many professionals, their physical environments often change, so they need to develop good problem solving and be equipped with adaptable tools.

Font Characteristics and Availability of Alternative Media

Once goals for treatment of reading problems have been developed, the occupational therapist should establish the media and formats in which the reading material is available (Table 15-2). For example, most bills, checks, legal documents, and many magazines and books are available in large (2M or 16- to 18-point) print. Often, financial information may be available in nonvisual formats. For example, telephone companies and utilities must provide information by phone at no additional charge if a client can certify his or her disability. Automated teller machines (ATMs) have jacks for headphones so users can hear as well as see the display.

Books, magazines, and daily newspapers are available in braille, on tape, or on CD by services such as Learning Ally and the NLS. Learning Ally has a membership fee which can be waived based on financial burden; NLS services are free. Radio reading services read the newspaper and other publications according to a consistent schedule, while NFB-Newsline is a free resource that allows users to listen to the newspaper when they want to and at their own pace. For the many newspapers available, visit www.nfb.org/audio-newspaper-service. The user navigates through the newspaper via the telephone number pad and has the ability to bookmark his or her place; however, the voice is robotic and may be problematic for the hearing impaired or non-English-speaking client. Major newspapers and magazines are available on the Web and are accessible by Web browsers equipped with software that reads the display aloud, magnifies the print, and improves contrast.

Font characteristics must be considered. Print size is expressed in N notation (points) or M notation. The M scale refers to the test distance in meters, where the lowercase letter (eg, x or m) with no descender like p or y subtends 5 minutes of arc on the retina—approximately the distance where the print is barely seen with normal vision. N notation refers to the printer's standard for sizing print, where 1 point equals 1/72 of an inch; however, the actual print size in points varies from font to font because it dates to the days when lead type was set and refers to the slug size, not the letter itself. Mehr and Fried's[1] survey of fonts found N8 (8 pt) lowercase and N5 (5 pt) uppercase to be approximately equivalent to 1M. Print characteristics also influence reading.

Font characteristics include type of font (eg, Times New Roman, Arial), font size, boldness, spacing between characters, and spacing between lines. Font characteristics significantly affect the visibility of individual letters (Figure 15-1). Unfortunately, the earliest research on the effects of font characteristics on visibility of print did not report how distance was controlled, if at all. Controlled research has revealed one general finding: increasing letter spacing increases the visibility of individual letters.[2-5] Different font types can be categorized as serif and sans serif (no serif). Serifs are little enhancements in letters. The text in this book is printed with a serif font; the section headings use a sans serif font. The effects of using serif vs sans serif fonts have not been found to consistently affect the visibility of print, although as with the use of colored filters, we have found strong individual preferences. Figure 15-1 also demonstrates how the same size font (in points) can have different visibility by varying font characteristics.

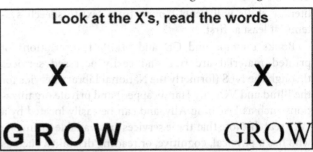

Figure 15-1. Fixate the Xs and attempt to read the word below. Font characteristics in san serif (Arial Bold) with heavy stroke width and increased print spacing (left) are more visible than with regular serif font type (Times New Roman) and typical spacing.

Tablet computers, smart phones, and personal computer systems have screen magnification applications or features that allow font size, type, and contrast to be modified (see Chapter 14). APHont is a font specifically designed for persons with low vision and is available for free through the American Printing House for the Blind at www.aph.org/products/aphont/.

Reading Task Demand

The visual requirements for reading vary depending on the fluency demands.[6] The performance goal might be categorized as spot, low-fluency, and high-fluency reading. Reading a few words such as a label or short passage requires spot reading—reading about 40 words per minute (wpm). Reading a longer passage such as a letter or instructions requires fluent reading of 80 wpm (low fluency). Highly fluent reading of 160 wpm is an average sixth-grade reading rate. A student would be expected to achieve normal reading rates of approximately 250 wpm or greater.[7]

One must consider the required reading rate, endurance, and comfort. Reading for pleasure requires that a person read comfortably for a relatively long time, requiring endurance. Speed is an individual preference. Students and many professionals often also need to read for long periods and at speeds consistent with normal visual reading. Some may need to skim and scan for critical information, such as a purchasing agent scanning Web pages for products. Others may wish to read slowly and carefully, such as an actor memorizing lines or someone reading poetry. People, even older individuals with moderate hearing loss, can read from slower to normal reading rates, quickly and comfortably, with text-to-speech (listening to someone with normal vision or a computer read a newspaper).[8]

Nonvisual Options

For someone with vision impairment, fast, comfortable "reading" is usually easily achieved by listening to passages being read. Sighted readers should be considered if the client is socially isolated. People with long-standing visual impairment often have not read for a long time and have lost basic literacy skills from disuse. People with poor literacy skills will benefit more from text-to-speech systems, at least at first.

Books on tape and CD and braille transcriptions of printed material are free and easily accessed services through the NLS (formerly the National Library Service for the Blind and Visually Handicapped) and private organizations such as Learning Ally, and can be easily located by a Web search. Note that these services are available to anyone who has a physical, cognitive, or reading disability, such as dysexia, that might prevent visual reading. Special players are required to play the recorded books, which are distributed by mail or via the Internet.

Sometimes clients resist recorded books, especially if this option has been presented later in a session after a visual option has been less successful. For this reason, we at least mention recorded books before visual options are attempted. Resistant clients can be reminded that normally sighted people often listen to books on CD, and these options can be used as an addition to visual reading, not a substitution.

Although the focus of this book is on vision rehabilitation with people who have usable vision, federal law requires that one consider nonvisual options such as braille for younger people who are unlikely to acquire fluent reading visual. Braille reading has become an important rite of passage into the culture of the blind. The goal of associations and federations of the blind is to fortify people who have "different" rather than "low" vision with a network of friends, leisure activities, employment opportunities, and a sense of pride. Introduction of braille to a client requires specialized certification as a certified vision rehabilitation therapist or a certified teacher of the blind/visually impaired. The occupational therapist, however, should have a sample of the braille alphabet and numbers in order to assess whether a client with hand impairment or cognitive impairment might have the capacity to learn braille. Hadley School for the Blind has the following sequential braille courses: (1) Tactile Readiness, (2) Learning the braille Alphabet, (3) Uncontracted/grade braille, and (4) Contracted braille/grade 2. These courses are free and good for the independent learner. Braille is typically read by lightly moving the fingertips over the raised braille dots, moving left to right, and primarily using the index fingertip to "read" and the 2nd and 3rd fingertips to maintain one's place and increase speed. . Good tactile sensitivity and stereognosis are required. Very adept braille readers read with both hands simultaneously.

Advanced Evaluation of Visual Requirements

The evaluation by an eye care provider (see Chapter 7) and functional vision therapy evaluation (see Chapter 8) should provide sufficient information to accurately estimate optimal light, magnification, and type of device with a minimum of trial and error. When working in the practice model, described in earlier chapters, in which an occupational therapist works along with a low vision optometrist, magnification for reading may have already been recommended for a client. What follows is a brief review with a focus on special considerations for a reading assessment. The therapist must know or measure the reading acuity, letter contrast sensitivity, and visual fields in order to undertake reading rehabilitation (see Chapters 7 and 8).

Visual Acuity and Critical Print Size Assessment

Reading speed with different print sizes should be measured with this prescribed device using a reading acuity test such as the MNREAD[9] (see Chapter 8). If, after training, the device does not provide the predicted magnification (see Chapter 13), or if visual acuity tends to fluctuate, as it does with diabetes, then reading acuity and critical print size should be re-evaluated.

When the therapist evaluates functional reading with a properly designed continual text reading test (see Chapter 8), the evaluation should give the following information:

- Maximum reading rate with size magnification alone. This is the expected reading rate with a magnification device.

- Critical print size(s). This is the smallest print or range of print sizes that produces the most fluent comfortable reading. Print size is in M units, and test distance is specified in centimeters, as well as whether reading is optimal with one eye occluded or both eyes.

- Reading acuity threshold. This is the smallest print that can be read.

Instruction should begin with print that is a line or two above critical print size. If a properly designed reading chart is not available, or if a patient has reading difficulty for nonvisual reasons, critical print size can be estimated as 3 lines above the print size at acuity threshold[10]; however, either method of estimating critical print size can vary considerably, so the best strategy is to use an appropriate chart and both the direct method and 3-line-above-acuity-threshold estimation methods.

Contrast Threshold Assessment

For reading, contrast sensitivity should be measured with a letter contrast chart. For functional reading testing, the most relevant results are measured with the test distance chosen so that letter size is at about 2× to 4× acuity threshold (see Chapter 8). Table 15-3 indicates the contrast of typical reading that we have measured in a survey and the contrast threshold requirements to read these different materials. In the cases of more advanced atrophic macular degeneration, glaucoma, or diabetes, often contrast

TABLE 15-3: TYPICAL PRINT CONTRAST AND CONTRAST THRESHOLD REQUIREMENTS[6]			
CONTRAST THRESHOLD REQUIREMENTS			
Text Contrast of Reading Material	*Uses*	*Severe Loss* *(10:1 Contrast Reserve) Cannot Fully Compensate*	*Moderate Loss* *Can Usually Fully Compensate With Optimized Lighting*
>95%	Computer and CCTV display with no reflections	Greater than 10% contrast threshold	5% to 10% contrast threshold
85% to 95%	Good quality print	Greater than 8% contrast threshold	4% to 8% contrast threshold
60% to 70%	Newsprint, telephone directory, paperback books	Greater than 5% contrast threshold	2.5% to 5% contrast threshold
50%	Cash register receipts, US paper money	Greater than 2.5% contrast threshold	1.2% to 5% contrast threshold

sensitivity is impaired as well as acuity, indicating a need for higher-contrast print and careful evaluation of lighting.

Assessment of Field of View

The field of view is critical for reading. Indeed, it has been argued that field of view, the number of characters a person can see in one glance, is the primary visual limiting factor.[11,12] One of the best ways to evaluate how field loss impacts reading is to observe the pattern of reading errors. Clients with a restricted right field of view will tend to spell words or hesitate or omit the end of longer words, or miss the last letters on a line when reading a near visual acuity chart. People with left field restrictions will tend to miss the first words on lines or the beginning of words. Those with inconsistent fixation, such as someone with a central scotoma who has not developed stable eccentric viewing, will miss different parts of words or words almost at random. The Pepper Visual Skills for Reading Test[13] and SKREAD[14] were designed to enable users to measure reading speed with different word lengths and score errors to estimate field restrictions and scanning problems. With a cooperative client, field of view can be directly measured by having the client tell how many letters can be seen when looking at the first letter of the word or end of a word. It is important to select the font size the client intends to read.

The Visual Requirements for Reading

The visual requirements for each reading rate depend on both the client's visual function and characteristics of the print. For example, for spot reading, the print size needs only to be about one line on an acuity chart above acuity threshold. If someone wants to read at a highly fluent level, print needs to be at least 2 to 3 times acuity threshold, close to critical print size. Acuity reserve is a ratio of the actual print size being read divided by the print size at threshold. Typically, if a person with 20/20 acuity (0.4/0.4) reads 1M size newsprint, the print is 2:5 times acuity threshold. This is called a 2.5:1 acuity reserve. A 2:1 acuity reserve means that the print size is twice the threshold. If someone with low vision can barely read regular newsprint, he or she likely has an acuity threshold of 1M (8 point) at 40 cm (16 inches); reading large print, 2M (16 point), provides an acuity reserve of 2:1, usually sufficient for fluent reading (see Table 15-2). If a logarithmic acuity chart is used, reserve can be specified more simply in terms of lines on the chart. With a 2:1 acuity reserve, a person is reading a print size that is 3 lines above threshold. Table 15-2 indicates the acuity reserve requirements for different reading rates. It indicates an approximation of the visual acuity requirements to read different common print sizes. In general, someone can read slowly and with difficulty print that is either at threshold or one line above acuity threshold. If a client needs to read fluently, the print size should be at least 3 lines or more above threshold, or a 2:1 acuity reserve. Critical print size is generally 3 to 4 lines above acuity threshold—twice acuity threshold plus a line.[10] We have found significant individual differences, however, with some individuals requiring more acuity reserve and some less acuity reserve and recommend critical print size be directly measured by changes in reading rate as well. Critical print size can then be transformed into equivalent power, indicating the magnification required for maximum reading rate (see Chapters 6, 8, and 10).

Not everyone can read fluently with magnification alone. Adequate contrast and field of view are necessary as well. Table 15-3 indicates the contrast threshold required for different reading rates. For fluent reading, print contrast must be at least 10 times contrast threshold (>10:1). For reading high-quality print with about 90% contrast, contrast threshold must be better than 9%. With print contrast

TABLE 15-4: THE VISUAL REQUIREMENTS FOR READING[6]

THE VISUAL REQUIREMENTS FOR VARIOUS READING RATES

Visual Factor		Reading Rates		
	Spot (40 wpm)	Low Fluency (80 wpm)	High Fluency (160 wpm)	Maximum (normal 250 wpm)
Acuity Reserve	1:1 (0 lines)	1.25:1 (1 line)	1.5 to 2.5:1 (2 to 4 lines)	2:1 to 3:1 (3 to 5 lines)
Contrast Reserve	3:1	4:1	10:1	>30:1
Field of View	1 character	2 to 5 characters	5 to 6 characters	16 to 20 characters
Scotoma Size	No limit defined	<22°	<4°	No scotoma

Adapted from Whittaker SG, Lovie-Kitchin JE. Visual requirements for reading. *Optom Vis Sci.* 1993;70:54-65

enhanced closer to 100% with an electronic magnifier (EM), print contrast threshold can be as high as 10%.

A surprising finding in our review of the research on vision and reading is that people can read fluently with a rather narrow 5- to 6-character field of view.[6,12] This assumes that the client is reading by scrolling text, slowly moving the line of print from right to left while looking straight ahead, rather than scanning left to right with typical eye movement patterns. When reading with a higher magnification, people are forced to move text from right to left in front of the narrow field of a magnification device or under an EM. People with central scotoma from macular degeneration learn to read with the steady eye technique (see Chapter 9), holding the eye in an eccentric position with the scotoma displaced so it does not eclipse the text, then moving the text so it is in the area where they can see whole words. The 2 major problems created by a more restricted field of view are difficulty scanning a page for relevant information, and losing one's place when reading. Once the line of text is found, however, it can still be read fluently as long as acuity and contrast reserve are high enough. Based on this concept, electronic and computer-based devices have been developed that scan several lines of text and present it as one continually scrolling line (like a marquee) in front of the eye so that the client does not have to look from line to line. These devices are discussed in Chapter 14.

Central field loss, generally resulting from macular degeneration, has a particularly devastating effect on visual reading. Although most people with any level of central field loss can recover visual spot reading sufficient for activities of daily living (ADL) with appropriate magnification, recovery of highly fluent reading cannot be recovered with significant central scotoma unless nonvisual reading strategies are used.

The visual requirements for reading are summarized in Table 15-4. Clients with visual impairment generally read better with too much, rather than too little magnification. Increased magnification enables the acuity reserve and contrast reserve requirements to be met, usually without approaching the field-of-view limitations of a few characters. As described later, clients can be taught to compensate for a narrower field of view resulting from higher magnification, but cannot progress to faster reading if inadequate magnification is prescribed. Clients with central field loss larger than 4 degrees (about 2 to 3 fingers' width at arm's length) cannot recover highly fluent visual reading and must use text-to-speech or braille to read fluently.

Case Examples

After some time had passed, Ms. Tuttle was having difficulty reading again even with appropriate lighting. Testing was conducted at 40 cm using the 2.5-D bifocal addition in her reading glasses with the MNREAD acuity chart on a table and a task light to help maintain the test distance and control lighting. She read the largest print fluently. She read successive lines of smaller print at about the same speed until at the 1.6M print size, when her reading speed declined and she started to stumble over the words. The critical print size, therefore, was 2.0M at 40 cm (0.4/2.0M) because 2M was the last line read at the maximum reading rate. Ms. Tuttle continued to read slowly and missed 2 words at 0.8M print. The reading acuity threshold, therefore, was 0.8M at 40 cm (0.4/0.8 M). The therapist quickly estimated that to read the 1M newsprint, an equivalent power of 5 diopters (D) was required. This was estimated by first dividing critical print size, 2M, by the print size in newspaper, 1M (2M/1M) to calculate the required enlargement ratio (ER = 2). The formula for equivalent power in D (see Chapters 8 and 13) is $D = ER * 100/d$, where d is the test distance of 40 cm. Using this formula, an ER of 2× was multiplied by 2.5 D to calculate 5 D of equivalent power. Because fluent reading was achieved with print magnification and the critical print size was about 3 lines above acuity threshold, typical of normal reading, the therapist concluded that no other visual impediments existed. Since fluent reading was achieved with print magnification alone, additional visual testing other than a lighting evaluation was unnecessary. Ms. Tuttle needed over 600 lux to achieve this level of vision. Now the decline in vision could have been due to refractive error or some correctable change in vision. As a result of this one session evaluation, the therapist referred Ms. Tuttle to her optometrist with the findings. Her optometrist checked her refraction and prescribed +5 reading glasses.

She returned 1 to 2 years later with a complaint of difficulty reading even with +5 glasses. The reading acuity test was performed with her new habitual 20-cm (8-inch) working distance and revealed that critical print size had increased to 4.0M and her reading speed had progressively slowed until reading acuity was achieved at 1.6M, although she could make out a few words at 1.2M. This result indicated a reduction in visual acuity and a need to test for the other possible visual impediments to reading, such as impaired contrast sensitivity or a central scotoma. In the vision evaluation, a central scotoma was found, but it was not absolute. With lower light levels, Ms. Tuttle often missed letters and words when reading, and the clock face method (see Chapter 9) indicated a central scotoma. With higher light levels and light yellow absorptive lenses to reduce glare, or white on black contrast with an electronic magnifier (CCTV), the scotoma was no longer apparent and did not interfere with reading. She could see whole words and recovered fluent reading with central fixation, and critical print size decreased from 4.0M to 2.0M and acuity improved to 1.0M. Now this was at a 20-cm (8-inch) working distance, with an equivalent power of 100/20 = 5 D. Ms. Tuttle wished to read the newspaper (1M font), which required an enlargement of 2× to reach critical print size, increasing the required overall magnification in equivalent power to 5 * 2 =10 D. Again, the occupational therapist referred the client to her optometrist, but with a concern that although Ms. Tuttle could read high-contrast print fluently, she would reject the 10-cm (4-inch) working distance and would still struggle with the lower contrast of newsprint (see Table 15-3). Many options exist to achieve this level of magnification; the challenge was finding the option that fit into Ms. Tuttle's lifestyle.

Jerry presented with similar visual acuity, also requiring 10 D of magnification for a maximum reading rate. Because he was used to close working distances, he easily tolerated 10 cm and accepted the reading glasses prescribed by his optometrist because they made reading much more comfortable. Jerry, however, had an absolute central scotoma that limited his maximum reading rate to about 120 wpm. The challenge with Jerry was figuring out a way he could read over 250 wpm required for school.

Possible Nonvisual Impediments

There are other nonvisual requirements for reading. Good motor skills are required to precisely move the text and position the devices. These requirements depend on the device being used (see Chapters 13 and 14). The cognitive and linguistic requirements are certainly a consideration, and these aspects are often the focus of treatment by educators of college and high school students, as well as speech therapists for adults treated in medical rehabilitation settings. As mentioned, people with long-standing visual impairment often have not read for a long time and have lost basic literacy skills from disuse. If it has been established that someone must read visually, a reading evaluation requires that one establish premorbid literacy and the cognitive ability to read. This can be easily done with larger, high-contrast print that is easy for the client to see.

Evaluation of Reading Performance

Performance is evaluated before and during treatment and as part of an ongoing evaluation of intervention strategies. The key to motivating a client is to use the actual materials a client wishes to read. The client should be encouraged to bring in materials of interest. A well-equipped low vision service must include samples of common reading tasks like medication bottles, bills, menus, activity schedules from retirement centers, directions on food packages, church bulletins, a regular and large-print Bible and other spiritual readings, a recent magazine and newspaper, and paperback and hardback books. The collection of reading materials should also include other languages common in the area of practice. One can determine reading efficiency with computerized text-to-speech by playing and timing passages and then testing comprehension.[8] The Pepper Visual Skills for Reading Test is valuable for a standardized reading[13] evaluation (see Chapter 8). This test uses unrelated words that increase in length and line spacing. It has exceptional test-retest reliability, has been validated, and might, therefore, be used to document changes in reading performance as a benchmark for documenting the efficacy of devices and therapeutic intervention. The test also has diagnostic value in revealing scanning difficulties in people with central field loss. A more quickly administered alternative is the SKREAD. For older students and adults in vocational programs that address literacy, the Morgan Test of Reading Comprehension (www.lowvisionsimulators.com) allows one to document literacy limitations using an instrument validated for people with low vision.[15] Otherwise, a test should be selected that measures vocabulary and comprehension separately from reading speed, which is more affected by vision.

Finally, one might need to compare reading performance with optical devices and electronic devices. It becomes essential to provide objective performance data to agencies or insurance companies to justify purchase of devices. One compares reading speed after the devices have been configured for maximum reading performance. Since devices often must be purchased with justification before instruction on use of the device can commence, the therapist should assist the client to ensure performance is only limited visually, not by his or her familiarity with the device, which will improve with training. In the online appendix (www.routledge.com/9781617116339), we have included a continual text reading test that allows one to compare reading with text-to-speech with print reading using paragraphs.[8] To evaluate text-to-speech reading, one must play a recording of the MP3 files. The different paragraphs are of approximately the same visual and phonological length and linguistic difficulty (fifth- to sixth-grade level). The recording will read the paragraph at increasing speeds until the client incorrectly answers 2/3 questions. Likewise, clients read paragraphs silently as quickly as possible, with comprehension validated at the same level or higher. The Pepper Test is recommended to compare visual reading using a test with better sensitivity to small changes in performance.

Strategies for Meeting the Visual Requirements for Reading

Once performance-limiting factors have been identified, one must develop treatment plans to address these impediments to reading.

Magnification

The most common method to increase acuity reserve involves a magnification assistive device. An assortment of optical and EM devices are available to magnify print (see Chapters 13 and 14), including handheld devices and strong reading glasses that enable relative distance magnification. Under the more common practice management model, the low vision optometrist may have already recommended or even prescribed optical devices. Ideally, devices are recommended, but not prescribed until after the occupational therapy evaluation has been completed and instruction has begun. If magnification (acuity reserve) appears inadequate, then the therapist should compensate by first enlarging the print. After instruction with a device, the client might improve in the ability to read smaller print with the recommended magnification. If reading larger print is faster than smaller print, then more magnification is indicated. If critical print size has been exceeded, then increasing the print size will not affect reading rate and more magnification is not indicated. Electronic devices have the advantage of producing higher magnification with greater comfort as well as enhanced contrast (see Chapter 14) and increasing contrast reserve. Newer electronic devices also have document scanning and reading features. If the desired reading task cannot be met with the recommended optical device, the client should be referred back to the low vision optometrist. However, many optometrists prefer that the therapist evaluate different devices and magnification levels and make recommendations. In any case, the optometrist must prescribe the optical device. Table 15-5 lists the different types of electronic devices and optical devices and the range of usual magnifications we have found patients tolerate. In the absence of an evidence base for the best range of magnification for different devices, these recommendations are based on a survey of the subject matter expert committee of the Academy for Certification of Vision Rehabilitation & Education Professionals (ACVREP) (www.acvrep.org) and are just useful as a general guideline. Also included in Table 15-5 are advantages and disadvantages of each device. We have found the best solutions often involve both an optical device and electronic magnification on a personal computer, tablet computer, or e-reader. For example, if a client finds a 10-cm (4-inch) distance with 10 D of reading addition uncomfortable, then the prescribed magnification can be reduced to 5 D, increasing the working distance to 20 cm (8 inches) and the print size enlarged to 2× to achieve equivalent magnification (Figure 15-2).

Inadequate Contrast Reserve: Lighting and Print Contrast

Contrast reserve can be improved by improving contrast sensitivity (threshold) or increasing print contrast. Both visual acuity and contrast sensitivity can be improved by optimizing lighting (see Chapter 12).[16,17] Retinal pathology and optic nerve degeneration appear to have variable, often unpredictable and idiosyncratic, effects on performance. Glare should always be minimized. Although people with low vision vary in their sensitivity to glare, glare always impairs visual acuity and contrast sensitivity. Directing light from the side and using a typoscope (a black plastic card with a window cut out for the print—Figure 15-3) decreases reflection off a white page. Reversing contrast to light letters on a dark background reduces glare as well (see Chapter 14). One should carefully evaluate the work setting to ensure glare does not interfere with the client's performance. The therapist can sit where the client sits to determine if there are reflections off screens, shiny surfaces, bright windows, and improperly positioned lights. If optical devices are used, lights often reflect off the lenses, producing disabling glare as well. With an EM (CCTV), the light used to illuminate the page being viewed can also become a glare source.

In cases where strong illumination is required, an absorptive lens (sunlens) evaluation is indicated (see Chapter 12). We prefer light yellow and orange tinted absorptive lenses or tints in reading glasses and do not recommend colored overlays because sunglasses are more convenient to use and reduce glare from other sources as well. Note that although most people with low vision perform best with increased directional light, some perform better with decreased light. A lighting evaluation should always be performed (see Chapter 8) to determine optimum light levels and then reproduced during the functional reading evaluation and treatment. The easiest and most effective way to modify light levels is to vary the distance of the light source rather than change the wattage of the bulb. Instructional strategies for lighting are in Chapter 10. A handout for clients and family to use for glare management is included in the online appendix (www.routledge.com/9781617116339).

TABLE 15-5: MAGNIFICATION DEVICES FOR READING

DEVICE	CONTRAST ENHANCED	SPEECH	MAXIMUM* MAGNIFICATION (EQUIVALENT D)	DEVICES CAN BE COMBINED TO INCREASE MAGNIFICATION**	ADVANTAGES	DISADVANTAGES
Handheld magnifier	No	No	20 to >32 D 5X to 8X	With reading add if held against lens.	Available with light, portable, for spot reading, low cost.	Not for fluent reading.
Stand magnifier	No	No	25 to >36 D 5X to 9X	With reading add only at a closer prescribed distance from magnifier lens.	Available with light for higher magnification. Easier to maintain focal distance. Can be used for fluent reading.	Challenging ergonomics. Some models too large for easy portability >8D, not suitable for writing.
Half-eye reading addition***	No	No	8 to 12 D (2X to 3X)	With handheld magnifier against lens or with any electronic device at prescribed distance.	Easily combined with smaller screen electronic devices for fluent reading.	Prone to binocular interference unless one eye is occluded. May need reading stand at higher add. Lighting difficult. Not suitable for writing.
Monocular reading addition*** (full-field microscope)	No	No	10 to >20 D (2.5X to 5X)	With handheld magnifier against lens or with any electronic device at prescribed distance.	Easily combined with smaller screen electronic devices for fluent reading.	>10D will require reading stand/support. Lighting is difficult. Not suitable for spot reading or writing.
Loupes	No	No	10 to 16 D (2.5X to 4X)	With handheld magnifier against lens or with any electronic device at prescribed distance.	For spot reading small print. Increased working distance for writing and nonreading near tasks.	Some are difficult to store and easily broken.
Flip-up addition	No	No	4 D	Adds power to current reading addition, or with any electronic device at prescribed distance.	Ideal to use with reading addition for people who usually read large print but occasionally need to read smaller print.	Often a handheld device is a more convenient alternative.

(continued)

TABLE 15-5 (CONTINUED): MAGNIFICATION DEVICES FOR READING

DEVICE	CONTRAST ENHANCED	SPEECH	MAXIMUM* MAGNIFICATION (EQUIVALENT D)	DEVICES CAN BE COMBINED TO INCREASE MAGNIFICATION**	ADVANTAGES	DISADVANTAGES
Tabletop electronic magnifier (CCTV)	Yes	Yes	4X to > 20X enlargement (10 to > 50 D at 40 cm)	Adds power to current reading addition.	Additional magnification with larger screen, increased portability with smaller device and screen. With higher magnification most comfortable for fluent reading.	Requires that user sit at a table.
Handheld electronic magnifier (CCTV)	Yes	Yes	4 to 8X (10 to > 20 D at 40 cm)	Combines with reading addition.	Can be used for writing, ideal for spot reading	Less suitable for fluent reading than a tabletop device
PC with without extra programs	Yes	Yes	2X to 4X enlargement (5 to 10 D at 40 cm)	Combines with near addition if a reading stand is used.	Additional enlargement with a larger screen. Very basic screen magnifiers are now available at no additional cost.	No additional cost except for reading stand. Font magnification is not consistent with all programs. Need additional optical magnifier in these cases.
PC screen magnifier/ screen reader	Yes	Yes	4X to 12X enlargement (10 to > 30 D at 40 cm)	Combines with near addition if an adjustable monitor stand is used.	> 2X magnifier easier to use than native PC magnifier/ screen reader. Can be customized to special applications.	Additional cost. Screen readers require additional training.
Tablet computer/ e-reader	Yes	Yes	2X to 4X enlargement (5 to 10 D at 40 cm) limited by screen size.	Combines with near reading addition.	Accessibility best via text-to-speech.	Magnification awkward because of small screen.

(continued)

TABLE 15-5 (CONTINUED): MAGNIFICATION DEVICES FOR READING

DEVICE	CONTRAST ENHANCED	SPEECH	MAXIMUM* MAGNIFICATION (EQUIVALENT D)	DEVICES CAN BE COMBINED TO INCREASE MAGNIFICATION**	ADVANTAGES	DISADVANTAGES
Smart phone	Yes	Yes	1.5× to 3× enlargement (4 to 8 D at 40 cm) limited by screen size	Combines with near reading addition.	Accessibility best via text-to-speech.	Magnification awkward because of small screen.

* Lower number in the range is usual maximum accepted by patients; the higher number indicates potential maximum with acceptance unusual. For electronic devices, maximum may be more or less depending on the size of the screen.

** Equivalent powers of both devices are additive.

*** Reading addition is in terms of accommodative demand (based on viewing distance); actual addition depends on age and refractive error.

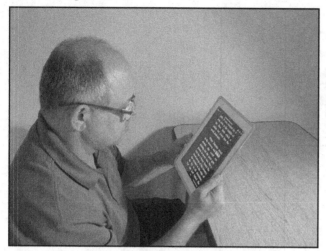

Figure 15-2. By combining 2× print enlargement on an e-reader with higher reading addition (5 D), a higher magnification (an equivalent power of 10 D) and contrast enhancement can be achieved using more common consumer products rather than more expensive low vision devices.

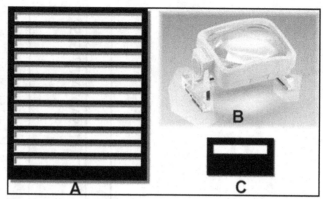

Figure 15-3. Picture of writing devices: (A) Writing guide. (B) Low-power stand magnifiers with lens that can be tilted. (C) A typoscope or signature guide. (Photo B printed with permission from Eschenbach Optik of America.)

Increasing print contrast also will generally improve acuity and, as a result, acuity reserve. For clients who present with restricted visual fields, often due to advanced glaucoma, retinitis pigmentosa, or laser-treated diabetic retinopathy, increasing acuity reserve by magnification of print will decrease field of view. Electronic systems that enhance contrast and reverse print contrast should be considered for these clients (see Chapter 14). As many of the conditions that lead to restricted fields progress to total blindness (see Chapter 4), these individuals benefit from computer systems where the display contrast is enhanced and maybe magnified slightly, but also with text-to-speech screen readers that will become more functionally significant as vision deteriorates. People with restricted visual fields should be referred for a new and careful refraction because even a 1- or 2-character increase in field of view can significantly enhance reading performance.

Central Field Loss and Eccentric Viewing

When people with normal vision read, they use the fovea/macula area of the retina in which visual acuity is at its highest level. People who have lost more than about 4 to 5 degrees of central vision lose the ability to read at rates approaching normal fluency with their residual vision (see Table 15-4). Nonvisual modalities should always be considered in cases of central field loss.

People with central field loss must be taught eccentric viewing and then the scrolled reading technique (see Chapter 10). Reading becomes a critical therapeutic activity in meeting a number of goals with people who have central field loss. Recovery of spot reading is common.

Peripheral/Unilateral Field Loss

Following stroke, field loss is associated with reading disabilities.[18-22] People with central sparing rarely have difficulty reading unless they also have impaired visual acuity that requires print magnification. They may have difficulty scanning a page for information because they cannot see the whole page. People with a split central field will only see half of what they look at and will usually have reading problems and might even have difficulty recognizing characters because they only see half of the character.

Right Visual Field Loss

If a client has a split central field with right field loss or positions a central scotoma to the right, reading is severely compromised because of a restricted field of view. It has been known for years that typically readers fixate the beginning of words.[23,24] Using this habitual fixation pattern, the person with a right field loss will not see the end of words. Reading is slow and often involves spelling words. We have found that clients recover reading by learning to look at the end of words rather than the beginning. This can be facilitated by having the client direct a pointer at the end of words while reading. One approach that has sometimes been effective involves reorienting reading material so the client is reading vertically or at an angle. For a right field loss, the client learns to rotate the page clockwise so the beginning of the lines should be on top (Figure 15-4). The client is reading down and to the left. In addition, the therapist must teach the client to eccentrically view to the right of the letters being read so the entire word can be visualized. If the patient has unilateral field loss with a split central field, often acuity is reduced 1 to 2 lines from normal. This may be because the client is now eccentrically viewing. In any case, acuity will be reduced and print must be enlarged slightly to 1.6M (14 pt). If the client holds the text and scrolls from right to left in front of the eye, the field-of-view requirements for fluent reading will decrease and reading sometimes is better than when stationary text is read. There is little evidence in favor of these reading strategies; however, we have found improvements in reading stationary text if clients have central field cuts but not linguistic alexia from a stroke. Another approach that requires specialized equipment involves scrolling print from right to left in front of the eyes "marquee style." This has been shown to effectively increase reading speeds.[21]

Left Visual Field Loss

With left central visual field loss from a unilateral field loss or central scotoma with left eccentric viewing, the client often loses his or her place when reading and has difficulty finding the beginning of a line of text. A commonly used strategy is to place a brightly colored straight edge along the left margin of the page. The client will know that he or she has to make a saccade back to the bright line when making the return sweep. An even more effective technique is to use a sandpaper or a Velcro strip along the left margin. The client places a finger on this strip and can "feel" the left margin. The client quickly learns to use this tactile awareness as a cue for the required eye movement at the end of each line. Retrace strategies described earlier for eccentric viewing will also help someone read with a left unilateral or overall field loss.

Case Examples

Ms. Tuttle wished to read the newspaper, spiritual materials, and paperback novels, which had become increasingly difficult even with higher illumination. Before any visual devices were introduced, Ms. Tuttle was introduced to the NLS recorded books for novel reading and a player was ordered. Recall that the reading acuity test indicated a critical print size of 2M at 20 cm (5 D), which required an enlargement of the 1M print by 2×, increasing the required overall magnification in equivalent power to 5 D * 2 = 10 D. The therapist anticipated that when introduced to this power of magnification, Ms. Tuttle would be able to read high-contrast print fluently but she would reject the 10-cm (4-inch) working distance and would still struggle with the lower contrast of newsprint (see Table 15-3). The EM was the device of choice for optimum reading because of its reverse-contrast capability with white letters on a black background and the possibility of increasing magnification as her visual acuity further declined. Ms. Tuttle may be reluctant to sit at a table to read because she had been reading seated in her recliner for the past several years. The therapist demonstrated a smaller EM that she could use on a table while sitting in her favorite chair. Comparing the EM with her old device sitting at the table, Ms. Tuttle immediately appreciated an improvement in reading speed and comfort while reading the newspaper and mail. Using large, 2M-printed reading materials, she could continue to read her spiritual materials and even

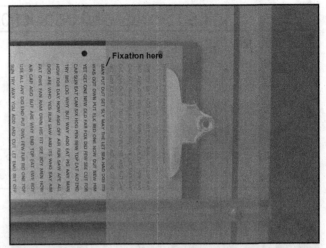

Figure 15-4. The client's view of text being read using the vertical scrolling technique. The client has a right field cut and would normally not see anything to the right. The client has been instructed to fixate to the right of the letter (eccentrically viewing) to see the entire letters and to read from top to bottom. Try reading this way. Vertical reading is relatively easy for someone with good reading ability.

books in her chair with 5-D reading glasses. It was expected that as her vision continued to decline, Ms. Tuttle would transition all of her visual reading to the electronic viewer and listen to her novels. She also liked to eat out, so for spot reading (menus), she was introduced to a 10-diopter, illuminated, handheld magnifier, which her optometrist prescribed. Handheld EMs would have been a possible option as well, but Ms. Tuttle had difficulty handling the devices with the curved pages in books.

Jerry needed to read quickly to keep up in school. Reading was possible with text-to-speech, which enabled the 250-wpm reading rate. He immediately accepted a version of an electronic magnifier (CCTV) that was portable, was hooked into his personal computer, and could work even under marginal lighting conditions. This EM had a remote camera that could be directed at the white board and projection screen in class and could capture and store images for review later so that he could follow along in class. The character recognition software could analyze the stored documents so they could be read aloud much faster than visually. He had a standalone electronic device like Ms. Tuttle's viewer in his dorm room for faster, more fluent reading, but it was not easily portable. Since Jerry still could focus his eyes, he used relative distance magnification and could see his iPad tablet computer with 2× magnification and had learned to become proficient using VoiceOver, the text-to-speech system, so he could make do without magnification. He also used his iPhone as a handheld magnifier and the apps for a host of other functions, such as a barcode reader to read products in the store and many signs. Another app could scan and store business cards. The greatest challenge for Jerry was to encourage him to learn braille. Fortunately, he was required to learn rudimentary

TABLE 15-6: READING INSTRUCTIONS WITH MAGNIFICATION DEVICES

1. Teach setup for reading.

2. Use text easy to see and read. Assist with device.

3. Teach how to use the device.

4. Teach how to scan successive lines of text.

5. Begin home-based exercises.

6. Grade the text being read from larger and easier to understand to smaller and more difficult.

7. Teach localization and scanning techniques.

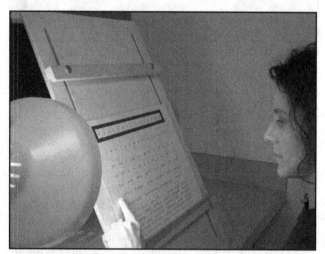

Figure 15-5. Improved visual-motor control is achieved by using adaptive finger pointing strategies to keep her place and a reading stand for good ergonomics while testing with the Pepper Visual Skills for Reading Test.

braille in school. His visual condition was progressive, and his visual reading would likely be severely disabled as he entered his 40s, presumably at a critical time in his professional development. He was encouraged to join the National Federation of the Blind, a blind advocacy group that strongly promotes braille and to develop his braille literacy in an immersion summer program.

Advanced Treatment: Instructional Strategies

These strategies are used in a traditional low vision setting where the only disability is vision. Clients who have not read in a long time are thrilled and highly motivated and often can complete the following steps quickly, even within one session. However, for clients requiring higher magnification, learning to read with low vision can be difficult and stressful. Recovery of reading resembles recovery of ambulation after a stroke. At first, the client is insecure and compensation for this insecurity can significantly impede

progression and recovery of normal movement patterns. Readers often skip words when reading a passage.[7] People relearning to read after recent vision loss often regress to painstaking, word-by-word reading. The reader with a lower frustration tolerance might also overreact emotionally to every stumble. If this occurs, the therapist should first instruct the client on relaxation strategies and then provide frequent rest breaks. When practicing at home, these clients should have assistance if possible. A good strategy is to schedule shorter treatment sessions with frequent rest breaks. Recommended graded steps for reading instruction are summarized in Table 15-6.

Reading With a Focus on Good Ergonomics

Ergonomics has a significant effect on performance as well as perceived comfort.[25] Reading instruction should proceed from a carefully controlled, ideal ergonomic situation to a setting more typical of the natural environment in which the reading activities will occur. Watson et al[25] described ideal ergonomics in detail in their study. Reading instruction with optical devices or electronic devices like EMs (CCTVs) should begin with the client seated at a table with feet firmly on the floor. A reading stand and chair-height adjustment that ensure posture appropriate for the client (usually 90 degrees at ankles, knees, and hips) should be used with the eyes approximately the same distance from the top and bottom of the page. The client should be instructed in how to identify and correct lighting problems. Refer to Chapters 12 and 13 for additional information about environmental setups for optical and electronic devices. The ideal reading surface should be a stand with a lip on the bottom edge against which the reading material rests (Figure 15-5) and which allows the page on a clipboard to easily slide left and right along a straight horizontal line. During this instruction, if reading in the natural environment is inadequate, the therapist should demonstrate how easy it is to read under the new method. Such demonstrations may convince the client to allow environmental modifications.

Use Easy-to-Read Text and Assist the Client With the Device

If a client has a low frustration tolerance or is easily fatigued, do not begin reading instruction with complicated training on how to use the assistive optical devices. The therapist should set up the device and provide hand-over-hand assistance so that the reader is using the device correctly and immediately starts instruction by reading something. A good starting point is to use text that is easy to understand, with single sentences written at a third-grade level and more than 2× the visual acuity level. Examples that are included in the online appendix (www.routledge.com/ 9781617116339) can be printed in different font sizes. More advanced exercises, in a progression of easier to see and understand to smaller print and higher grade levels, are provided by the Learn to Use Your Vision (LUV) reading series workbook.[26] With a more typical client, the difficulty of reading materials may progress quickly, but to be safe, easier is better at first. In general, especially with reluctant clients, the treatment should advance to readings of interest to the client. This text uses exercises that are engaging and that make the otherwise tedious practice enjoyable to most clients. Large-print *Reader's Digest* often has good starting material.

Teach Use of the Device

Rather than start with lower magnification, which is easier to use, and progressing to higher magnification, the better method to grade difficulty is to provide hand-over-hand assistance with the expected full magnification and then withdraw assistance gradually and as needed. The instructional methods for optical and electronic devices depend on the device and are described in Chapter 13 and Chapter 14. Even experienced device users may use poor technique, so a quick hand-over-hand demonstration to start is better than a lot of verbal instruction. If a success-oriented approach is used, the therapist starts the client with reading single sentences, providing as much assistance as necessary. After the client has read successfully, the therapist shows the client the size of the material he or she successfully read without the magnifier to demonstrate the effectiveness of the device. Physical assistance then is unobtrusively withdrawn while the client is reading without saying anything. If a client persists with a incorrect procedure, stop and demonstrate the difference between correct and incorrect handling with verbal instruction. For example, with a higher magnification optical device, pull the device too far away from the object, then too close, and finally at the correct distance so the client can see and learn to recognize the problem and correct it. For cognitively impaired clients, avoid verbal cuing during reading because verbal cuing is often distracting and disrupts reading comprehension. Do not correct reading errors unless necessary for comprehension. Generally, with the success-oriented approach, setup

is taught last. For many who have no cognitive problems or are already familiar with the devices, brief verbal instruction and a single demonstration often will suffice.

Teach Scanning Successive Lines of Text

With stronger magnification devices, only a word or 2 can be seen at a time. One of the first skills a client must master is staying on the line being read and scanning back to the beginning of the next line. Sliding or moving the text horizontally on a reading stand facilitates staying on a line. To find the beginning of a line, use of a ruler or having the client position his or her finger at the beginning of the line being read provide effective cues. A retrace technique involves having the client first read a line, then follow the end of the line backward to the beginning, and then move down to the next line to continue. Finally, if a reading stand is not available at home, the client should learn to read multiple lines while the material is on a table or by holding the reading material.

Home Exercises and Transition to the Goal Task

Once the client has been prescribed the device, he or she must practice at home. Setup for reading, including use of devices and lighting that will be used at home, should be included during practice. The graded exercises described next are used for home-based practice.

At this point, the client should be able to identify and correct a problem with the setup for reading, poor lighting, poor positioning of the material being read, or improper use of a device. Once these obstacles have been overcome, the client can practice alone or with distance supervision. With additional practice, the client can progress rapidly through the rehabilitation process.

Grade the Text Being Read

If a client quickly completes the previous steps, the therapist may simply transition to text that the client brings or material that is of high interest to the client. If the client struggles with the steps, the progression of practice reading has traditionally started with single word identification. Tasks include searching for words or categories of words, such as counting or circling the names of plants or sports on a page. Then the client should be presented with simple sentences. An excellent method that is often used at this stage in therapy is a traditional reading instructional approach called the *cloze strategy*. The cloze strategy is a technique in which a person tries to read a sentence with some words or parts of words missing. For example, "You can lead a horse to water but you c___ make him drink." To succeed, the individual must rely on grammatical and linguistic cues. This is useful with clients with central scotomas because the scotoma causes parts of words or whole words to disappear. To use the cloze strategy in vision rehabilitation treatment, the client is taught to skip words not immediately understood and rely more on context to understand the content. Using this strategy, clients can still read with better than 90% accuracy. Reading then progresses to smaller print and longer passages with questions about content. The reading difficulty of the material can be advanced as well. These exercises, written for adults, are available in workbook form.[26] In general, it is most engaging for the client to transition to the preferred reading material as quickly as possible.

Localization and Scanning Skills

Finding the starting place to begin reading with high magnification can be difficult because readers depend on a large field of view to know where to fixate. When a reader uses a high-power magnification device that allows the words to be recognized and read, the device often restricts field of view, sometimes to just 1 to 2 words. Localization techniques should be used to compensate for restricted field of view and enable the client to locate the starting position for reading. The reader first views the unmagnified or minimally magnified page and then estimates where he or she wishes to read (the target) by the general layout of the text. The reader positions the text so the target will be centered under the magnifier and magnifies the text to read the individual words, or places the magnifier in front of the eye while looking at the target. For example, a reader can see where lines begin and end without a magnifier. The page is repositioned so that the beginning of the line is directly in front, and while continuing to look at the beginning of the line, the magnifier is positioned in front of the eye. This increases magnification so the reader can recognize the word. These specific techniques for spotting and navigating with high magnification are described for each magnification device in Chapters 13 and 14.

Reading as a Multidisciplinary Effort

In clients with multiple disabilities, reading rehabilitation often should be a multidisciplinary effort, if possible. In a typical medical rehabilitation model, the occupational therapist focuses on environmental modifications, adaptations to social roles, use of assistive devices, ergonomics, and the mechanics of reading. Speech therapists, if available, may work on developing reading strategies such as the cloze strategy, as well as providing an opportunity for practice. The eye care provider understands the optics, a person's refractive error, and how the visual factors interact.

Writing Strategies

Handwriting with low vision is often problematic. People who have been writing or typing their whole life can still do so without vision. However, 2 common problems occur: (1) locating where to write on a form or page, and (2) staying on a line or within an allotted space. Other issues may include

crossing the letter "t" and dotting the letter "i," managing descending letters (p, g, y, q, j), and how to avoid or compensate for stopping in the middle of a word or sentence.

Evaluation

The Low Vision Writing Assessment[27] is a standardized test with exceptional test-retest reliability. This assessment evaluates the most common handwriting activities: (1) writing a grocery list, (2) filling out a check, (3) writing a short descriptive narrative, (4) filling in a medical form, (5) writing a note to oneself. This assessment allows for visual and nonvisual strategies, as well as use of computer-aided devices. Once again, we prefer to focus on specific goal tasks identified by the client. For those who need to write frequently, such as Jerry, writing speed can be measured or the baseline and outcome can be stated as one of the following: (1) did not perform, (2) required assistance, (3) performed with reported difficulty, (4) performed with modified independence. The therapist can find appropriate evaluation materials such as forms and lined paper in most settings. Bold lined paper for writing can be purchased as well.

Interventions

First-Response Interventions

- Use of a black bold line pens, bold line paper, and large print/raised line checks.
- Signature guides or typoscopes (see Figure 15-3) are flat templates, made in plastic, metal, or cardboard, with a cutout for a signature or a few words. People with low vision often sign their name and write without seeing what they are writing. Use of a signature guide requires sighted assistance to select the correct spot to place the guide. Signature guides are inexpensive to purchase, but also easy to fabricate. These should be available in any clinic for general accessibility. People need to practice writing in the middle of the space with these devices. Sighted users tend to use the bottom edge as a line and cannot move the pen beyond this edge for letters like y and g that have lower descenders.
- Use of pay-by-phone services can substitute for check writing.

Advanced Interventions

- A person who loses vision later in life and retains good motor coordination will be able to write extensive passages or fill out a check by hand without seeing as long as she or he has a guide to help stay on the line (see Figure 15-3). Like signature guides, other writing guides are designed to fit over checks or typing paper. The person stays on the line within the cutout spaces to, for example, fit over a check, envelope, or piece of paper. The client feels or can see the space in which he or she can write by feeling it with the other finger while writing. Since the overlays are black, the white paper can be more easily seen through the window of the overlay, so often the client can see the space in which he or she must write. Standard writing pens are used with writing guides as bold pens will fill in the space too much. Additionally, guides were designed to allow the user to locate where to write but not necessarily to read what is finally written. It is the person receiving the document that must be able to read it so the desired visibility is determined by the recipient.

- Large-print checks are available from banks and provide 1.5× to 2× enlargement.

- Some devices such as lower-power stand magnifiers, handheld magnifiers, optical and electronic, devices, and telemicroscopes (see Chapter 13) provide magnification for someone to guide writing visually while maintaining a sufficient working distance. Sometimes stronger magnifier or handheld electronic viewers can be angled to make room for a pen. However, visual distortion will result. The device should be lined up with the eye and angled against the page.

- People can also write near-normal-size lettering using an EM (CCTV) (see Chapter 14).

- Computers are the ideal device of choice for writing correspondence and paying bills. For an individual with low vision who needs to write long letters and passages, the best option is to learn to touch type. Most people can master this process practicing 15 minutes a day for a few weeks. Programs like Talking Typing Teacher (MarvelSoft Enterprises, Inc) have been developed that teach people who are blind to type on a computer.

- The accessible tablet computers and smart phones with voice recognition and control have been a boon for those who have weak typing skills. These devices have the capacity to enable the client to keep notes, maintain a calendar, and write e-mails. An external Bluetooth-enabled keyboard is available for these devices and is recommended for faster typing. The devices are able to use standard computer monitors that will enable magnification of the screen as well.

Instructional Materials

The materials for reading include a chair, table, and reading stand with adjustable height so the client's posture can be optimized. A variety of directional lights should be available, including fluorescent, standard incandescent, and a spectrally balanced light. The low vision rehabilitation therapist needs to have a computer equipped with adaptive software and an EM (CCTV), preferably one that allows color contrast to vary. Black overlays with cutouts, paper with bold lines and extra-wide spacing between lines,

black felt-tip pens, and signature guides should be available to give to clients.

Evaluation materials should include a continual text reading chart like the MNREAD Chart, the Pepper Visual Skills for Reading Test, and a workbook with reading exercises.

SUMMARY

Reading is often the focus of therapy in low vision rehabilitation programs in optometric practices. The occupational therapy treatments should involve much more than optical devices. Using computer-based devices with EMs, visual enhancement, and text-to-speech devices, a person with any level of vision loss can now read and write as efficiently as someone with typical vision. A variety of optical and portable electronic devices provides the therapist with many options to enable reading and writing goals. The 2 cases, one an elderly woman, another a young college student, were used to illustrate how 2 people with similar visual acuity would require substantially different devices, environmental modifications, and a different therapeutic approach depending on nonvisual factors. Reading rehabilitation requires a partnership. The eye care provider specializing in low vision contributes an understanding of the optics, a person's refractive error, accommodative ability, and the interaction of the many visual factors. The therapist contributes an understanding of context; task demand; and other psychosocial, physical, and cognitive abilities and disabilities. A speech therapist, reading specialist, or teacher will better understand the linguistic aspects of reading. Key to cost-effective service delivery the evaluations enable both the therapist and eye care provider to narrow in on the appropriate devices and required magnification with a minimum of trial and error.

REFERENCES

1. Mehr EB, Freid AN. *Low Vision Care*. Chicago: Professional Press; 1975.
2. Chung ST, Li RW, Levi DM. Crowding between first- and second-order letter stimuli in normal foveal and peripheral vision. *J Vis*. 2007;7:10, 11-13.
3. Leat SJ, Wei L, Epp K. Crowding in central and eccentric vision: the contour interaction and attention. *Invest Ophthalmol Vis Sci*. 1999;40:404-512.
4. Liu L, Arditi A. How crowding affects letter confusion. *Optom Vis Sci*. 2001;78:50-55.
5. Yu D, Akau MMU, Chung STL. The mechanism of word crowding. *Vis Res*. 2012;52:61-69.
6. Whittaker SG, Lovie-Kitchin JE. Visual requirements for reading. *Optom Vis Sci*. 1993;70:54-65.
7. Carver RP. *Reading Rate: A Review of Research and Theory*: Academic Press: San Diego; 1990.
8. Hensil J, Whittaker SG. Comparing visual reading versus auditory reading by sighted persons and persons with low vision. *J Vis Impairment Blindness*. 2000;94:762-770.

9. Legge GE, Ross JA, Luebker A, LaMay JM. Psychophysics of reading. VIII. The Minnesota Low-Vision Reading Test. *Optom Vis Sci.* 1989;66:843-853.

10. Cheong AC, Lovie-Kitchin JE, Bowers AR. Determining magnification for reading with low vision. *Clin Exp Optom.* 2002;85:229-237.

11. Lovie-Kitchin JE. *Reading Performance of Adults With Low Vision.* Ph.D. thesis. Brisbane, Queensland: Queensland University of Technology; 1996.

12. Legge GE. *Psychophysics of Reading in Normal and Low Vision.* Mahwah, NJ: Lawrence Erlbaum Associates; 2007.

13. Watson GR, Whittaker SG, Steciw M. *Pepper Visual Skills for Reading Test (revised).* Milwaukee, WI: Fork in the Road Vision Rehabilitation Services LLC; 1995.

14. MacKeben M, Nair UKW, Walker LL, Fletcher DC. Random word recognition chart helps scotoma assessment in low vision. *Optom Vis Sci.* 92:421-428.

15. Watson GR, Wright V, Long SL. *Morgan Low Vision Reading Comprehension Assessment (LUV Reading Series).* Lilburn, GA: Bear Consultants; 1996.

16. Fosse P, Valberg A. Lighting needs and lighting comfort during reading with age-related macular degeneration. *J Vis Impairment Blindness.* 2004;98:389-409.

17. Fosse P, Valberg A. Contrast sensitivity and reading in subjects with age-related macular degeneration. *Vis Impairment Res.* 2001;3:111-124.

18. Rowe F, Wright D, Brand D, et al. Reading difficulty after stroke: ocular and non ocular causes. *Int J Stroke.* 2011;6:404-411.

19. Aimola L, Lane AR, Smith DT, Kerkhoff G, Ford GA, Schenk T. Efficacy and feasibility of home-based training for individuals with homonymous visual field defects. *Neurorehabil Neural Repair.* 2013;28:207-218.

20. Sheldon CA, Abegg M, Sekunova A, Barton JJS. The word-length effect in acquired alexia and real and virtual hemianopia. *Neuropsychologia.* 2012;50:841-851.

21. Ong Y-H, Brown MM, Robinson P, Plant GT, Husain M, Leff AP. Read-Right: a "web app" that improves reading speeds in patients with hemianopia. *J Neurol.* 2012;259:2611-2615.

22. Mennem TA, Warren M, Yuen HK. Preliminary validation of a vision-dependent activities of daily living instrument on adults with homonymous hemianopia. *Am J Occup Ther.* 2012;66:478-482.

23. Rayner K, Inhoff AW, Morrison RE, Slowiaczek ML, Bertera JH. Masking of foveal and parafoveal vision during eye fixations in reading. *J Exp Psychol.* 1981;7:167-179.

24. Rayner K, Bertera JH. Reading without a fovea. *Science.* 1979;206:468-469.

25. Watson GR, Ramsey V, De L'Aune W, Elk A. Ergonomic enhancement for older readers with low vision. *J Vis Impairment Blindness.* 2004;98:228-240.

26. Wright V, Watson GR. *Learn to Use Your Vision for Reading (LUV Reading Series).* Lilburn, GA: Bear Consultants; 1996.

27. Watson GR, Wright V, Wyse E, De L'Aune W. A writing assessment for persons with age-related vision loss. *J Vis Impairment Blindness.* 2004;98:160-167.

16

Basic Self-Care

This chapter begins a series of chapters devoted to techniques that promote return to occupational performance including: self-care; managing the home; leisure, recreation and sports; and community activities. Since people who are totally blind can use adaptive techniques for most self-care and activities of daily living (ADL) it was somewhat surprising to find a correlation between disabled ADL and level of vision impairment.[1] Included are some basic adaptive techniques and strategies for people with low vision usually involving a combination of visual, non-visual, optical and electronic interventions that have been discussed previously in this book. The occupational therapist can introduce the strategies described in this and the following chapters but should refer to a Vision Rehabilitation Therapist (CVRT) for more advanced training, if such training exceeds the occupational therapist's area of expertise or knowledge base. These services and, often adaptive equipment, are usually provided through the Veteran's Administration, state and non-government agencies. With additional education, occupational therapists are eligible to obtain certification as a CVRT (www.acvrep.org, www.aerbvi.org).

In a recent research review[2] Liu, Brost, Horton, Kenyon, and Mears concluded "Older adults living with visual impairment need more than low vision devices to perform ADLs and IADL's. To maintain their daily occupations at home, they need a set of skills to deal with day-to-day challenges. The intervention must cover knowledge of low vision, use of low vision devices, problem-solving strategies, and community resources."[2] Although there is very little research on the specific techniques discussed in this chapter, fortunately, the devices and adaptive techniques can be quickly evaluated on a case-by-case basis. Many of the specific strategies described in this chapter are based on techniques that come from the field of vision rehabilitation therapy[3-6]; others from our own experience or taught to us by our clients. In addition to describing adaptive techniques and devices, the chapter also presents a problem solving approach to teach clients so they will be able to continue to develop adaptations to their vision loss for commonly experienced challenges faced by adults with vision impairment. Further, we will provide information about community resources that are available to the therapist and persons with vision loss.

The general strategy used to organize a treatment plan for these activities includes 4 areas: **E**nvironmental Modification, **P**rocess Adaptation, **I**ntroduction of Equipment, or **C**hange of End-Product/Task Simplification—the **EPIC** Framework. Table 16-1 describes the EPIC Framework in detail, which includes examples of functional applications related to locating food on a plate.

Whittaker SG, Scheiman M, Sokol-McKay DA.
Low Vision Rehabilitation: A Practical Guide for Occupational Therapists,
Second Edition (pp 301-308).
© 2016 Taylor & Francis Group.

TABLE 16-1: THE EPIC FRAMEWORK

1. **E**nvironmental Modification—Place darker food on light, non-patterned plate; incorporate portable task lamp; cover glossy table with matte-finished tablecloth.

2. **P**rocess Adaptation—Have food locations described according to clock positions or right/left/top/bottom; consistent locations of foods on plate.

3. **I**ntroduction of Equipment—Use fork tines or tip of knife to tap around plate in organized manner to determine locations of different foods; use sectioned plate.

4. **C**hange of End Product/Task Simplification—Select easier-to-detect version of food/food group desired (carrot slices vs peas, fried egg on toast instead of fried egg with toast on the side).

TABLE 16-3: LOW VISION PRINCIPLES

1. Lighting—Use backlit watch.

2. Contrast and color—Use watch or clock with white numbers/hands on black background or vice versa; use digital bedroom clock with bright red numbers.

3. Glare control—Use a clock without a glossy cover, proper positioning of light near clock to avoid glare.

4. Organization—Use timepiece with talking hourly chime; use talking timer with automatic time announcement.

5. Relative size magnification—Use watch or clock with enlarged numbers and large, distinguishable hour and minute hands.

6. Relative distance magnification—Bring watch close to eye, bring clock down to eye level and step closer to it.

TABLE 16-2: THE EPIC CONTINUUM OF ADAPTATION FROM VISUAL TO NONVISUAL

Use a sharpie marker to mark the top of the shampoo cap with a large, bold "S"; and the top of the conditioner with a large, bold "C."

↓

Tie a brightly colored non-fray bow on one container and not the other.

↓

Put a standard rubber band on one bottle and not the other.

↓

Put the shampoo in the front of the shower/tub and conditioner in the back. Containers placed in order of use—front to back. (If a spouse is involved, they would need to agree to the system.)

↓

Substitute an all-in-one shampoo and conditioner product. (May not be an option if client likes current products.)

The 4 different aspects of intervention contained in the EPIC Framework provide the therapist with a platform from which to expand the options that a client can choose among. Each of these interventions includes nonoptical devices and adaptive techniques, as well as "low vision" interventions that both facilitate use of residual vision and utilize sensory substitution and nonvisual cues (Table 16-2).

Low vision principles of lighting, contrast/color, glare control, organization, and relative size and relative distance magnification can also assist the therapist in developing a potential selection of adaptive devices and techniques.

Table 16-3 includes examples focusing on accurately keeping track of time and demonstrates these principles.

Please refer to Chapter 12 on environmental modifications that maximize functional vision, as well as facilitate use of nonvisual strategies. Commonly used nonoptical assistive devices and adaptive techniques throughout this chapter will be introduced, with reference to specific tasks with some discussion of their basic features, use, and variations. These devices will be discussed generically because new, but often similar, products are always coming onto the market. Some adaptive products that have proven popular, are widely used, and are anticipated to remain on the market may be identified by name. Some products can be made at home, but the therapist has to evaluate the trade-off comparing the cost of the time it takes to create a product versus the cost for the client to purchase a similar item. Even in terms of a basic guide to write signatures, it is less expensive to have the client purchase one than try to produce one of equal quality. The therapist might consider buying inexpensive items like signature guides in bulk and simply giving them to clients. Many of these nonoptical devices and techniques have advantages and limitations, and these may be discussed briefly. Many times, a client will have to choose a product that best meets his or her needs but still needs to be adapted or requires training to use, and the therapist might need to have samples available for demonstration and training, such as talking watches and clocks. Nonoptical assistive devices are often products located in specialty catalogs, but there are times when a client's needs can be met with a product available on the commercial market, either out of the box or with adaptation. Products in specialty catalogs may include large-print phone and address registers, raised/large-print timers, talking weight scales, braille watches, and writing guides, while items on the general market can include digital food timers, large-print medication boxes, insulin pens, nested/contrasting measuring cups and spoons, and digital recorders. Refer to Table 16-4 for major specialty catalog providers furnishing ADL equipment for use by clients with low vision or blindness.

TABLE 16-4: LOW VISION ACTIVITIES OF DAILY LIVING PRODUCT CATALOGS

- LS&S Products: www.lssproducts.com
- Maxiaids: www.maxiaids.com
- Independent Living aids: www.independentliving.com
- American Printing House for the Blind: www.APH.org
- Mattingly Low Vision: www.mattinglylowvision.comindex.cfm

SELF-CARE

The basic ADL realm and a variety of low vision and nonvisual interventions are available and chosen based on best fit for the client and his or her situation. These tasks include the areas of bathing and showering, personal hygiene and grooming, dressing, personal device care, and self-feeding. Some of these areas may be further subdivided into smaller components. The category of eating may include locating food on the plate, locating dinnerware on the table, cutting food, spreading condiments, seasoning foods, pouring hot and cold liquids, bringing a reasonable amount of food to the mouth, and eating neatly. Dining in one's home, even with company, is considerably simpler than dining in a restaurant, where even more challenges will be addressed in other chapters.

Bathing and Showering

Distinguishing containers. One of the most common difficulties with bathing and showering is distinguishing bathing products like shampoo from the conditioner. Several possible interventions were provided earlier in Table 16-2. Location can be used to differentiate shampoo from conditioner only if the person lives alone or others in the family follow this approach as well. Changing the end product by purchasing a combination shampoo and conditioner eliminates this difficulty, again if it meets the needs of those living in the household as well. Transferring shampoo and conditioner into more visible or differently shaped containers is an option, but requires more effort. In this situation, or when marking only one container, as with a rubber band, the client should choose the option that is most meaningful and thus more memorable to him or her.

Transfers and setting up the bath. Another component of bathing and showering affected by vision impairment is safety entering and exiting the bathtub and shower. Many adaptations revolve around enhancing visibility in the bathing area—using high contrast, brightly colored non slip strips can be wrapped around grab bars, a contrasting towel placed on a lightly colored shower seat or tub bench, or a

dark bath mat on the tub floor. A contrasting, nonskid bath mat can be used in the shower stall after creating a drainage hole, or one can be draped over the entry side of the tub to make the height of the side more visible when stepping in. The water height can be monitored via a contrasting strip on the inner side of the tub edge or a contrasting floating object.[3]

Locating items. Locating the soap may pose difficulty at times. A bat mitt with a soap pocket can be used. Using liquid versus bar soap may prove helpful. A wall dispenser assists with a number of bathing products, such as for soap, shampoo, and conditioner. The location of the dispensing buttons, front to back, may indicate order of use. The raised dispensing buttons may be color coded to their respective bottles; marked with a bold line Sharpie marker with "1 or B" for body wash, "2 or S" for shampoo, "3 or C " for conditioner, or raised markings can be placed on the buttons 1 mark representing body wash, 2 marks indicating shampoo, etc. Soap placed in a full-length stocking of sufficient length can be tied around the neck, wrist, or a fixture. This is not only an inexpensive option, but also an economical one in that a new bar can be added before the old one is used up.

Personal Hygiene and Grooming

Dental. Applying toothpaste to a toothbrush requires placing the correct amount in the proper place. Another consideration is keeping the toothpaste confined so it does not soil the bathroom sink. The simplest of modifications is to incorporate contrast by placing a light-colored toothbrush on a dark washcloth and/or switching to dark or striped toothpaste to further contrast with the bristles of the toothbrush. Generally one-half to one inch of toothpaste is sufficient, and this amount can be measured out by squirting the toothpaste on the tip of the index finger; then the toothpaste can be applied to the toothbrush bristles or directly into the mouth.[5] Placement of the toothpaste can be facilitated by holding the bristles between the thumb and index finger to gauge where and how much toothpaste

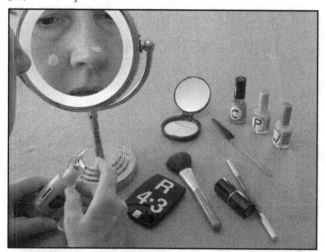

Figure 16-1. Using the dot technique for foundation application, the counting technique for blush application, and magnifying makeup mirror for visual feedback.

to apply. The simplest but most novel nonvisual approaches entails squirting the toothpaste into the palm and scooping it up with the bristles or, if the client lives alone, merely squirting the toothpaste directly into the mouth. A consideration with toothpaste as well as other products with caps is not losing sight of the cap. The easiest solution is to put the cap in a "memorable place"—this is a concept that will be repeated throughout upcoming chapters. Another solution to the misplaced cap problem is to "palm" the cap while using the product. Toothpaste, however, is a product that can be purchased with a hinged/attached cap, thus eliminating the problem altogether.

Makeup, shaving, and mirror use. Use of a magnifying and/or lighted magnifying mirror may be of help during makeup application, although some distortion may be present. These mirrors come in standard and compact form, and up to 10X magnification is commercially available. One challenge with mirror use is lighting. Typical bathroom lighting, which has many reflective surfaces, results in considerable glare (see Chapter 12). The best lighting is a handheld wide beam flashlight because it can be directed on the area of interest and positioned to minimize glare. Electronic magnifiers with remote/flex arm cameras (see Chapter 14) can be directed to the face and hands for those with more severely reduced acuity. Cameras can be set to "mirror mode," reversing the images just like a mirror. Some lighted makeup mirrors are also available.

Magnifying mirrors are the same as magnifiers in that the stronger the power of the magnifier, the smaller the field of view, or the less of the face that is seen and the larger any blemishes appear. The advantage of an electronic magnifier is the capacity to "zoom"; the disadvantage is that display colors do not match real colors. Makeup should be subtle (easier to blend, mistakes less obvious), consistent with coloring of the complexion, and used sparingly. Sometimes, applying compact foundation or blush by finger

vs applicator gives the user more control. Using a reliable friend or obtaining guidance from the makeup consultant at a makeup counter will help in this area. Finally, smart phones and tablet computers can be used to take snapshots and then the picture zoomed in to check makeup.

Several popular nonvisual makeup techniques will be discussed next. The objective of these techniques is to ensure that the quantity, location, and application of makeup are appropriate. One method for foundation is to apply a small dot to the forehead, nose, chin, and each cheek and to blend and smooth the foundation upward and outward in a systematic manner to ensure adequate coverage (Figure 16-1). Another nonvisual method is to count the number of brush strokes needed on a cake of blush or eye shadow and the number of strokes above the base of the cheekbone or over the eyelid and extending to its outer corner. Counting helps to determine the amount of makeup applied, while the cheekbone and outer corner of the eyelid serve as landmarks for appropriate delineation of location.[4] Overlapping strokes when applying eye shadow will ensure consistency—and it is a principle that can be generalized to other daily activities.

A sighted observer can provide feedback to determine how much makeup is enough, both in the beginning and when changes in brand, color, and method of application or applicator change. Putting foundation and nail polish in the refrigerator will provide a tactual cue—the coldness—to aid in application. A styling salon can also assist with nail care, shaping of eyebrows, and other areas. An optometrist or ophthalmologist should be consulted as to safe use of mascara.

Shaving with limited vision poses few problems for men. The key difficulty during shaving is obtaining full coverage of the face when using a razor blade or electric shaver. Three key behaviors to attain this objective include using landmarks, overlapping strokes, and tactile monitoring. For example, the finger of the nonshaving hand can be placed at the base of the sideburn—this would serve as a landmark, to which the shaver can then be guided. Overlapping strokes, reshaving at a 90-degree angle to the original strokes, and checking shaved areas with the fingertips ensure that no area is missed.[4] Maintaining a mental picture of the face and areas shaved or shaving one half of the face at a time is also helpful.

Dressing

Matching clothing. The major difficulty in dressing is identifying and matching clothing. Sunlight, a full-spectrum bulb/lamp, and newer light-emitting diode (LED) 200-lumen or greater flashlights provide appropriate color rendition and assist in visual color identification of clothing. Cleaning out closets and drawers of unused clothing, storing seasonal clothing in another area, and separating casual from dressier clothing all work toward maximizing overall organization. Clothing not worn in a year should be given or thrown away. Products for organization can include drawer dividers, hanging shoe racks, garment bags with shelves, and other commercial organizers. Techniques for organization include hanging outfits together, and, for women, accessories can be placed in a plastic bag hung around the neck of the hanger. Clothing can also be grouped by color, category (skirts, pants, so on), or placement/location. Labeled shoeboxes can be used to store and differentiate shoes. When buying clothing, consider purchasing clothes that are color coordinated and then mix and match. For other ADL tips, refer to "A Self-Help Guide to Non-Visual Skills" written by Dan Roberts and available free in large-print or downloadable format at www.lowvision.preventblindness.org/publications/a-self-help-guide-to-non-visual-skills.

A lot of clothing can be identified by the design, texture of the fabric, types of fasteners and their location, the style of the collar, neckline, sleeves, and any decorations. The blue sweater may have a round neckline and buttons up the front, whereas the yellow sweater buttons up the front but is ribbed, with a turtleneck. Shoes can also be differentiated by style or shape or the pair kept together by use of a clothespin. Socks can be paired together using diaper pins or specifically designed products called sock locks or sock savers. The socks can be laundered and stored in the sock lock/saver. Some sock locks will allow the user to notch the plastic device for color identification: no notch equates to black, one notch equates to blue, and so on.

Large print can be used for labeling the garment directly, using a laundry marker, or indirectly on an index card pinned to the garment or hung on the clothes hanger using a rubber band. Raised print on a file card can provide a multisensory label by combining large print, color, and tactual cues. Labels such as these require the client to remember what label goes with what garment until the clothing is laundered and relabeled.

One of the most popular tactual labeling techniques for clothing is the use of rustproof safety pins. Safety pins can be varied by number and position—no safety pin indicates black, one horizontal safety pin indicates blue, one vertical safety pin indicates brown, and two crossed safety pins indicate green. No marking is placed on the clothes article that the client has the most of (in this example, black pants). Beads can be added and locations varied as long as the pins are placed in locations (pocket or hem) that are not visible and do not cause discomfort. Another strategy is to put one safety pin on all the clothes that match each other. So, for example, place a single safety pin on a green-and-blue striped shirt, a blue plaid blouse, a blue sweater with snowflakes, and a blue skirt that all these tops match.[4] Tactual labeling includes small aluminum braille tags that are sewn or pinned onto the clothing care label of the garment. Each label is just 2 or 3 letters that can be recognized by touch by knowing the 26 letters of uncontracted braille.

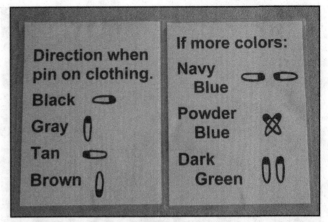

Figure 16-2. Labeling options for clothing.

These tags permit up to 21 light and dark colors and several common patterns.

Auditory labeling systems also now exist that can be used on clothing. These systems consist of adhesive washable labels that can be attached directly to the garment. Information regarding the clothing color, pattern, style, and even care instructions is recorded on the label by the client or a caregiver using the handheld recording/playback device. Colors of clothing can also be identified by an electronic color identifier/detector, which speaks the color aloud when you hold it against the garment. Color detectors/identifiers and color-identifying apps for the iPhone should be tried to ensure the accuracy level meets the client's needs—we find accuracy is often a problem. Lighting plays a big factor in realistic color rendition so a consistent and sufficient level of lighting should be used each time these products are used. Figure 16-2 illustrates a labeling strategy for clothing.

Scheduling. One of the primary tasks within this basic ADL category includes telling time—both calendar and clock time. Keeping track of appointments and other important events often requires the use of a large-/giant-print calendar. These are available in low vision specialty catalogs, and most are large and wall mount in nature. A bold line pen can be used to place entries on the calendar itself if sufficient space is available. If space is inadequate for an entry such as an appointment or special event then a symbol or sticker can be placed in the appropriate date box on the calendar and the associated information placed in a bound notebook accompanied by the same symbol or sticker. An eternal talking calendar is available for those who cannot access a large-print calendar. Tactual adaptation and some cognitive skill are required to access the buttons due to the calendar's flat panel, but it allows many appointments to be recorded, even multiple appointments on one day. Smart phones and personal organizers are often used to keep a calendar and to tell time as well (see Chapter 14).

Many options are available to tell time via a clock or watch. Several considerations in watch choice depend on

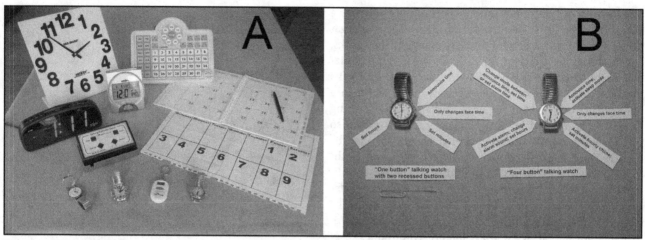

Figure 16-3. (A) Products for adaptive time keeping. (B) One- and 4-button talking watches. (Products courtesy of LS&S—see LS&S QR Code in catalog for video instruction.)

the features desired—4 buttons vs a single button, alarm, alarm sound options, hourly chime, male/female voice, volume control, availability of calendar time, language availability, style, and complexity of resetting, among others. Although many watches come in male and female sizes, a large face male watch permits greater spacing on the watch face often making it easier to see or feel its' features whether it is a low vision, braille or tactile watch. Often, a watch, like jewelry, is an expression of one's personality, so one size does not fit all.

Generally, resetting a talking watch or clock is more difficult than the single press of a button required for the timepiece to announce the time. Several newer talking models minimize the need to manually change clock settings. An atomic time piece will reset itself once the appropriate time zone is set. An interactive clock responds voice responses/commands include but are not limited to, telling and changing the time, telling or changing the alarm time, and other settings. A braille or tactile watch is also an option for a client who prefers a silent timepiece. A braille watch is a tactile timepiece, often a cover that is opened to reveal the watch face. It does not use braille characters, but instead uses a pattern of raised dots, lines, or both that substitute for the numbers and are placed at increments around the clock face. To determine the time, the client uses the fingertips to feel the hands of the watch in relation to the raised markings placed at increments around the clock (Figure 16-3).[5] A new tactile watch has emerged on the market that has raised markings at 12, 3, 6, and 9 o'clock positions and time is indicated by 2 ball bearings, 1 ball bearing on the side indicating hours and one on the face indicating minutes.

Smart phones with text-to-speech options and voice recognition now can be used for timekeeping, calendars, reminders, and memos using built-in applications and adaptive features. With the iPhone, the applications are supplied with the operating system. The voice recognition system is called Siri and can be used to request information, input calendar entries, create messages, and, to a limited extent, e-mail in speech form. Special applications such as Talker and Voice Brief specialize in reading e-mail or summarizing news, weather, and other information on the phone. When purchasing add-on software, one must always ask if the user with low vision can easily start, set up, and control the program. Many are designed for people to use while driving or walking and assume the person can visually start and set it up (Table 16-5). Some iPhone/iPad apps can provide a large print, high contrast digital time display (see Figure 12-2).

EATING AT HOME AND IN A RESTAURANT

Clock positions can describe the location of food on the plate as well as location of utensils and other containers of food and beverages at the place setting and on the table in general. The "locating technique" is used when a client desires to locate an item on the table in a discrete, careful manner without knocking items over. This technique encourages the client to explore the tabletop in a deliberate and methodical manner by first locating the table edge in front of him or her. The hands are curled slightly and are moved in a circular pattern away from the edge, locating objects with the backs of the fingers and skirting around others (Figure 16-4).

Cutting and scooping food. Cutting food can present difficulty and therefore it is suggested that foods such as meat be placed at the 6 o'clock position. Locate the edge of the meat with the knife and insert the fork tines pointing downward about 0.5 to 1 inch from the edge of the meat, and then slide the knife along the tines of the fork to guide the cut, creating a bite-sized piece (Figure 16-5). A "pulling

TABLE 16-5: KEEPING CURRENT

Learning and keeping up with adaptive equipment is a challenge. Here are a couple of suggestions to help you along the way:

- LS&S QR codes are next to a number of products in their catalog. The free QR Reader app is downloadable on the iPhone. Just scan these codes to obtain verbal instructions and videos on how a product is used.

- Search AFB's online *AccessWorld* for product reviews and evaluations. See www.afb.org/aw/main.asp.

- View free videos at www.lowvisionchef.com and on YouTube.

- Some companies will provide either verbal instructions on the phone or, in some cases, will provide written instruction sheets prior to purchase.

- Performing an online search for products can be a problem because search terms are often common. To narrow in on adaptive products for people with vision impairment, add the term *blind*. Also add the phrase *low vision*. Put the phrase in quotation marks for a more exact search, or use advanced search features of the search engine.

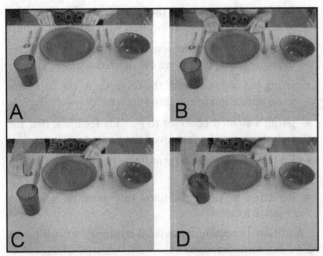

Figure 16-4. (A) Using locating technique at mealtime: sit perpendicular to edge of table. (B) Locate edge of plate using curled fingers. (C) Move hand forward, fingers curled, to locate cup. (D) Grasping cup with hand.

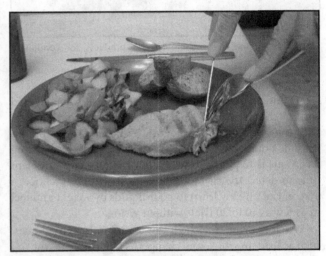

Figure 16-5. Using technique for cutting bite-sized piece.

sensation" indicates the meat has not been fully severed. In a restaurant setting, the client can ask to have meat deboned and/or cut when ordering. Loose foods like corn can be scooped up by pushing the full utensil against a "buffer," which could be the knife, mashed potatoes, or a piece of bread.[4] A high rimmed plate, a plate with sectional dividers or plate guard can be purchased and snapped onto the edge of the plate.

Spreads and condiments. Condiments such as butter can be placed in the center of the bread and spread in an outward fashion or placed in the upper-right or upper-left corner of the bread and spread from top to bottom in an overlapping fashion. The slickness of the bread as gauged by the knife indicates coverage. At home, the index finger, when placed under the rim of a salad dressing or catsup bottle, can detect the flow of condiment. Portion-controlled spouts can be purchased to place on containers with

vinegar, oil, and other such liquids (Figure 16-6). In a restaurant setting, a client can ask to have such condiments in a small cup on the side. If the client desires to further limit the dressing on the salad, the fork can be dipped into the dressing before the lettuce is pierced. Practice and attention to subtle cues are required to be able to gauge the presence and size of a piece of food on a utensil by noting its weight. The client should discreetly feel the location of the food around the edge of the plate and move it toward the center of the plate. This prevents food from slipping off the plate and allows the client to more readily locate remaining food.

Pouring. There are a wide range of devices and techniques to accomplish the task of pouring hot and cold liquids (Figure 16-7). Pouring can be enhanced by using contrasting cups and mugs (eg, black coffee in a white mug). Clear glassware should be avoided when possible. A fingertip inserted just inside the rim of a cup with the second joint resting on the rim can be used to detect the height of the liquid being poured. The same fingertip will

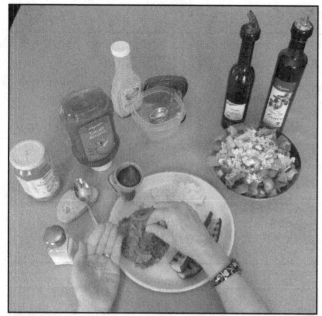

Figure 16-6. Adaptive techniques and products for condiment application.

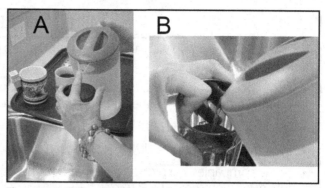

Figure 16-7. (A) Pouring over sink—locating and centering spout over cup with forefinger. (B) Pouring over sink—checking for water level with forefinger.

locate and guide the spout (spout at 9 o'clock when aligned with pitcher handle at 3 o'clock) to the center of the glass, with the spout touching the inside rim but not resting on it, while pouring. One of the critical aspects of this pouring technique is to pour slowly to allow the fingertip sufficient time to detect the rising fluid. With structured practice, a person can quickly learn to pour liquids by weight and feel in as few as 10 to 20 trials without vision.[7]

When pouring, the client can attend to nonvisual cues, such as listening for sound changes as liquid reaches the top of the cup, as well as noting changes in weight and temperature on the side of the glass. A "count" can be developed for a specific-sized glass. Colored ping pong balls and ice cubes float and can be used as a cue that the fluid has reached the desired level. A product called a liquid level indicator (LLI) can be used to detect liquid level height. This device is hung over the rim of the mug or glass with the prongs placed inside the rim of the cup. The prongs emit a nonvisual cue (beep, music, vibration) when they detect hot or cold fluid.

SUMMARY

A variety of techniques and adaptive devices of both a low vision and nonvisual nature have been presented, as well as several frameworks from which to expand the interventions available in the area of basic ADL. It is important at this point to summarize several of the key nonvisual strategies that will continue to emerge in upcoming chapters. These include the following:

- Using overlapping strokes to ensure that an area is entirely covered

- Using a mental image of an object to know where one is and where one needs to be

- Marking a location with the finger of one hand in order to bring a object to that location with the other hand

- Counting or timing to determine the number of increments required to achieve the desired goal

- Using the distance from the fingertip to the first joint as an indication of roughly 1 inch

- Using a sighted observer to provide feedback that the technique used has achieved the desired outcome

- Putting an object in a memorable place that has meaning to the client

- Referring to clock positions to determine where an object is located

Additional common nonvisual strategies will be introduced in future chapters.

REFERENCES

1. Haymes SA, Johnston AW, Heyes AD. Relationship between vision impairment and ability to perform activities of daily living. *Ophthal Physiol Opt.* 2002;22:79-91.

2. Liu C-J, Brost MA, Horton VE, Kenyon SB, Mears KE. Occupational therapy interventions to improve performance of daily activities at home for older adults with low vision: a systematic review. *Am J Occup Ther.* 2013;67:279-287.

3. Duffy M. *Making Life More Livable.* New York: AFB Press; 2002.

4. Ponchillia PE, Ponchillia SV. *Foundations of Rehabilitation Teaching With Persons Who Are Blind or Visually Impaired.* New York, NY: American Foundation for the Blind; 1996:3-21.

5. Inkster W, Newman L, Storm Weiss D, Yeadon A. *Rehabilitation Teaching for Persons Experiencing Vision Loss.* 2nd ed. New York: CIL Publications and Audiobooks of VISIONS; 1997.

6. Yeadon A, Grayson D. *Living With Impaired Vision: An Introduction.* New York, NY: American Foundation for the Blind; 1979.

7. McSweeney MS, O'Hare F, Deverell L, Ayton L. The role of vision with drink pouring and other daily tasks. In: Lovie-Kitchin J, ed. *Vision 2014 Abstract* 2014:26.

Home Management

17

This chapter introduces some basic adaptive techniques and strategies pertaining to home management for people of have low vision usually involving a combination of visual, non-visual, optical, and electronic interventions that have been discussed previously. The focus in this book is on performance; getting the job done using whatever technique works and is acceptable to the client. We will emphasize vision because research has found a correlation between level of vision impairment and disability[1] and we find patients prefer using vision. Research supports using a mix of techniques as well as problem solving strategies.[2] The occupational therapist can introduce the strategies described in this and the following chapters but should refer to a Vision Rehabilitation Therapist (CVRT) for more advanced training if such training exceeds the OTs area of expertise or knowledge base.

Many of the specific strategies described in this chapter are based on techniques that come from the field of vision rehabilitation therapy[3-6]; others from our own experience or taught to us by our clients. Further, we will provide information about community resources which are available to the therapist and persons with vision loss.

Home management skills consist of a broad range of tasks, many of which require reading in some format, thus making the activity more challenging to achieve with vision loss. Home management skills can separate those clients able to live on their own from those who do not live on their own. The same frameworks suggested in Chapter 16 on basic self-care can be applied here. Table 17-1 is an example focused on slicing vegetables for a cooking activity.

This chapter will focus on the major homemaking skills of communication, financial management, meal preparation, household management, and shopping. Management of health, medication, physical activity, and mobility within the home and out in the community will be addressed in the remaining chapters due to the volume of information available.

Communication Skills

Writing

Communicating information is a vital necessity, whether it is by written format, the telephone, or keyboarding. Writing strategies are generally discussed in Chapter 15. One might not expect people would have difficulty just learning to write larger, but we find some do. The therapist might need to develop a program of graded instruction to teach a person to write larger.

Size magnification strategies. The client should be taught to write just big enough to read several days later.

Whittaker SG, Scheiman M, Sokol-McKay DA.
Low Vision Rehabilitation: A Practical Guide for Occupational Therapists, Second Edition (pp 309-322).
© 2016 Taylor & Francis Group.

Table 17-1: The EPIC Framework—Slicing Vegetables

1. **E**nvironmental Modification—Slice vegetable on contrasting surface.

2. **P**rocess Adaptation—Slice round vegetable in half to stabilize it when cutting; use claw position vs extended finger position when holding vegetable prior to slicing; use the "bridge" technique.

3. **I**ntroduction of Equipment—Use knife with a guide; use slicing guide.

4. **C**hange of End Product/Task Simplification—Use precut fresh, frozen, or canned vegetables.

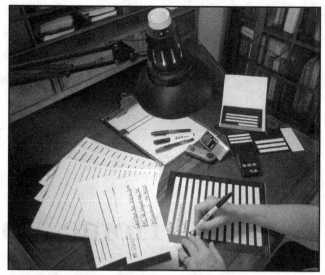

Figure 17-1. Adaptive writing aids and audio recorders.

However, the larger the writing, the more space is taken up, so being concise is the key. On a large-print calendar a client might write "Dr. P, 9:30,"—it is not necessary to write down the full name of the doctor, location, to bring medication list and insurance card (these should be routinely brought), or a.m./p.m., as these are known factors. The client will write differently if someone else is going to read it. For personal use (recipes, address book), abbreviations can be used more frequently, but such shorthand methods should be avoided if the writing needs to be read by others (envelopes, Christmas cards) or both (shopping list). One common mistake is to use all capital letters. The use of uppercase and lowercase letters makes it easier to visually identify words.

Low vision writing tools. Tools can include bold line paper and bold line pens. Bold line paper is available in various line thickness, space widths, bindings, and color in order to meet the specific visual strengths and needs of the client. Bold line envelopes are now available. The thickness of bold line pens varies, the most popular of which is the 20/20 pen, which is 1 mm in width. It is also helpful to try pens of widths above and below this parameter. The most beneficial bold line writing pen is black, felt, or gel tip and designed for writing, as it does not bleed through. This is an important feature when desiring to write on the back of a page or the next page.

Writing typical size and filling out forms. People with acquired vision loss generally can write legibly using the size and style of handwriting before vision loss even if they cannot see what they are writing. These individuals often benefit from writing guides or templates when normal print size is needed.[4] A basic writing template is generally a piece of black plastic with rectangles cut out in which a signature, numbers, or a few words can be written, as on a signature line on a form, a check, or an envelope. In teaching the use of any guide, it is important that the client be taught to "mark" the beginning edge of the rectangle, a common strategy described in Chapters 10 and 16. The pen tip is brought to the fingertip (and the inner edge of the rectangle) when beginning to write so as to optimize use of the space available.

The client uses a thin line (ballpoint) rather than a bold line pen to avoid letters running together. The client practices signing at first, then writing a few words. If using vision, clients will tend to write using the bottom of the opening as a line. This will prevent writing descenders (letters with tails like y, g, and p), and most will quickly learn to write above the bottom edge of the rectangle. For those who struggle writing in the upper part of the window of a signature guide, a special signature guide with an elastic cord attached across the length of the cut-out should be tried. In this situation the client writes on the elastic cord and pushes the cord down with the pen tip to make the tails of a letter. Clients with brain injury and spatial perceptual impairments like spatial neglect may have difficulty with this task even with otherwise normal visual acuity. If the client cannot successfully use a signature guide, then use of any other guide will not be realistic. When writing typical size print, as with a guide, the client should be instructed to finish words and lines, and if there is a need to stop, then a finger should be used as a place marker (Figure 17-1).

Braille. If the client has significant vision loss, a referral should be made to a CVRT for instruction in braille and alterative systems of reading and writing. A client can learn to use just grade 1 braille, which is only the alphabet, numbers, and punctuations marks. This may be helpful if the client wants to write items that only he or she needs to read—grocery lists, phone numbers and addresses, labels, recipes, and messages. Grade 2 braille consists of grade 1 braille and nearly 200 "contractions," which represent groups of letters or whole words. This is the grade of braille that books are published in.[4] For those with tactile sensitivity issues, braille also can be written in jumbo format (enlarged braille cell); however, books are generally published in the smaller standard size braille cell.

Telephone Use

Telephone use may require relative size magnification using the many large-numbered keypads on standard table/wall-mount, cordless, and cell phones. Although it is easier for a person with recent vision loss to use large-numbered phones, a person can be taught a tactile technique to dial a phone, which is more useful to someone who might use a phone other than his or her own. Maintaining the 3 middle fingers on the home row (4, 5, 6) allows the client with vision loss to locate other numbers from this central row. This is a common strategy on keypads. Many telephones have a raised dot or slash on the number 5, which can also aid the client in maintaining orientation to the keypad. Either the home row or the number 5 can be further marked with more visual and tactile markings.[5] Speed and voice dialing (phone company service or phone feature) minimize the amount of dialing required.

Adaptive cell phones include the Jitterbug, which is a low vision phone that has been on the market for several years, in differing versions. The iPhone has both a magnification feature and a screen reading program called Voice Over installed that allows the user to access the flat screen keypad and any other information on the touch screen. These features on the iPhone can not be used simultaneously. Additional publications for iPhone use are available through National Braille Press' yearly Catalog of Publications in a variety of accessible formats (www.nbp.org). These publications include *Getting Started with the iPhone in iOS 7, Twenty-one Apps We Can't Live Without, Twenty-two Useful Apps for Blind iPhone Users (2013)*, and others. For more resources on accessible applications for the iPhone visit www.applevis.com. Phones in the Android family either have a screen reader that is built in or one must be purchased from the Android Market. The website www.andreashead.wikispaces.com discusses numerous Android applications for persons with low vision or blindness. The use of smartphones and their applications both equalize people with vision loss and make their everyday activities appear no different then their sighted counterparts. By applying a raised dot on the 5 of a mobile phone with a keypad and programming the phone to speed dial an available family member, a mobile phone can be turned into an emergency call system.

In 2014, 2 fully accessible talking cell phones came on the market through Odin Mobile: the Odin VI, which has a standard keypad, and the Nexus, which has a touchpad (as well Internet access). Information regarding phone purchase, accessibility features, coverage areas, carrier services, instructional videos and podcasts, as well as downloadable manuals, are available on the website, www.odinmobile.com. Accessible phones are available in each states' Specialized Telecommunications Assistance Program, which will pay for or significantly discount the cost of the phone depending on the model chosen. Check your state website under "telecommunications assistance."

Accessing telephone numbers can be achieved in a variety of ways. Large-print phone and address books, preprogrammed phones, and operator assistance (which often may be free to people with vision impairment) are all options. Several varieties of large-print address/phone books are commercially available with line spacing at about half an inch. A binder with large-print dividers in landscape format can be made for clients who require print larger than that permitted in commercial address records.

Accessing the phone book to contact a plumber or other service, for example, can be achieved through the directory assistance exemption program. This program provides operator assistance at no charge. The therapist can keep application forms required by local telephone companies on file that are needed to obtain this service. Requirements may vary between providers of telephone services.

Financial Management

Money Identification

Financial management ranges from the identification of coins and bills to maintaining financial records. Coins can be identified tactually by their edges. The 2 lower-denomination coins—the penny and nickel—have smooth edges, while the 2 higher-denomination coins—the dime and quarter—have "milled" or ridged edges. The edges can be felt with the finger pad or heard when scratched by the fingernail. A client usually requires structured practice to learn to discriminate change by feel. Paper money has larger, darker denomination numbers on a light background in the lower-right corner of the new $5, $10, $20, and $50 bills, as well as distinct color schemes. Paper currency of other countries and the new US $100 dollar bills have tactile markings. Coins of other countries are often shaped and sized differently as well. Bills are usually managed through a folding system, with more folds in less frequently used denominations. A common system is keeping $1 bills open, $5 bills folded crosswise, $10 bills folded lengthwise, and $20 bills receiving 2 folds. Variations of bill folding exist in the literature, and it is best to choose what is most memorable or meaningful for the client.[3]

Persons with low vision may develop a backup system to organize folded bills within their current wallet ($1 bills in front, $5 bills behind on the left in first bill compartment, $10 bills in second compartment, with $20 bills behind on the right). Four-pocket billfolds are commercially available, as well as different coin organizers. Using specific denominations, such as $10 or $20 bills, for purchases and keeping these separate from the change received will allow the client to sort and reorganize money upon returning home. Using bills and coins closest to the purchase price will minimize

SIDEBAR 17-1: GOVERNMENT PROGRAMS FOR MONEY IDENTIFICATION

The Bureau of Engraving and Printing of the U.S. Treasury has developed several alternatives for currency identification for persons with vision loss. As of September 2014 they began distribution of free iBill money readers through The National Library Service for the Blind and Physically Handicapped (NLS) to its patrons. Non-NLS patrons must submit an application signed by a "competent authority" (which includes occupational therapists and many other health care, social work, and blindness professionals) who can certify eligibility. Instructions will be provided on an audio CD. The reader has a volume control and 3 modes: speech, tone, and vibration for people who are hearing impaired or deaf and blind.

In addition 2 apps are now available for bill identification: the Eyenote for the iPhone and the IDEAL Currency Identifier for the Android phone. The U.S. Treasury reports this is a stopgap measure until at least 2020 when accessible currency can be released. Accessibility features are expected to include a new raised tactile feature and continued addition of large, high-contrast numerals and different colors to each denomination. For more information and applications, visit www.bep.gov and click on U.S. Currency Reader Program.

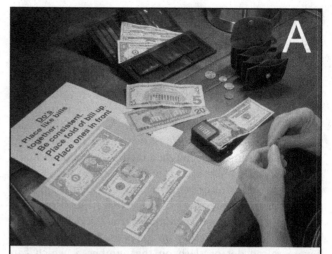

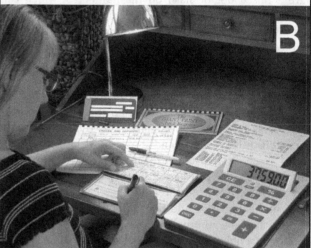

Figure 17-2. (A) Currency and coin management, including Bureau of Engraving iBill reader. (B) Financial management with a desk lamp, large-print documents, and calculator. (Products courtesy of LS&S.)

sorting of change. Talking handheld currency identifiers are available. MoneyReader is an application compatible with most mobile devices, including older versions of the iPhone, iPod, and iPad (Figure 17-2[A]). See Sidebar 17-1 for government programs for currency identification.

Paying Bills

Bill paying can be completed through the use of large-print/raised-print checks, a standard check and check guide, online, through smartphone banking applications, or directly through the bank. A standard check guide must be paper-clipped to the check to keep it in place, while a book-style guide enfolds the check, thereby maintaining its position. Large-print checks can be obtained through many, but not all, banks at no additional charge and include a larger check register. If more space is required, larger version check registers are available in low vision catalogs. Large-print, braille, and recorded statements may also be obtained through the bank. Money Talks (www.aph.org) is software that enables the user to print checks, print/emboss check registers for all bank accounts, and import transaction information from the user's bank to reconcile his or her check register. A free demo copy can be downloaded by visiting American Printing House for the Blind's website.

Talking automated teller machines (ATMs), available at many major banks, have raised tactile or braille symbols on the keypad and function keys and an audio jack that accommodates any standard headset or earphones (Figure 17-2B).

Maintaining Records

Recordkeeping begins with isolating documents that need to be saved—this begins with regular sorting of mail and other paperwork received or generated in the home. The following example provides some general guidelines. Organizing records may begin with location, for example, placing records in a standalone 2-drawer file cabinet with the top/easier accessed drawer containing records that need to saved up to 1 year and requiring more frequent access (utility bills, bank statements, cancelled checks, insurance policies, etc). The bottom drawer is divided into front and back sections, with records saved for 3 years in the front (medical bills) and the back reserved for records that need to be saved for up to 7 years (tax records and supporting documents, records of satisfied loans, passports, medical records, etc).

The documents in the drawers may be further organized by color-coded folders or may be labeled in large print or with barcodes (recorded labels) that can be read with apps like LookTel (www.looktel.com) that not only recognize barcodes but also allow the user to print labels. A fireproof, locked safe box can contain items never thrown away (marriage license, birth and death certificates, homeowners and life insurance policies, deeds, wills, etc). Appliance and device manuals and warranties may be placed on a pantry shelf for easier access, while current bills up to the last 3 months and receipts can be stored in expandable alphabetical files. Recordkeeping must be based on the person's individual needs and organizational style. A client willing to purchase extra software and a document scanner will generally find it easier to use the computer to store and access documents (see Chapter 14). A therapist should have sample equipment available and learn to demonstrate use of a computer with adaptive software for recordkeeping, as well as financial management and written correspondence.

MEAL PREPARATION

Introduction and Reading Recipes

Meal preparation consists of setup (reading directions/recipe, identifying food products), food preparation (slicing, peeling, measuring), and cooking (setting appliance dials, centering pan, turning and transferring food, determining food doneness, timing food). Recipes can be placed in the client's preferred print size or in a recorded format. A recipe can be recorded on a label from one of the several pen-shaped labeling devices, as the labels themselves do not have a time limit, but the recording device does. A binder or recipe box can be used to categorize recipes by typical categories (salads, soups, entrees, desserts, etc) and then employing various combinations of labeling techniques suggested in recordkeeping. Recipes can also be stored on a computer or electronic device and later enlarged or read out loud when needed.

Food Identification

Refrigerator and pantry organization are both key in identification of food products. Reduced clutter can be achieved by adhering to expiration dates and discarding products that have not been used in the last 12-month period. Everyday storage bins, handmade dividers, and commercially available kitchen organizers for wall, cabinet, or drawer storage can be used. Foods can be further organized by similarity (fruits, pastas, condiments), location (fruits on left upper shelf, pastas on right upper shelf), time of use (breakfast items on first shelf, lunch items on second shelf), common use (store meat, cheese, and associated condiments together in refrigerator), and alphabetically (basil, cinnamon, cloves, garlic).[7]

Many food products and their packaging have unique features or characteristics that can aid in distinguishing one product from another. For example, clear soup and clear salad dressing, when shaken, make a sloshing sound, while cream soup and dressing make a thud sound. A container of breadcrumbs and a container of powdered drink mix have the same size and shape, but powdered drink mix has greater weight. The shape of a container can aid in identifying condiments such as mustard, ketchup, and tartar sauce. Sometimes different senses can be used to differentiate products in the same family: brown sugar smells different, granulated sugar sounds different, and confectioner's sugar feels different.

A basic food labeling system can be implemented with rubber bands or hair bands (no rubber band on cans of fruit and one on cans of vegetables), but if the client likes to make chili, for example, a second rubber band may be placed on beans. Generally, no more than 3 singularly wrapped rubber bands should be used, so this system is good for discriminating some basic food categories but not for specific identification. Magnetic letters, which are bright in color, can be half-hitched to a food container by a rubber band ("C" on cans of corn or boxes of chocolate cake mix). MagneTachers, available from the American Printing House, comes in a 1-inch width and is a magnetic strip with nonsmearable, matte finished paper on one side on which a label can be written in permanent marker. En-Vision America sells a handheld talking barcode scanner with a multimillion-item database that will not only identify an item such as Hamburger Helper, but will also provide nutritional information, ingredients, preparation directions, and more. Apps are now available for the iPhone for performing these basic functions (Figure 17-3). One of note is TapTapSee (www.taptapseeapp.com) which recognize products and generic objects. Further information on labeling techniques and products is in Chapter 12.

Cutting, Slicing, and Peeling Foods

Food preparation tasks can include, but are not limited to, cutting/slicing/dicing, peeling, measuring, mixing, and opening packages and cans, as well as spreading and pouring, which was covered in the last chapter. Slicing, although covered in the framework at the beginning of this chapter, can be explained in a little more depth. Protective attire such as cut-resistant gloves and knife guards, which protect the backs of the fingers when cutting, are available as an added precaution if someone has tactile insensitivity or motor impairments. Such attire may not be necessary, however, and may interfere with efficient performance of these functions. Generally, the best strategy is to have structured training on use of an adaptive technique.

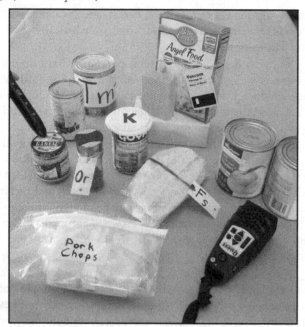

Figure 17-3. Food-labeling devices and techniques.

SIDEBAR 17-2: HEALTHY EATING AND OCCUPATIONAL THERAPY

During adaptive meal preparation, education occupational therapists should focus on how food is being prepared *and what is being prepared,* as well as adaptive food preparation techniques. Occupational therapists should focus on a healthy lifestyle and a healthy way of eating in keeping with eye health and health in general. Sandra Young, OD, has written a cookbook titled *Visionary Kitchen: A Cookbook for Eye Health* (published 2013), which includes 150 healthy recipes and sections on essential micronutrients for the eyes (including lutein, zeaxanthin, beta-carotene, omega 3 and omega 6 fatty acids, and others) and their primary food sources. It is available at www.visionarykitchen.com. The back of the book has several pages of evidenced-based articles and research on the 4 major eye diseases and the required nutrients, which support her recipes. It can truly be said, "You are what you eat."

Many vegetable and fruits have nutritive properties for eye health. Occupational therapy practitioners can make their clients aware of this during adaptive food preparation activities. It is not a myth a myth that carrots contribute to eye health. For more information and recipes see Sidebar 17-2.

Cutting requires keeping the fingers out of harm's way while achieving the desired food size. A color-contrasting cutting board may be used—slicing onions on the black side and carrots on the white side, for example. Controlled cutting can be achieved by a technique where curled fingers act as a backstop for the knife: (1) place the slightly curled fingers on top of the food item, (2) slide the fingers away from the end of the item to the desired slice thickness, (3) slide the blade of the knife along the surface of the food item until the flat side is against the backs of the curled fingers, (4) back the fingers away from the knife while holding the food in place, and (5) then cut the food item (Figure 17-4[A]).

An alternative approach is the bridge technique described by Ponchillia and Ponchillia[4] in which the fingers are used as guides for the width of the slice: (1) The knife is placed at the edge of the item to be sliced. (2) The knife is then moved away from the edge of the item to the desired width. (3) The thumb and forefinger are placed on either side of the knife from above, thus forming a bridge. (4) The cut is made. The forefinger can move back and forth to help judge the size of the slices from above while remaining out of the way of the blade (Figure 17-4[B]).

With either cutting technique mentioned, periodically handling the slice after will allow the client to judge thickness and can also confirm success. Safe, tactile cutting technique usually requires repeated practice with a variety of food products.

The issue that generally arises when peeling vegetables is ensuring that there is no peel remaining on the vegetable or fruit. Peeling in an overlapping, organized fashion is a commonly used strategy. Peeling half of the vegetable at a time can also make the task easier. Using a peeler instead of a knife often provides more control related to the amount peeled. Different styled peelers such as an enlarged grip or palm peeler may also enhance ease and control. After rinsing the vegetable and fingers, tactile cues are used to check performance, with peeled areas having a moist, smooth feel and the unpeeled portion having a rough texture.

Many vegetables and fruits have nutritive properties for eye health. Occupational therapy practitioners can make their clients aware of this during adaptive food preparation activities. It is not a myth that carrots contribute to eye health. For more information and recipes see Sidebar 17-3.

Measuring Foods

Measuring liquid and dry ingredients is an underlying task in even the most basic of cooking tasks. Color-contrasting black and white measuring cups and spoons may be helpful. It is also important to note that dry measuring cups provide the same accuracy as a liquid measuring cup, except that a dry measuring cup needs to be filled to the top, thus resulting in overflow. Overflow can easily be caught by a receiving container and returned to the original container with a funnel. Some clients prefer cups to be labeled as to the quantity each measures.

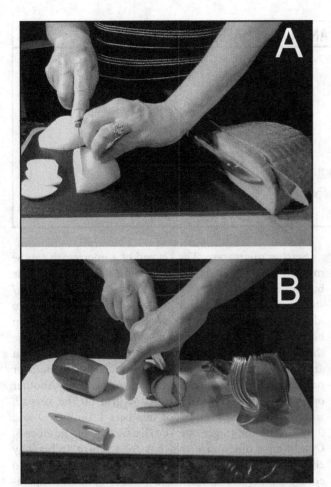

Figure 17-4. (A) Curled finger cutting technique with reverse contrast cutting board (black and white) and knife with variable slicing guide. (B) Bridging technique with reverse contrast cutting board and tomato in slicing guide. (Products courtesy of LS&S.)

SIDEBAR 17-3: THE LOW VISION CHEF

The owner of www.lowvisionchef.com was a career chef with 28 years in the food industry who happened to develop macular degeneration and is legally blind. In addition to a plethora of food preparation and cooking products (kitchen safety, peelers and knives, bowls and colanders), the website offers a wide range of cooking tips (use a piece of bread to soak up meat fat), as well as a range of videos (knife skills, knife guard choices). The owner leads training sessions and sponsors the "Out of Sight Cooking Club." She uses a number of her own website products, and is a great resource for therapists and consumers when it comes to understanding the features of products and how they can fit an individual's needs.

Although large-print or color-coded measuring cups are available, the "nesting" feature of measuring cups allows easy recognition—a 4-cup set has a quarter-cup as its smallest measurement and 1 cup as its largest. Measuring cup handles can also be notched, with a quarter-cup with 4 notches to 1 cup with 1 notch. For an alternative to standard horizontal measuring spoons, metal measuring spoons can be bent into ladles, and common liquids like oil and vanilla can be transferred to a wide-mouthed jar. This allows the client to dip the ladle-like measuring spoon into the jar of liquid, where it will self-level, and then can be brought directly over the receiving bowl to empty.

Cooking Food

Stove and oven use. Cooking food requires setting the temperature on the stove, oven, or toaster oven or the time on a microwave. Getting close to the dials on the front panel of a stovetop/oven, leaning over to access dials on a back panel, or using a magnifier are to be avoided, so techniques employed are often nonvisual in nature. Often,

turning the dial to the 6 o'clock position on a standard stovetop will set the burner on medium, and a return to the off position at 12 o'clock is accompanied by a "click" sound. Clock positions can be used on the oven dial as well. On a digital oven, the temperature button typically defaults to 350 degrees, and a single press on an up/down button (if present) corresponds to 5 or 10 degrees increase/decrease in temperature. Tactile markings, in any case, can be used to locate the buttons on the flat pad of the digital oven. A notched wooden spoon (to gauge distance from edges of stovetop) or a corner template can be used to center a pot on a flat-top cooking surface. A hand can be circled about shoulder height (may be adjusted depending the client's height) above the burner to detect heat leakage indicating the pan is off center. In addition, it is important that safety measures be followed during the client's use of these appliances.

Gas and electric stoves and ovens. Several differences exist between an electric and gas stove. If an option is available, the pros and cons of each must be presented to the client. Gas burners turn on and off immediately, the range of adjustment is continual, adjustments are immediate, and the flame is both visual and tactile in nature. Gas, however, has an open flame, is toxic, and has no detectable odor. Electric burners have precise increments of adjustment, have a closed source of heat, and have a more defined burner area. The cons of electric stoves include being slow to heat up and cool down, heat adjustments take longer, and the burner lacks visual and auditory cues that it is off. Finally, the broiler on an electric stove is part of the upper part of the oven, while in a gas stove the broiler is underneath the oven floor, thus requiring bending. Self-cleaning capability may also be an issue.

Use of a stovetop and/or oven inherently involves moderate or high levels of heat and the potential for serious burns. In view of the hazards, the writer has included a list

TABLE 17-2: STOVETOP AND OVEN SAFETY TIPS
1. Place pot on cold burner; turn off burner before removing pot.
2. Place slightly filled teapot on hot burner.
3. Turn pot/pan handles to 3 o'clock or 9 o'clock position.
4. Match burner to pot size.
5. Put food in cold oven.
6. Use nonflammable oven mitts, preferably elbow length; use oven rack guard.
7. Always pull out oven rack when inserting/removing food.
8. Vent oven slightly to release heat and stand to side to remove food.

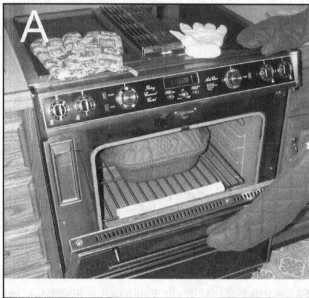

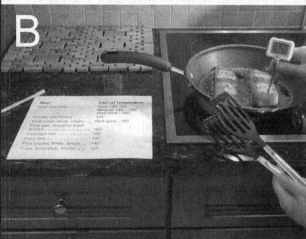

Figure 17-5. (A) Techniques and devices for cooking safely in the oven. (B) Cooking salmon, with pan handle at 9 o'clock and fillets at 3 and 9 o'clock, and large-display thermometer and double spatula.

of stovetop and oven safety tips in Table 17-2, some of which are demonstrated Figure 17-5.

Setting microwave. The keypad of a microwave can be marked with raised and/or high-contrast markings on the buttons required for key functions such as start and clear/stop. Color coding, another strategy, can assist the user to identify the start button with a green marking and the stop button with a red marking. Some clients may prefer to have the 1-minute button marked and just add minutes to heat an item, while others may want full access to the number pad through marking of the home row (4, 5, 6). Another option is a high-contrast tic-tac-toe grid on the keypad, which defines the location of numbers 1 through 9 and 0 by sliding the finger one key distance below number 8. Obtaining a microwave that has food sensor technology eliminates reading labels and inputting cooking times to ensure food is heated sufficiently and to optimal temperature. A talking microwave allows full accessibility. For more information on marking, see Chapter 12.

Determining food doneness. Ensuring that food is cooked to desired doneness can be achieved through 3 primary avenues: texture, timing, and temperature. For example, "The carrots feel done (when pierced)," "This fish is perfectly done (when flakes with a fork)," and "Those cookies smell like they are getting done," are all typical statements used by a cook. Texture and other sensory cues have always been used to determine foods are cooked to desired level.[4] Large-print/high-contrast, large-display, and talking timers are available in low vision catalogs and provide a more concrete method of gauging when food is fully cooked.

The old-fashioned dial timer is easiest to use and is relatively inexpensive and available with adaptations for low vision (see Chapter 16 and online appendix [www.routledge.com/9781617116339]). Some digital timers provide auditory feedback in the form of beeping sounds—a beep occurs with each press of the hour or minute button and that corresponds to a 1-hour or 1-minute increment in time set on the timer (Figure 17-6). Counting beeps is a common strategy with buttons or digital controls, but, unfortunately, is not always available. Another strategy is to look at the order of the buttons—often they reflect order of use or another feature. A client who mostly reheats food can mark on the food item package in large numbers how many minutes are required to heat it.

Internal temperature is a third and the safest way to determine doneness of foods, particularly meats. Large-display, tactile, and talking food thermometers can be obtained from major specialty catalog suppliers (see Chapter 16) (see Figure 17-6). Be aware that not all products that "talk" may be usable by a person with vision loss—some devices in this category may announce the result (meat is done), only after some settings are set visually (the desired internal temperature). The iDevices kitchen thermometer interfaces with multiple Apple devices through their app and provides auditory and large print temperature readings of cooked foods through use of a flexible probe.

A common and often effective intervention for anyone with functional vision is to optimize lighting, because inspecting for doneness or spoilage by the appearance of food requires optimization of contrast sensitivity (see Chapter 12). Use of movable tabletop lamps can be easy to implement and used to optimize illuminance and minimize glare. Overhead lights are rarely effective unless the fixture is replaced with spotlights and track lighting that direct light onto work areas from above. Under-cabinet lighting is often useful, as are pendant lights suspended from the ceiling over island counters.

Handheld magnifiers (see Chapter 13) are often used in the kitchen to read recipes and labels and inspect food for appearance and spoilage. An alternative way to avoid spoilage is to label food with the date on which it is stored in the refrigerator or freezer, or mark the item with expiration dates in accordance with food safety standards. The more serious cook who attends to food presentation often finds a telemicroscope or mounts for an illuminated handheld magnifier useful because these devices free both hands for the task at hand.

Cooking courses such as "Crock-Pots: Slow and Easy Cooking," "Microwave Magic," and "No-Cook Cooking" are available to clients through Hadley School for the Blind at www.hadley.edu/Findacourse.asp. If the cook has very little functional vision, more advanced training focused on nonvisual cues, techniques, and equipment for cooking and baking may be provided by a CVRT. Certified vision rehabilitation therapists will also work on use of small cooking appliances such as a countertop grill or an electric skillet.

HOUSEHOLD MANAGEMENT

Laundry Care

Maintaining and repairing clothing requires setting washer and dryer dials, threading a needle, and performing basic hand and machine sewing.

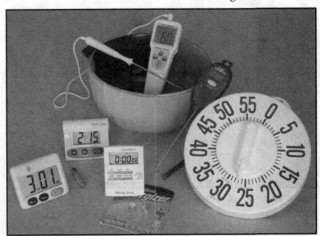

Figure 17-6. Adaptive timers and food thermometers.

Dials. Adaptive techniques for operating the dials range from keeping a dial preset, attending to any tactile/auditory cues that are present when turning the dial to a setting, and marking each dial at a specific setting. Presetting washer dials on cold temperature, load size on medium or large, and wash cycle on regular will cover most washing needs. Some dials click when turned to a setting, and the settings are in a logical order, so clicks can be counted to obtain the desired setting—for example, the water temperature dial might be first/leftmost click, cold; second click, cool; third click, warm; and fourth/rightmost click, hot. Clock positions can also be used—the 3 o'clock position on the dryer might represent 40 minutes drying time.[5] Stains are difficult to detect and may be done so tactually by marking with a safety pin or by obtaining reliable sighted assistance. Stain removal sticks and individually wrapped stain treatment towelettes permit more immediate treatment.

Stains. Because laundry care requires inspections for relatively low-contrast stains and matching colors, lighting is critical (see Chapter 12) and generally requires movable light sources, as well as some lower-powered magnification. The work environments should include equipment required for labeling and matching clothes. Strategies for premeasuring detergent and additives are useful as well. A standard black dry measuring cup can be used for lightly colored powdered detergent, while a similar white cup can be used for darker colored liquid detergents. In substitution for measuring liquids, one can purchase premeasured products like detergent pods and fabric softener sheets. A handheld high-intensity flashlight (150 lumens or greater) is essential if someone has impaired contrast sensitivity. The client will need to be instructed on how to position the light with magnifiers (if needed) to avoid glare and maximize contrast. With more severe vision loss, clothes should be professionally laundered periodically or sighted assistance is needed.

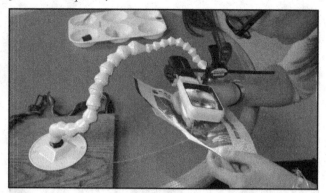

Figure 17-7. Use of a high power optical device for needlework or sewing.

Sewing

Sewing presents a particular challenge because clients often require about the same level of magnification required for reading small print and, in addition, need to optimize contrast enhancement. Even adults with typical vision often use lighting and magnification aids for needlepoint, fine sewing, and quilting. A good starting point is to use an adjustable floor lamp that can be positioned for various work settings, such as when using a sewing machine or sitting and performing hand sewing. The larger, commercial magnifying lenses available in sewing stores often are not strong enough for a person with even a moderate loss in acuity. Prescribed optical devices are often used instead (see Chapter 13) (Figure 17-7).

Stronger illuminated stand magnifiers (up to as high as 8 D) are available. Loupes, mounted on eyeglasses, allow up to about 8 D of add to be achieved while maintaining a sufficient working distance, and telemicroscopes with caps designed for about a 15-cm working distance can be used to achieve the greatest magnification and binocularity, which is useful if someone can use both eyes. Telemicroscopes can be configured to over 20 diopters, but require training and ergonomic consideration to use effectively (see Chapter 13).

Organization is necessary to experience a successful sewing experience. Using a contrasting, lipped tray will increase visibility of the thread, keep small sewing supplies together, confine the workspace, and keep small and/or sharp items such as needles and straight pins from falling on the floor. A wristlet pin cushion will hold pins and needles, a length of yarn or a chain can hold a pair of scissors, while thread spools can be organized and labeled in pill bottles that are slightly larger than the spool itself. Darker spools of thread can consistently be placed in the bottom of the bottle, lighter colored spools on top.

Needle threading can be achieved by large-eyed needles, adaptive needles (top self-threading needles and side self-threading needles), loop or hook needle threaders, and threading devices (Figure 17-8). Some of the options are only feasible for long/large-eyed needles, while others can

accommodate small-eyed needles as well. The choice of device or technique is based upon the preferences, abilities, and goals of the client—a former sewer may prefer using small needles for finer stitchery, while a client with sensorimotor issues may need a larger, more tactual needle and needle threader to sew up a seam. Thread is easier to manage if it contrasts against the task background, if it is coarser in nature, and if beeswax is used to give it more texture and stiffness during threading activities.

Sewing machine adaptations include self-threading sewing machines, self-threading needles or needle threaders, high-contrast or tactile seam guides, small crochet hooks to thread the machine, and bobbin mates that keep the matching bobbin and spool together (see Figure 17-8). Some needle threaders can be used without vision. A sewing store clerk or sighted assistance may be used to locate the end of the thread on the spool, which is located in a notch under the paper label. After locating the end of the thread, the spool is placed in a pop-cap medication vial, with the end of the thread hanging outside the vial, and the vial cap is then closed. The vial or cap may then be labeled in large print with the color of the thread.

During mending activities, pins are used to secure a hem in place and to align a seam, as well as localize where the sewing will occur. When a button is to be replaced, its relocation is determined by the previous threads, and then clock positions can be used to identify where the holes are (2-hole button, 12 and 6 o'clock; 4-hole button, 2, 4, 8, and 10 o'clock).[5] When sewing on a 2-hole button, the thumb detects the needle as it comes up through the 12 o'clock hole, and later the thumb is used to mark and confirm the location of needle placement at the second hole at 6 o'clock prior to inserting the needle into the button. The following examples are ways to avoid sewing by altering the end result. The Buttoneer Fastening System uses a small handheld device and fastener to reapply the button. A garment can be hemmed professionally for a nominal fee by many drycleaners. Sew No More Fabric Glue is a mending liquid that can make invisible repairs to clothing. A referral to a CVRT may be warranted, as these professionals are widely versed in adaptive sewing by hand and by machine.

Cleaning

Housekeeping presents a challenge because soil and dust are often lower contrast and are difficult to see. Having a portable light source such as a head-mounted lamp (available in camping supply stores) or a high-intensity flashlight often proves useful. A lighting evaluation should be performed for this and stain identification goals.

Helpful cleaning products for an individual who has vision loss might include multi-purpose cleaning wipes that are impregnated with a cleaning solution and static cleaning cloths and dusters that attract dust like magnets. Storing cleaning products in a bucket in their place of use

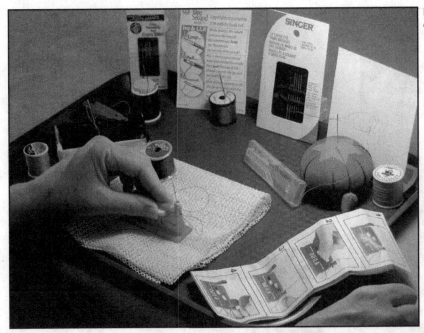

Figure 17-8. Sample needle threaders and sewing equipment.

(eg, tile cleaner in the bathroom, linoleum floor cleaner in the kitchen, each with other accessory cleaning items) will help keep items from being mixed up. Keeping a sponge at each sink will provide immediate help with spills.

An adaptive cleaning strategy used by people who are blind involves a systematic wiping technique where one wipes a surface, much like reading, from the upper left across as if one row at a time. One uses the nondominant hand to mark the row being wiped, wiping toward it and then moving down one row (Figure 17-9). Housekeeping with low vision includes several features to maximize the quality of the cleaning process. Preventative cleaning, such as always wiping down counters after preparing a meal, diminishes the amount of cleaning that needs to be done later on.

Tactile feedback can identify a greasy stovetop, but when tactile feedback is unavailable, a regular cleaning schedule is helpful, such as weekly cleaning of the toilet bowl. The above systematic, organized approach to washing, dusting, and sweeping, among other chores, may also include a recurrent strategy called overlapping strokes to ensure that an entire surface area is cleaned. Sometimes overcleaning is implemented, as in cleaning a bedroom mirror by wiping in overlapping strokes in one direction and repeating the same strokes perpendicular to the first. Larger areas to be cleaned, like the living room, can be broken down into smaller areas and landmarks; for example, a coffee table in the center of the room can be used to help maintain orientation to what has been cleaned. Making the bed is easier if safety pins are placed at midpoints of the bedding to ensure they are centered.[4]

SHOPPING

Visual challenges associated with shopping include visual clutter and lighting that can be excessive for those with glare sensitivity. Indoor glare-reducing absorptive lenses (sunglasses) are often recommended, especially for food shopping (see Chapter 12). Often, people with more severe vision loss require assistance in an unfamiliar store, but can learn to shop in familiar settings. Shopping can be completed by catalog, online, in person, home delivery, or a personal shopper. In-person shopping, banking, and other services that might require extra assistance are best done during the times when the store is least likely to be busy, avoiding rush hours. At a grocery store, this is likely to be in the morning early in the week. It is wise to call ahead if seeking assistance to shop such as at a grocery store or clothing department. If the client has an option an older female, being a more experienced shopper and cook, may provide the best assistance and advice. Being prepared and knowing in advance what one would like to purchase is important.

An aisle-by-aisle grocery list is helpful, whether shopping alone or using an assistant. A grocery list can be in large print, braille, or recorded format for the client and standard print for the assistant. It is helpful to write the grocery list in the same sequence as the shopper will encounter the products after he or she enters the supermarket, according to the store's own layout.[5] Handwritten or computer-generated labels identifying grocery items can serve as a grocery list and peeled off and placed on the food item by the client, avoiding placement over the barcode. A potentially less expensive method is to develop

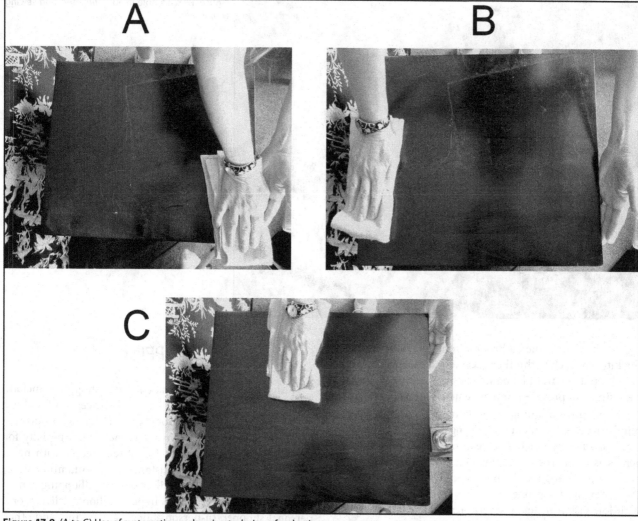

Figure 17-9. (A to C) Use of systematic overlapping technique for dusting.

reusable labels or index cards, as discussed Chapter 12, that then serve as a grocery list. The shopping bags themselves can be labeled to help in item identification. When using a shopping assistant, inform the assistant what type of help is required. If the client has specific products in mind, then he or she should be prepared to identify brand, size, quantity, grade, flavor, color, and price range. The client should handle and tactually or visually inspect each product before it is placed into the cart to confirm correct size, packaging, and quality. The client can assess the quality and ripeness of produce by using different senses. The assistant can also read and record cooking instructions, nutrition labels, and expiration dates.

If the client plans to shop independently, he or she may become familiar with the store layout ahead of time by obtaining a store map at customer service. Grocery store layout generally follows some basic principles. Produce is often located near the store entrance. Frozen foods are often located in freezer cases in the center of the store. Packaged baked goods are usually located near the dairy aisle (Figure 17-10[A]) More expensive items are usually placed near high-demand items and near the store entrance to encourage impulse buying. If the store has its own bakery, it is usually located in the rear or near the entrance. Fast-moving, high-demand items are usually located at eye level (Figure 17-10[B]) The shelf life of food purchases can be extended by selecting items at the rear of the shelf; foods with the shortest "use-by" dates are usually placed at the front.

Optical devices such as telescopes (see Chapter 13) enable the client to independently see signs and products at a distance. For reading labels, a client with less severe vision loss can use a handheld magnifier. Electronic handheld magnifiers and smart phones (see Chapter 14) have the capability of taking a picture of a label or product up close. The client can then enlarge the picture and view it.

Once at the checkout lane, the client can utilize several strategies during payment. The client should let the clerk know how much money is being handed to him or her so the clerk understands change is expected. Paying with the denomination just above the cost of the purchase or asking for change in ones will aid in bill identification. If the client's purchase is $12.30, for example, then giving the cashier a $10 bill and a $5 will allow the client to predict the change of two $1 and 70 cents, or a $20 bill would result in change of seven $1 bills and 70 cents. Requesting that the clerk count the change and identify each bill given back or requesting specific denominations can assist the client to track his or her funds. Indicating to the cashier that extra time is needed to reorganize or fold change will lead to a more relaxed transaction. A credit or debit card alleviates the need to manage bills and coins and is a widely used compensatory technique.

For information on online shopping, refer to "Untangling the Web—Let Your Fingers Do the Shopping: A Review of Seven Online Shopping Web Sites."[8]

CONCLUSION

Home management interventions using EPIC Framework include **E**nvironmental modification (alphabetizing the spice rack, placing garlic powder where it is used most often with roasting pans), **P**rocess adaptation (identify garlic by smell), **I**ntroduction of equipment (labeling the garlic powder lid with a large-print black "G" on a white label, using fresh garlic and a garlic mincer), and **C**hanging the end product (switch to minced garlic). In this same example, labeling is a low vision technique, while the sense of smell is a nonvisual technique in adherence to the low vision-to-nonvisual continuum. The third and final framework focused on low vision principles is also represented: relative size magnification and contrast in evident in use of black print on white background label, while organization is evident in the alphabetizing of the spices, including garlic. Let the frameworks expand therapeutic options that can be offered.

The following is a summary of additional low vision/nonvisual strategies introduced in this chapter:

- Use of home row for finger placement in order to find other numbers on a number/keypad.

- Incorporate color coding for object and function identification.

- Emphasize logical order of buttons to assist in memory.

- Use of landmarks to provide orientation to surroundings.

- Use of overlapping strokes to ensure an area is entirely covered.

- Use of a mental image of an object to know where one is and where one needs to be.

- Marking a location with the finger of one hand in order to bring an object to that location with the other hand.

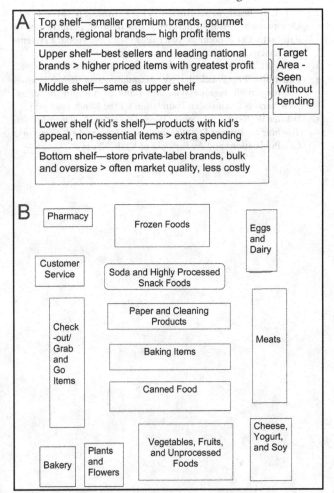

Figure 17-10. (A) Typical shelf product arrangement. (B) Typical grocery store layout.

- Counting or timing to determine the number of increments required to achieve the desired goal.

- Use of the distance from the fingertip to the first joint as an indication of roughly one inch.

- Use of a sighted observer to provide feedback that the technique used has achieved the desired outcome.

- Put an object in a memorable place, one that has meaning to the client.

- Refer to clock positions to determine where an object is located.

- Maintain a reasonable working distance if using mounted magnifiers, telemicroscopes, or loupes.

REFERENCES

1. Haymes SA, Johnston AW, Heyes AD. Relationship between vision impairment and ability to perform activities of daily living. *Ophthal Physiol Opt.* 2002;22:79-91.

2. Liu C-J, Brost MA, Horton VE, Kenyon SB, Mears KE. Occupational therapy interventions to improve performance of daily activities at home for older adults with low vision: a systematic review. *Am J Occup Ther.* 2013;67:279-287.

3. Duffy M. *Making Life More Livable.* New York: AFB Press; 2002.

4. Ponchillia PE, Ponchillia SV. *Foundations of Rehabilitation Teaching With Persons Who Are Blind or Visually Impaired.* New York, NY: American Foundation for the Blind; 1996:3-21.

5. Inkster W, Newman L, Storm Weiss D, Yeadon A. *Rehabilitation Teaching for Persons Experiencing Vision Loss.* 2nd ed. New York: CIL Publications and Audiobooks of VISIONS; 1997.

6. Yeadon A, Grayson D. *Living with Impaired Vision: An Introduction.* New York, NY: American Foundation for the Blind; 1979.

7. Sokol-Mckay D, Michels D. The accessible pantry: food identification tips, tools, and techniques. *RE:view.* 2006;38:131-141.

8. Ingber J. Untangling the web—let your fingers do the shopping. *Access World.* www.afb.org/afbpress/pub.asp?DocID=aw060605. Published November, 2005. Accessed on May 20, 2014.

Leisure, Recreation, and Sports

As occupational therapists, we often tend to focus on practical activities of daily living. Yet, leisure activities often determine a person's quality of life. An individual's passion often provides a sense of purpose and something to anticipate. Many leisure activities also sustain a person's physical and mental capacity, as well as directly affect health, wellness, and an ability to maintain independence. This is especially true for those activities that require some level of interaction by the client, such as playing a game rather than watching television. Occupational therapists are well aware that games can be used to turn the somewhat tedious repetition of some exercise into an enjoyable therapeutic activity. If games are used, it is essential that the therapist explain to the client the therapeutic value of the activity, or it might be dismissed as trivial.

This chapter will address a wide variety of activities that are done for enjoyment and diversion, individually or with a group, formally organized or not, in the home or in the community. There is overlap between these 3 categories. Sometimes these activities can be modified; other times, a replacement may need to be found. For competitive games, it is important to classify players according to their relative degree of visual impairment, as established by the International Blind Sports Federation (IBSA) and the

United States Association of Blind Athletes (USABA) in the "IBSA Visual Classifications."[1] In addition, the rules of the game may be adjusted based on level of vision loss, and in team sports, the teams themselves may be equalized (a bowling league of "teams" may be created that includes equal numbers of blind individuals on each team). The frameworks from the previous chapters continue to apply. Table 18-1 provides an example related to knitting.

LEISURE ACTIVITIES

A leisure interest inventory is a helpful way to delineate the client's areas of interest: past, present, and future. A very comprehensive leisure inventory can be viewed by Googling: "Georgia Mentor Leisure Interest Survey." The inventory was not designed for persons with low vision but can provide a starting point for assessment of this very important occupations. The activity categories included in this inventory are: team and individual sports, music, dance, arts & crafts, table games, outdoor leisure/social, community activities/entertainment, social clubs/organizations, literacy/continuing education and volunteer work. The inventory is as expansive as the possibilities.

Whittaker SG, Scheiman M, Sokol-McKay DA.
Low Vision Rehabilitation: A Practical Guide for Occupational Therapists,
Second Edition (pp 323-334).
© 2016 Taylor & Francis Group.

TABLE 18-1: THE EPIC FRAMEWORK— KNITTING
1. **E**nvironmental Modification—Use contrasting towel on lap behind knitting; paint tips of needles or hooks to contrast with yarn; use needles that contrast with yarn; use hands-free, lighted magnifier.
2. **P**rocess Adaptation—Work with your fingers close to the tips of the needles so dropped stitches can be more easily felt; count stitches dropping a coin or paper clip in a cup per stitch.
3. **I**ntroduction of Equipment—Use larger needles that produce larger, easier-to-feel stitches; use knitting/crocheting needles with lighted tips (www.anniescatalog.com for crocheting hooks; www.herrschners.com for knitting needles).
4. **C**hange of End Product/Task Simplification— Introduce color by using multicolored yarn instead of designs made with different colors; try round loom knitting (looms and project book available at www.loomahat.com/round-loom).

Cards and Board Games

Adapted tabletop leisure activities include playing cards, word games, and board games. Many versions of playing cards are available, from standard store-bought jumbo index playing cards with half-inch numbers, to card decks available from low vision catalogs that incorporate bold numbers up to one and a half inches in height. Other considerations when choosing a playing deck is the game the client desires to play (standard deck, pinochle, Uno, Skip-Bo), the visual clutter present, font simplicity, and the introduction of alternative colors and styles (EZC cards are reverse contrast) (Figure 18-1). Playing cards can now be labeled with adhesive labels that come with the pen-shaped talking labeling devices introduced in Chapter 12. Now that several of these labeling products come with earphones the card player can "read" his or her own cards privately.

Large-print playing cards are valuable tools in teaching eccentric viewing and scanning (see Chapter 10). Braille cards may be used to introduce braille reading and other tactile techniques. A standard braille playing deck only requires the client be able to tactually discriminate 2 braille symbols on each card, the first standing for the number and the second for the suit, with a total of 17 different single braille characters (2-10, J, Q, K, A, D, H, S, C) and not the entire braille code.[2] Toodle Tiles: Emmy's Town Software from American Printing House for the Blind, is a computer game based on the matching card game of Mahjong and

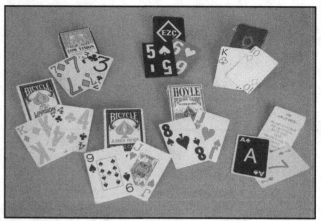

Figure 18-1. Alternative styles of playing cards. The lighter numbers are vivid colors that are quite visible. Lighter is usually red. The LoVISION Bicycle cards use different colors to differentiate hearts from diamonds and clubs from spades. Otherwise, the lighter color is red.

features bright, high-contrast colors and simple designs, as well as audio cues and feedback, each time a tile is chosen; this may be used as a graded visual scanning with feedback activity to teach a person to compensate for field loss (see Chapter 11).

Tabletop games are available in a variety of formats. A checker game designed for those with low vision or no vision could have a variety of adaptations, including brightly colored, tactually different checkers (round/square), a board with raised and recessed squares that contrast with each other, and the checkers or the board may have peg holes to hold pieces in place. Other games such as chess, Monopoly, cribbage, dominoes, Scrabble, Bingo, etc, come similarly adapted through low vision catalogs (www.lssproducts.com) and are excellent therapeutic activities for teaching eccentric viewing (see Chapter 10) and compensatory scanning (see Chapter 11).

By far the most popular are playing cards and Bingo. Several very large print Bingo cards are available in specialty low vision catalogues or can be made on the computer. With the EZ Read Fingertip Bingo cards the fingertip slide number covers eliminate the problem of knocking into and displacing chips. If the client cannot see the numbers then he or she can memorize them and then reuse the adaptive card.

Because it does not require a lot of memorization, a popular game among those who cannot see the numbers is tactile dominos, played on a magnetic surface (available at www.lssproducts.com). Scrabble can be adapted by placing large adhesive black letters on the backs of the original tiles and keeping tiles to be chosen from in a bag. Several 3- to 5-inch 3D tactile brainteaser wooden puzzles are available in low vision specialty catalogs, as well as a Rubik's Cube that has both bright colors and raised tactile markings (circles, triangles, dots).

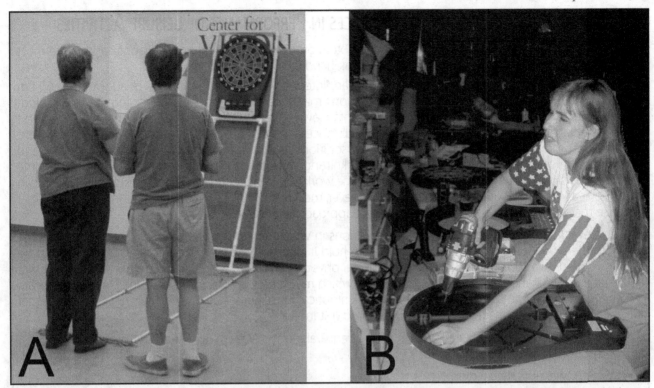

Figure 18-2. (A) Customers throwing darts at AudioMaster dartboard. (Reprinted with permission of Center for Vision Loss.) (B) Sam Jasmine (owner of Audio Dartmaster, product developer, and entrepreneur, [www.audiodartmaster.com]) assembling Audio Dartmaster.

Puzzles

Word puzzles are excellent therapeutic activities to help develop higher-level scanning skills that can be problematic in cases of spatial neglect or hemianopia with cognitive impairment (see Chapter 11). A variety of large-print word puzzle books are available in low vision catalogs and on the commercial market. However, often puzzles labeled "large print" on the commercial market may be less than the minimum 14-point size to qualify as large print. S&S Worldwide (www.ssww.com/about) has several spiral-bound word search, crossword, and Sudoku books in 16-point print on 100-pound paper. A wide variety of themed word search puzzles and freeform crossword puzzles are free for downloading at www.qets.comcrossword.htm (point size Unknown) and www.puzzles.ca/large_print_word_search.html (22 Arial Bold). This provides the option of printing them on any preferred color-contrasting background. Talking word puzzle software for crossword and word search puzzles is available through American Printing House for the Blind in CD-ROM and digital form, including a free sample demonstration.

Darts and Targeting Games

A person who has recently developed low vision or blindness may be surprised that he or she can still play games that involve throwing at a target. Two examples of adapting targeting games darts and horseshoes illustrate the techniques that can be used with any such game. A dart board game comes in a fully accessible audio version from www.audiodartmaster.com. The game gives specific directions as to where the dart has landed by combining clock positions with point values (eg, 1 o'clock equals 18 points) and indicates when a dart hits inside or outside of the double or triple ring. The audio dart master tells the player when to remove his or her darts and then announces the next player up. There are audio "clicks" or "pings" to help a player line up a shot and "scream" sound effects during the dart game "Killer"[3] (Figure 18-2). Several game options are available, as well as a spoken manual. For people with low vision, dart type games can be adapted using light-emitting diode (LED) lights, high-contrast reflective tape on the targets, and/or the use of telescopes (see Chapter 14).

The United States Blind Horseshoe Association has suggested game modifications for visually impaired and blind players. In addition to moving 10 feet closer (from 40 to 30 feet), visually impaired players may use highly visible white paint on stakes, horseshoes, and pitching boundary lines and a white towel over the backstop to enhance targeting. Blind players can use a pitching area tactually marked with a rubber mat, install a beeper behind the backstop to improve targeting, and employ a pitch partner to assist and provide feedback on the opponents' pitches and adjustments to the player's pitch to improve performance.[3]

SIDEBAR 18-1: USE OF OPTICAL DEVICES IN PERFORMANCE OF LEISURE ACTIVITIES

Important: Because the client must relearn visual motor control while working under magnification, care must be taken with sharp or dangerous tools such as knives, hand tools, and power tools.

Arts and crafts activities typically are performed at an "intermediate" working distance of about 40 to 60 cm (16 to 20 inches). The distance is determined by a person's magnification needs, the distance required to manipulate the objects and tools, and ergonomic requirements. Devices that are effective for reading may not be appropriate for a craft activity because the lens-to-object distance is too close to hold a tool, or may require the client to bend over too close to see something. The best solutions are a combination of nonvisual adaptations and visual devices. For example, if someone is an expert, knitting can be, and often is, done by feel even by people with typical vision. The person must, however, view the work from time to time to check for errors. Checking can be done at a very close distance. The beginner, however, must view what he or she is doing and now requires a distance that allows room for the needles. The best approach is as follows:

1. First, evaluate ergonomics under typical conditions in which an activity will be performed. Can someone hold the work in their lap (knitting), or can they hold it close to their eyes, or does the activity need to be performed on a table or easel (painting)? Consider physical conditions such as hand tremor or weakness that might require hand support, or back problems, which may require certain postures. One can now estimate the required object-to-lens distance and select an optical (see Chapter 13) or electronic device (see Chapter 14) that will provide magnification at the required distance.

2. Magnification requirements can be estimated in equivalent power by magnifying an object on a computer or electronic magnifier (see Chapter 13, Figure 13-2).

3. Lower power (less than 6 diopters).

    a. Stand magnifiers or mounted handheld magnifiers (see Figures 13-12, 13-13, and 13-14) allow a comfortable eye-to-lens distance, but increasing magnification limits the lens-to-object distance.

    b. Loupes (see Figure 13-10) and telescopes (see Figure 13-15) allow a greater eye-to-object distance than a full-field microscope or strong reading glasses. Telescopes allow the greatest eye-to-lens distances, but with decreasing field of view.

    c. Electronic magnifiers are rarely needed at this level of magnification.

4. Intermediate power (6 to 16 D). A stable work surface is required for tool use while viewing.

    a. Loupes are available, but are useful only for spotting or work with small tools when greater than 10 diopters.

    b. Telemicroscopes can be effective up to about 16 diopters, but field of view becomes very limited and a closer working distance (30 to 40 cm, 14 to 16 inches) becomes necessary at greater than 16 diopters.

5. Higher magnification requires the use of an electronic magnifier (see Chapter 14, Figure 14-2). Detachable cameras or remote cameras with tablet computers can be used.

6. Nonvisual strategies become more practical and can actually be safer as magnification requirements increase. People can learn to check stitching and work by feel as well as vision.

Arts and Crafts

Arts and crafts are a common leisure pastime. Optical devices can play an important role in leisure activities. See Sidebar 18-1 for some considerations and suggestions regarding their incorporation Lighting that mimics daylight and provides true color rendition may be helpful for those with some functional vision where the project involves color discrimination. Color vision testing under different types of illumination becomes an important part of the vision evaluation. The Farnsworth-Munsel D15 is the test of choice, where the client places 15 disks with different hues in an order. It has been adapted for low vision with larger disks (www.richmondproducts.com, www.precisionvision.com). A scoring chart allows the therapist to identify color confusion. The therapist can address confusion with different types of lighting and sunlenses.[4] Many specific craft projects can be modified with adaptations further refined under a low vision simulator or blindfold. Low vision simulation and blindfolding allow the therapist to experience the vision loss and develop successful adaptations and techniques that both persons who are totally blind or who have vision impairment can utilize.

Craft items may be organized in traditional organizers designed for the purpose or in small tackle boxes, toolboxes, multidrawer storage units, pegboards, small sandwich baggies, plastic containers with secure lids, and pill vials with screw caps. Trays from restaurant supply stores can provide a high-contrast, well-delineated workspace. These are available in a wide array of colors, several sizes, and with a lipped edge to prevent small/sharp items from getting away. A lipped cookie sheet can work in a pinch if contrast is not an issue.

A good resource for pre-adapted craft activities is "Craft Adaptations for Adults With Vision Impairments" by Stephanie Van, which is available in Word or PDF format (send an e-mail to VIPKrafter@gmail.com). Some of Stephanie's craft tips include using glue sticks instead of liquid glue; when using a scissors, cut slowly using small strokes; set up supplies in order of use; clean up as you go; and be specific in instructions ("use 3 swipes of glue stick" rather than "use a small amount of glue").[5] Any group craft benefits greatly from an exact replica of the project to be completed for crafters to explore and accessible instructions in large-print, recorded, or digital format.

Painting and Visual Arts

Painting might be made easier by switching from oils to watercolors or pastels, focusing on the use of broader brush strokes rather than finer strokes, painting more flowing landscapes or more abstract, less defined subjects rather than precise portraits and other objects. Clay provides a tactual medium, but does not require uniformity and precise detail. Pottery can be created from coils or slabs of clay or by pinching a solid ball of clay; sculpture can be created from mental images of objects. Masklike sculptures can be made by molding clay over a face covered by newspaper. Glaze may be applied by dusting, spraying, dipping, trailing, or brushing and can provide both tactual (crawling glaze) and visual interest (a crackle glaze).

A visual artist, especially one who does detailed representational work, might be encouraged to experiment with changing his or her style that reflects the new view of the world. To show our clients who are artists how style can change with vision, we keep a copy of Marmor and Ravin's examples of artists with low vision,[6] or samples of their work can be found on the Web. One notable visually impaired artist is Degas, who became legally blind toward the end of his career. Others include Mary Cassatt, Camille Pissarro, Georgia O'Keefe, and Paul Henry, also notable 19th- and 20th-century artists.

Beading is a tactile activity that can have a planned pattern or be freeform. Shapes, textures, and colors can be more important than size. Hands-free magnification in spectacle format and head-mounted lighting can be used by those with functional vision. According to craft suggestions from www.visionaware.org, a square of corrugated cardboard with the ridges exposed will allow the beads to be lined up as the design is being formed and will prevent beads from rolling away.[7] Beading wire also does not require threading, but allows a nice drape in any jewelry designed.

Needlework

"Needle Arts With Vision Loss" is a series of books on adaptive blind techniques for various needlework crafts. The books are available through www.smashwords.com or searching for the author, Shireen Irvine Perry. Her first 2 books on making braided rugs and needle felting have been published; books on machine sewing, knitting, crocheting, ribbon work, and beading are for future publication. The books are available for purchase in various formats, including downloading to a computer, e-reader, or an Apple product.

The Touch of Yarn is a beginners' guide to knitting with vision loss and is available in standard-print, large-print (18-point), braille, and electronic format at www.touchofyarn.mybigcommerce.comcategories/books. It is written by Davey Hulse in simple yet descriptive text, including techniques for correcting mistakes once you have knitted past them.

Bargello, a type of yarn needlepoint embroidery consisting of upright flat stitches, can be a successful craft, particularly for making pillow fronts. An easy-to-thread, large-eyed plastic needle can be used in conjunction with canvas material that has large holes that are made more visible against a contrasting background. A horizontal ripple-style pattern consisting of varying-length vertical stitches allows for a less precise and more freeform style. Alternating rows in contrasting colors of yarn can also increase the ease of the task for an individual with functional vision.

Woodworking

Woodworking ranges from creating a small shelf to building furniture to making home repairs or remodeling. Measurements from one-sixteenths of an inch to one-sixty-fourths of an inch can be performed with a large-print, raised-print, braille, or talking tape measure or specialized tools such as the Click Rule or a RotoMatic, which rely on fine tactile sensitivity and/or hearing to count thin threads on a rod, small turns of a nut, or clicking sounds. Marking the board can be completed by incising a line with a knife and marking the edge of the incised line with masking tape. Both are tactile, but the wider, raised tape can lead the woodworker to the thinner, recessed line. According to Larry Martin from Woodworking for the Blind, Inc at www.ww4b.org/index.php, enhanced safety using power tools can be accomplished through the use of push blocks, featherboards, and special-purpose jigs with appropriate hold-downs for gripping a work piece securely while shaping it (Figure 18-3). Jigs should have handles for positioning and keeping hands away from danger.[8] Woodworking can be quite dangerous, and careful instruction and practice are required as part of a rehabilitation program.

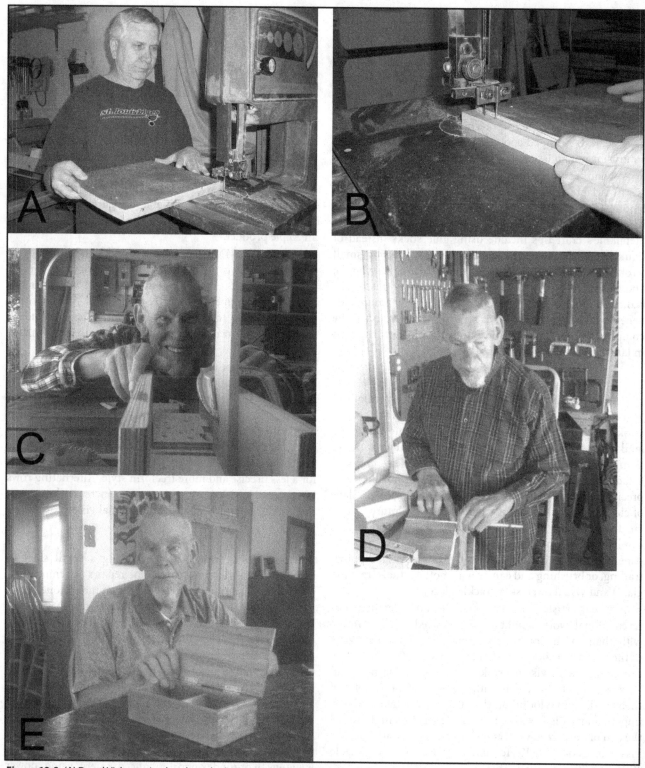

Figure 18-3. (A) Darrel Vickers using bandsaw duplicator pin to cut a straight line following a guide template. (B) Close-up of Darrel using bandsaw duplicator pin. (C) Gil Johnson setting table saw jig for cutting finger joints. (D) Gil in his shop using a click rule. (E) Gil shows finished box in red oak with finger joint construction.

Woodworking for the Blind, Inc provides recordings of several woodworking magazines, including descriptions of photos and project plans that accompany the magazines. Their *Manual for Blind Woodworkers* was updated in 2014. These resources are available in CD or MP3 format or for download by members from their website (www.ww4b.org).

Membership is free and is available to persons who cannot read or access standard print and to organizations serving those individuals. Members can communicate via their listserv (blindwoodworkers@yahoo.com).

Gardening

Gardening can be adapted to any level of vision loss. A contrasting border of white flat flagstone, painted rocks, or crushed seashells will make a garden stand out and yet not present a tripping hazard. A wind chime, colorful bird bath, or other sensory element can function as a landmark for orientation within the garden. Consider choosing plants that are more easily seen, have interesting textures, or are fragrant. To achieve proper spacing, the gardener can use a rope knotted at consistent intervals (such as 12 inches for low-growing marigold seedlings) or seed tapes, which are commercially produced fine paper tapes with seeds sandwiched between layers at regular intervals. High-contrast gardening tools can be purchased, or current tool handles wrapped with high-contrast duct tape, which comes in many highly visible colors.[9] Large-print labels on tongue depressors can aid in plant identification.

A tool apron placed around a pail or a sectioned bucket with a handle provides areas for tools and for garden waste. Getting to know plants and flowers tactually in different stages of growth will enable the gardener to discern plants from weeds and flowers in the height of bloom from those that have become passé (now wilted or having a crunchy sound). Placing plants in a line with regular spacing and labeling them will also help identify surrounding weeds. Weed-suppressing fabric can help to minimize weeding. A previous measuring strategy, using the distance from the fingertip to the first joint, can help achieve a one-inch depth of mulch. One-handed shears for pruning permits the gardener to feel the plant with one hand while the other hand works the shears. These and other additional tips are available at the Thrive website (www.thrive.org.uk). "Carry on Gardening" and "Getting on With Gardening" are 2 helpful publications that are free in PDF format or, for a nominal fee, in large print and braille by contacting info@thrive.org.uk or by calling +118-988-5688 between 9:00 AM and 5:00 PM, UK time.[10] A gardening webinar with these suggestions and more is also available through Hadley School for the Blind at www.hadley.edu.

Television and Home Movies

Watching television is one of the most common leisure activities. The best magnification for television watching should be approximated by relative distance magnification. Halving the distance of the chair from the television from 6 feet to 3 feet increases the image size by 2× using the concept of relative distance magnification. Since magnification of a screen often includes size, distance, and use of telescopes, putting these types of magnification together requires a formula discussed in Chapters 13 and 14. An alternative approach to accessing television programs and home movies is through descriptive DVDs or Descriptive Audio (formerly Video) Service available on the television through regular broadcast networks and cable and satellite networks. Descriptive Video adds a narrative component to visual elements that might otherwise be missed by a person with vision impairment, including facial expressions, costume design, scenery detail, and "sight gags." These extra descriptions are seamlessly inserted into natural pauses in the dialogue. Descriptive Video apps can be downloaded for smart phones by searching using the terms *descriptive video* and *low vision*.

Over 300 DVDs with this additional feature are listed at www.acb.org/adp/dvdsalpha.html. DVDs may be available for loan, rent, or purchase depending on the organization or resource. The exact process of accessing these audio-described programs depends on whether the client receives the signal over the air, through cable or satellite, or through a converter box. In general, the Second Audio Program (SAP) is the option chosen. The federal 21st Century Communications and Video Accessibility Act, Public Law 111-260, signed into law on October 8, 2010, mandates audio description, at least for the largest networks in the largest population areas, although changes are to occur progressively over a 10-year period. A summary of the act is located on Federal Communication Commission (FCC) website at www.fcc.gov/guides/21st-century-communications-and-video-accessibility-act-2010; the full text of Public Law 111-260 can be viewed at www.gpo.gov/fdsys/pkg/PLAW-111publ260/html/PLAW-111publ260.htm. For more information and updates on the Audio Description Project (ADP), visit www.acb.org/adp/index.html.

Currently, the biggest challenge to accessible television is the complexity of the remote controls, which are difficult to navigate even without vision loss. Programmable remote controls exist (www.lssproducts.com) to simplify access by reducing the number of choices to a few channels that a client almost always watches, but currently, these devices may not control the recording and on-demand services provided by cable companies. Remote controls with dozens of buttons remain difficult to navigate for our older clients, who are more familiar with a cable provider remote. Currently, we often use tactile markings on a familiar remote to guide the client to frequently used controls. Remotes adapted for low vision vary widely in the features that they offer. Some remotes are very simple, consisting only of volume and channel up/down buttons. Other such remotes have illuminated/tactile/enlarged buttons. a programming feature or the ability to control other devices such as cable/satellite or a DVD player. One large service provider, Comcast, is reported to have a voice guidance feature which speaks what is on the screen to help viewers decide what to watch and also audio description of programs that viewers are watching.

Music

Although one might assume that playing music does not require vision, a musician usually must read music to succeed professionally. Reading music is much like reading print, and many of the same devices and approaches can be used (see Chapter 15), with one difference. In our research on evaluating a device for reading music in an unpublished study, we found musicians could generally read music fluently if the staff (the 5 lines) on sheet music is about 5 times the size of the smallest print that they can read at the same distance with the same magnification device. For a typical musical score, a person who can read 0.8 M print can read most musical scores, but some smaller-print scores may need to be enlarged to where the staff is 5 X 0.8M or 4M in size.

The challenge for musicians is sight reading—that is, reading music and playing at the same time. Except for vocalists, musicians usually require 2 hands to play and a working distance of about 50 cm (18 inches). People with low vision have been able to use up to about 2× to 3× telemicroscopes (see Chapter 13), but this provides only up to about 6 diopters of magnification. Use of a standard closed-circuit television (CCTV) type electronic viewer (see Chapter 14) requires the assistance of a sighted helper. We found a recently developed computer-based electronic viewer specifically for reading music, the Lime Lighter (www.dancingdots.com), which enables sight reading music without sighted assistance. The musician advances the score on the screen with a foot pedal. Music is scanned into the Lime Lighter using a standard document scanner or by download and then converted into a format that can be edited and reformatted to fit on the screen. The touch screen also allows the musician to make notes on the score, just like other members of the orchestra. As with other electronic viewers, the Lime Lighter enables sight reading for those with significantly greater magnification needs. We found that most of those who could use telemicroscopes found the Lime Lighter more comfortable.

OUTDOOR RECREATION AND SPORT

Fishing

A person who is legally blind is entitled to a free fishing license. An application may be obtained from the Department of Fish and Game and requires a signature from the eye care physician. Another common strategy is that sometimes "less is more," as the more there is to choose from, the harder it is to choose. To that end, tackle should be minimal, well organized, and kept in a central location at the fishing spot. Lures should be placed in a specific order, or labels should be placed above the compartments of the tackle box. A darning hook can be used to fish line through larger eyes on lures. A low vision or audible bite indicator is available through fishing and tackle stores. For safety, the fishing hook should be placed in a safe, memorable place. When a fisherman can't see where his or her lure lands, he or she can learn to compare auditory measurements, such as counting seconds between castings and hearing the line hit the water, with visual distances estimated by their guide.[3]

Although nonvisual strategies are generally preferred, many like to have a handheld magnifier or may use a loupe or telemicroscope to set up their hooks and lures to use in a pinch, such as with a tangled line or broken reel. In general, the people with low vision who fish quickly learn to do as much as possible prior to the fishing trip, such as setting up tackle, in the comfort of their home with all their magnification devices available (see Sidebar 18-1).

Bowling

The American Blind Bowling Association (ABBA) has a website (www.abba1951.org), a publication that comes out 3 times a year, and a chat group. There are about 90 active leagues throughout the United States, and tournaments are held throughout the year. A bowling team generally consists of one sighted and one or more totally blind players, with the sighted player calling hits and pins for each team and keeping score. The website has a detailed "Instructional Manual for Blind Bowlers" in online, audio, and downloadable format. The primary adaptive device is a portable bowling guide rail, a 12- to 15-foot rail positioned alongside the first board outside the width of the lane and extending back from the foul line (Figure 18-4). Sometimes a tactile marker on the floor, such as a carpet strip, can also help the bowler line up with the center of the lane and approach the foul line squarely. Bowlers recognize their balls by the weight, color, and grip, which includes hole configuration, span between holes, and hole depth, which varies from bowler to bowler. The photographs in Figure 18-4 are members of the long-established Allentown Blind Bowlers League; Sidebar 18-2 is a brief discussion of the league and one of its members.

Golf

The website www.blindgolf.com leads to the home page of the United States Blind Golf Association (USBGA). The USBGA has visually impaired and totally blind divisions and several tournaments throughout the United States. Golf is played with sighted assistance of a coach who gives the golfer course description, correct yardages, and helps with club selection and proper alignment. The established rules of golf are followed, with the exception of being able to touch the club to the ground in a hazard and having the coach stand behind the golfer when lining up a putt, who

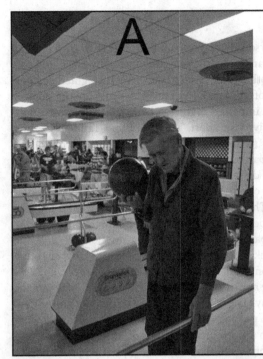
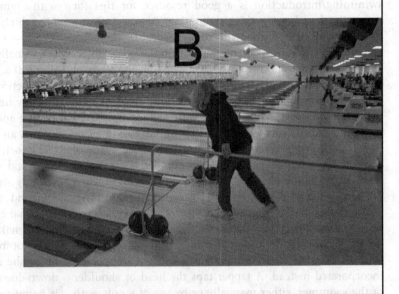

Figure 18-4. (A) John focuses on position before making the shot. (B) Terri at the rail after release.

SIDEBAR 18-2: A BOWLER'S STORY

Terri is 63 years old and has been an avid league bowler for 26 years. When she first started bowling, Terri had residual vision and was able to play on a sighted league and able to distinguish her orange ball among the others. As her vision continued to decline to light perception only, she felt she could not compete with a league of fully sighted members and joined the Allentown Blind Bowlers League, which was formed 65 years ago in 1950. In order to continue bowling, Terri had to adopt new techniques to do what she formerly used vision to do. She placed a large "X" made of duct tape on her orange ball for a tactile cue and was able to locate her ball on the return rack by eliminating balls with rubbers inserts and different finger hole sizes and depths. She was also no longer able to position herself accurately with respect to the bowling lane, so she began to use a bowling rail. When relying on the rail for direction, Terri needed to manage her ball with her right hand only. Her ball proved to be too heavy for single-handed use so she reduced its weight from 12.5 to 10.5 pounds. Sighted members of the team cue members with vision loss when it is their turn up and call out numbers of specific pins missed or their general location (ie, left side).

Terri has been president of the Allentown Blind Bowlers League for 16 years. Like any other league, there is also a vice-president, secretary, and treasurer. As president, Terri seeks to educate and market to the sighted and visually impaired community regarding the opportunity to continue bowling. Despite the week-to-week challenge of obtaining transportation, members faithfully participate in the typical 30-week season. The league is self-sustaining and self-funded. It breaks down the membership into 4 teams, including equal numbers of several sighted members on each team. Each season, new teams are formed, equalizing teams by using a computerized tracking system for obtaining averages and determining handicaps.

The comradery and playful competition are evident when the Blind Bowlers League is bowling. Sighted and visually impaired members are side by side, young and old (the oldest member is 91 years of age). Terri states that bowling is her night out, a time to have fun. It gives her a sense of independence and a feeling of belonging to the community. The sound of Terri's laughter when bowling is the league's best advertisement.

can provide verbal cues. The coach also stands next to the hole to provide a larger target. Chromax (www.chromaxgolf.com) has developed high-visibility golf balls in a multitude of colors. Marking the "sweet spot" on clubfaces with colored tape may also help golfers with low vision.[11] Wearing a visor or tinted glasses may provide sun and glare protection when out on the green.

Swimming

The website www.britishblindsport.org.uk/vi-friendly-swimming/introduction is a good resource for tips for recreational and competitive swimming. Both swimming near the wall or in a pool with ropes separating the lanes can aid in maintaining orientation within the pool. Color-contrasting lane markings may be located on the floor of the pool, or can be in the form of brightly colored floatation markers attached to the ropes dividing the lanes. By starting with the back against the wall, a commonly used technique called "squaring off," the swimmer can be positioned in the right direction to maintain a straight line of travel. The swimmer can count the number of strokes it takes to cover the length of the pool to determine when the end of the pool is nearing. In recreational swimming, a bright red marker/floatation device or a radio/beeping device can be placed on the wall at the end of the lane to notify the swimmer of the lane's end. For national competition, an external visual aid cannot be used. A "tapper" is incorporated instead. A tapper taps the head or shoulder of the swimmer, either manually or by use of a pole with a tennis ball tip, to indicate that the lane is ending.[11] The United States Association of Blind Athletes website offers information on accessible swim programs, information on qualification requirements, and adaptations permitted for each blindness classification.

Tennis

Adapted tennis is played on a badminton or smaller tennis court using shorter rackets (22 inches or shorter, or a junior racket) and a high-contrast or audible ball. String, such as baling twine, is affixed to the outer boundaries of the court with masking tape and can be felt easily through thin-soled sneakers.[3] Balls can be either black or fluorescent green to give maximum contrast with the color of the playing area. Players who are totally blind are allowed 3 bounces, while partially sighted players are allowed 2 bounces. The players verbally announce when they are ready to serve, receive, or play the ball. Rules exist as to who can volley to whom when sighted, low vision, and blind players are playing together. See www.metroblindsport.org/index.php?pageid=25 or www.hanno.jp/matsui/rules.html for the complete rules for adapted tennis. Audible tennis balls with a bell inside can be purchased at www.braillebookstore.comsearch.php. The American Printing House for the Blind (www.aph.org) has developed a product entitled *30-Love: Tennis Guidelines for Players With Visual Impairments*, which includes 2 rackets, 6 sound-adapted tennis balls, and a manual on the guidelines in large print or braille.

Cycling

Some persons with low vision can ride their own bicycle, with a human guide (sighted guide) wearing a brightly colored shirt; others ride tandem cycles with a sighted partner. The types of cycles and partners depend on the goal of the visually impaired cyclist—whether it be for recreation, physical activity, or sport. The U.S. Blind Tandem Cycling Connection (www.bicyclingblind.org) connects blind and visually impaired cyclists with sighted cyclists for tandem cycling and disseminates information about cycling clubs, events, and opportunities. Tandem cycling is a collaborative effort. The sighted "captain" or "pilot" in front must be clear and specific in his or her communications with the visually impaired "stoker" or "copilot" in the back. Both the pilot and stoker need to develop a system of verbal or tactile cues that communicate when to start, stop, speed up, slow down, make a turn, and handle an emergency. For example, the pilot may state "Coming to an intersection" to indicate he or she is purposely slowing down rather than slowing down due to a steep incline. Not indicating an intersection is being approached may lead the copilot to pedal harder as if anticipating a hill. Even mounting a tandem bike is a team effort. Often the pilot straddles and stabilizes the bike while the stoker mounts. Further information can be found at the U.S. Blind Tandem Cycling Connection website.

Cross-Country/Downhill Skiing

Ski for Light is an all-volunteer organization that hosts an annual weeklong program that teaches classic cross-country skiing to adults who are visually impaired. Many major ski areas now provide adaptive instruction in alpine skiing as well. Vests are worn that identify the visually impaired skier and guide to prevent other skiers from attempting to ski between them (Figure 18-5[A]) The person with vision loss may learn to ski with a tether connecting him or her to the instructor and advance to skiing with a human guide (sighted guide) preceding or behind. Continuous communication occurs between the guide and skier, sometimes delivered using 2-way personal radios. The human guide (sighted guide) may relay information according to the clock method—"the tree is at 11 o'clock" or the grid system, with the guide calling "2, 2, 1, 2," with the left zone being 1, the middle zone 2, and the right zone 3 (Figure 18-5[B]). A safety word is established to avert danger; when shouted by the guide, the skier drops to the ground.[3] The American Blind Skiing Foundation (www.absf.org) plans skiing events for visually impaired skiers.

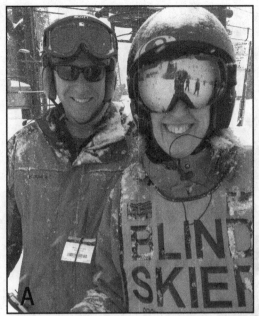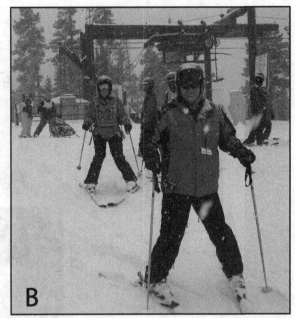

Figure 18-5. (A) Skier with vision loss wearing orange identifier vest and guide, using Eartec Simultalk 24G radio. (B) Guide in lead, providing verbal instruction using wireless radio.

Beep Baseball

The game differs from baseball in a variety of ways. Teams consist of a sighted catcher, pitcher, and 1 or 2 spotters. All other players, including the batter, play under blindfold. Only first and third base are used, and each consists of a 4-foot padded cylinder with speakers and a sounding unit that gives off a buzzing sound when activated. When the ball is hit, the base operator activates one of the bases. The batter must run to the buzzing base before the ball is caught by the opposing team. To enable the batter to hit the ball, the catcher sets the target where the batter normally swings, while the pitcher attempts to place the ball on the hitter's bat. To cue all players, the pitcher announces when he or she is ready to pitch and then says "pitch" when the ball is thrown. The field is divided into defensive positions 1 through 6 (first base, right field, etc). The spotter calls the number indicating the general direction the ball is traveling (Figure 18-6). The defensive player only fields the beeping ball, often diving to trap the ball. Beep baseball is a competitive sport with 30 leagues nationally. This information and more is available at the National Beep Baseball Association website (www.nbba.org).

Hiking and Other Sports

An alternative large hook-shaped tip for the long cane called a Bundu Basher can help with negotiating areas with tall grass. Yoga mats may be purchased with tactile raised shapes identifying the center of the mat and various locations on the mat for placing hands and feet in performing yoga positions. Adaptations for kayaking include navigating by the voice of the guide or using a tandem kayak. Some experienced kayakers paddle alone, depending on their residual vision, or may use a sound source such as a radio or remote-activated beeper that can be utilized to guide them on their return to shore.[12] An available resource is *Canoeing and Kayaking for People With Disabilities*, written by Janet Zeller of the American Canoe Association.[13]

The Blind Judo Foundation will identify instructors interested in working with clients with vision impairment, whether the goal is self-defense, recreation, or competition. Assistance may be provided to enter and exit the mat and to find the starting mark. Referee hand signals are also simultaneously spoken.[12]

Information about other competitive sports can be obtained by visiting the USABA website at www.usaba.org/index.php/sports.

SUMMARY

Sports and leisure activities may not only be goals by themselves, but also may be effective therapeutic activities to teach eccentric viewing, scanning, and use of devices. When games are used as therapeutic activity, always explain to the client the rationale so the treatment is taken seriously. Keep the following tips in mind:

- Simplify; sometimes less is more, as the more there is to choose from, the harder it is to choose.

- Squaring off will provide direction straight ahead.

- Focus on the broader picture rather than the small details (especially in crafts).

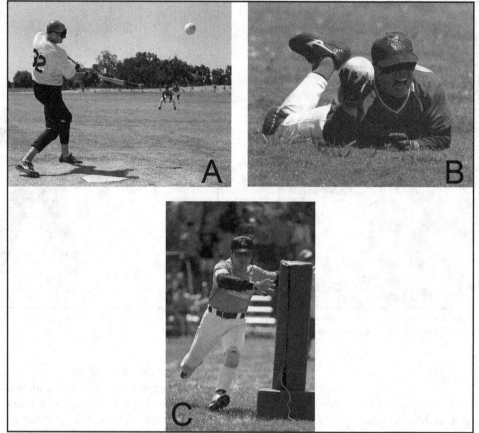

Figure 18-6. (A) Batter with vision impairment hitting beep baseball under blindfold. (B) Outfielder with vision loss fielding a ball under blindfold. (C) Scoring in Beep Ball World Series. (Reprinted with permission of John Lykowski.)

- Use a restaurant tray for task organization.

- Be specific when giving instructions, such as, "You can locate the discard pile at the 2 o'clock position."

- When a game says "large print," call and ask for the specific print size.

- Use a sound source as a target.

- In games where vision might produce an advantage, make sure others are blindfolded or have the same visual access as the person with low vision.

REFERENCES

1. International Blind Sports Federation. *IBSA Classification Rules and Procedures*; 2012.
2. Ponchillia PE, Ponchillia SV. *Foundations of Rehabilitation Teaching With Persons Who Are Blind or Visually Impaired*. New York, NY: American Foundation for the Blind; 1996:3-21.
3. Leibs A. *The Encyclopedia of Sports and Recreation for People With Visual Impairments*. Charlotte, NC: Information Age Publishing, Inc; 2013.
4. Schwartz SH. *Visual Perception: A Clinical Orientation*. 4th ed. New York: McGraw Hill; 2010.
5. Van SS. *New Independence! Craft Adaptations for Adults With Vision Impairements (Revised)* Mohegan Lake, NY: Associates for World Action in Rehabilitation and Education; 2007.
6. Marmor M, Ravin JG. *The Artist's Eyes: Vision and History of Art*. New York: Abrams; 2009.
7. VisionAware. *Beadwork After Vision Loss*. www.visionaware.com. Accessed November 3, 2014.
8. Martin L. *Woodworking for the Blind Incorporated*. www.ww4b. org/index.php. Accessed November 1, 2014.
9. *Harvest the Benefits of Gardening* (seminar transcript presented by Hadley School); 2014.
10. George V, Morrell L, Spurgeon T. *Getting On With Gardening: A Guide for Blind and Partially Sighted Gardeners*. Beech Hill, Reading, UK: Geoffrey Udall Centre; 2007.
11. MacGregor A, Furber C. Visually Impaired (VI) Friendly Swimming. A Guide for Supporting Visually Impaired Adults and Children in the Pool. *British Blind Sport*. www.britishblindsport. org.uk/vi-friendly-swimming/introduction. Accessed November 3, 2014.
12. Lieberman L, Ponchillia P, Ponchillia S. *Physical Education and Sports for People With Visual Impairments and Deafblindness: Foundations of Instruction*. New York, NY: American Foundation for the Blind Press; 2013.
13. Zeller J. *Canoeing and Kayaking for People With Disabilities*. Fredricksburg, VA: The American Canoe Assn; 2009.

Community Activities and Mobility

Being involved in activities outside the home promotes socialization with others, enjoyment, increased activity, a sense of competence, a feeling of belonging to something larger than oneself, and an expansion of one's world. Vision loss, both in and of itself and in combination with aging, can needlessly diminish this involvement. If the functional vision evaluation (see Chapter 8) reveals a person requires bright light, has glare sensitivity, or has impaired contrast sensitivity, the therapist should look for mobility problems, especially under dim light conditions, and, as a result, reduced community participation where lighting is difficult to control. Several common "community activities" are presented here with a variety of low vision and nonvisual adaptations to facilitate successful participation. The ability to move around on one's own independently is critical to involvement in both the home and community. A variety of adaptive mobility options will be described, many of which can be taught by the low vision therapist or referred to a certified orientation and mobility specialist (COMS). Table 19-1 describes the EPIC Framework applied to reading a menu at a restaurant. The first step is to instruct a client and, if needed, family on how to optimize light levels and avoid glare when they do not have control over lighting by using body position, hats, and sunlenses (see Chapter 10).

COMMUNITY ACTIVITIES

Eating in a Restaurant

Eating out at a restaurant is a popular form of socialization outside of the home. Reading a menu and face recognition are common problems among people with mild to moderate vision loss; seeing food and eating neatly may become problems with more severe vision loss. To read a menu is a common goal that is often achieved with illuminated handheld magnifiers, either optical (see Chapter 13) or electronic (see Chapter 14). Recognizing faces and seeing food are usually addressed by a lighting evaluation (see Chapter 8) and instruction so the client can learn to locate a seat and use discrete techniques to optimize lighting and avoid glare (see Chapter 10). A request can be made to be seated in a well-lit area (see Chapter 12) or near a restroom, if the client feels easy access to the restroom is necessary. If a client is glare sensitive, he or she should sit so that a bright window or light is to the client's side rather than in front.

Clients sometimes become conscious of eating in a more public venue and observing social niceties. One easy and effective strategy for people with vision impairment is to select food that is easier to see and eat neatly. For example,

Whittaker SG, Scheiman M, Sokol-McKay DA.
Low Vision Rehabilitation: A Practical Guide for Occupational Therapists,
Second Edition (pp 335-346).
© 2016 Taylor & Francis Group.

TABLE 19-1: THE EPIC FRAMEWORK— READING A MENU

1. **E**nvironmental Modification—Use a flashlight; ask if large print is available.

2. **P**rocess Adaptation—Contact restaurant ahead regarding menu accessibility or overview of food categories; access menu from website to read ahead.

3. **I**ntroduction of Equipment—Use KNFB Reader application on iPhone; use iPhone and magnification feature to access menu.

4. **C**hange of End Product/Task Simplification— Narrow choice of meal category desired and ask companion or waitress to read those options on menu.

more compact pasta, such as rotelle, might be easier to eat than spaghetti. Sometimes spaghetti, salad, and even deboned meat can be cut using a grid pattern to ensure that pieces are more bite sized. Requesting meat to be deboned or cut, a lettuce wedge to be cut or replaced with chopped romaine, having salad placed in a bowl instead of a plate, or having vegetables placed in a separate bowl or on the main plate are all simple requests that the kitchen can meet. Since people often avoid devices and interventions that draw attention, nonsighted techniques (see Chapter 6) are often preferred over lights and devices. A condiment such as salad dressing can be placed on the side in a small cup and spooned out and applied in a circular pattern over the lettuce or can be lightly applied to the salad in the kitchen. The salt shaker can be discerned from the pepper by its heavier weight or smell. A small amount can be shaken into the palm of one hand so regular amounts can be pinched and applied evenly over the food by following a consistent pattern. It is best to start using condiments sparingly at first—more can always be applied later. Neat eating strategies are discussed in Chapter 16.

Visiting Public Attractions, Movies, Theater, and Sports Events

Enjoying museums, theaters, and other cultural institutions is another popular community activity, but generally one that requires some advanced planning to determine and/or request accessibility. *Project Access* is a project of Art Beyond Sight/Art Education for the Blind and is dedicated to increasing accessibility to the arts. Their database of 180 accessible art institutions lists them by city and state at www.projectaccessforall.org/institutions. Museum accessibility features might include tactile tours, handling sessions, verbally descriptive tours that focus on visual

features (color, texture, facial expressions, positioning of people), touchable replicas, tactile or raised line drawings, and artwork designed to be touched. Use of distance viewing devices (see Chapter 13) should be addressed in advance, as they may be viewed by museum employees as cameras, which are often prohibited. A sighted assistant may be necessary to use the audio tour cassettes, while some advance automatically at the exhibit as it is approached.

Since screen sizes are quite large, seeing the action in a movie theater is usually preferred to watching movies at home for people with low vision. Audio description is increasingly available for first-run movies—some as downloadable apps on an iPhone—and more and more movie theaters are being built or renovated with the necessary equipment to offer the description track to patrons. Likewise, many live theaters have special shows with audio description. When paying for the ticket, the client should learn to ask for an audio description headset; make sure it is for audio description, not assisted listening devices for people who are hearing impaired.

A good resource on audio description is entitled "The Visual Made Verbal: A Comprehensive Training Manual and Guide to the History and Applications of Audio Description."[1] This resource, written by Dr. Joel Snyder, is available for purchase at www.acb.org/adp. Shelley Rhodes, MA, CVRT, has suggested 2 websites to locate audio-described movies: www.mopix.org lists theaters equipped with the technology to provide audio-described films and www.captionfish.com allows users to search for accessible theaters by zip code and lists show times. Shelley also indicated that many of the DVD and Blu-Ray versions of popular movies also have an optional Descriptive Video Service (DVS) track on the language menu; for a complete listing, go to www.describedmovies.org.

In any venue with a stage (theater, concert hall, sports arena), seating can be requested closer to the event. Distance magnification devices (see Chapter 13), such as spectacle-mounted telescopes, are prescribed for people with low vision and can be combined with closer seating to achieve the magnification required to see facial expressions. Bioptic mounts are particularly well suited for dance, sports, and live theater. During a sports event, for example, the client can quickly move from a magnified view of an individual player through the telescope to a full-field, unmagnified view of the positioning of the other players through the carrier lens. For sports events, people with low vision listen to simultaneous radio broadcasts for a verbal description of the action.

Volunteerism

Volunteering in community activities and organizations is essential to the backbone of society; it is a way of giving back to the community and gaining purpose in one's life. Kendra Farrow, CVRT and Research and Training

Associate at the National Research and Training Center on Blindness and Low Vision, reports a lack of research on this very important topic, but suggests that one of the biggest challenges is determining the client's areas of interest related to volunteering and then narrowing down those interests by finding a location that is not too difficult to reach by walking or by using transportation options in the community. Adults can volunteer at church, senior centers, literacy programs, preschool programs, and in organizations that they received service from, like not-for-profit blindness agencies.

In this day and age, many organizations lack the staff and funding to continue to provide much-needed community services. Newspapers may advertise volunteer opportunities. For example, a simple online search of "volunteer opportunities in Allentown, PA" brought up 44 nearby opportunities related to advocacy and human rights, animals, arts and culture, and board development. The advanced search feature on the same site located 14 volunteer opportunities related to "children and reading." To spend a treatment session calling these various agencies and inquiring about accessibility would be a productive therapeutic activity that would address many aspects of functional communication (telephone use, making and reading notes, looking up information, etc), as well as apply problem-solving therapy (see Chapter 6) in cases of emerging depression.

Travel

The use of a white cane becomes quite valuable as a sign that a person has vision impairment when interacting with strangers, and he or she may receive accommodations without asking. In addition, traveling, whether near or far, requires extensive planning via mail, the Internet, or a travel service. It is important to look for access-specific information related to the city that will be visited. Airlines should be informed at the time of booking of any accommodations that are required, such as assistance traveling to, from, and between gates and preboarding. The Transportation Security Administration (TSA) officer must be informed of the kind of assistance required for the screening process. A collapsible long cane must undergo x-ray screening.

A COMS can provide orientation to the local airport and techniques that can help with becoming acquainted with other airports. It is important to keep travel information in an accessible medium and program a cell phone with all necessary numbers of the airlines, hotels, and tour operators. Luggage should be very distinct visually and/or tactually so that it can be easily described to others or more easily located. Some visual and/or tactile markings should be packed should anything require marking, like a rubber band around the hotel room door. A talking global positioning system (GPS) or GPS app on an iPhone is helpful for local travel upon arrival at one's destination.

When a client has multiple disabilities, collaborative treatment between an occupational therapist and a COMS is generally most effective. Many techniques can be suggested by the occupational therapist, but referral should be made to a COMS for advanced techniques. *Use of a white cane should only be introduced and taught by a COMS.*

ORIENTATION AND MOBILITY

Mobility is a critical skill underlying all other activities, be it with or without an ambulation or mobility device, including a car. Equally important are the destination and the activity performed at the destination. The definition of mobility, what it involves, adaptive techniques and equipment, and additional resources will be provided in this section. It begins by providing an informal screening tool that can be used to initially identify candidates for mobility training (Table 19-2). This is intended to reveal some basic difficulties in the home and community environment and could include both client observation and patient report. Depending on the scope of the practice, intervention may be provided by the low vision occupational therapist or the COMS (see Chapter 1).

Table 19-3 includes an example of the EPIC Framework related to an indoor mobility activity—the client walking from the bedroom to the kitchen.

Mobility generally includes use of sensory skills to detect an object of desire or to avoid obstacles. People with field loss can achieve more independent mobility using habitual compensatory scanning (see Chapter 11). Some people with just acuity loss and intact visual fields have sufficient vision to walk, and even drive, without devices, or perhaps a telescope to read signs. For those with more severe vision impairment, different mobility options exist for independent travel, such as a long cane, special low vision and nonvisual techniques, use of a guide dog, or use of electronic travel aids and GPS systems. A certified orientation and mobility specialist will address the above area and help determine if a client would benefit from a dog guide and would refer a client to a dog guide school The client needs to be able to choose the option that fits his or her level of residual vision, the activity he or she would like to engage in, and the environment in which he or she is traveling.

One client might prefer a human guide (sighted guide) to go to the movies with a friend, but prefer a long cane when going to the nearby store on his or her own. A long white can be used simultaneously with a straight cane, walker, wheelchair, and possibly an adaptive scooter. The speed of a scooter should be slow enough to allow the user to preview the path ahead and avoid obstacles. The services of a COMS should be sought in these situations, especially if any mobility device is necessary. For people with multiple impairments, the occupational therapist works with the COMS—for example, addressing mobility issues so a

TABLE 19-2: OCCUPATIONAL THERAPY MOBILITY SCREENING TOOL

	YES	NO	WHERE
Hesitant gait			
Bumps into or misses objects right, left, overhead, floor level			
Shuffles feet			
Trips or stumbles			
Looks down at feet			
Holds on to walls and furniture			
Veers			
History of falls			
Uncomfortable with physical assistance provided by others			
Others grab, push, pull, or walk arm in arm to provide assistance			

Adapted from Riddering AT. Evaluation and intervention for deficits in home and community mobility. In: Warren M, ed. *Occupational Therapy Interventions for Adults With Low Vision.* Bethesda, MD: American Occupational Therapy Association, Inc; 2011:269-300.

TABLE 19-3: THE EPIC FRAMEWORK— WALKING FROM BEDROOM TO KITCHEN

1. **E**nvironmental Modification—Incorporate sufficient and even ambient lighting throughout hallway; ensure contrast between carpet and baseboard/wall; cover shiny hallway floor or use low-gloss polish.

2. **P**rocess Adaptation—Trail hand along wall; listen to hum of refrigerator to serve as guide to kitchen.

3. **I**ntroduction of Equipment—Put an air freshener in the bathroom, which is midway between the bedroom and the kitchen.

4. **C**hange of End Product/Task Simplification— Keep a travel cup of water on the nightstand to avoid nightly trips to the kitchen.

person has a free hand for a long cane, or learning scanning techniques in a case of spatial neglect.

Orientation refers to a person's use of sensory cues to navigate in familiar and unfamiliar settings. In familiar environments like their own home, often people who have learned to adapt to total blindness navigate without devices, as the environments have been memorized. Significant others and visitors have learned to be avoid clutter and moving furniture, except in special circumstances and only after telling the person with vision loss. Many times, these are used in combination. In an unfamiliar environment, judg-

ing travel distance is a kinesthetic skill that must be honed through practice and repetition. To learn the distance of a chosen route (distance from bedroom to bathroom or from elevator to a treatment area, for example), the client must begin at the same starting point and finish at the same end point, his or her pace must be consistent and without interruptions, and he or she must travel this route a number of times before kinesthetic awareness of the distance can be established. Human guide (sighted guide) travel is useful for introducing this skill, as these features can be controlled. Having a guide will help the client establish a point of reference for judging distances traveled.[2]

Using Landmarks and Clues

Using vision to get around is enhanced by use of eccentric viewing (to read an aisle sign in the supermarket) and scanning (to see the displays of fruit and avoid people in the pathway). Traveling can be augmented or hampered by lighting, contrast, organization, and glare (see Chapters 10 and 12). The client with low vision can be taught to use all the senses to orient him- or herself in order to travel safely and effectively through an environment. According to Dona Sauerburger, MA, COMS,[3] 2 key elements in both the indoor and outdoor environment are landmarks and clues—landmarks are permanent; clues are temporary information. Landmarks and clues can be visual, auditory, tactile, or olfactory.

A landmark that can help the individual with residual vision in moving from the dining room to the kitchen, for example, could be a set of large red pillar candles on the dining room table to the bright green teapot on the stove;

a clue would be the intermittent light coming through the kitchen window. A nonvisual landmark might be a change in floor texture from carpet to linoleum; a clue would be the frequent scent of flowers on the dining room table in the dining area to the sound of the icemaker in the refrigerator in the kitchen. Learning to pay more attention to environmental landmarks and clues in the home can be generalized to the outdoors and new environments when orientation and mobility training begins.

Sighted/Human Guide

A sighted guide, also known as human guide, is a technique that enables a person with vision loss to use someone with sight as a guide to get from one location to another in a safe, efficient, and respectful manner. This is a technique that occupational therapists should know if they are working with clients with low vision. They should be able to offer it as an option if a client needs to come to the treatment room or to locate the restroom, among other circumstances. This technique should also be taught so that clients can teach significant others how to guide them when it is desired, such as under poor visibility conditions, in new environments, or in the face of unanticipated obstacles (construction, for example). Not everyone needs a sighted guide, as the client may have sufficient vision or familiarity within the environment to see his or her way, or can follow the therapist's voice. The client may have independent mobility with a cane. If unsure as to what the client needs, just asking, "How can I help you?" will indicate respect for each other and a collaborative effort.

Human guide (sighted guide) technique involves 2 people working in concert, with both actively involved in the mobility process. The guide gives verbal and physical cues through his or her movement while the individual being guided follows the cues. If the client is led through a door, he or she is also required to hold it open, or if both parties are attempting to squeeze between 2 restaurant tables, the client is cued to assume a single-file position. The other responsibilities of the client are to determine the walking pace and the preferred arm of the guide he or she wishes to hold. The 2 most important aspects of the human guide (sighted guide) technique include the following:

1. The client grasps the guide's arm at the elbow or places a hand on the client's shoulder; the guide should not grab or hold onto the client. Grabbing a person unannounced may startle and disturb a person's balance; it is also discourteous, even dangerous.

2. To initiate sighted guide, the guide should always first ask the person with vision impairment if he or she needs assistance. If the visually impaired person agrees, the guide should ask which arm (or shoulder) the client prefers. The guide will lightly contact the client's preferred arm to let the client know it is available.

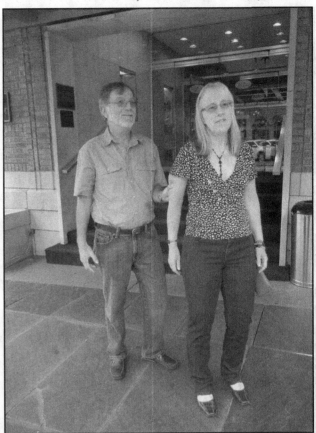

Figure 19-1. Basic human guidance (sighted guidance) position.

Clients should be taught how to instruct others on human guidance (sighted guidance) and to be politely assertive in asking a guide to adjust his or her pace. If a client and guide are walking side by side, or the client is being pulled or pushed, then additional instruction is needed.

The basic human guide (sighted guide) position requires that the person with vision loss firmly grip the guide's arm, usually just above the elbow, or on the shoulder if the visually impaired person is taller (Figure 19-1), with 4 fingers on the inside and the thumb on the outside. The guide's arm should remain close to the side of the body, and the client should remain half a step behind the guide by positioning his or her elbow at about a 90-degree angle. On the side where the client holds the guide's elbow, the guide's shoulder is in front of the client's shoulder, resulting in a position almost the width of 2 people. This basic position is usually modified to suit the environmental situation, whether it be going through a doorway, up or down steps, through a narrow space, in and out of an elevator, or when taking a seat. The key in all modifications is that there is never a loss of physical contact between the guide and the person being guided. With practice, the person being guided should eventually be able to sense the changes in the guide's body movements in preparation for a variety of environmental features and obstacles.

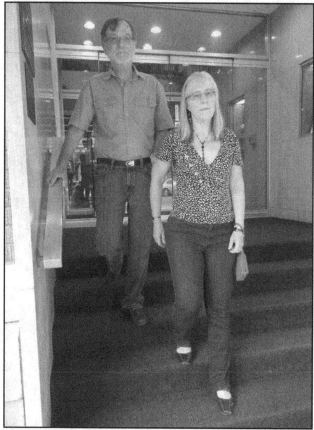

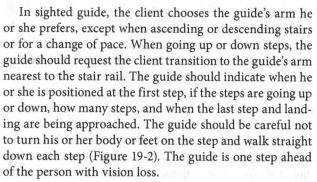

Figure 19-2. Descending stairs with human (sighted) guide.

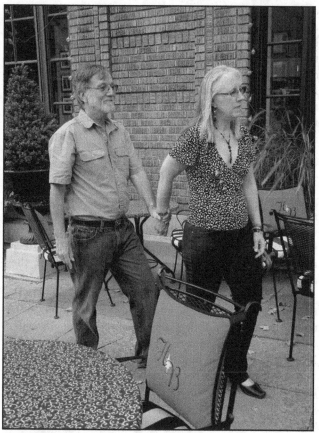

Figure 19-3. Navigating a narrow space with a human (sighted) guide.

In sighted guide, the client chooses the guide's arm he or she prefers, except when ascending or descending stairs or for a change of pace. When going up or down steps, the guide should request the client transition to the guide's arm nearest to the stair rail. The guide should indicate when he or she is positioned at the first step, if the steps are going up or down, how many steps, and when the last step and landing are being approached. The guide should be careful not to turn his or her body or feet on the step and walk straight down each step (Figure 19-2). The guide is one step ahead of the person with vision loss.

Crowds and tight spaces require an approach that places both the guide and the client in single file. The guide places his or her guiding arm behind the back in a diagonal position and extended toward the client. This will indicate to the person being guided to fully extend the gripping arm, slide the gripping hand down to the wrist of their guide, and step directly behind the guide, resulting in the client being one full step directly behind the guide (Figure 19-3). Resuming the standard human guide (sighted guide) arm position tells the client that he or she is now out of the narrow space. A beginner-level video in human guide (sighted guide) by Dr. Whittaker can be viewed at www.youtube.comwatch?v=vMgRd_IxO6M. An intermediate-level video

by Mary Jessica Chandler, COMS, TVI, can be viewed at www.youtube.comwatch?v=CbuufiLZSmY.

The human guide (sighted guide) technique can be varied, depending on the client's mobility needs and other factors. If the client needs a little support, the guide can interlink his or her arm with the client's or have the client rest his or her hand on the forearm of the guide. If the client needs the support of a walker, a "reverse sighted guide" technique may be used. This modification permits the client to maintain hold of the walker with both hands while receiving tactile signals from the guide's hand placed on the client's back, elbow, or hand. For example, if the guide places his or her hand lightly on the client's back between the shoulder blades, no pressure means continue straight ahead, pressure toward the right shoulder blade means turn right, pressure toward the left shoulder blade means turn left, and a hand on the shoulder means stop.[2]

Independent Mobility Techniques

Independent mobility techniques focus on ways to get around an indoor setting when vision is limited in one's own residence, an assisted living facility, a nursing home, or office building.

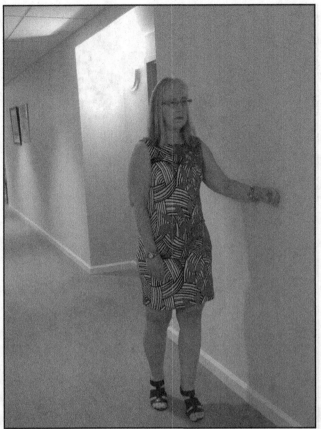

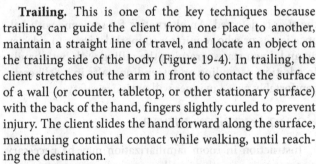

Figure 19-4. Trailing technique using parallel alignment.

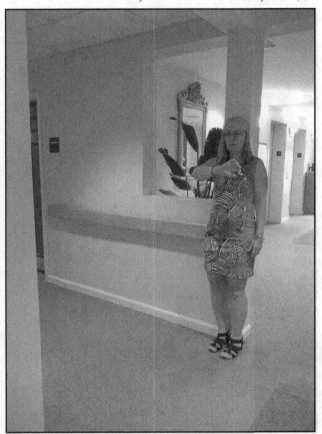

Figure 19-5. Squaring off (perpendicular alignment).

Trailing. This is one of the key techniques because trailing can guide the client from one place to another, maintain a straight line of travel, and locate an object on the trailing side of the body (Figure 19-4). In trailing, the client stretches out the arm in front to contact the surface of a wall (or counter, tabletop, or other stationary surface) with the back of the hand, fingers slightly curled to prevent injury. The client slides the hand forward along the surface, maintaining continual contact while walking, until reaching the destination.

Trailing with an ambulatory device. Trailing with a cane, walker, or wheelchair is also possible. Walking near the wall with the walker or contacting the wall with an elbow may help maintain a straight line of travel. For a manual wheelchair, the user may push the wheelchair several times and then contact the wall with the nearest hand to check that the distance has been maintained, resulting in a straight line of travel. Alternatively, if the user is strong enough, he or she may propel the wheelchair by the wheel rim with the hand farthest from the trailing surface and simultaneously propel with the nearest hand, thus mobilizing and monitoring distance from the wall at the same time. Curb feelers or semiflexible wire attached to the vertical post of the front wheel of the wheelchair or walker leg can provide auditory feedback, and when positioned at a 45-degree angle backward, will not scratch the wall.[2]

Squaring off and aligning. These are techniques that help establish and maintain direction or a straight line of travel, particularly when crossing open areas. Squaring off (Figure 19-5) requires the client stand perpendicular to a straight surface (wall or table), while aligning (Figure 19-6) requires a parallel stance next to a straight surface. In both situations, the client can use the straight surface to project a straight line of travel across a room. To combine these techniques, the client may align him- or herself with the side of a bed, for example, to walk straight across the room to contact the wall, trail the wall out the bedroom door, and continue trailing down the hallway to the kitchen, using kinesthetic memory to gauge distance, and place his or her back against the refrigerator to cross the room in a straight line to end up at the sink. These techniques also help to instill confidence in movement.

Protective techniques. Independent mobility techniques also consist of upper and lower body protective techniques when the potential for accidentally contacting an object exists (Figures 19-7 and 19-8). The arm serves as a bumper to prevent self-injury to the part of the body being protected. The upper body technique requires that the forearm be positioned in front of the opposite shoulder with the palm facing out. This position will protect the head and shoulders from open cabinet doors and when retrieving a dropped item from the floor. The lower body technique

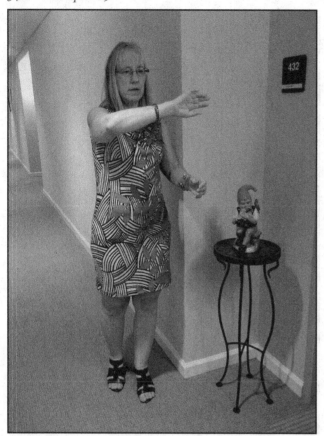

Figure 19-6. Checking parallel alignment and initiating upper body protective technique before crossing an open space.

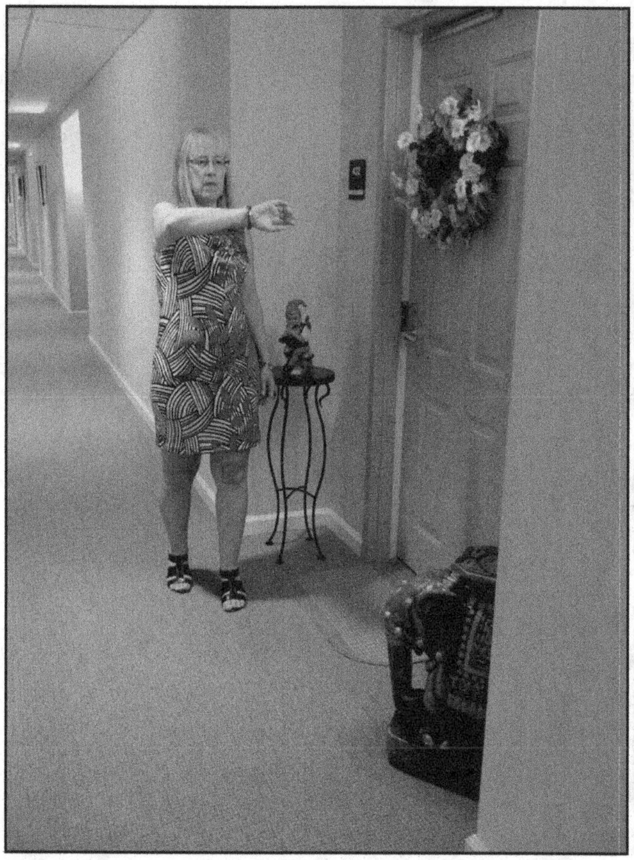

Figure 19-7. Walking across an open space using upper body protective technique.

requires that the forearm be positioned in front of the opposite thigh, the hand about 1 foot from the thigh, and palm facing the body. This position will help protect the body from sharp table and counter edges and chair backs. In both positions, as in trailing, the fingers are relaxed and slightly curled to prevent injury.

Stair climbing. Standard building codes require that steps all be the same size, so once a person makes the first and last steps, stepping in between is automatic and does not require vision. The therapist, however, should be careful to look for irregular steps, as an inconsistent rise can be particularly hazardous because of people's expectations. Patterned carpeting makes it more difficult to judge the edge of steps. Stairs to a cellar or basement may lack any contrast and may blend together easily. Insufficient lighting or glare may be an issue; glare may be present if the lighting consists of a bare bulb, as is often the situation on the wall of a staircase or ceiling of a basement. Several adaptations can be implemented to make the stairs more visible or tactually accessible (see Chapter 12). Shine a spotlight at the top and bottom steps, or place a tactile marker on the handrail.

Mobility instruction should be provided on approaching steps squarely and never at an angle, grasping the handrail, and locating the first step by sliding one foot forward until

the step is detected. An alternative for someone with balance issues or who requires a support device is to sidestep up and down stairs, grasping the railing with both hands. In addition, ascending or descending stairs in a deliberate, comfortably paced manner will optimize safety.

Room Familiarization

Instruction in room familiarization may be necessary if someone is recently visually impaired or moves to a new residence, including an alternative independent living situation, personal care home, or nursing home. Room familiarization is a systematic and structured exploration of the environment to gather spatial information necessary to develop a mental/cognitive map of the room. The guide has the client stand at the entrance to the room and this serves as the "home base," or reference point, for exploring the room. The guide may orient the client to the room according to the clock method, as in "the dresser is at 9 o'clock" or by naming the walls: "the dresser is on the left wall."

The client can be taught to visually scan (if possible) and listen for information about the environment, for example, locating the bright red chair in the far-left corner of the room or hearing the street from different positions in the room. Then the client walks the perimeter of the room and

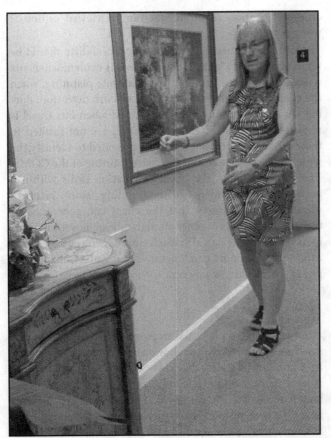

Figure 19-8. Trailing using lower body protective technique.

SIDEBAR 19-1

While waiting for the services for evaluation and white cane training by a COMS, there is much an occupational therapist can do if someone has multiple impairments:

- If mobility impaired, try to enable a person to use a support cane rather than a walker to free up a hand for sighted guide, protective technique, and white cane use.
- Evaluate tactile, proprioceptive, kinesthetic, and spatial perception and motor function, and treat impairments or develop compensations for effective cane use.
- Collaborate with the COMS in compensating for other disabilities.
- Help the client accept mobility devices.
- Teach introductory human guide (sighted guide) and protective techniques.
- Teach simple trailing, room familiarization, and use of visual stimuli to orient in a room.
- Adapt walkers with white and red tape, or recommend the client use a white support cane.
- Perform lighting evaluation and instruct client on how to optimize lighting and adapt to poor lighting.
- Teach clients to use telescopes and other optical aids.
- Adapt environment to facilitate mobility.

identifies landmarks around the edge. The center of the room is explored in a grid fashion. A final component of this instruction would be to switch the home base and have the client repeat walking or to just identify to each critical object along the walls to gain a different spatial perspective within the room and to help solidify the mental map.[2]

The White Cane

Many individuals with low vision may benefit from using a long white cane. Occupational therapists should not recommend or provide such a cane, but should refer to a COMS. However if the client desires to identify him- or herself as visually impaired, an occupational therapist can mark any other mobility device such as a walker or support cane by ordering the white and red reflective tape (available at www.ambutech.com). If the client is agreeable, cards placed in the spokes of the large wheel on the wheelchair can serve as an auditory indicator of the user's movements to others around; a softened card will be audible but less noisy. A red and white flag may accomplish the same purpose, but will provide less advance notice (Sidebar 19-1).

If the client lacks the strength to use the long white cane effectively, an exercise program may be provided to enhance upper extremity strength, range of motion, and coordination. The occupational therapist may make

recommendations to adapt the mobility device or cane grip, and provide a program to maximize the individual's wrist and hand functioning. Sugru (available at www.sugru.com) is a moldable product that come in many highly visible and contrasting colors and can be used to modify "grips" of all type including canes. When using the standard grip, the hand is held in much the same way as it is when one offers to shake hands.[2] Other purposes of the long cane include alerting the user to objects in the pathway, detecting surface changes or curb drop-offs, and protecting the lower body.

Low Vision Techniques

People who have inferior peripheral field loss are often prone to mobility problems. Those with an inferior quadrantopia, for example, will miss lower obstacles that could pose tripping hazards. With an hemianopia, not only will the client be prone to missing tripping hazards, but might also miss people walking toward him or her, or even vehicles on the affected side. Chapter 11 describes in detail techniques for evaluating and treating people with peripheral field loss, attention deficits, and spatial-perceptual impairments. The treatments include the use of a field expansion prism and habitual compensatory scanning, where a client is taught to develop a habit of looking in the direction of the field loss to see on the affected side. People with central field loss, especially inferior central field loss, may be prone to tripping hazards, especially in cases of dry macular degeneration, where reduced contrast sensitivity puts a person at risk for missing a step-off or curb.

Treatment for impaired visual acuity and contrast sensitivity begins with a focus on lighting and on marking possible obstacles in settings where a person can modify the environment. An effective low vision intervention might be as simple as a high-luminance flashlight or mobility lamp. For orientation, reading signs, and seeing landmarks, telescopes may be prescribed (see Chapter 13). A person can be taught to stop and spot with a handheld telescope or more quickly spot with a bioptic spectacle mount, allowing the client to quickly glance from the carrier lens to the telescope. These are even used for driving. Smart phone apps include a talking GPS for navigation, and even use of the camera for telescopic use. To read a sign, a user can first snap a photograph of the scene and then enlarge the view, eliminating the need to stabilize the telescope during viewing.

Scope of Practice

Scope of practice is an important issue. Anne Riddering, OTR, CLVT, COMS, has developed a scope-of-practice framework that helps to define what interventions occupational therapists can provide with respect to home and community mobility and when to refer to a COMS. Some home mobility areas that can readily be addressed by occupational therapists include locating furniture, ascending and descending stairs, avoiding obstacles, locating light switches and doorknobs, safe transport of items from one location to another, and human (sighted) guide. Community mobility interventions include, but are not limited to, use of a monocular, glare control, walking around the yard or the block (no street crossings required), scanning, asking for help, and education in driving retirement/transportation options.[4] The feasibility of an occupational therapist providing intervention in these areas is highly dependent on both the advanced training and knowledge of the therapist and the occupational therapist's comfort level, the client's level of residual vision, the predictability and characteristics of the outdoor environment (slope, steps, terrain changes, sidewalk, lighting, weather conditions, obstructions and hazards such as roots uplifting the sidewalk, and foot traffic, among other things. Occupational therapists are eligible to seek and obtain the education and certification to become a COMS. The Academy for Certification of Vision Rehabilitation & Education Professionals (ACVREP) spe-

cific certification requirements can be viewed online at www.acvrep.org.

Certified orientation and mobility specialists should be referred to when a significant field loss is evident when any street crossings are present, to teach route planning, when the client has difficulty in drop-off or curb detection, during rural travel without sidewalks, and when bus travel is required. Reasons to refer to a COMS are not limited to these circumstances, but the list is provided to identify the wide scope of practice and extensive training of the COMS. The COMS teaches the client orientation skills within a particular environment (office building, store, airport), usually with the intent that the client can generalize or transfer these skills to other similar, or even novel, environments. The COMS can also teach simultaneous use of a long cane with a support cane, hemiwalker, walker, manual or power wheelchair, or scooter.

Driving

Some people with visual impairment, even legal blindness due to acuity loss, are allowed to drive in certain states. In a number of states, driving with reduced visual acuity is legal if the person uses an assistive device known as a bioptic telescopic system (BTS). The BTS is a type of eyewear that is composed of the carrier lenses, which typically has the client's prescription, and the telescope(s), which is mounted into or upon the carrier lenses. During general driving, approximately 90% to 95% of the time, the client looks through the carrier lenses. Once an object, such as a traffic sign, is sighted in the carrier lenses, the telescope is used to gather further information/detail (ie, wording on a sign). The telescope is used much like a rearview mirror, with the driver glancing in the telescope from time to time (Figure 19-9).

A low vision occupational therapist can have several roles when working with a client who is interested in pursuing driving with BTS and meets his or her state requirements. First, the occupational therapist needs to know the laws in the state regarding the visual requirements for driving. Driving laws vary state by state with respect to acuity and visual field requirements, restrictions (ie, daylight driving only), who and how it is determined that the client qualifies, whether bioptic telescopes or prism glasses are allowed/required, and other factors. As of August 2009, 39 states allowed a person with low vision to drive with a BTS. This information can be located in an alphabetized listing of states at www.ialvs.comdriving_regulations.html#!dmv-laws-by-state/c9ba.

According to Pam Bartle, OTR/L, a certified driver rehabilitation specialist (CDRS) and a certified driving instructor (CDI), one of the roles of low vision occupational therapists working with clients who qualify for driving with a BTS can be to provide the initial education and training in a nondriving capacity. The therapist can educate the client on the basic principles and spotting techniques using the BTS. Treatment sessions should start in the clinic with the client practicing spotting nonmoving targets while stationary and then spotting moving targets while stationary. Treatment would advance to dynamic activities with the client spotting stationary targets while moving and then spotting targets in motion while moving. Sessions would progress to practical applications in the community using the BTS for instrumental activities of daily living (IADL), such as community mobility/walking and grocery shopping.

The low vision occupational therapist can also work with the client to develop compensatory strategies for dealing with common glare/sun issues typically experienced when driving (ie, use of different-colored sun filters, wearing baseball cap). By working with the client in a nondriving capacity, the therapist can be instrumental in preparing the client for referral to a driver rehabilitation program with a specialty in low vision for in-vehicle training. The low vision occupational therapist can find local driver rehabilitation programs and driver rehabilitation specialists at www.aded.net, the website for the Association for Driver Rehabilitation Specialists (ADED). Program listings include subspecialties such as low vision driving.

Low vision occupational therapists who are working with clients with a progressive eye disease should help them plan for driving retirement. This includes identifying alternative transportation resources in their community. Some resources regarding driving alternatives include the following:

- *Community Mobility Driving and Transportation Alternatives for Older Persons* by William Mann (2012)

- *Finding Wheels: A Curriculum for Nondrivers With Visual Impairments for Gaining Control of Transportation Needs* by Anne L. Corn and L. Penny Rosenblum (2000)

People with visual impairment sometimes continue to drive even though their vision does not meet the state requirements. The occupational therapist should discuss with the client the legality and potential safety issues of continuing to drive and refer the client to a low vision optometrist for a low vision evaluation and optical devices if permitted by the client's state of residence. In addition the occupational therapist should inform the client's physician if the person continues to drive. The ability to drive or return to driving is a sensitive issue that should be addressed by the low vision optometrist and reinforced by the low vision occupational therapist. A discussion focusing on the questions in Table 19-4 will begin the conversation as to the feasibility of continuing to drive.

The Low Vision Centers of Indiana (www.biopticdrivingusa.com/how-bioptics/) has numerous links for low vision driving. This includes information on different aspects of vision testing, an introduction to driver training, a listing

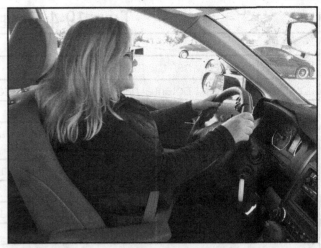

Figure 19-9. Driver with vision loss using BTS optical system.

of pertinent articles, and an 8-minute client-focused video on bioptic driving that explains the concept of bioptic eyewear, the fitting process, the training required, and the rules for bioptic driving in Indiana.

If drivers compensate by driving more slowly, mild to moderately reduced visual acuity (20/100) presents a measurable but relatively small risk for drivers, unless there is also a loss in contrast sensitivity.[5] Field restrictions and decreased peripheral attention create a high risk for driving with hemianopia, presenting a significantly higher risk than quadrantanopia.[6] Another important predictor of increased risk for driving is decreased peripheral visual attention, which is often associated with older drivers.[7] A recent review of the research on interventions for driving rehabilitation[8] did not find evidence that training alone decreased crashes; using a different outcome, such as staying in one's lane and reading signs with bioptic telescopes, did improve performance. The same training protocol with prisms for hemianopic vision loss for driving (see Chapter 11) was not effective. In the view of the writers, the best general strategy is to encourage legal drivers with vision impairment to take on-road driving tests by a CDRS to evaluate fitness to drive rather than depend solely on state criteria.

Advanced low vision occupational therapists with an interest in driving rehabilitation need to consider obtaining additional training in driver rehabilitation. Three publications for occupational therapists interested in driving include the following:

- *Driving and Community Mobility: Occupational Therapy Strategies Across the Lifespan* edited by Mary Jo McGuire, MS, OTR/L, FAOTA, and Elin Schold Davis, OTR/L, CDRS (2012)

- *Driver Rehabilitation Across Age and Disability: An Occupational Therapy Guide* by Sue Redepenning, OTR/L, CDRS (2006)

TABLE 19-4: DRIVER SCREENING TOOL

	YES	NO
Does the driver see when the traffic light changes?		
Can the driver detect potential hazards, such as traffic cones and flashing road-crew signs?		
Can the driver read street signs or recognize a neighbor across the street?		
Does the driver have additional conditions, such as advanced age, cardiac issues, or arthritis, that cause difficulty turning the head?		
Does the driver take medications that can affect visual and cognitive performance?		
Does the driver have reduced contrast sensitivity?		
Can the driver clearly and rapidly read the dashboard panel display?		
Can the driver keep up with the traffic flow?		
Does time of day or lighting conditions (such as cloudy days or bright sunlight) affect the driver's ability to see?		
Has the driver had any near-miss incidents (close calls) or do other drivers frequently honk at him or her?		

Reprinted with permission from Corn AL, Erin NJ, eds. *Foundations of Low Vision: Clinical and Functional Perspectives.* New York: American Foundation for the Blind Press; 2010:777-778.

- *Driving With Confidence: A Practical Guide to Driving With Low Vision* by Eli Peli and Doron Peli (2002)

In addition, ADED has developed a pathway for the occupational therapy practitioner to become a CDRS. Included is information on education and experience requirements, as well as self-study activities, to prepare an individual to sit for the certification examination. The ADED also has an extensive listing of educational offerings, including online courses, related to driving.

REFERENCES

1. Snyder J. *The Visual Made Verbal: A Comprehensive Training Manual and Guide to the History and Applications of Audio Description.* New York: American Federation for the Blind Press; 2014.
2. Wiener WR. *Foundations of Orientation and Mobility* 3rd ed. New York: American Federation for the Blind Press; 2010:831.
3. Sauerburger D. Indoor movement and orientation with vision impairment. *VisionAware.* www.visionaware.org/section.aspx?FolderID=8&SectionID=115&TopicID=515&DocumentID=5800. Accessed October 23,2014.
4. Riddering AT. Evaluation and intervention for deficits in home and community mobility. In: Warren M, ed. *Occupational Therapy Interventions for Adults With Low Vision.* Bethesda, MD: American Occupational Therapy Association, Inc; 2011:269-300.
5. Higgins KE, Wood JM. Prediciting components of closed course driving performance from vision tests. *Optom Vis Sci* 2005;82:647-656.
6. Racette L, Casson E. The impact of visual field loss on driving performance: evidence from on-road driving assessment. *Optom Vis Sci.* 2005;82:668-674.
7. Clay O, Wadley VG, Edwards JD, Roth DL, Roenker DL, Ball KK. Cumulative meta-analysis of the relationship between useful field of view and driving performance in older adults: current and future implications. *Optom Vis Sci.* 2005;82:724-731.
8. Justiss MD. Occupational therapy interventions to promote driving and community mobility for older adults with low vision: a systematic review. *Am J Occup Ther.* 2013;67:296-302.

Managing Diabetes and Medications

Debra A. Sokol-McKay, OTR/L, SCLV, CDE, CVRT, CLVT

DEMOGRAPHICS

Diabetes is a major national health issue. According to the 2014 National Diabetes Statistics Report, diabetes affects 29.1 million people in the United States, or 9.3% of the population. While an estimated 21 million people were diagnosed in 2012, 8.1 million (27.8%) are unaware that they have the disease. Prediabetes affects 86 million people and is a disease in which an individual demonstrates high blood glucose levels, but not high enough to be diagnosed with diabetes. Almost 1.7 million new cases of diabetes were diagnosed in people aged 20 years or older in 2012.[1] If trends continue, one study projected that as many as 1 out of 3 U.S. adults could have diabetes by 2050.[2]

Diabetes is a systemic disease for which there is no cure, and its complications affect every major system of the body. Stroke is 1.5 times higher and heart attacks 1.8 times higher in persons age 20 and over with diabetes than in those without diabetes. In adults with diabetes aged 40 and over, 4.2 million, or 28.6% of people, have diabetic[3] retinopathy that may result in loss of vision. Forty-four percent of the new cases of kidney failure can be attributed to diabetes. More than 60% of nontraumatic lower limb amputations in the United States occur among persons with diabetes.[1]

According to the American Diabetes Association, in 2012, the total direct and indirect costs of diabetes in the United States was $245 billion, with direct medical costs of $176 billion and indirect costs of $69 billion, including disability, work loss, and premature mortality. Average medical expenditures were 2.3 times higher for people with diabetes than for people without diabetes. In the United States, care for persons diagnosed with diabetes accounts for more than 1 in 5 health care dollars.[1] The financial costs are rivaled by the overwhelming physical and psychosocial toll that diabetes places on those who have it and their loved ones. Depression is 2 times higher in persons with diabetes than without.[4] The course of depression is generally chronic; even after successful treatment, depression will recur in as many as 80% of people with diabetes.[5]

Two premier studies, the Diabetes Control and Complications Trial (DCCT)[6] and the United Kingdom Prospective Diabetes Study (UKPDS),[3] have demonstrated the benefit of tight blood glucose control on the reduction in the development and progression of chronic complications. The results of the DCCT (1983 to 1993) showed a reduction in risk of complications (eye disease: 76%; kidney disease: 50%; nerve disease: 60%; cardiovascular disease: 35%) when persons with type 1 diabetes were treated with an intensive management regimen consisting of 4 injections/day or use

Whittaker SG, Scheiman M, Sokol-McKay DA.
Low Vision Rehabilitation: A Practical Guide for Occupational Therapists,
Second Edition (pp 347-378).
© 2016 Taylor & Francis Group.

of an insulin pump and blood glucose monitoring 4 or more times/day.[6]

The Epidemiology of Diabetes Interventions and Complications (EDIC) study was a follow-up study to the DCCT study, and 95% of the original DCCT participants were included. The EDIC study began in 1994, with results obtained in 2005, 11 years later. Thirty years since the DCCT was initiated, the EDIC study has also demonstrated the consistent beneficial effect of intensive management on the development of both macrovascular and microvascular complications. Risk reduction has declined somewhat over time; however, a lingering benefit has persisted over the past 2 decades since the end of the DCCT.

The UKPDS (1977 to 1991)[3] showed the importance of intensive blood glucose control to persons with type 2 diabetes. It reported that better blood glucose control through intensive antidiabetic therapy resulted in a 25% reduction in microvascular complications, including retinopathy, and a 35% reduction in early kidney damage. In addition, improved blood pressure control through medication in persons with high blood pressure and diabetes resulted in reductions in stroke (33%), death from the long-term complications of diabetes (33%), and serious deterioration of vision (33%).[3]

INTRODUCTION TO DIABETES AND ITS IMPACT ON VISION

Diabetes mellitus is a group of metabolic diseases characterized by hyperglycemia, or high blood glucose. It occurs when the body cannot use the glucose in the blood because the pancreas is not able to make or release enough insulin, the insulin that is made is not used effectively because of resistance of the cells to receiving it, or both. The symptoms of acute hyperglycemia include frequent urination, excessive thirst, extreme hunger, blurred vision, fatigue, headache, poor wound healing, and muscle cramps.

The 2 major types of diabetes are type 1 (formerly juvenile-onset, type I, or insulin dependent) and type 2 (formerly adult-onset, type II, or noninsulin dependent). The other 2 forms of diabetes include gestational and secondary. Type 1 diabetes affects 5% to 10% of persons with the condition and most often develops before age 30.[7] Persons with type 1 diabetes require an external source of insulin to sustain life, due to autoimmune destruction of the insulin-producing cells of the pancreas. Environmental factors such as viral infections and diet contribute to type 1 diabetes.

Type 2 diabetes affects about 90% to 95% of persons with diabetes. It is usually diagnosed after 30 years of age; however, it is becoming increasingly more prevalent in young children and adolescents. Both insulin deficiency and insulin resistance are present in persons with type 2 diabetes, although how much of each is present is

variable. Type 2 diabetes is strongly genetically linked, and environmental factors also play an important role. Major risk factors for the condition include age (high prevalence in older adults), ethnic background, positive family history of type 2 diabetes, high physical or emotional stress, lack of exercise, and obesity. Type 2 diabetes may be treated with weight loss, diet, exercise, oral medications, noninsulin injectable diabetes medication, and insulin. Some endocrinologists and diabetes professionals are trying to preserve pancreatic function by introducing insulin early in the treatment of diabetes.

Two additional diabetes diagnoses have been proposed for individuals who do not neatly fit the type 1 or type 2 categories. A diagnosis of latent autoimmune diabetes in adults (LADA) describes an individual who appears to have type 2 diabetes but is gradually undergoing the autoimmune destruction of insulin-producing cells that is indicative of type 1 diabetes. These individuals may or may not require insulin at first, but eventually will. Maturity-onset of diabetes of the young (MODY) occurs in adolescence or early adulthood and often can be treated with oral medications that are typical with type 2 diabetes.[8]

Diabetes can contribute to a multitude of conditions affecting the eyes, including diabetic retinopathy, macular edema, cataracts, glaucoma, ocular palsies, and fluctuating vision. In addition, the incidence of macular degeneration, although unrelated to diabetes, is also strongly related to increased age and thus another prevalent eye condition in persons with type 2 diabetes. Eye disease is 25 times more common in persons with diabetes than in the general population. From 1997 to 2011, the number of adults with diagnosed diabetes who reported visual impairment—that is, trouble seeing even with their glasses or contact lenses—increased from 2.7 million to 4.0 million.[9]

Diabetic retinopathy (see Chapter 4), the most common eye condition, is often detectable within 5 years of diagnosis. Twenty-one percent of persons with type 2 diabetes already have retinopathy at the time of diagnosis. Ninety percent of people with diabetes who are diagnosed with the disease (either type 1 or type 2) and are less than 30 years of age will develop nonproliferative retinopathy within 20 years after initial diagnosis, and 50% will progress to sight-threatening proliferative retinopathy. The number of people with diabetic retinopathy and sight-threatening diabetic retinopathy is expected to triple by 2050 to over 16 million people.[8]

Diabetic retinopathy can occur in a mild to very advanced form, from nonproliferative (formerly background or pre-proliferative) to the proliferative stage. The nonproliferative stage is further broken down into mild, moderate, severe, and very severe. Mild nonproliferative diabetic retinopathy (NPDR) occurs when the microvasculature of the retina becomes weakened and begins to leak fluids. Small deposits are formed on the retina and tiny hemorrhages appear. Often, no vision loss is noted at this stage. During moderate to very severe NPDR, further vascular damage occurs, resulting in capillary closure and retinal ischemia; however, persons at this stage may not detect changes in vision.

In the final stage, proliferative diabetic retinopathy (PDR), new blood vessels begin to grow in the retina in response to the hypoxia. However, these vessels are fragile and will rupture, causing pre-retinal and vitreous hemorrhages. At this stage, vision impairment may range from mild blurring to severe vision loss. Persons experiencing bleeding may report a veil, cloud, or streaks of red material within their field of vision. In addition, the fibrous scar tissue that develops between the vessels, retina, and vitreous can contract and pull on the retina, causing retinal tears and detachment. A retinal detachment can cause total blindness in the affected eye. If neovascularization occurs in the optic disc, the risk for major vision loss is high.

Diabetic macular edema (DME) can be present in NPDR or PDR and it may impair central vision. The impact on vision may vary from mild blurring to severe loss. Fluctuating vision may arise from swelling in the lens of the eye as a result of high and low blood glucose levels, or it may be in response to postural changes, environmental conditions such as lighting, eye fatigue, or general fatigue.

A major treatment for severe to very severe NPDR and PDR is panretinal photocoagulation, or laser surgery, which is applied in a scatter pattern to the peripheral retina. This treatment does not target the new abnormal blood vessels themselves, but is thought to halt their proliferation by destroying enough tissue that the demand for oxygen is decreased.[10] A vitrectomy may be performed when hemorrhages into the vitreous of the eye do not resolve or when retinal detachment has or may occur. During vitrectomy, the vitreous contents are removed and replaced with a clear solution. Clinically significant macular edema is treated with focal photocoagulation to seal leaking blood vessels. The goal of these treatments is to reduce vision loss. Avastin (bevacizumab), used off-label, and Lucentis (ranibizumab), its Food and Drug Administration (FDA)–approved counterpart, are anti-vascular endothelial growth factor (anti-VEGF) drugs that are used to treat diabetic macular edema and neovascular glaucoma. Eylea (aflibercept), introduced in mid-2014, is the first VEGF inhibitor approved for dosing on a less than monthly basis for the treatment of DME.

The functional vision in persons with diabetic eye disease is quite variable, ranging from mild blurring and irregular patches of vision loss in the central or peripheral field of vision to severe vision loss or total blindness. Vision loss may vary between both eyes. It is not uncommon for a person with diabetes and vision loss to have a preferred, better-seeing eye. An eye report may be helpful to provide visual acuity and visual field measurements within a clinical setting; however, it is also important to obtain a sense of what a client can see during functional activities in a natural environment. Fluctuating vision is common in people with diabetes and can affect the usefulness of residual vision, especially if vision fluctuates throughout the day and is needed during a time of day when it's at its worst.

An individual's subjective acuity, or personal experience of his or her vision loss, is just as important as objective acuity, or results from an eye chart, especially with respect to low vision. The client's performance of activities requiring vision may be better than acuity suggests, or in some cases, worse. Two clients with diabetic eye disease and similar visual acuity changes may use their residual vision differently. A client may well have, through experience, discovered areas of usable vision, which may not appear consistent with actual acuity measurements. Because complications of diabetes may affect several aspects of vision, a thorough functional vision evaluation should be performed, including near reading acuity, contrast sensitivity, a lighting evaluation, and central field testing (see Chapter 8).

CHRONIC COMPLICATIONS OF DIABETES AND GENERAL PRECAUTIONS

The chronic complications of diabetes usually take a long time to develop—often years—and usually after years of high blood glucose. On many occasions, by the time diabetes is diagnosed, complications may have been present for a long time, resulting in permanent damage. Treatment may result in some improvement; however, the damage cannot be eliminated. Regular screening for diabetes may prevent complications by allowing early diagnosis and treatment. To prevent these complications, it is important to monitor for early signs in order to reverse them. Early signs can be detected with regular eye and foot exams; monitoring of blood pressure, weight, blood lipids and hemoglobin A1c; assessment of kidney function, etc.

Prolonged hyperglycemia is the cause of the many chronic and systemic complications of diabetes. These complications affect both the large and small blood vessels in the body and therefore are divided into 2 major categories: microvascular and macrovascular. The microvascular conditions include retinopathy, neuropathy, and nephropathy. Twenty percent of persons with type 2 diabetes will have microvascular complications upon diagnosis. Macrovascular complications include coronary artery disease, cerebral vascular disease, and peripheral vascular disease. These complications contribute significantly to the morbidity and mortality associated with diabetes, particularly in persons with long-standing diabetes.

Retinopathy that has advanced to the proliferative stage carries with it a number of precautions to prevent retinal bleeding. These include avoiding the following behaviors: lifting objects heavier than 5 pounds (or limit as determined by physician), bending so the head is lower than the waist, engaging in activities that raise blood pressure in the eyes, moving suddenly, and straining. A primary care provider and ophthalmologist should be consulted before engaging in any strenuous activities.

Diabetic neuropathy, another microvascular complication, can be diffuse, affecting both the peripheral and autonomic nervous systems, or it can be focal, affecting a single nerve or group of nerves. Peripheral neuropathy is the most prevalent form. It is chronic and progressive in nature. Symptoms can include a "pins and needles" sensation in the hands and feet, pain, numbness, the inability to detect temperature or position, and inability to feel feet when walking. Precautionary measures include proper use and disposal of sharp objects, avoiding exposure to and handling of hot items, and implementing proper foot care. Autonomic neuropathy involves nerves that control automatic body functions and affect mostly internal organs. This form of neuropathy tends to occur later in the course of diabetes. Fifty percent of persons with diabetes who have peripheral neuropathy also have autonomic neuropathy. Autonomic neuropathy may affect many systems, including genitourinary, gastrointestinal, cardiovascular, and sudomotor (responsible for the body's temperature regulation, ie, through sweating).

Cardiovascular effects of autonomic neuropathy are noteworthy. They include postural hypotension, which can cause lightheadedness, dizziness, and weakness. Precautions include slow positional changes and transitional movements. Cardiac denervation syndrome, a fixed heart rate that does not change in response to stress, exercise, breathing patterns, or sleep, may be present. In later stages of cardiac denervation, a silent or painless myocardial infarction (MI) can occur. Other typical symptoms of an MI, such as nausea, shortness of breath, sweating, and vomiting, may be present. These symptoms require immediate medical attention. Stress testing should precede any type of exercise program.

Focal neuropathy is generally acute and time limited, with pain often being the primary symptom. The most common form of focal neuropathy is carpal tunnel syndrome, which is 3 times more common in persons with diabetes than among the rest of the population.[11]

Nephropathy is the final microvascular complication. End-stage renal disease may result in symptoms of nausea, vomiting, dyspnea, lethargy, hypertension, and fluctuating blood glucose levels. 95% of persons with diabetic nephropathy have some retinopathy, with 50% experiencing significant vision loss. This syndrome is called renal-retinal syndrome. Monitoring blood pressure by use of a large-display or talking blood pressure monitor may be required.

Macrovascular complications are responsible for 80% of the mortality of adults with diabetes. These complications are characterized by both arteriosclerosis and atherosclerosis. Coronary artery disease can lead to congestive heart failure (CHF) or a heart attack. It is critical to monitor fluid retention. A person with low vision can monitor weight gain from CHF-related fluid retention by use of a large-display or talking scale.

Cerebral vascular disease can lead to a stroke. Symptoms such as dizziness, slurred speech, numbness or weakness in an arm or leg, or sudden loss of sight may occur. Ability to access emergency medical services is important. Peripheral vascular disease can lead to lower leg and foot ulcers and the need for amputation. Symptoms can include pain with standing, walking, or at rest. Guidelines may include remaining seated during tasks, incorporating rest periods into standing/walking activities if pain is relieved by rest, and seeking medical attention if pain interferes with standing and walking activities or is reported at rest.

ACUTE COMPLICATIONS OF DIABETES

Acute complications can arise from diabetes itself or its treatment. They are short term and may take only minutes, hours, or maybe days to develop and can also be resolved relatively quickly. Hypoglycemia (low blood glucose) arises from the treatment of diabetes with medications that increase pancreatic insulin production. Diabetic ketoacidosis (DKA) and hyperosmolar hyperglycemic state (HHS) are both characterized by pronounced hyperglycemia (high blood glucose), the former due to insulin deficiency and the latter due to extreme dehydration. All 3 of these conditions require immediate attention and are life threatening.

Hypoglycemia

The major acute complication of diabetes is hypoglycemia, or low blood glucose, which is defined as a blood glucose level of less than 70 mg/dL. Hypoglycemia is not a result of diabetes itself, but is a consequence of its treatment. Typical causes relate to the amount and timing of (1) insulin or certain antidiabetes medications (but not all), (2) physical activity, and (3) food or carbohydrates eaten. Medications such as Lopressor (metoprolol tartrate) used for treating secondary medical conditions can also cause low blood glucose. Because physical activity might bring on hypoglycemia, this condition commonly occurs in a general rehabilitation facility. Common symptoms can include sweating, shakiness, difficulty concentrating, blurred vision, dizziness, weakness, or trouble performing a routine task. Severe hypoglycemia can result in pronounced confusion, seizures, coma, and death.

Hypoglycemia is treated with carbohydrate-containing foods or beverages such as juice, soda, honey, or commercially made products such as glucose tablets or gel. If possible, the person should check his or her blood glucose level to determine the amount of carbohydrates required to raise his or her blood glucose to a safe level. Regardless of whether or not the person is able to test, the symptoms should be treated as soon as possible. A person with hypoglycemia symptoms should consume 15 grams of carbohydrate (4 ounces juice or regular soda, 1 tablespoon honey, or 3 to 4 glucose tablets), wait 15 minutes, and then retest blood glucose to determine if additional treatment is required. This is known as the 15/15 rule. If a meal is not planned within 1 to 2 hours of treating a hypoglycemic reaction, then a snack containing 15 to 30 grams of carbohydrate should be consumed to prevent another episode of hypoglycemia.

Several safety measures and adaptations can be implemented to assist the client with vision impairment to avoid or manage hypoglycemia. Persons with diabetes should always wear diabetes identification and carry a blood glucose monitor and a readily available carbohydrate source at all times. Commercially preportioned 15-gram carbohydrate sources, such as glucose tablets, glucose gel, and small 4- to 5-ounce cartons of juice, or home-portioned baggies containing 2 tablespoons raisins, 7 Life Savers, or 9 SweeTarts will prevent overtreatment and a resulting high blood glucose level. Products high in fat such as chocolate candy bars, cake, and potato chips should be avoided, as they are absorbed too slowly and increase weight.

Physical activity that might lower blood glucose should be scheduled 1 to 3 hours after mealtime, when the food from the meal is still supplying glucose to the body. The individual with diabetes should be referred to a physician or diabetes educator if (1) he or she is not able to recognize the symptoms of low blood glucose, (2) an episode of low blood glucose occurs in which the person is unable to care for himself or herself, or (3) if blood glucose levels are very low for 3 days in a row at the same time of day.

Hyperglycemia

Diabetic ketoacidosis occurs most frequently in persons with type 1 diabetes and is commonly caused by omitted or inadequate insulin or a severe stressor such as illness. Blood glucose levels of 250 mg/dL and higher are noted and dehydration is present. The client may complain of weakness, fatigue, dizziness, or achiness. Symptoms may progress to nausea, vomiting, abdominal pain, breathing of a gasping nature, and "fruity" smelling breath indicative of moderate to large ketones.

A mild form of DKA can be treated in an outpatient fashion if both blood glucose and ketone levels can be determined, the client is able to drink and retain fluids, and supplemental insulin can be provided to lower blood glucose levels. The physician should be contacted for guidance. Currently, however, there are no fully accessible forms of ketone testing. Urine ketone test strips require subtle differentiation of pastel colors to determine the level of ketones present. Only 2 meters, the Precision Xtra (Abbott Laboratories) and the Nova Max (Nova Biomedical), test

blood ketone levels, but require reading of a liquid crystal display (LCD) display. More severe DKA is characterized by an inability to retain fluids and mental status changes. Diabetic ketoacidosis then becomes a medical emergency requiring hospitalization.

Hyperosmolar hyperglycemic state is more common in elderly persons with type 2 diabetes whose diabetes is left untreated or severely undertreated, which may occur in nursing homes. Severe physical stressors resulting in HHS may include infection, fluid loss, and cardiovascular events. Hyperosmolar hyperglycemic state is characterized by blood glucose levels of 600 mg/dL and greater and the presence of severe dehydration. Decreased fluid intake may result from diarrhea, fever, and impaired thirst mechanism, among other precipitating factors. Hyperosmolar hyperglycemic state may occur over several days and may result in both impaired mentation (confusion and lethargy) and neurologic changes that resemble a stroke. Any episode of HHS is considered severe and a medical emergency requiring immediate hospitalization.

Summary

It is essential that blood glucose levels be measured if hypoglycemia or hyperglycemia is suspected. However, states' licensure requirements or the policies of medical rehabilitation facilities often prohibit occupational therapists from measuring blood glucose or dispensing diabetic medication. For this reason, clients with diabetes should be encouraged always to bring their blood glucose meter, any medications, and a carbohydrate source with them to treatment sessions. The client or a caregiver may perform the testing and administer the medication under the supervision of the occupational therapist. If the client has hypoglycemic symptoms and is unable to check his or her blood glucose, than the client should treat himself or herself with 15 grams of carbohydrate until symptoms subside. Activity needs to be discontinued, in part, due to inability to confirm blood glucose levels are within a safe range to continue activity. *Hypoglycemia is a life-threatening condition. If in doubt, contact emergency services.*

DEFINITION OF DIABETES SELF-MANAGEMENT EDUCATION AND THE ROLE OF THE LOW VISION THERAPIST

Managing diabetes successfully requires a broad range of habits and behaviors. Diabetes self-management education (DSME) is the ongoing process of facilitating the knowledge, skill, and ability necessary for diabetes self-care. The overall objectives of DSME are to support informed decision making, self-care behaviors, problem

TABLE 20-1: THE AADE7 SELF-CARE BEHAVIORS

AADE7 SELF-CARE BEHAVIOR	SAMPLE BEHAVIORS
Healthy eating	Eating at restaurants, reading labels, measuring serving size or portion
Being active	Being physically active in the home, at work, in the community, tracking physical activity
Monitoring	Blood glucose monitoring, tracking blood pressure, weight, and foot health, as well as the number of steps walked throughout the day (to ensure enough physical activity)
Taking medications	Identifying medications, tracking medication administration, rotating sites for insulin injection
Problem solving	Managing low blood glucose, illness, travel
Reducing risks	Smoking cessation, self-inspection of feet, maintaining up-to-date personal health records, having regular eye, foot, and dental exams
Healthy coping	Dealing with emotional issues, keeping track of and following instructions from one's health care team

TABLE 20-2: THE EPIC FRAMEWORK—INSULIN MEASUREMENT

1. **E**nvironmental Modification—Use task lighting, including models worn on the head; use white contrasting background behind syringe so the black dosage numbers and plunger stand out.

2. **P**rocess Adaptation—Change from vial and syringe to insulin pen or an alternative insulin delivery system.

3. **I**ntroduction of Equipment—Use an insulin measurement device that incorporates the syringe.

4. **C**hange of End Product/Task Simplification—Use a different size syringe (if taking 40 units with a 100-unit syringe, switch to a 50-unit syringe).

solving, and active collaboration with the health care team and to improve clinical outcomes, health status, and quality of life. Recent education research endorses the inclusion of practical problem-solving approaches, collaborative care, psychosocial issues, behavior change, and strategies to sustain self-management efforts.[12]

According to a model developed by the American Association of Diabetes Educators (AADE) in 2003, there are 7 key behaviors that define a healthy lifestyle with diabetes; these are known as the AADE7 Self-Care Behaviors. They are (1) healthy eating, (2) being active, (3) monitoring, (4) taking medications, (5) problem solving, (6) reducing risks, and (7) healthy coping (Table 20-1).[13,14] Many of these tasks and behaviors overlap and are interrelated, and each poses a unique challenge to a person with vision impairment. Using the AADE framework allows for easy communication and treatment planning between occupational therapists and diabetes educators, as well as a focus on meaningful behaviors and functional outcomes. For more in-depth information on the 7 self-care behaviors visit www.diabeteseducator.org/DiabetesEducation/PWD_Web_Pages/Learn_about_AADExs_Seven_Self-Care_Behaviors.html for a podcast on each behavior, available in English and Spanish. A consumer-oriented worksheet can be downloaded, placed in accessible format, or used as a topic in a diabetes support group.

Table 20-2 is an example of the EPIC Framework as applied to one facet of diabetes self-management—measuring insulin dose.

The basic role of the low vision therapist is to provide support, reinforcement, and referral. This role requires knowledge of diabetes, its complications, functional implications, and precautions, in addition to knowledge of professionals in the field of diabetes. Clients often present with chronic complications of diabetes and secondary physical disabilities such as peripheral neuropathy, stroke, arthritis, and Parkinson disease/tremor, which are barriers to performance of diabetes self-care behaviors. Occupational therapists can provide important adaptations and techniques to overcome those barriers.[15] In an advanced role, the low vision therapist provides (1) general training in low vision and nonvisual skills and environmental modification related to organization, contrast, lighting, and magnification; and (2) specific training in the tools and techniques of adaptive diabetes self-management. This advanced role requires in-depth, current knowledge of all facets of diabetes and diabetes self-management, as well as practical knowledge of low vision tools and techniques relative to diabetes management. More specific guidelines are as follows:

- The low vision therapist who is not a certified diabetes educator (CDE) should not provide initial instruction on aspects of diabetes self-management. This is the responsibility of the physician, physician assistant, nurse practitioner, or other primary diabetes care provider, such as nurses and dieticians who are CDEs. If a client has not received such instruction, the client should be referred back to the primary diabetes care provider to arrange for such instruction.

- The role of the low vision therapist is to reinforce or adapt instruction provided by the CDE and primary diabetes care provider, who generally provide written instructions that can be followed by the low vision therapist.

- The low vision therapist may adapt some techniques to better accommodate vision disability, for example, use of magnification devices or improved lighting for reading medications, blood glucose monitor use, or skin checks, with follow-up skill confirmation by the CDE or primary diabetes care provider recommended.

As of 2015, occupational therapy remains among the qualifying professions established by the National Certification Board for Diabetes Educators (NCBDE) for medical professionals seeking to obtain certification as a diabetes educator. Although one of the writers is a CDE, her anecdotal experience is that there are very few occupational therapists holding the CDE, the certification examination is suitably difficult, and there is ample need for occupational therapists properly trained as CDEs to provide adaptive tools and techniques for clients who have physical disability and/or vision loss to better address their diabetes self-management needs.

MEMBERS OF THE DIABETES SELF-MANAGEMENT TEAM AND THEIR ROLES

It is important to be aware of members of the diabetes management team, each member's role, reasons to refer to these other health care providers, and resources for reimbursement for their services. The core diabetes team should consist of the client, a physician, a nurse diabetes educator, a dietician, an ophthalmologist, and a low vision optometrist. Persons with diabetes should be educated as to the availability and roles of these team members.

A physician or other primary diabetes care provider should guide the treatment team. An endocrinologist, a physician who specializes in endocrine disorders, including diabetes, should manage the diabetes care for everyone with type 1 diabetes. Many persons with diabetes, particularly uncomplicated type 2, can have a primary care provider such as an internist, family physician, or other primary care provider to effectively manage their condition. An endocrinologist may be recommended for an individual with type 2 diabetes if he or she is following an intensive self-management program requiring 3 or more insulin injections a day or is using an insulin pump. Other circumstances that may warrant follow-up by an endocrinologist include blood glucose levels consistently higher than desired, one or more diabetes complications, other medical conditions that make diabetes management more difficult, or an individual's desire for a change in his or her care plan. Routine follow-up visits should be scheduled every 3 to 6 months, or more frequently if the client has difficulty keeping blood glucose levels under control, is experiencing complications, or becomes ill.[16]

The nurse diabetes educator provides comprehensive training in diabetes, as well as basic and more advanced diabetes self-management tasks. Referral for initial or follow-up training by a nurse diabetes educator is recommended when an individual lacks information or has misperceptions about what diabetes is and its effects on the body, has not received basic diabetes self-management training, or has difficulty with at least one diabetes-related task. A diabetes nurse educator should also be consulted when a client needs information about using a medication; doing blood glucose monitoring and using the results; incorporating physical activity into his or her self-management program; or planning for managing travel, stress, or illness.

A dietician provides training in healthy meal planning and develops individualized meal plans, taking into account many variables, including caloric requirements, food preferences, and cultural background. Referral to a dietician is recommended when an individual does not know what to eat or how much to eat, feels restricted by his or her meal plan or makes unhealthy food choices, lacks or has an outdated food/meal plan, or has not seen a dietician in several years. Dietitians can also provide meal plan modifications when complications such as renal failure or CHF exist or if the client would like to lose weight or pursue a plant-based nutrition plan.

An ophthalmologist is necessary to diagnosis eye disease(s), monitor disease progression, and provide medical treatment inclusive of prescription eyewear, medications, and eye surgery. This team member is especially important when diabetic retinopathy, macular edema, glaucoma, or even macular degeneration are already present in order to maintain optimum eye health and visual functioning. All persons with diabetes should receive routine dilated eye exams at least every year, or more frequently depending on the presence and degree of eye disease. It is recommended that persons with proliferative retinopathy receive an ophthalmologic exam every 3 to 4 months or more frequently.[17]

The optometrist determines whether a change in the traditional eyeglass prescription might be of benefit. An optometrist specializing in low vision performs a detailed evaluation of distance and near visual acuity, contrast sensitivity, assessment of central scotomas, and the peripheral visual field (see Chapter 7). Based on the results of this evaluation and the case history, the optometrist begins the process of determining the magnification needs of the patient for various activities of daily living (ADL) and selects and prescribes appropriate low vision optical aids. To be most effective, the optometrist and occupational therapist should work together to determine the appropriate optical devices for a patient.

The occupational therapist/low vision therapist may be the person to coordinate overall care of a person with low vision because the occupational therapist considers the whole picture, while the others focus more on specific parts of the picture. The occupational therapist should perform a detailed functional vision evaluation (see Chapter 8) to supplement the optometric evaluation, as well as an evaluation of occupational performance, psychosocial status, social environment (see Chapter 6), and physical environment (see Chapter 12). Optometrists or the occupational therapist will often evaluate and address lighting, contrast, and glare in general. Usually, the occupational therapist will determine how these issues affect diabetes self-management skills and occupational performance in general (see Chapter 9). Because accurate diabetes self-management can literally be a matter of life and death, and because many advanced devices and adaptive techniques are necessary, an occupational therapist should have advanced training and certification in low vision or blindness rehabilitation to manage the adaptive visual aspects of diabetic management. First-response (see Chapter 1) interventions are not sufficient. The AADE's Disability Position statement recognizes the important role of the occupational therapist as a member of the diabetes self-care multidisciplinary team.[18]

Other potential members of the diabetes self-management team may include, but are not limited to, a pharmacist; dentist; psychologist, social worker, or other mental health professional; podiatrist; and nephrologist. Many issues related to these professionals may come to light during the ADL component of the functional low vision assessment and may prompt the occupational therapist to make a referral.

Most insurance plans pay for diabetes self-management training provided by a nurse or a dietician who is a diabetes educator and who is affiliated with a health care setting or medical office. Outpatient diabetes self-management education is reimbursable under Medicare and includes up to 10 hours of one-time initial training within a continuous 12-month period, and 2 hours of follow-up training each year thereafter. A physician must order these services. The approved providers must meet the National Standards for Diabetes Self-Management Education and Support (www.care.diabetesjournals.org/content/37/Supplement_1/S144.extract) and be an accredited program provider. The Centers for Medicare and Medicaid Services (CMS) recognize 2 accrediting agencies: the American Association of Diabetes Educators Diabetes Education Accreditation Program (DEAP at www.care.diabetesjournals.org/content/37/Supplement_1/S144.extract), and the American Diabetes Association Education Recognition Program (ERP at www.professional.diabetes.org/HomeDiabetesEducationAndRecognition.aspx?hsid=4). In January 2002, Medicare added a new Part B benefit for medical nutrition therapy (MNT). Eligible persons with diabetes can receive 3 hours of initial MNT and up to 2 hours annually thereafter in addition to the hours for basic DSME.

In 2011, CMS implemented the competitive bidding program for mail-order diabetes testing supplies (monitors, test strips, control solution, lancing devices, and lancets). The mail-order suppliers (23 at time of this writing) chosen must be used in order to maximize Medicare reimbursement for testing supplies; clients can locate their preferred blood glucose monitor or a similar model on CMS's website at www.medicare.gov/SupplierDirectory/. The most critical issue is usually not payment of the blood glucose monitor, but reimbursement of test strips, which is the most costly element of ongoing testing. When contacting any supplier, mail order or brick and mortar, it is important to confirm that the supplier accepts assignment, which prohibits the supplier from charging the client for the amount in excess of Medicare's reimbursement.

Private insurers may limit the level of coverage and an individual's choice to specific models within their formulary. However, many plans have a process through which a patient's physician or other provider can request a nonformulary product through documentation of medical necessity. The rehabilitation professional can assist the person with visual impairment in providing information to his or her prescriber, so a letter documenting medical necessity for a talking blood glucose monitor and the strips to go with it can be written on his or her behalf.

Under Medicare and many third-party payers, an individual must be declared legally blind to qualify for a fully speech-capable blood glucose monitor. This diagnosis change supersedes the 5-year waiting period. Insurance coverage of a monitor and supplies requires a physician's prescription.

According to the CMS, under Medicare Parts A and B, "Syringes and insulin aren't covered (unless used with an insulin pump) unless you join a Medicare Prescription Drug Plan." Many prescription drug plans under Medicare Part D may include coverage for insulin, syringes, and insulin pens. The client needs to consult with his or her insurer concerning available coverage. Both insulin and insulin pens require a physician's prescription. Some manufacturers have patient assistance programs that are income based.

In July 2002, Medicare Part B and Medicaid approved coverage for biannual foot exams for persons with peripheral neuropathy and loss of protective sensation.[10] A Medicare recipient under Part B may qualify for therapeutic shoes (depth-inlay shoes, custom-molded shoes, and shoe inserts or shoe modification) with a physician's prescription and if certain conditions are met. With continuing changes in the health care environment, occupational therapists need to keep abreast of changes in reimbursement issues.

EVALUATION

The evaluation of a person with diabetes and vision loss has numerous components. It is important to initially determine whether the client has had basic DSME and what are the daily self-care tasks that the person needs to perform in order to manage diabetes with vision loss. It is never too late to refer the client to a CDE for basic DSME. The equipment and resources with which the person with diabetes is familiar should be determined. It is critical that the individual have a basic foundation of knowledge and skills before adaptive diabetes education can be initiated.

It is important to know the outcome of an eye exam and if the individual will be or has recently undergone eye surgery, as the level of vision currently present may change. The assessment should include information on whether visual decline has been gradual or sudden, its stability, and what the primary and secondary eye conditions are, as these will vary in their functional implications and, therefore, the intervention techniques and tools chosen will vary also. The low vision therapist should also determine if the individual has been diagnosed as legally blind.

Functional vision must also be assessed to determine if residual vision is sufficient to safely and accurately complete daily diabetes self-management tasks, irrespective of the environment (work, home, recreational facility, restaurant) (see Chapter 8). If a functional vision evaluation indicates vision impairment, the client should be referred for an optometric low vision evaluation. It is important that the therapist prepare the individual with diabetes and vision loss for the low vision exam by explaining what will occur and how it differs from a conventional eye exam. Encouraging the individual to make a list of activities he or she wishes to accomplish and bringing samples of items or materials that need to be viewed or read is critical; these may include a syringe, medication/food labels, a blood glucose monitor instruction manual, or an insulin pump with a digital display.

If the low vision optometrist recommends optical devices, these may be incorporated into diabetes self-care. Training in the use of optical devices, as well as adaptive visual scanning (see Chapter 9), may be required to optimize use of residual vision for diabetic management or other aspects of occupational performance. Sometimes, the occupational therapist may suggest a different device if it can be used for several activities that may not have been considered when the device was first recommended. In the letter of referral, the low vision optometrist should be told about possible needs for magnification and devices for diabetes management.

In accordance with adult learning theory it is important to ask the client the following questions in order to provide intervention that is of most interest and immediate need to them.

- What is the hardest part of having diabetes?
- What concerns you most about your diabetes?
- What are you hoping to get out of our time together?

As occupational therapists it is important to hear our client's story first. For sample diabetes self-management questions refer to Table 20-3.

The therapist should frequently retest visual acuity. This will enable the client and the therapist to better understand if vision is reliable or if it fluctuates day to day or throughout the day, which will occur with low or high blood glucose levels, eye fatigue, postural changes, ambient lighting, or general fatigue.

Physical impairments secondary to or independent of diabetes need to be taken into consideration. These may include weakness, decreased or altered sensation, and coordination deficits related to the complications of diabetes, such as peripheral neuropathy, carpal tunnel syndrome, and stroke. Additional diagnoses that may require further adaptations include arthritis, tremors, and hearing loss. Often, vision loss necessitates the use of other senses for task completion, including sense of touch and hearing. The ability to localize touch; detect position, movement, texture, pressure and pain; and discriminate temperature is necessary.

Cognitive functioning needs to be assessed in the areas of concentration, ability to follow multiple-step directions, problem-solving skills, ability to form mental images, capacity to learn new information, and memory. Learning adaptive diabetes self-management often requires that the individual interpret and integrate information, perform mathematical computations, and implement simple algorithms. Psychosocial functioning is important to assess due to the high rates of depression, anxiety, and burnout in persons with diabetes. Social, emotional, and physical support systems; insurance coverage and/or financial resources; and level of independence and support the client desires should all be noted. One of the major barriers to performance with clients who have diabetes is endurance, both physical and cognitive. One needs to take care to provide rest breaks and monitor fatigue, scheduling more challenging therapeutic activities earlier in the session.

TABLE 20-3: SAMPLE ASSESSMENT QUESTIONS

MONITORING

Blood Glucose Monitoring

- Do you monitor your blood glucose? If so, how often?
- Have you received formal training in using a blood glucose monitor and from whom?
- What blood glucose monitor do you use?
- Can you consistently read the display?
- Do you have difficulty or require assistance in any aspect of using your blood glucose monitor? Inserting the strip, locating the blood sample on the finger, placing the blood drop on the test site of the test strip?
- Do you rotate your lancing sites?
- Can you and do you record your blood glucose results? Who uses these results and how?
- How do you discard lancets?
- What pharmacy do you use for your supplies?

Other

- Should you monitor your weight or blood pressure, and if so, are you able to?

TAKING MEDICATIONS

Medication Management

- Are you able to accurately and consistently identify your medications? If so, describe your method?

Insulin Measurement

- Do you use insulin? If so, what type(s) of insulin, their dosage(s), and time(s) of day taken?
- What brand/size of syringe do you use?
- Are you able to accurately and consistently able to see the dosage lines on your syringe? If so, describe your method?
- How do you know when your insulin vial or pen is empty?

HEALTHY EATING

- Have you ever received instruction in how and what to eat with diabetes? How long ago did you receive this instruction and from where?
- Do you have special guidelines or a meal plan to follow? If so, describe.
- Are you able to read your meal plan, food labels, and other nutritional information?
- How do you determine portions and measure food quantities?
- Do you prepare your own meals? If you have difficulty or receive assistance, identify in what tasks? Setting stove and oven dials, determining when food is done, cutting food?
- Have you ever burned yourself? If so, describe how?

PROBLEM-SOLVING

Hypoglycemia

- Do you experience low blood glucose and if so how frequently?
- How do you know when your blood glucose is low?
- How do you treat it?

(continued)

TABLE 20-3: SAMPLE ASSESSMENT QUESTIONS (CONTINUED)

PROBLEM-SOLVING

Illness

- Can you readily access emergency phone numbers or emergency assistance?
- Do you have a sick day plan? If so, are you able to read it?
- Do you have a sick day kit that you can readily access?
- Can you take your temperature when you are not feeling well?

REDUCING RISKS

Foot and Skin Care

- Are you able to bathe your feet and don socks and shoes?
- Do you inspect your feet? If so, how often and by what method?
- Do you have your physician inspect your feet every visit or do you regularly see a podiatrist?
- Do you have numbness or tingling in your hands and feet?
- Do you cut your nails? If so, how?
- What do you do if you have an injury to your foot or a foot infection?

Other

- Do you maintain up-to-date personal health records and if so how?
- Do you have regular eye and dental care exams?

HEALTHY COPING

- Are you coping with your diabetes, and if so how?
- How do you to access and maintain instructions from your healthcare providers?

BEING ACTIVE

- Do you have an exercise program or are you interested in beginning one?
- Do you have any difficulty getting around indoors or outside?
- Does your vision prevent you from engaging in physical activity? Describe what activities.
- How do you track your progress in your physical activity?
- Have you ever been instructed in exercise related precautions?
- Do you wear a diabetes identification tag?

AREAS OF INTERVENTION IN ADAPTIVE DIABETES SELF-MANAGEMENT

General Intervention Strategies

Many persons with diabetes and vision impairment will want to utilize their residual vision to complete diabetes self-management tasks. The low vision therapist's role is to ensure the client achieves accurate, safe, consistent results when incorporating remaining vision. Methods to maximize use of residual vision include modification of the task environment through lighting, organization, and contrast; use of optical devices; and labeling and marking techniques. Both general and specific applications of these principles will be provided. Depending on the extent and type of vision loss, the client may achieve varying degrees of success in a diabetes self-care task utilizing vision and may need to also supplement performance with nonvisual techniques or devices.

Lighting, Contrast, and Organization

Lighting often is the most essential environmental consideration to enable a person with low vision to use his or her remaining vision (see Chapter 9), but optimal lighting varies considerably among people with diabetes. The

Figure 20-1. Blood glucose monitoring setup with environmental adaptations, market test strip port on large display monitor, and marked depth setting on lancing device.

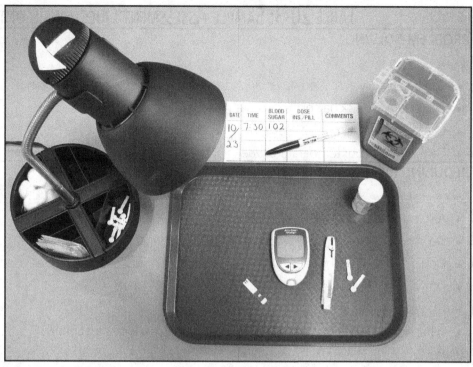

lighting assessment component in the functional vision evaluation will indicate optimal light levels, glare sensitivity, and the need for contrast enhancement (see Chapter 8). If additional lighting is beneficial, then it is important to incorporate a flexible-arm task lamp so that illumination of the work surface and glare can be carefully controlled by changing the distance and position of the light. The task lamp needs to be positioned nearest the better-seeing eye or opposite the person's working hand in order to avoid casting shadows on the immediate work surface. Various forms of lighting worn on the head are now available, but may cause reflective glare. An environmental evaluation should be performed (see Chapter 12). For example, glare from the work surface, such as the table, or from the equipment, such as the blood glucose monitor display, needs to be minimized by a covering in the former example and repositioning the lamp in the latter.

Organization can include reduction in clutter, advanced preparation, and consistency in placement of task materials. Keep like equipment together. Using a tray with a lip will organize task equipment, help the user maintain orientation to supplies, define the workspace, and prevent materials from "getting away" from the user. The latter is especially important where "sharps," such as lancets or syringes, and liquids from measuring beverage portions can drop or be spilled onto the floor. Advanced preparation is helpful so that a diabetes task can be completed in a sequential, timely fashion with a minimum of stress. Assembling a lancing device before turning on a blood glucose monitor or having beverages labeled to enable the user to discern noncaloric

from caloric items are both examples where prior preparation is beneficial (Figure 20-1).

Contrast enhancement can be achieved by placing light-colored supplies on a dark surface and vice versa. The background should be solid in color to avoid having items "lost" in busy patterns. Placing a syringe against a white background permits the black plunger tip and syringe markings to stand out, while a dark blood glucose monitor and dark test strips will be more visible on a light tray.

Optical Devices

Optical and electronic devices can be incorporated into many diabetes self-management tasks, although each type of device has its benefits and limitations and must be tailored to the individual and the task (see Chapter 13 and Chapter 14). The low vision optometrist and the low vision therapist work together as a team to educate the individual with diabetes and vision loss regarding devices that are available, their features, and their applications. Portable optical devices allow the user to perform a task such as blood glucose monitoring or nutrition label reading away from the home. Spectacle format magnification and stationary electronic magnifiers (closed-circuit televisions, or CCTVs) allow both hands to be used during a task such as insulin measurement.

Special precautions need to be observed when measuring insulin when the syringe is placed in a horizontal fashion under the CCTV. Optical magnification, however, will not resolve the decreased contrast present in blood glucose monitor and insulin pump LCDs, but electronic magnifiers will enhance contrast. Relative distance magnification can also be used by bringing the eye closer to the task (using prescribed near spectacle correction) (see Chapter 13). Blood glucose monitors with speech output are also available.

Marking and Labeling Techniques

Marking can also be incorporated to bring attention to features of objects that are less visible to a person with diabetes and vision impairment. Markings can be visual, focusing on high-contrast, bright colors; they can be tactile, emphasizing textural properties such as raised or rough markings; or they can combine elements of both. The features that can be marked include indiscernible elements such as a test strip port on a blood glucose monitor or weight markings on a food scale. Due to potential contact with blood, marking materials should be durable, permanent, and washable and include colored bump or touch dots, raised markings made with brightly colored fabric paint, or even rubber bands.

General Teaching Strategies

Provide choices and alternatives to clients, outline the benefits and limitations of a piece of equipment or a technique, and provide guidance to elicit safe choices. Remember always that retinopathy and other forms of eye disease, as well as diabetes, are all progressive, and the client needs to be aware of other equipment that may be available to satisfy his or her future needs. In general, electronic magnifiers are preferable to optical magnification because the magnification of these devices can be adjusted to fluctuations in vision and progressive vision loss. Adaptive diabetes self-management techniques and devices must be tailored to individual needs. It is up to the client to determine what is most suitable and workable for his or her own needs. The following is a list of general teaching strategies that will enhance the learning experience for the person with diabetes and vision loss:

- Allow for visual and tactile exploration of equipment and its setup.

- Be very descriptive and specific in the explanation, relying on low vision, tactile, and auditory cues.

- If beneficial, provide information on what might be seen so that the person with vision loss would know what a sighted person sees.

- Establish agreement on spatial positioning and directional concepts, such as front and back, right and left.

- Have the client decide where to place or how to position an object, or explain positioning in established frames of reference, such as clock or cardinal positions.

- Always establish a point of reference to guide orientation to other objects around it.

- Establish a common terminology, introducing new terms as desired or needed by the client.

- Allow the client to direct his or her own learning experience by working through a process as independently as possible, providing feedback as needed. Build on the client's knowledge and experience.

- Encourage the client to make suggestions regarding problem-solving approaches.

- Let the client know what is being done at all times and why in order to provide a complete and integrated experience.

- If a client has depression, low frustration tolerance, or a cognitive disability, one should start with activities that are expected to be generally easy for the client and use a success-oriented approach (see Chapter 6) to introduce devices and adaptive strategies that the client might consider.

Process and Outcomes

A high degree of accuracy in performing the tasks of diabetes self-management is necessary. Therefore, the following is strongly recommended:

- Any adaptations or techniques chosen must be effective when the user's vision is at its lowest. Fluctuating vision is likely to occur when a person has low or high blood glucose and needs most to test blood glucose levels, measure food, or administer insulin.

- Accurate insulin measurement and blood glucose monitoring should be observed on at least 3 separate occasions, or 2 times each on each of 2 separate occasions.

SPECIFIC AADE7 INTERVENTION STRATEGIES

Healthy Eating

Medical nutrition therapy is an important component of successful diabetes self-management, not only to control blood glucose levels, but also blood lipids, blood pressure, and overall health. There is no such thing as a general "diabetic diet"; eating with diabetes means eating in a healthy manner. A person with diabetes should have an individualized food/meal plan developed for him or her by a registered dietician, preferably one who is a CDE.

Persons with type 2 diabetes who do not take any diabetes medication, ie, whose diabetes is controlled by diet and exercise, are encouraged to spread food, especially those containing carbohydrates, throughout the day, eating 3 meals or smaller meals with snacks, although generally they can eat according to their own schedule. When persons with type 2 diabetes also take oral medications or

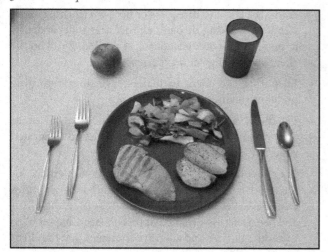

Figure 20-2. Plate method of portion control.

injectable medications that are not insulin, meals need to be kept small to moderate in size, with snacks for persons on specific medications that can cause hypoglycemia. Meal times and carbohydrate content of meals need to be consistent. These approaches are designed to help stabilize blood glucose levels.

Persons with type 1 or type 2 diabetes who are on a fixed-dose insulin regimen need to be consistent in the times meals are eaten and the carbohydrate content of meals in order to maintain a balance between insulin and food. Timing and amount of insulin taken are determined by timing and frequency of meals and their carbohydrate content. Persons on a flexible-dose insulin regimen can determine their insulin dose based on the carbohydrate content of meals that they have eaten or plan to eat. This approach helps to maintain a flexible balance between insulin and food. Timing and frequency of meals and carbohydrate content of meals are based on the person's own schedule and food preferences. Insulin is integrated into usual eating habits. This information should be provided by the physician or CDE.

Several common methods for teaching nutrition management and meal planning include the following: food pyramid, plate method, diabetic food list (formerly "the exchange lists"), and carbohydrate counting. The food pyramid provides basic nutrition information but generally does not address issues specific to persons with diabetes. The plate method provides a good set of general guidelines for relative quantities of each food group at each meal, based on a 9-inch plate (eg, one-quarter of the dinner plate consists of meat, one-quarter of the plate contains starch, and one-half of the plate contains low-carbohydrate/non-starchy vegetables, with one fruit serving and one milk serving completing the meal). It is a good way to begin to learn about appropriate portion sizes and balanced meal planning. This technique may be sufficient for persons with early type 2 diabetes (Figure 20-2).

The food lists for diabetes identify groups of measured foods that have about the same nutritional value. Foods in each list can be substituted (exchanged) for other foods in the same list. An individualized meal plan will identify when and how many choices from each food group are to be eaten for each meal and snacks. Two new consumer resources that may be used by many dietitians is *Choose Your Foods: Food Lists for Diabetes*, available in both English and Spanish from the American Diabetes Association or www.diabetes.org and *Eating Healthy With Diabetes: Easy Reading Guide* from Academy of Nutrition and Dietetics and American Diabetes Association or www.eatright.org. The latter guide purports to offer large-print format, numerous photos, and very little text and is designed for persons with limited reading skills or impaired vision. Accessibility appears limited based on described features (use of photos) and print size used.

The method of meal planning most useful to persons with diabetes who need detailed portion control focuses on counting carbohydrate choices or grams. This approach focuses on the total carbohydrates in food being eaten (total starch plus sugar, not just sugar), with a carbohydrate choice consisting of 15 grams. In basic carbohydrate counting, each meal is allotted a certain number of grams of carbohydrates or carbohydrate choices. Reading food labels or using a nutrition guide is essential to determining carbohydrate content of foods. A sample meal would be about: 1 large slice of toast (18 grams of carbohydrate) + 4 ounces of orange juice (15 grams of carbohydrate) + one 5.5 ounce, 6-inch long banana (23 grams of carbohydrate) + 1 soft boiled egg (protein) = 56 grams of carbohydrate or about 4 carbohydrate choices.

More advanced methods of carbohydrate counting, which involve matching units of insulin to carbohydrate grams, are also used, but are beyond the scope of this chapter. The *Complete Guide to Carb Counting*, 3rd edition, written by Hope S. Warshaw, MMSc, RD, CDE, BC-ADM, and Karmeen Kulkarni, MS, RD, CDE, BC-ADM and published by the American Diabetes Association (2011) will provide more extensive information, including deciphering food labels, how to eat at restaurants, tips and tricks for accurate portions, and using carb-to-insulin ratios.

Many low vision and nonvisual techniques and adaptations will assist a person with vision loss in nutrition management and meal planning. The following areas should be addressed: making a grocery list and locating needed items in grocery store; identifying and labeling food products; measuring food and portion sizes; safe food preparation and cooking; and accessing meal plans, cookbooks, nutritional information, and food labels. Some of these areas will be discussed next.

Optical devices (see Chapter 13) and (see Chapter 14) sighted assistance (a friend or store clerk) can be used to identify food products in the store. Additional independent methods of food identification when storing products at home include organization (locate all cans of fruit together), by other senses (cream soup sounds different when shaken than broth soup), or by labeling (large print, raised letters, rubber bands, audio labels such as the talking can lid or auditory labeling systems). A labeling system needs to be designed for a person's specific needs and should be sustainable by the client and/or significant others.

The low vision therapist should check to make certain the client can read labels with any necessary assistive devices. Handheld electronic magnifiers are often useful for this task because nutritional labeling is often smaller than 1M (8 point) font in size. Nutrition information can be accessed via the Internet, using computer software that enlarges or provides speech to the content on the screen, or via smart phones with accessibility features. See Chapter 12 regarding Digit-Eyes, an app that accesses a label through it's bar code. A portable bar code reader with speech is also available for reading nutrition labels. Both access the internet to maintain an updated database but each can be tailored to meet personal needs by adding items.

Measuring food amounts and determining portions are prerequisites to using any of the mentioned meal planning methods. For people who use the plate method, divided plates with raised tactile dividers are readily available for purchase. Using contrasting plates, cups, and bowls that hold particular portion sizes may assist some persons in using their remaining vision to estimate portions. For example, a color contrasting 1.5-cup cereal bowl may be used to estimate a 3/4 cup, one carbohydrate choice of lightly colored cornflakes cereal when the bowl if 1/2 full. A food template or food model can also be utilized to tactilely estimate a portion of cake or baked potato. More specific measurement of solid or liquid foods and beverages can be obtained by using nested, large-print, color-coded, or tactilely marked measuring cups. In the cereal example above, a 3/4 cup measuring cup could be stored in the cornflakes cereal box. Portion-controlled serving utensils for hot foods can be purchased from restaurant supply stores and resources for specialty kitchen products. A large-display, talking, or tactilely marked scale can be used to measure foods by weight such as a 4 ounce apple or 3 ounce potato (Figure 20-3).

People also need access to written meal plans and information about the nutrition content of foods. Large-print meal plans can be developed or nutrition information may be enlarged on a copier, but maintaining contrast and clarity becomes difficult. A meal plan can be reformatted and customized in a print size/font specific to each individual. Some general guidelines when reformatting a meal plan into large print include the following: use black print on white or yellow paper that has a dull finish; choose a plain, sans serif instead of a fancy font; increase spacing between lines of print; left justify print; use headings that are larger and bolder than regular large print; and avoid columns and charts. Any hospital-driven nutrition guide

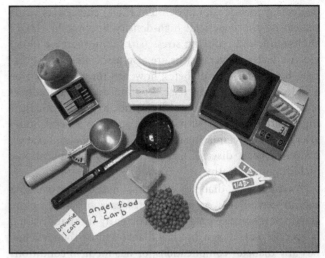

Figure 20-3. Tactile, talking, and large display food scales; food portion control and measurement devices; and food templates and models.

should follow the same principles, but also include a table of contents so that the user can more efficiently locate the information desired.

A decision must be made as to how many pages of the client's preferred print size a meal plan is and at what point an audio recording may be considered a more reasonable alternative. Reformatting material in audio by means of a digital recorder or other voice recording device may be required. It is beneficial to become familiar with any material to be audio recorded so that the process proceeds at a natural but even pace; scripting may be helpful.[19] A special program through the National Library Service allows downloading of recorded material such as books from a computer onto a cartridge designed for use with the digital talking book machine. Cartridges and special downloading cables can be purchased through a number of sites listed at www.loc.gov/nls/cartridges/index.html.

There are also a number of iPhone/Android apps with nutrition information, including CalorieKing and CarbFinder. More general fitness apps such as Track 3 and My Fitness Pal also have extensive carbohydrate and nutritional information databases. My Fitness Pal is a website that works in tandem with apps for iOS, Android, and Windows Mobile. A product evaluation of My Fitness Pal was completed by *Access World* in May 2014 and can be viewed at www.afb.org/afbpress/pub.asp?DocID=aw150505. It concluded that the iOS app was mostly accessible and the website manageable in terms of the bulk of information.

Being Active

The role of exercise and physical activity in maintaining and improving health is well known. Additional benefits to the person with diabetes include improving blood glucose control, allowing muscles to use insulin more effectively, assisting in controlling blood pressure, decreasing low-density lipoprotein (LDL) cholesterol while increasing the beneficial high-density lipoprotein (HDL) cholesterol, and reducing stress (stress can increase blood glucose levels). Several risks are also associated with exercise in persons with diabetes; however, these risks can be avoided with proper exercise program design and adherence to precautions. These risks include hypoglycemia during or after physical activity/exercise (even several hours after), hyperglycemia (usually in type 1 diabetes), exacerbation of heart disease, and worsening of complications, including retinopathy.

Anyone with diabetes who has not been exercising should consult his or her diabetes care provider before starting an exercise program, particularly if the individual is over 35 years of age, has had diabetes more than 5 years, has any diabetes complications, or has medical conditions such as heart disease or breathing difficulties. General exercise guidelines that apply to everyone include maintaining hydration; incorporating stretching, warm-up, and cool-down exercises; avoiding vigorous exercise in extreme environmental conditions; and beginning an exercise program slowly. Exercise should be stopped if pain, lightheadedness, or shortness of breath occurs.

Additional guidelines should be implemented when an individual has diabetes. Exercise precautions such as wearing diabetes identification, exercising with someone who is familiar with diabetes, wearing proper shoes, and inspecting feet after exercise are all important. A range of safety measures should be implemented during exercise to avoid or manage hypoglycemia. The safest time to exercise is 1 to 3 hours after a meal. Body areas that are likely to be involved in the exercise should be avoided as injection sites when planning to exercise immediately after insulin administration.

Blood glucose levels should be monitored before and after exercise, as well as during if symptoms of low blood glucose are experienced. Persons with diabetes should always carry a fast-acting source of carbohydrates at all times. Exercise should be avoided when blood glucose levels are greater than 250 mg/dL and urine testing reveals ketones are present. Although not a typical occurrence, it would be more likely to occur in a person with type 1 diabetes.

An ophthalmologist should be consulted when a person wants to engage in exercise and has diabetes and vision loss, especially more advanced retinopathy. Proliferative retinopathy requires avoidance of the following activities[17]:

- Activities that raise the blood pressure in the body or head (doing resistance exercises with weight machines, lifting free weights, or using rubber exercise bands).

- Bending the head forward below the level of the heart/waist (toe touches, sit-ups, some yoga exercises).

- Holding breath or straining (as when tightening abdominal muscles and lifting legs).

- Activities that jar or involve bouncing of the head (jogging, contact sports).

- Strenuous, high-impact activities (high-impact aerobic dance, racquet sports, intense competitive sports).

- Strenuous arm exercises (rowing or arm bike exercise).

- Activities involving severe atmospheric pressure changes (diving, mountain climbing).

With these precautions, an individual with proliferative retinopathy should be able to participate in moderate-level physical activity.

Various adaptations are available to enable persons with diabetes and vision loss to participate in physical activity and exercise. A walking program is an easy and readily accessible form of exercise. Walking can be done by means of a treadmill or in familiar areas using points of reference such as walls and furniture. Walking with a friend (using the human guide [sighted guide] technique) (see Chapter 19), a guide dog, or using a mobility cane is also an option but requires training by a certified orientation and mobility specialist (COMS). A guide wire, rope, or railing can be used to mark off an area such as a yard or indoor track.

The American Printing House for the Blind (www.aph.org) has a Walk/Run for Fitness Kit that includes a guidebook (large print and braille), 2 talking pedometers (to encourage a buddy system), an adjustable tether, and a 22-foot guide wire system. Persons with vision impairment can use a tandem or stationary bike for cycling. Swimming can be a year-round activity requiring minimal adaptation. Alternatives include swimming near a wall of the pool, using lane markers, or participating in water aerobics. American Printing House for the Blind also has a Jump Rope to Fitness Kit that includes different styles/3 lengths of jump rope, including a "talking" ropeless jump rope, an orientation antishock mat, and guidebook in large print and braille. See Chapter 19 for additional physical activity suggestions and adaptations.

According to Lieberman, Ponchillia, and Ponchillia,[20] many exercises can be done with a fitness or exercise ball. They outline 10 different fitness ball exercises in their book, *Physical Education and Sports for People With Visual Impairments and Deafblindness: Foundations of Instruction.* Exercise balls and exercise ball CDs can be located on the Internet. Several free Wii games can be downloaded through www.vifit.org, including Wii Bowling, Wii Tennis, and Pet n' Punch. These games require a Wii remote and Windows PC and provide vibrotactile and audio cues for participation.

Safety measures should be implemented when participating in aerobic exercise. The floor area should be checked for hazards and obstacles. Positioning near a wall or chair helps to maintain orientation. Exercise can be performed in a seated position. Videos for use by persons with vision loss should include initial instruction and practice in movements before music is added. Instruction should use analogies and be very specific, as in, "Make your legs in the shape of a 'v'" or "Bring your right elbow to your left knee."[20]

Exercise programs designed for those with vision loss can be purchased at www.blindalive.com. These at-home fitness programs fully describe each movement and position for the participant. They are available in digital download or CD format. A sample of the detailed verbal descriptions provided for the various movements is available on their website, as are several half-hour to one-hour podcasts discussing fitness, types of fitness, and fitness and nutrition. Currently there are 2 types of programs available: sculpting with weights and cardio. The weight sculpting program utilizes hand weights and an exercise mat and comes in 2 versions, one more intense than the other. The cardio programs come in 2 versions: a low-impact and a faster-paced version, and incorporate a chair for balance. Samples of level 1 in each category are available at the Blind Alive YouTube channel.

Talking pedometers and large-print exercise records can be used to track and record exercise progress. The Fitbit Flex, a wristband-based exercise tracker, is accessible when used in conjunction with the iOS or Android app. Like a pedometer, it can track steps taken, minutes exercised, or calories burned, among other parameters. Many advanced features and settings are discussed in an *Access World* review dated August 2014 and accessed at www.afb.org/afbpress/pub.asp?DocID=aw150804.

Monitoring

Blood Glucose Monitoring

Blood glucose monitoring is a vital tool in diabetes self-management. It determines the effectiveness of medication, diet, and physical activity in normalizing blood glucose levels; it guides adjustment of treatment; and it helps the person with diabetes prevent and detect hypoglycemia. Guidelines from the American Diabetes Association (ADA) recommend that persons with type 1 diabetes self-monitor blood glucose (SMBG) 3 or more times daily, while persons with type 2 diabetes treated with insulin should SMBG "as needed." The ADA has not provided testing frequencies for those treated with oral medications or nutrition therapy.

Alternative guidelines defined by the American Association of Clinical Endocrinologists (AACE) suggest 3 or more blood glucose tests a day for persons with type 1 diabetes, more than 2 tests a day for persons with type 2 diabetes on insulin or oral medications, and 1 test a day if treated with nutrition therapy. Diabetes educators find SMBG valuable so clients can make informed decisions and adjustments to their therapy regimen and lifestyle based on their blood glucose readings. Ultimately, the treating physician should be consulted on the client's desired testing frequency and timing based on the guidelines/

SIDEBAR 20-1: RECOMMENDED BLOOD PLASMA GLUCOSE LEVELS

The ADA recommends blood plasma glucose target ranges between 70 and 130 mg/dL preprandial (prior to a meal) and < 180 mg/dL postprandial (1 to 2 hours after start of a meal). The AACE recommends less than 110 mg/dL preprandial and less than 140 mg/dL postprandial.

factors stated earlier.[8] These goals apply to most persons with diabetes; however, each person needs to have specific goals set by his or her physician that takes into account not only the previous guidelines, but also age, comorbid diseases, or other unusual circumstances or conditions.[8] (Sidebar 20-1.)

A blood glucose monitor is a device that measures glucose in the blood by a chemical change or an electric current that is produced when blood comes in contact with the test site of the test strip. The lancing device used to obtain the blood sample is spring loaded and resembles a refillable pen. A small, sharp lancet is placed in the lancing device and should be removed after each use. Generally, the blood sample is obtained from the finger, although many monitors now on the market are approved to test alternative sites. The fingertips have more nerve endings, so the fingertips may hurt more than other sites with fewer nerve endings.

Alternative sites may include the palm, forearm, upper arm, and thigh, but specific guidelines need to be followed when using such a site for blood glucose monitoring. Because of circulatory physiology, there is a wide difference in blood glucose levels between the fingertip and alternative sites when glucose levels are rapidly changing. The alternative site may lag behind significantly, which could result in blood glucose levels that appear within range when they are actually low, resulting in undetected hypoglycemia. Alternative sites can be used during routine testing before meals, when fasting, and near bedtime at least 2 hours after eating.

The following alternative sites should not be used:

- During hypoglycemia, after exercise, during illness, within 2 hours of a meal, when blood glucose levels are either rapidly increasing or decreasing

- If a person has hypoglycemic unawareness, which is an inability to detect the warning signs of low blood glucose levels

Continuous glucose monitors (CGMs) are blood glucose monitoring devices that provide readings frequently, typically every 1 to 5 minutes. The 2 that are currently on the market in the United States require a thin wire or sensor to be inserted under the skin and test the glucose in the interstitial fluid. Both of these devices provide blood glucose readings that are calibrated with and used to supplement finger-stick measurements, not replace standard blood glucose testing. They are used to detect and track patterns in glucose levels. These devices have a small display and are generally not accessible to persons with vision loss.

Many steps are involved in the maintenance and use of a standard blood glucose monitor. Maintenance issues include keeping track of expiration dates of test strips and glucose control solution, coding or calibrating the monitor (now only a few monitors require this), setting the time and date, performing glucose control solution check, accessing monitor memory, cleaning the monitor, replacing the battery, and accessing the instruction manual or resource person when in need of assistance. Generally, all of these steps are performed on an as-needed basis. Many monitors have extra features such as computer download capability, blood glucose averaging, and flagging events such as episodes of hypoglycemia.

Coding or calibrating a blood glucose monitor is required to match the test strips being used to the monitor, and therefore is done each time a new bottle or box of strips is opened. Many monitors now have automatic calibration/coding or a no-code feature, some require the manual insertion of a code key, and some continue to entail reading a number from the test strip container and manually inputting it into the monitor. A second important maintenance task is performing a glucose control solution test. This is performed to ensure the monitoring procedure is being done correctly and that the monitor and strips are working properly. Opening a new bottle of strips, obtaining blood glucose results higher or lower than expected, and leaving the test strip bottle open all warrant a glucose control solution check. This test is performed by applying control solution rather than blood to the test strip.

Numerous steps are also required in daily use of a blood glucose monitor. These steps include assembling and using a lancing device, opening the strip bottle/foil, knowing if there is one or multiple strips in the hand, properly orienting and inserting the test strip, attaining and identifying a sufficient blood sample, determining the location of the blood sample on the finger, achieving proper placement of the blood sample on the test strip, and reading the monitor display. Assembling a lancing device and removing the lancet is a multistep task in and of itself.

A variety of tools, adaptations, and techniques can assist a person with mild vision loss to continue to use a LCD monitor. A number of monitors have large displays and bold numbers, contrast or reverse-contrast displays, or backlighting. A person with vision loss needs to try out different models to see which is best for him or her. Providing or enhancing task lighting and contrast, as well as incorporating different forms of optical and nonoptical magnification, may also prove beneficial.

Many steps in blood glucose monitoring, such as inserting a lancet into a lancing device and placing the blood sample on the test site, usually require use of both hands.

Use of an electronic magnifier such as a CCTV or a hand held magnifier in combination with a double ended clamp are both helpful options within the home, but lacks portability if a blood glucose monitor needs to be used in the community, such as in a restaurant or when taking a walk for exercise. Portable spectacle magnification may be advantageous but n requires working distance that a client might not find comfortable. Hand held optical devices (Chapter 13) and electronic devices (Chapter 14) are very useful for reading expiration dates and code numbers as they are steps that are only occasionally done and can be performed in the home setting.

Many monitors are designed to be brought to the blood sample, so they also can be picked up and brought closer to the eye. Blood glucose meter charts can be located through the Diabetes Forecast Buyer's Guide available at www.diabetesforecast.org/landing-pages/lp-consumer-guide.html (for listing of meters, including those that have audio capability and backlighting), www.diabetesforecast.org/files-legacy/images/extras/v66n01_p41-47_1.pdf (for actual meter chart), and www.diabeteshealth.commedia/pdfs/PRG0113/BloodGlucoseMeters.pdf (for chart with pictures of meter displays).

Visual and tactile features of test strips (underside of strip is white or solid colored; combined light and dark areas on topside with shiny electrodes at one end; raised or recessed areas; square or rounded ends; smooth vs textured surfaces; and positioning within test strip bottle) may aid in proper orientation of the test strip prior to insertion into the port. High-contrast or tactile markings with fabric paint can be placed on salient features of a monitor or lancing device to highlight the location of buttons, settings, or openings. Producing a larger, more visible blood drop or using a white towel for contrast will help to discern and obtain a sufficient blood sample.

Currently, a number of blood glucose monitors (Figure 20-4) with speech capability are available for persons with low vision in the United States, as indicated in Table 20-4. Some meters, such as the OneTouch Verio Sync (Life Scan, Inc), can be synced with an iPhone, iPad, or iPod touch and then results can be accessed via the Voice Over feature. Several speech capable, integrated blood glucose monitors (one that internally contains the lancets and tests strips) have been developed in the past but none have come to fruition.

When evaluating a talking blood glucose monitor, some beneficial features to look for include full speech capacity for memory, setting time, low battery, and errors; either no coding or automatic coding; sufficient time to apply blood; reasonable blood sample size required; ability to apply more blood; a repeat function; moderate strip size; uses common batteries and highly tactile buttons and test strip ports. Accessible manuals are desirable, either in CD format or downloadable. Some talking monitors are combined with a blood pressure monitor. (These are generally wrist

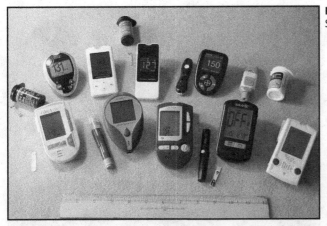

Figure 20-4. Blood glucose monitors. First row: 5 talking monitors. Second row: 2 with backlighting, 2 with reverse contrast.

TABLE 20-4: TALKING BLOOD GLUCOSE MONITORS

MONITOR NAME	WEBSITE	MANUFACTURER/ SUPPLIER	SPEECH CAPABILITY	
			Full	*Partial*
Advocate RediCode	www.dsosi.com	Diabetic Supply of Suncoast	X	
Easy Max Voice 2nd Generation	www.oaktreeint.com	Oak Tree Health		X
Element V	www.infopiausa.com	Infopia		X
Embrace	www.omnishealth.com	Omnis Health		X
Fora V20	www.foracare.com	Fora Care	X	
G Mate Voice	www.gmate.com	Philosys		X
Glucocard Expression	www.glucocardusa.com	Arkray		X
Prodigy Voice	www.prodigyvoice.com	Prodigy Diabetes Care	X	
SolusV2	www.solometers.com	Biosense Medical Devices	X	

monitors, which are not usually considered very accurate.) When vision is insufficient, additional nonvisual techniques may be required. Tactile features on monitors, strips, or lancing equipment can aid in locating and identifying key parts, or equipment can be adapted with raised markings. Features such as notches or cutouts and smooth or textured surfaces can aid in properly orienting and inserting the test strip or locating the test site.

Knowing if there is a blood drop on the finger or a sufficiently sized blood sample is often one of the major challenges. Specific techniques can be employed to promote increased blood flow to the fingertip, thereby more consistently achieving a sufficiently sized blood sample. These include the following:

- Vigorously wash hands in warm water.
- Hang arm down by the side for 30 seconds so blood pools in fingertips.
- Shake hand down as if shaking down a thermometer.

- Massage or "milk" finger from knuckle toward fingertip before lancing.
- Before lancing, use a rubber band as a small tourniquet: wrap a double-thickness of rubber band around the middle segment of the finger to make the blood fill the end segment. After lancing, remove the rubber band (Figure 20-5[A]).
- After lancing, milk the finger in a press/release fashion to facilitate blood flow.
- Make sure lancet is pressed against finger.
- Change depth setting of lancing device so puncture is deeper.
- Change lancet device to one with a larger point.
- Rotate sites.
- Use lotion to keep skin supple.

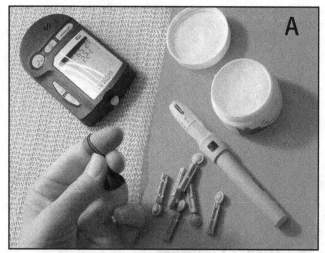

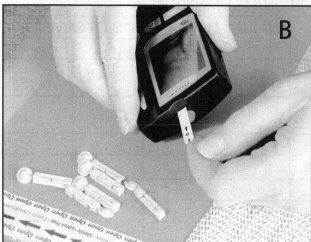

Figure 20-5. (A) Getting enough blood on the strip—the rubber band method. (B) Putting blood on the strip (note adaptation for inserting strip directly below it).

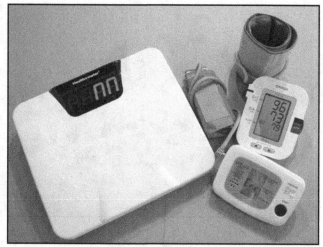

Figure 20-6. Large-display or talking blood pressure monitors and scale.

- At times, sighted assistance may be necessary to determine the number of times a finger needs to be milked before an adequate blood sample is achieved.

Making a mental map of where the puncture is made on the fingertip may help the user to locate the blood drop on the finger after lancing. Usually, the sides of the fingers and thumb, and possibly the fingertips, are used to obtain a blood sample. When lancing, the finger pads should be avoided for 2 reasons: they hurt more, and they are needed for tactile sensitivity for many tasks, including reading braille.

Many physicians and endocrinologists are often unaware of the availability of talking blood glucose monitors and would benefit from similar education. A prescription must be written by the physician treating the individual's diabetes in order for a blood glucose monitor to be covered by insurance. The prescription should include the following information: the name of the blood glucose monitor, the diagnosis code, the testing frequency, and the quantity of test strips and lancets desired beyond that provided by the starter kit. If a talking model is being sought, a statement of legal blindness should also be included on the prescription. A corroborating eye report from the eye care physician may be required by the pharmacy, the insurance company, or the medical physician to support the diagnosis of legal blindness.

The self-care behavior "monitoring" also includes keeping track of blood pressure, weight, and other health parameters.

In 2015 the American Diabetes Association recommended a blood pressure of < 140/90 for people with diabetes, regardless of age. The client should consult their physician for a more individualized goal. According to the American Heart Association a weight gain of more than 3 pounds in a day is a warning sign of heart failure.

With respect to health monitoring devices, the following guidelines should be considered. Large LCD devices should be evaluated by the individual with diabetes and vision loss to ensure that they can consistently be read; getting close to the display may not be an option, such as in a weight scale. When suggesting any talking device, many voice-related features need to be considered before recommending a specific model. These include voice clarity, volume, speed, pitch, and accent. In many cases where a hearing impairment is present, a male voice may be preferable due to the lower pitch (Figure 20-6).

Taking Medication

Being able to identify, track, and administer medications, whether in oral, injectable, or any other form, is a critical component of diabetes self-management and health management overall. Most adults diagnosed with diabetes take oral medication, insulin, or both to manage their condition. According to the Centers for Disease Control

(CDC), between 2010 and 2009, 14% of the adults diagnosed with diabetes (type 1 or 2) took insulin only, 15% took both insulin and oral medications, 57% took oral medications only, and 16% did not take either insulin or oral medication.[21] Clients may initially be treated with a single medication, progressing to combination therapy wherein 2 or more oral agents, or an oral agent and insulin, may be used. It is important to have some fundamental knowledge about the different kinds of oral medications and insulin, as well as some of their key properties/characteristics. As we learn more about the many underlying physiological reasons that people develop type 2 diabetes, an ever-increasing number of both oral and injectable medications is being developed and used to normalize blood glucose levels. The dose, frequency, the time(s) of day, and whether it is taken before or with food vary with each medication (Table 20-5).[7,21]

In addition to the primary medications that are used to treat the actual diabetes, there are commonly used secondary medications that can have a side effect of causing hyperglycemia or hypoglycemia. Many times, clients are not aware of this side effect, and sometimes health care professionals also are equally unaware (Table 20-6).

Adaptations for Oral Medications

A wide array of adaptive techniques and equipment is available that incorporate low vision and/or nonvisual features to enable independent identification and tracking of oral medications. Task lighting, a contrasting background, optical magnification, and pill vial magnifiers all can assist a person to use remaining vision to identify medication. Several national pharmacies such as Walgreen's and Rite Aid will provide large print. Pill containers can be labeled in large print, or a color-coding system can be implemented. When vision is insufficient, wooden or plastic letters can be used as tactile labels, or small adhesive-backed raised dots can be applied to the container representing the number of pills to be taken (Figure 20-7).

Many of the visual and tactile labels convey only a limited amount of information, such as a medication's name or how many pills are to be taken; however, auditory medication labels are capable of recording additional label information. A basic auditory label, such as the Tel-Rx, consists of a small recording device that attaches to each medication bottle and provides 20 seconds of recording time. These labels are reattached at the time of refilling and may be initially labeled by the client or the pharmacist by request. Walgreens sells a similar recording product, the Talking Pill Reminder, that attaches to the medication bottle cap, can record for 30 seconds, and has a beeping interval timer. See Chapter 12 for more advanced generic labeling systems that can be applied to medications.

En-Vision America offers a multifaceted medication labeling program that can provide large print, braille, and auditory or talking labels. The large print labels are high-contrast, 18-point print presented in a booklet-style format, containing the same information as on the regular label and is attached directly to the medication bottle. A 2D barcode is also printed on the label and may be scanned with a smartphone using the ScripView app to audibly access the detailed drug information. For those without a smart phone, a ScripTalk playback station can be obtained that will read the label that is programmed with all the printed information. Because the data is stored in the label itself, it can be used on any size bottle, box, vial, tube or other prescription container. This service is offered by several mail order pharmacies including CVS, Caremark, Kohl's, and Walmart. More information, an audio demo, and a state-by-state list of participating brick and mortar pharmacies can be viewed at www.envisionamerica.com.

Several methods are also available to enable a person to track his or her medication usage. One technique is to apply elastic bands to the bottle equal to the number of daily doses, remove one band after taking each dose, and then reapply all bands after taking the last dose. The Take-n-Slide, is very similar to the rubber band technique, but is a device that is attached to the bottle. One version consists of a strip of 4 sliding buttons corresponding to the 4 times a day pill are taken; each time a pill is taken its button is slid to the right. Large-print and braille pillboxes are also popular alternatives. Such pillboxes are available in different shapes and sizes, ranging from 1×/day to 4×/day. Many pillboxes come in different colors so that a color can be associated with the time of day a medication is taken.

Some pillboxes come equipped with timers and auditory alarms, such as the e-pill Multi Alarm system, to remind the client to take his or her medication. Verizon's "Answer Call" system is a reminder service that calls the patient at his or her home telephone number at the time he or she has specified (2 options for regular reminders: Monday through Friday or 7 days a week). When the patient answers, he or she hears a reminder message that is either self-recorded or recorded by a significant other. An additional fee applies.

Some free smart phone apps that can assist in tracking medications are My Medication Schedule, which allows creation of a medication schedule and sends text/e-mail reminders to take the medication and to refill (available free at www.mymedschedule.com). MedSimple (free for both iPhone and Android) can track and monitor medications all in one place, set reminder alarms for reordering specific medications, and even access coupons. MedCoach (free Android and iPhone apps) refills prescriptions online with most pharmacies and has medication and refill reminders. MediMemory, available at www.medimemory.comgetting_started.html#product_comparison has 2 versions: MediMemory Lite and MediMemory, with the fee dependent on the version purchased.

A number of automated medication management systems are currently on the market. The Philips Medication Dispensing Service is an automated pill dispenser that has alerts for dispenser errors and missed doses.

TABLE 20-5: MEDICATIONS USED IN TREATMENT OF DIABETES, THEIR ACTION, AND POTENTIAL TO CAUSE HYPOGLYCEMIA

CLASS/ROUTE	ACTION	COMMON NAMES	OTHER
Sulfonylureas/Oral	Works on pancreas to increase release of insulin	Glucotrol, Amaryl	Can cause hypoglycemia, timing not meal related, weight gain
Meglitinides/Oral	Works on pancreas to increase release of insulin	Prandin, Starlix	Can cause hypoglycemia, before meals, weight gain
Biguanides/Oral	Enhances glucose transport into fat and skeletal muscle; reduces production of glucose by liver	Metformin, Glucophage	Does not cause hypoglycemia, prior to meal(s), possible weight loss
Thiazolidinediones (TZDs)/Oral	Enhances glucose transport into fat and skeletal muscle; reduces production of glucose by liver	Actos, Avandia	Does not cause hypoglycemia, taken with main meal(s) of day, weight gain
Alpha-glucosidase inhibitors/Oral—not used much	Works on small intestine to reduce rate of carbohydrate digestion and glucose absorption	Precose, Glyset	Does not cause hypoglycemia, first bite of each meal, weight neutral
DPP-4 Inhibitors/Oral	Prevents breakdown of naturally occurring compound in body called GLP-1; GLP-1 reduces blood glucose	Januvia, Onglyza, Tradjenta	Does not cause hypoglycemia, with or without food, weight neutral
SGLT2 Inhibitors/Oral	Works in kidneys; blocks SGLT2 from absorbing glucose; causing excess glucose to be eliminated in urine	Invokana, Farxiga	Does not cause hypoglycemia, first meal of day/in morning, possible weight loss
Combinations drugs/Oral	Combined mechanisms	Metaglip, Glucovance, Janumet,	Potential for hypoglycemia, timing and weight gain depend on combination
Amylin Analogs/ Injectable	Assists insulin to lower post-meal glucose levels	Symlin	Does not cause hypoglycemia, before major meal(s), possible weight loss
Incretin Mimetics/ GLP-1/ Injectable	Stimulates glucose-dependent insulin release	Victoza, Byetta, Bydureon	Does not cause hypoglycemia, timing depends on particular drug, possible weight loss
Dopamine Receptor Agonists/Oral	Unknown mechanism	Cycloset	Does not cause hypoglycemia, with first meal of day, weight neutral
Insulin/Injectable	Works directly on lowering blood glucose	See Table 20-6	Can cause hypoglycemia, timing depends on type of insulin, weight gain

Table created using reference 7.

Adaptations for Injectable Medication

Insulin is the medication most often associated with diabetes. It is currently used in an injectable form and as of 2015, an inhalable form. At present, 3 companies manufacture injectable insulin in the United States: Lilly (brand names Humulin and Humalog), Novo Nordisk (Novolin, Novolog, and Levemir), and Aventis (Lantus and

TABLE 20-6: NONDIABETIC MEDICATIONS THAT MAY AFFECT BLOOD GLUCOSE LEVELS

MEDICATIONS THAT CAUSE HYPOGLYCEMIA	MEDICATIONS THAT CAUSE HYPERGLYCEMIA
• Aspirin, in large doses	• Sudafed
• Coumadin	• Lasix
• Chantix	• Lipitor
• Lopressor	• Lopressor (both)
• Dilantin	• Prednisone
• Prozac	• Abilify
• Timoptic	• Albuterol
• Sulfa medications such as Bactrim	• Glucosamine
	• Hydrocortisone
	• Synthroid
	• Niacin

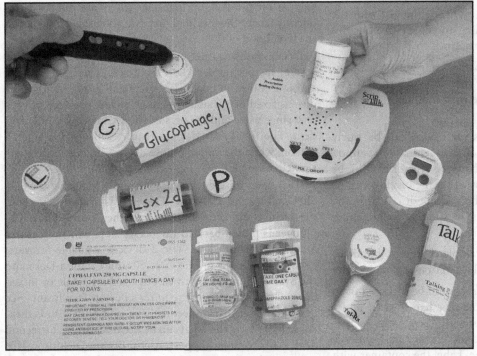

Figure 20-7. Selective low vision and auditory medication management adaptations and devices.

Apidra). Insulins are classified according to their speed of onset of action, peak effect, and duration of action. Several premixed insulins are also available (70/30, 50/50, and 75/25). Some insulins are clear, colorless solutions, while other insulins are suspensions, which should be evenly cloudy. For a comprehensive list of the many different insulin formulations, their actions, and more, visit www. diabetesincontrol.comimages/issues/2014/07/insulin_comprehensive_review_20140709.pdf.

Frequency of insulin dosing is dependent on many factors: the type of diabetes, level of insulin deficiency or resistance, timing and carbohydrate content of meals, physical activity, and waking and sleeping patterns. Common dosing frequencies include a single daily injection administered in the morning or at bedtime or a 2-injection regimen with insulin administered in the morning before breakfast and before the evening meal or at bedtime. Intensive insulin therapy ranges from 3 to 4 times a day, with a 4-injection regimen requiring one injection in the morning and one at each mealtime. Some persons take a fixed dose of insulin that is set by their physician. Others take a variable dose, which is a dose that can be altered by the individual, taking into account his or her current blood glucose level, carbohydrate amounts just eaten or about to be eaten, and recent or imminent physical activity, among other factors.

Many steps are required for safe insulin use. They include insulin storage, identification (if more than one is taken), insulin/vial preparation, measurement, mixing (if more than one is taken), air bubble management, administration, injection site management, determination of quality and quantity of vial contents, and sharps disposal. Specific information regarding insulin itself can be obtained from the manufacturer's guidelines. Low vision therapists should adhere to standard procedures for preparing, mixing, and drawing up insulin and can begin to familiarize themselves with these basic procedures through educational materials available through syringe manufacturers such as Becton-Dickinson or through each insulin manufacturer. Following are some basic principles:

- Suspended (cloudy) insulins should be rolled between the palms to resuspend the contents in the vial. This step is not necessary for clear insulins.

- Pressurize the insulin vial by filling the vial with the amount of air corresponding to the desired insulin dose prior to drawing out insulin.

- If drawing 2 insulins into the same syringe, always pressurize both vials first. Then draw the shorter-acting insulin into the syringe first and then the longer-acting insulin.

- While some combinations of insulin can be safely mixed in the same syringe, other combinations cannot. If your client takes more than one type of insulin, be sure that he or she knows whether the insulins can be safely mixed. If the prescriber did not discuss this, the pharmacist can answer this question, as well as other questions about medications.

- Always ensure the vial is completely inverted and the syringe and vial are vertical when drawing out insulin.

- Sharps (needles and lancets) should be disposed of in a purchased sharps container or a hard plastic, puncture-proof opaque container with a screw cap, such as detergent bottles and plastic juice containers. Reinforce the lid with heavy-duty tape. Label the container with the word *sharps*. Specific state-by-state laws can be located at www.safeneedledisposal.org.

Many low vision and nonvisual techniques and devices are now available to assist in insulin management. All insulin bottles are the same size and shape, except for those manufactured by Aventis, such as Lantus and Apidra, which are taller and thinner. To distinguish 2 similar vials, a rubber band can be placed around one of the vials, or commercially-made insulin vial sleeves that come in different highly visible colors and different sizes can be used.

A wide range of visual and nonvisual devices can be used for insulin measurement. The primary method of insulin delivery is the vial and syringe. It is important to be aware of the features of a syringe, which include syringe/barrel size, needle gauge (width), and needle length. For visual accuracy in dosing, the syringe size is matched to the insulin dose to be injected as follows:

- 0.30 cc or 3/10 cc (for doses < 30 units)

- 0.5 cc or ½ cc (for doses < 50 units)

- 1 cc (for doses 50 to 100 units)

In addition to the environmental modifications and optical devices identified earlier in this chapter, several magnifiers are made specifically to fit on the syringe, and they may enable a person with very mild, stable vision loss to read the dose markings on the barrel. These include the clip-on syringe magnifier, the Becton-Dickinson Magni-Guide, and the Insul-eze. The syringe magnifiers will fit any syringe and provide up to 2× enlargement They vary in their features, which may include a holder for the insulin vial, the plunger, or the syringe barrel, all of which will assist the user to align the syringe needle with the rubber stopper on the vial. Syringe magnifiers are not used frequently due to the minimal magnification they provide and the likelihood of fluctuating vision.

When choosing a nonvisual insulin measurement device, several factors need to be considered. These include the amount of insulin taken (large or small dose); whether the dose is fixed or variable, single or mixed; the current type of syringe used; and the person's desire to be fully independent. The fixed-dose devices require setting by a sighted person, while the variable-dose devices do not require any sighted assistance.

Two fixed-dose devices are currently available: the Safe Shot and the Inject Assist. These measuring devices hold the syringe and can be preset for either 1 or 2 doses. The plunger is pulled back to the preset stop, which measures a specific insulin dose. The 2 devices available for variable insulin doses are the ½ cc/50 unit Count-a-Dose and the Syringe Support. Both can be used for single or mixed doses. The Count-a-Dose requires a Becton-Dickinson ½-cc syringe with a ½-inch needle. Each unit of insulin is measured by a single click that can be felt and heard. The second device, the Syringe Support, uses a Becton-Dickinson 1-cc syringe. The device is set by a calibrated screw that has a raised white marking. A single turn of the screw measures 2 units of insulin. All of these devices except the Safe Shot have a syringe and vial holder that lines up the syringe needle with the rubber stopper on the insulin vial. For the Safe Shot, the Center-aid and the Insul-cap will guide the syringe needle into the rubber stopper; the latter device also holds the syringe firmly to the vial (Figure 20-8[A]).

Although the procedure for using each insulin measurement device differs, the nonvisual technique for removing air bubbles in the syringe and knowing when the insulin vial is empty is universal. Removing air bubbles is critical because air bubbles take up space that insulin should

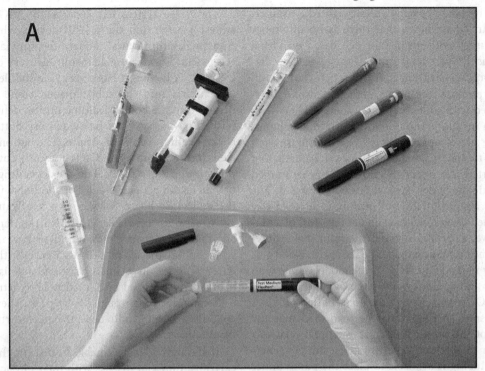

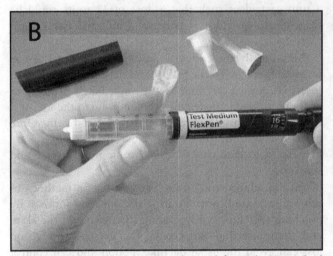

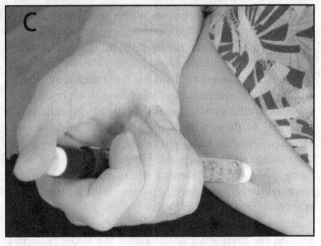

Figure 20-8. (A) Insulin measurement devices, left to right: Magni-Guide magnifier, Safe-Shot with Insul-Cap; Count-a-Dose; Syringe Support; various insulin pens. Includes application of pen needle to insulin pen. (B) Dialing up insulin pen. (C) Demonstration of self-injection with insulin pen.

be occupying and therefore the insulin dose will be less. Expelling air bubbles is performed by drawing insulin into the syringe, pushing it back into the vial at least 3 times, and then filling the syringe with the desired dose on the fourth time. Tapping the syringe will help release air bubbles too.

It is important to avoid using an almost empty insulin vial, as air can be drawn in instead of insulin. Using no more than 950 units out of 1000-unit vial will ensure that there is sufficient insulin in the vial at all times. Always determine how many doses an insulin vial contains without using the last 50 units. For example, if a person took 50 units each day from a 1000-unit vial of Lantus, one vial would last 19 days (950/50=19). The person should set aside

19 syringes and start a new vial when these are used. A second technique is to mark off each successive day on a calendar that a dose is taken (in this case 19 days), using different marking symbols for each 19-day period.[21]

Insulin pens, another method of insulin delivery, can be operated nonvisually, although most are not endorsed by the manufacturer for this use. A pen is available for each insulin type. Some pens are reusable and require refilling with insulin cartridges; other pens are prefilled and disposable. Depending on the model, pens can deliver insulin in ½-, 1-, or 2-unit increments. An audible and tactile click is noted for each increment when dialing a dose using the dosage knob. Insulin pens come with a disclaimer regarding use by visually impaired persons without sighted assistance; however, research has shown that there is no difference in dosing accuracy with an insulin pen based on visual status.[21] An insulin pen chart can be located at www.diabetesforecast.org/2014/Jan/images/insulin-pen-chart-2.pdf.

The insulin pump, a continuous method of insulin delivery, can be used with some success by some persons with vision loss. An insulin pump is a miniaturized, computerized device the size of a pager that delivers insulin through flexible plastic tubing to a small needle or soft cannula that has been inserted just under the skin. It is programmed to closely mimic the body's normal release of insulin. The pump releases a steady trickle of insulin 24 hours a day (preprogrammed basal rate/dose), and at the press of a button it can deliver a specific amount of insulin (bolus dose) calculated by the pump user to handle the rise in blood glucose caused by meals and snacks. Some models come with tactile buttons and audio features for programming bolus insulin doses. Often one press of the bolus button provides one unit of insulin. A CCTV may be used to change the basal dose(s) of the pump which are modified relatively infrequently or to check other settings or features—generally sufficient tubing is available to place the pump under the CCTV camera.

Candidates for the insulin pump must meet specific requirements under Medicare guidelines, including but not limited to, already successfully using daily carbohydrate counting, multiple blood glucose checks, and mealtime insulin dosage adjustment. Insurance may require additional documentation of need from the prescriber to cover an insulin pump. Currently there is no insulin pump accessible to those with vision loss. Some pump screens can accommodate a cell phone magnifier. Sufficient flexible tubing can be incorporated to permit placement of the pump under a CCTV camera. Alternatively, the client can learn to briefly disconnect the pump while the pump screen is accessed under the CCTV.

A new disposable insulin delivery device is now available on the market for adults called the V-Go (Valeritas, Inc), sometimes also known as a patch pump. It is an option that can take the place of insulin pens or an insulin pump. The V-Go uses rapid-acting insulin and is currently cleared for use with Humalog and Novolog. The V-Go is marketed for use in persons with type 2 diabetes because the amount of insulin used at meals can only be adjusted in 2-unit increments and persons with type 1 diabetes generally require smaller adjustments in insulin dosing. It is a disposable insulin delivery device that is worn for a 24-hour period. The V-Go administers a preset basal rate of insulin (20, 30, or 40 units) via continuous infusion over the day. In addition, a bolus or meal-time amount of insulin can be delivered at the press of a button as determined by the user to cover a meal or snack. Unlike an insulin pump, there are no batteries, electronics, tubing, programming, or a screen to read.

The V-Go system has 2 parts: the V-Go device with adhesive patch and the EZ fill device, which is used to transfer insulin from a standard insulin vial to the device receptacle. The disposable insulin delivery device is about 2 ½ by 2 ¼ inches. It has a very fine stainless steel needle that inserts into the subcutaneous tissue to administer insulin into the body. Mealtime insulin delivery is accomplished by pressing the bolus delivery button, 1 press or click equaling 2 units of insulin. The buttons can be operated through clothing. V-Go is currently covered both as a prescription and a medical device depending on individual patient health plan coverage. For additional information on the V-Go visit, https://www.go-vgo.com/training.

Afrezza, an inhalable insulin in powder form, is now approved for persons with type 1 or type 2 diabetes and is an option the client can discuss with their physician. Afrezza comes in a small cartridge and is administered using a whistle-sized oral inhaler. The cartridges come in a 15-cartridge see through blister pack. The blue cartridge contains a 4 unit insulin dose, the green cartridge an 8 unit insulin dose.

If the individual is unable to discern the color of the cartridge they can discuss with their physician only using 4 unit cartridges such that a dose of 12 units could be three 4 unit cartridges versus one 4 unit and one 12 unit cartridge.

Additionally the cartridge only fits in the inhaler one way and there are tactile features on the cartridge to aid in insertion. A used cartridge can be immediately disposed of or if not. it has tactile features that indicate to the user if it is empty. The insulin used is rapid acting and is therefore used to cover mealtimes only. Contraindications to use of Afrezza include clients with chronic lung disease and smokers.

Insulin administration itself may focus on methods to achieve increased control during the injection process. By pinching the skin, gently placing the needle on the skin, and then inserting the needle, the person with vision loss can avoid the usual dartlike motion and can control where the needle is inserted.[17] Also insulin should only be injected subcutaneously. Using the appropriate length needle will control the depth of the needle injection. Shorter needles are more widely used for this reason. The client should speak to their physician or educator to ensure they are using the appropriate needle length on their syringe or pen.

Insulin measurement devices that are used in conjunction with syringes are available through the several specialty low vision catalogs listed at the end of this chapter under "Resources." Many can also be purchased directly from the manufacturer and some from select pharmacies. These devices are paid for out of pocket. Insulin pens and pen needles are obtained and billed for by a pharmacy and require a physician's prescription. General medical physicians may need to be educated regarding the benefits and feasibility of insulin pens for persons with vision loss; however, a general prescription is sufficient.

Problem Solving

Managing diabetes poses many challenges. Simple schedule changes, like eating an extra piece of birthday cake, losing track of time and forgoing lunch due to a busy schedule, and more complicated disruptions like catching the flu, being hospitalized for hip surgery, or traveling on vacation to a far-away location all present challenges in how diabetes is managed and require the use of problem-solving skills. Problem-solving skills are taught by the CDE, but can be addressed by the low vision therapist in terms of low vision or nonvisual adaptations. Many of these adaptations have already been addressed elsewhere in this chapter. For example, eating an extra piece of birthday cake can be planned for by reducing carbohydrates at the meal when the birthday cake was served, or after the fact may require an increase in medication/insulin or additional physical activity to normalize blood glucose levels. Portion control, adaptive insulin measurement, and adaptive physical activity have already been addressed.

Low Blood Glucose

Low blood glucose as a result of missing a meal may require low vision, talking, or tactile timepieces that will enable clients with vision loss to ensure timeliness of meals and medications. Large-print or recorded blood glucose records will allow the person with diabetes and his or her physician to determine any event that may have contributed to low blood glucose. Nondiet/regular soft drinks can be marked with a rubber band ("R" for regular) to distinguish them from those that are noncaloric/counterparts. Immediate access to emergency phone numbers is critical and several possible adaptations include a large-print, pre-programmable telephone and speed or voice dialing. Low vision and nonvisual methods for blood glucose monitoring, measuring insulin, and obtaining desired portions of carbohydrate foods were addressed earlier in this chapter.

Sick Days

Illness is perceived as a stressor by the body and may increase blood glucose levels. The emotional stress from being ill can add to it. In addition, loss of appetite that sometimes accompanies illness may upset the balance between food eaten (or not), medication, and activity level, which may cause blood glucose levels that are too high or too low. Every person with diabetes needs to have a sick day plan prepared with a diabetes educator, but if the individual is visually impaired, then this plan also needs to be in a readily accessible format. General sick day guidelines focus on continuing to take medication or insulin even if the person is not eating because blood glucose goes higher when a person is ill, even without food; following their normal meal plan; and maintaining hydration (drinking 4 to 8 ounces of calorie-free fluid every hour). The primary diabetes care provider should be contacted if the client cannot tolerate any foods or fluids or cannot take diabetes medicines. This plan may also include information such as amounts and types of foods and fluids and when to eat and drink them, how frequently to test blood glucose levels, target blood glucose goals during illness, and when to call the doctor.

Talking thermometers (oral, rectal, underarm, and ear) are available to use when a fever is suspected. They should be purchased ahead of time so they are available when needed. Ketone testing may be required in persons with type 1 diabetes. Direct urine testing with ketone test strips is a highly visual task requiring discriminations of gradations of color and therefore may require sighted assistance. One blood glucose monitor, the Precision Xtra, has a blood ketone testing feature with visual display meter. An adaptive timer or watch with an hourly chime would be helpful to remind the client of the need to drink fluid on a regular basis. People with diabetes and vision loss need to be more prepared for a potential sick day than their sighted counterparts. It may be beneficial to have several small bins labeled in the client's preferred format and dedicated to nonperishable sick day foods and beverages, one consisting of some easily tolerated carbohydrate foods and liquids and protein-rich foods, and another bin for calorie-free beverages and foods (Table 20-7).

Finally, the client's treating physician, endocrinologist, or diabetes educator should be on speed dial or programmed into the client's phone as an emergency contact. Also a readily accessible form of transportation, particularly a family member or friend, should be in place.

Reducing Risks

Foot Care

Regular and thorough foot care is essential for avoiding or minimizing lower extremity complications in persons with diabetes. Foot and skin care becomes an extremely important task in light of peripheral neuropathy and vascular complications. In the United States, according to the Centers for Disease Control, in 2010 there were about 73,000 non-traumatic lower limb amputations every year due to diabetes; this is about 60% of all lower limb amputations. About 60% of people with diabetic retinopathy have had foot problems. It has been shown that in persons with diabetes careful foot care and proper education has reduced the amputation rate associated with diabetes to 50%. Foot care includes basic hygiene, proper foot inspection, appropriate footwear, and special precautions. Many techniques and devices are available to assist the person with vision loss to perform these tasks safely.

TABLE 20-7: SICK DAY FOODS

Easily tolerated carbohydrates	Cooked cereal, crackers, applesauce, containers of premade regular Jell-O, vanilla wafers
Easily tolerated protein-rich food	Peanut butter, powdered milk
Carbohydrate-containing liquids/almost liquids if cannot eat	Boxed juices, containers of premade regular pudding, cans of creamed and chunky soups
Calorie-free beverages and foods to maintain hydration	Sugar-free powder drinks, cans/cubes of bouillon or broth, tea, diet/calorie-free soda, sugar-free Jell-O

Basic hygiene includes washing the feet daily with mild soap and warm water, drying between the toes, and avoiding foot soaks. Lowering the water temperature on the water heater, using a scald-free adapter, or a low vision or talking bath thermometer may be helpful to ensure bathwater temperature is within a safe range (98 to 100 degrees Fahrenheit). Applying alcohol-free moisturizing lotion to the feet (but not between toes) prevents dry, cracked skin. Cutting or using chemical corn or callus removers should be avoided; however, if at low risk and approved by the physician, a pumice stone may be used for smoothing purposes. Sighted assistance for cutting nails should be obtained from a reliable friend or family member. A podiatrist should be consulted when thick, hard nails or foot problems are noted. An emery board may be used to file and smooth rough edges of toenails. Toenails can be periodically checked with fingertips to ensure they are filed straight across and not too short.

A foot inspection should be done daily at a consistent time and place, such as after bathing or before bed. Visual techniques are to be used only if remaining vision is adequate and reliable. Visual methods may include incorporating appropriate lighting, a handheld magnifier, contrast (dark towel behind a light-skinned foot or light towel behind a dark-skinned foot), and magnifying/lighted mirrors. Handheld electronic magnifiers and even smart pads and smart phones can be used to photograph skin that is difficult to see. The image can then be magnified and the contrast enhanced with electronic magnifiers. However, sighted assistance should be obtained weekly or if a new problem is detected. In addition, a physician should perform a foot inspection every visit, and a podiatrist should be seen at least annually.

A tactile foot inspection is utilized when vision is insufficient. It requires intact sensation in the hand and fingertips. The fingertips are used to explore the entire foot in a careful, systematic fashion. The skin is inspected for cuts, blisters, swelling, new calluses, and other irregularities, with particular attention to any previous or existing foot problems. Changes in foot shape are noted, and the back of the hand can be used to feel for excessively cool areas (decreased circulation) or warm areas (possible inflammation) in comparison to other areas of the foot or the opposite foot. In addition, changes in foot odor should be noted, especially when removing socks and shoes. A bad or unusual foot odor can be sign of a fungal infection; often, a suddenly offensive or foul odor will be the first indication of an infection. Socks should be felt for wet or crusty areas that might be indicative of blood or discharge. If discharge has adhered to the sock, a sticking or pulling sensation may be noted during sock removal.

Research in 2012 by Dr. Ann Williams,[24] CDE has shown the effectiveness of a nonvisual foot examination in helping persons with diabetes and vision impairment find new foot problems when they are in early, easily treated stages. Dr. Williams concluded that "patients often are embarrassed to ask others to touch their feet or are reluctant to ask yet another 'favor' from people they already rely on for so much assistance." During the study, education in systematic nonvisual foot inspection resulted in more new foot problems found than when clients self-invented their own techniques. Persons who were taught to self-screen their feet did so a significant number of days out of the month and found the foot exam highly acceptable.

Following inspection, if a cut, blister, or sore has not begun to heal within a day, the physician should be contacted. A foot that is painful or swollen requires immediate medical attention. In addition to daily foot inspections, all clients with diabetes should have their feet inspected during each visit to their primary care physician. Clients should not be hesitant to take their socks and shoes off at the beginning of the visit as a reminder to their physician.

Socks and shoes should be worn at all times and socks should be changed daily. Socks should not be lumpy or mended, and they should be made of materials that "breathe" and keep feet dry (such as wool and synthetic blends). Shoes should be of a closed style and should fit well upon purchase. Similarly, they should be made of materials that allow air to circulate, such as canvas or leather. Persons with diabetes should feel inside their shoes before putting them on each time to make sure the lining is smooth and that there are no hidden objects, nail points, or rough areas. Additional precautions include avoiding artificial heat, such as heating pads and electric blankets; avoiding crossing the legs for extended periods; and avoiding wearing tight socks and garters, which hinder blood circulation.

Another aspect of reducing risks is tracking health parameters, including blood glucose levels, weight, etc. The memory feature of a monitor is not intended to replace the logbook, but rather to provide the option of recording readings at a later date. The minimal content of a blood glucose log should include blood glucose results with date and time taken, exercise, illness, special events, food eaten, and any other medications taken, all of which may impact a blood glucose result, as well as what medication (oral medication or insulin), how much, and when taken—especially if dosages are changed. Large-print blood glucose diaries or logs are commercially available, can be computer generated, or can be audio recorded. Diabetes Pal and My Glucose Buddy (both for Android and iPhone) can track blood glucose levels, food, medication, weight, and blood pressure (www. diatribe.org/issues/58/conference-pearls).

Healthy Coping

Diabetes can bring forth a multitude of emotions: guilt ("I just ate too much sugar"), anger ("Why me?"), anxiety ("I am always afraid my blood sugar will go low."), fatigue ("I can never take a break from my diabetes"), depression ("Is it worth all this trouble?"), and burnout ("It is just too much, I give up"). Diabetes is a disease that does not take a vacation, and self-care can be overwhelming and stressful. Adding vision loss to the picture can magnify its emotional impact—not only the loss of vision itself, but the need to learn a new way to do things ("Just when I thought I was getting a handle on it"). Depression is 2 times higher in persons with diabetes and higher in persons with vision loss. A therapeutic approach that has been shown to be effective as a treatment for depression is problem-solving therapy (see Chapter 6).

Explore coping by presenting the following questions and engaging the client in problem-solving behavior:

- Name 3 emotions that you feel when you think about your diabetes.

- Who can you talk to when you feel this way?

- Name 3 activities that will help you work through this emotion and feel better.

- What might prevent you from doing these activities?

- How can you overcome these obstacles?

Journaling can be an effective way to express thoughts and emotions related to diabetes in a thoughtful and productive way, and you may even be able to hash out and solve problems by writing about them. Bold line paper in spiral-bound format can be utilized, as well as a recording device (see Chapter 15). Meditation, yoga, and relaxation techniques can also help with management of these diverse emotions. Hadley School for the Blind (www.hadleyedu. org) has a course entitled "Stress Relief and Meditative Gardening" and webinars entitled "Stress Management," "Getting Healthy With Yoga," and "How Diabetes Saved My Life."

Yoga is widely practiced for health, relaxation, and well-being and entails a combination of breath control, simple meditation, and the adoption of specific body postures. Cindy Rogers, a certified yoga instructor who is blind, reports that yoga without sight allows breathing to be more audible and cultivates a greater sense of one's inner self and feelings. Yoga requires little adaptation—a tactile line placed lengthwise down the center of the yoga mat allows the participant to maintain their orientation to the mat while in positions and during movement (some positions are floor level, others are upright). Placing the mat near the wall allows the participant a source of external support as well as a means of orientation through the process of alignment and squaring off (see Chapter 19). Detailed verbal instruction is required to perform poses correctly and safely—this can be provided by an informed class instructor or by way of a CD or digital download (available through www.blindyoga.net/ or other sources). Tactile representations, called the Yoga Joes, are now available. Yoga Joes are a series of 9 three inch high figures demonstrating different yoga poses (Figure 20-9). The figures, which are representations of soldiers, were aimed at attracting more men including veterans into the practice of yoga. They can be purchased through www.yogajoes.com. Before pursuing yoga, the client should discuss precautions related to postures taught and eye safety with their eye care physician.

Guided imagery and meditation CDs are inherently accessible. A free 15-minute download of guided imagery is available at www.healthjourneys.com by Belleruth Naparstek, a licensed social worker and psychotherapist. Mindfulness meditation classes are proliferating—the local hospital may host a series, or they may be taken online. The founder of mindfulness-based stress reduction, Jon Kabat-Zinn, has developed several different series of CDs that can be purchased at www.mindfulnesscds.com. Shorter free guided meditations can be played or downloaded from www.marc.ucla.edu/body.cfm?id=22.

Several print resources for stress management exist that can be downloaded to an e-book reader or iPad, including *Stress Free Diabetes: Your Guide to Health and Happiness* by Dr. Joseph Napora (2010) published by the American Diabetes Association and *Diabetes Burnout: What To Do When You Can't Take It Anymore* written by William H. Polonsky, PhD (1999).

Joining a support group or chat room may be helpful. An online support group focused on persons with diabetes and vision loss is available by subscribing to blind-diabet-ics-subscribe@yahoogroups.com. The National Federation for the Blind has a discussion group called "Diabetes Talk for the Blind," which can be accessed through their website, www.nfb.org. Coping can be facilitated by learning more about diabetes; knowledge is power. Some accessible resources include *Diabetes Forecast* magazine (National

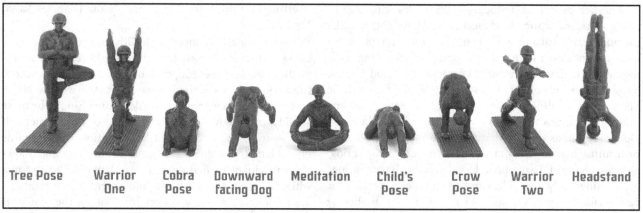

Figure 20-9. Yoga Joes. (Reprinted with permission of Mark Wickens Photography.)

Library Service), *Diabetes Self-Management* (English or Spanish read over the phone through www.nfbnewsline. org). Diabetes changes rapidly, so publications should not be much more than 5 years old.

Take a diabetes vacation. Maybe you say to yourself, "I will treat myself with a hot fudge sundae once in a while. I know I will have higher blood sugar later and will not beat myself, up over it. I will make sure to take a walk afterwards." Or how about a child-size sundae? Or settle for low-sugar/low-fat ice cream and hot fudge. Maybe fit the sundae into your meal plan. Have a salad, meat, and vegetable at your evening meal and skip 3 carb servings and eat a sundae instead. Seeking perfection is just adding another stressor. Instill in your clients that diabetes should not control their lives.

There are times when a licensed mental health professional should be consulted for serious mental health issues. Significant depression may reflect itself in poor self-care behaviors (related to general self-care or diabetes self-care), hopelessness, lack of energy, changes in appetite, feelings of worthlessness, and trouble concentrating, among other symptoms. Symptoms of severe anxiety may include but not be limited to restlessness, difficulty concentrating, sleep problems, and irritability. Referral to these professionals may also be helpful for a person who is adjusting to a new diabetes complication, a significant life loss or added stressor, or the burnout that can result from living with chronic disease and disability.

SUMMARY

Occupational therapists are ideal professionals to work with persons with diabetes. They work in diverse settings and currently provide rehabilitation to assist clients to maximize self-care with respect to chronic complications of diabetes (such as peripheral neuropathy and stroke) and other physical limitations. Occupational therapists with low vision expertise can enhance their role by providing

low vision interventions and adaptations for self-care in general and specific to diabetes self-management. The latter requires advanced knowledge and training and a commitment to continually update oneself with respect to changes in diabetes self-care. Occupational therapy's focus on function enhances collaboration with diabetes educators through the use of the AADE7 self-care behaviors framework. Multidisciplinary care is essential to empowering clients with diabetes and vision loss to successfully manage this systemic and potentially devastating disease.

RESOURCES

Educational Offerings

- American Association of Diabetes Educators (AADE) Career Path Program Certificate Program for Diabetes Self-Management Education: Designed to provide a structure for training and online education for health care providers involved in delivery of diabetes education and care. Interested parties should contact at 1-888-338-3633 or visit www.diabeteseducator.org.

- AADE's "Core Concepts: The Art and Science of Diabetes Education": A 3-day intensive course. For dates and locations, contact AADE at 1-800-338-3633 or visit www.diabeteseducator.org.

Organizations

- American Association of Diabetes Educators (AADE)— Disabilities Community of Interest; www.aadenet.org or 1-800-338-3633

- American Diabetes Association (ADA); www.diabetes. org or 1-800-342-2383

- American Dietetic Association; www.eatright.org or 1-800-877-1600

- National Library Service for the Blind and Physically Handicapped (NLS), Library of Congress; www.loc.gov/nls (publications in accessible formats)

- National Diabetes Information Clearinghouse of National Institute of Diabetes & Digestive & Kidney Diseases (NIDDK); www.niddk.nih.gov or 1-800-860-8747

Publications

Professional Publications

- Mensing C, Cornell S, Halstenson C. *The Art and Science of Diabetes Self-Management Education Desk Reference*, 3rd ed. Chicago, IL: American Association of Diabetes Educators; 2014 (can be purchased at www.diabeteseducator.org).

- Warshaw HS, Kulkarni K. *The Complete Guide to Carb Counting*, 3rd ed. Alexandria, VA: American Diabetes Association; 2001 (can be purchased at www.shopdiabetes.org/557-The-Complete-Guide-to-Carb-Counting-3rd-edition.aspx).

- Colberg S. *Exercise and Diabetes*. Alexandria, VA: American Diabetes Association; 2013 (can be purchased at www.shopdiabetes.org/1408-Exercise-and-Diabetes.aspx).

- Young-Hyman D, Peyrot M. *Psychosocial Care for People with Diabetes*. Alexandria, VA: American Diabetes Association; 2012 (can be purchased at www.shopdiabetes.org/1301-Psychosocial-Care-for-People-with-Diabetes.aspx).

- Scheffler N. *21 Things You Need to Know About Diabetes and Your Feet*. Alexandria, VA: American Diabetes Association; 2012 (can be purchased at www.shopdiabetes.org/1312-21-Things-You-Need-to-Know-About-Diabetes-and-Your-Feet.aspx).

- Chous AP. *Diabetic Eye Disease*. Auburn, WA: Fairwood Press; 2003.

- Sokol-McKay D. Vision rehabilitation and the person with diabetes. *Top Geriatr Rehabil*. 2010;26(3).

- Williams AS, Schnarrenberger PA. A comparison of dosing accuracy: visually impaired and sighted people using insulin pens. *J Diabetes Sci Technol*. 2010;4(3):514-521.

Consumer Publications

- Hayes C. I Hate to Exercise: A Book for People with Diabetes. 3rd ed. Alexandria, VA: American Diabetes Association; 2013.

- Sokol-McKay D, Cate Y. Diabetes. A "Living Life to Its Fullest Podcast" recorded by the American Occupational Therapy Association. Viewable as episode 14 at www.aota.org/en/About-Occupational-Therapy/Patients-Clients/Podcasts.aspx. 2009.

- Sokol-McKay D. Introduction to diabetes & diabetic retinopathy. www.Visionaware.org. Includes links to "What is diabetes," "Symptoms of diabetic eye disease," "Managing your diabetes," and other related topics. www.visionaware.org/section.aspx?FolderID=6&SectionID=111. 2014.

- National Federation of the Blind. *Bridging the Gap: Living With Blindness and Diabetes*. https://nfb.org/Images/nfb/Publications/books/BridgeGap_Diabetes.htm. 2009.

- Diabetes Association of Greater Cleveland. *Diabetes: The Basics* and *Living With Diabetes and Visual Impairment*. www.dagc.org or (216) 591-0800.

- *Diabetes Forecast*, a monthly publication available to ADA members. Publishes a yearly resource guide. Accessible format through NLS and NFB-NewsLine.

- Diabetes self-management. www.DiabetesSelfManagement.com or 1-800-234-0923.

- American Diabetes Association. *Count Your Carbs, Getting Started*. 2014. Available at www.diabetes.org or 1-800-342-2383.

- American Diabetes Association. *Choose Your Foods: Food Lists for Diabetes*. 2014. Available at www.diabetes.org or 1-800-342-2383.

- American Diabetes Association. *Choose Your Foods: Food Lists for Weight Management* 2014. Available at www.diabetes.org/ or 1-800-342-2383.

- Academy of Nutrition and Dietetics and American Diabetes. *Eating Healthy with Diabetes: Easy Reading Guide*. 2014. Available at www.eatright.org or 1-800-877-1600.

REFERENCES

1. American Diabetes Association. *Statistics about Diabetes*. Alexandria, VA: American Diabetes Assn.; 2014.
2. American Diabetes Association. Economic costs of diabetes in the U.S. in 2012. *Diabetes Care*. 2013;36:1033-1046.
3. Diabetes Trials Unit. Prospective Diabetes Study (UKPDS). University of Oxford, UK; 2002.
4. Anderson RJ, Freedland KE, Clouse RE, Lustman PJ. The prevalence of comorbid depression in adults with diabetes: a meta-analysis. *Diabetes Care*. 2001;24:1069-1078.
5. Lustman PJ, Griffith LS, Clouse RE. Depression in Adults with Diabetes. *Semin Clin Neuropsychiatry*. 1997;2:15-23.

6. NIH. Diabetes Control and Complications Trial. In: (NIDDK) NIoDaDaKD, ed. Washington D.C.: National Institutes of Health; 1994:1-2.

7. American Diabetes Association. What are my options? *American Diabetes Association*. http://www.diabetes.org/living-with-diabetes/treatment-and-care/medication/oral-medications/what-are-my-options.html. Published June 6, 2013. Updated March 3, 2015. Accessed June 7, 2014.

8. Mensing C, McLauglin S, Halstenson C. *The Art and Science of Diabetes Self-Management Education Desk Reference.* Chicago: American Association of Diabetes Educators; 2011.

9. Centers for Disease Control. Number of Adults Aged 18 Years or Older With Diagnosed Diabetes Reporting Visual Impairment. 2014.

10. Chous AP. *Diabetic Eye Disease.* Auburn, WA: Fairwood Press; 2003.

11. Funnell M, Feldman E. Diabetic Neuropathy In: Franz M, ed. *Core Curriculum for Diabetes Educators.* Chicago: American Association of Diabetes Educators; 2003:200.

12. Haas L, Maryniuk M, Beck J, et al. National standards for diabetes self-management education and support. *Diabetes Care.* 2014;37:S144-S153.

13. American Association of Diabetes Educators. *AADE7 Self-Care Behaviors Background.* Chicago: AADE; 2003.

14. American Association of Diabetes Educators. *AADE7: Self-Care Behaviors.* Chicago, IL: AADE; 2014.

15. Sokol-McKay DA. *Managing Diabetes with Physical Limitations. Diabetes Self-Management.* New York: R.A. Rapaport Publishing, Inc; 2013:8-13.

16. Williams A. Working with your diabetes team. *Voice of the Diabetic*: National Federation of the Blind; 2005:12-13.

17. Kiss S. Eye disease related to diabetes. In: Mensing C, ed. *The Art and Science of Diabetes Self-Management Education Desk Reference.* 3rd ed. Chicago, IL: American Association of Diabetes Educators; 2014:767.

18. Williams A, Sokol-McKay DA, Bartos, B, et al. AADE Position Statement: Diabetes and Disabilities. *The Diabetes Educator.* Thousand Oaks, CA: Sage Publications; 2012.

19. Kitchel E. Large Print: *Guidelines for Optimal Readability and APHont, A Font for Low Vision.* Louisville, KY: American Printing House for the Blind; 2004.

20. Lieberman L, Ponchillia P, Ponchillia S. *Physical Education and Sports for People With Visual Impairments and Deafblindness: Foundations of Instruction.* New York, NY: American Foundation for the Blind Press; 2013.

21. Centers for Disease Control. 2011 National Diabetes Fact Sheet. 2013.

22. Petzinger R. Adaptive medication measurement and administration. In: Cleary M, ed. *Diabetes and Visual Impairment: An Educator's Resource Guide.* Chicago IL: The American Association of Diabetes Educators Education and Research Foundation; 1994:129-130.

23. Williams AS, Schnarrenberger PA. A comparison of dosing accuracy: visually impaired and sighted people using insulin pens. *J Diabetes Sci Technol.* 2010;4:514-521.

24. Williams A. Nonvisual foot examination for people with visual impairment. Poster presented at: 50th European Association for the Study of Diabetes Annual Meeting; September 15-19, 2014; Vienna, Austria. http://www.easdvirtualmeeting.org/resources/19468. Accessed May 18, 2015.

Establishing a Low Vision
Rehabilitation Specialty Practice

Maxine Scheiman, MEd, OTR/L, CLVT and
Stephen G. Whittaker, PhD, FAAO, OTR/L, CLVT

Throughout this text, we have tried to establish the research and clinical basis for providing low vision rehabilitation as part of occupational therapy practice. We have emphasized that the ability to evaluate and treat low vision is necessary to meet the needs of many clients. Occupational therapists working with the adult population will encounter many clients with low vision, even if this is not the primary reason the client has been referred for occupational therapy.

The prevalence and incidence of low vision in the United States are high and experts predict a large increase over the next two decades because the prevalence of low vision increases sharply in persons older than 65 years. The prevalence and incidence of low vision in the United States were reviewed in Chapter 2, generally indicating that the prevalence of low vision is close to the prevalence of stroke. Nearly 20 years after Mary Warren wrote her seminal paper describing the role of occupational therapy in low vision[1] there remains a dearth of services for people with low vision whereas there are ample services for people with other disabilities such as stroke even though low vision is nearly as prevalent.

It is our hope that if you have reached this section of the book, you have a strong interest in becoming more involved in this new and exciting practice area of occupational therapy. If so, you are likely to be left with a number of important

questions about educational requirements, certification, practice opportunities, billing, and reimbursement.

Some of the important questions that need to be addressed include the following:

1. What are the educational requirements for an occupational therapist to provide low vision rehabilitation services?

2. Is certification necessary to provide low vision rehabilitation services?

3. How does the occupational therapist interact with other vision rehabilitation professionals?

4. What practice opportunities are available?

5. How do I market my services as a provider of low vision rehabilitation services?

6. Are low vision rehabilitation services provided by occupational therapists covered by Medicare and other insurance?

7. How do I properly bill insurance for low vision rehabilitation services?

8. Are optical aids and other devices covered by insurance?

9. What equipment do I need to get started in the field of low vision rehabilitation?

This chapter is designed to provide answers to these critical questions.

DIDACTIC EDUCATION/ CLINICAL TRAINING

Although information about the visual system is certainly part of every occupational therapy curriculum, the information provided is generally basic and introductory. Few programs are designed to prepare the entry-level occupational therapist for the practice of low vision rehabilitation, either from a didactic or clinical training perspective. Mary Warren states that "Although occupational therapists have been involved in the rehabilitation of persons with vision loss since the inception of the profession in 1917, we never played an extensive role in low vision rehabilitation."[2] Occupational therapists have indeed always played a role in low vision rehabilitation because nearly two-thirds of older adults with low vision have at least one other chronic medical condition that may interfere with activities of daily living (ADL) and require occupational therapy.[3] Thus, in the context of providing care for other chronic conditions, occupational therapists must routinely manage issues related to low vision in their elderly clients.

Entry-level occupational therapy program curricula have been changing to address the prevalence of low vision in the adult population. Many experienced occupational therapists need to gain additional information and clinical experience to feel comfortable practicing low vision rehabilitation at a sophisticated level, much as hand therapists seek specialized training. A useful guide to the core knowledge base required to practice low vision therapy is provided by the Academy for Certification of Vision Rehabilitation and Education Professionals (ACVREP) (www.acvrep.org) which we have taken care to cover in this book for adults.

Educational opportunities are now available for occupational therapists to receive this additional educational experience. These opportunities include graduate degree level programs, multiple-day continuing education workshops (both on-site and online), presentations from companies that sell and produce optical aids, home study courses, and of course, textbooks like this one.

While all registered/licensed occupational therapists are legally qualified and currently able to provide and bill for low vision rehabilitation services without any additional education or certification, most will need additional education and clinical experience to competently function as low vision therapists. The decision about how much additional educational experience and the nature of the educational experience is a personal one that each occupational therapist must make. Individuals vary in their preferred learning style. For an assertive, self-assured individual with strong independent learning skills, reading a book, taking a home-study course, and gaining some experience with optical aids from a manufacturer's workshop may be sufficient to develop the core knowledge base. Additional clinical practice supervised by an experienced low vision therapist is also recommended and is required for ACVREP certification. Some may prefer to enroll in a formal graduate program in low vision rehabilitation that includes clinical training. The various opportunities are listed with contact information in Table 21-1. We have tried to make this listing as complete as possible. Of course, organizations come and go and new programs are being developed. Thus, it is important to use this table as a starting point and be aware that new programs and educational opportunities will certainly be available after publication of this book.

Continuing Education Courses

It is common for occupational therapists to gain knowledge about new areas of practice through postgraduate, continuing education seminars and workshops. One- and two-day workshops are offered periodically for low vision rehabilitation. Some of the companies offering such workshops are listed in Table 21-1. These workshops generally cover information about epidemiology of low vision, diseases causing low vision, basic optics, the occupational therapy evaluation and low vision rehabilitation, billing for services, and hands-on experience with optical aids. After completing one or two of these courses most occupational therapists would feel comfortable providing basic low vision rehabilitation services to clients presenting with low vision as a secondary diagnosis. Some self-assured occupational therapists might feel comfortable enough to initiate a low vision service in a hospital setting, or provide home-based low vision rehabilitation services with clients presenting with a primary diagnosis of low vision.

Companies that produce and sell optical devices sometimes provide inexpensive continuing education for occupational therapists and these seminars offer an excellent opportunity to gain hands-on experience with microscopes, magnifiers, telescopes, closed-circuit televisions, and other video display technology. For example, Eschenbach Optik of America (www.eschenbach.comseminars.php) has been providing this service for many years and this company offers seminars in many cities around the country on an annual basis. The Eschenbach course is entitled *Low Vision Care...What's it All About?* This low vision care presentation for eye care and rehabilitation professionals is designed as an introduction to low vision care and optical devices.

The primary missing ingredient from short continuing education courses is clinical experience with clients. Gaining meaningful clinical experience is the greatest challenge facing the therapist who would like to be involved in low vision rehabilitation. Opportunities may exist in some communities for an interested occupational therapist to volunteer or find employment in a situation in which

TABLE 21-1: POSTGRADUATE EDUCATIONAL OPPORTUNITIES FOR EDUCATION IN LOW VISION REHABILITATION

NAME OF ORGANIZATION	TYPE OF EDUCATION	CONTACT INFORMATION
Salus University	Post Doctorate in Occupational Therapy with a specialty in Vision Rehabilitation or Certificate in Vision Rehabilitation	www.salus.edu
University of Alabama	Graduate level education and certification program	www.uab.edu/shp/ot/low-vision-rehabilitation-graduate-certificate
Vision Education Seminars	Live workshops, Webinars and online courses. Self study exams for CE credit for this textbook	www.visionedseminars.com
Lighthouse and Guild for the Blind courses	Live workshops and online courses	www.lighthouse.org
Eschenbach courses	Live workshops	www.eschenbach.com
AOTA home study courses	Home study courses	www.aota.org
The American Foundation for the Blind	Live and online courses	www.afb.org
The Hadley School for the Blind	Tuition-free individualized instruction for CE credit	www.hadley.edu/hsps.asp
Lions Research and Training Center at Johns Hopkins Wilmer Eye Institute	Online courses	www.emeraldeducationsystems.com
Cross Country Education	Live workshop	www.crosscountryeducation.com

low vision rehabilitation is already being provided by another experienced therapist. In any case, finding a setting to acquire supervised clinical instruction is a challenge. Recognizing this challenge, ACVREP will arrange supervision of applicants for certification from a distance using technological methods.

Home Study and Distance Education

In 1995, the AOTA devoted its entire October issue to the topic of low vision and in 1998 developed the AOTA Occupational Therapy Practice Guidelines for Adults with Low Vision. In 2000, Mary Warren edited a home study course entitled "Low Vision: Occupational Therapy Intervention with the Older Adult," published by the AOTA.[4] This self-study course was updated in 2008. These three documents provide a starting point for independent learning. In 2006, the AOTA published revised practice guidelines for a specialty certification in low vision (www.aota.org) There also is a home study course available to accompany this textbook (www.visionedseminars.com).

A recent trend in education is online or distance learning and many opportunities now exist for this type of education in the area of low vision rehabilitation. The Hadley School for the Blind (www.hadley-school.org) currently offers a number of online courses for professionals, including coursework in braille, low vision technology, introduction to low vision, self-esteem and adjusting to blindness, and macular degeneration. Some, but not all of these courses are provided without any tuition charge.

The Lions Vision Research and Rehabilitation Center at the Johns Hopkins Wilmer Eye Institute offers some exceptional distance learning opportunities and outstanding up-to-date information about low vision rehabilitation at their website (www.emeraldeducationsystems.com).

A course currently offered on this website is entitled "Understanding Visual Impairments and Functional Rehabilitation of Visually Impaired Patients." The course consists of several online courses lectures and supplemental material that cover the following topics: anatomy and physiology of vision, diseases of the visual system, optics and optical devices, functional and ADL assessments, visual skills training, rehabilitation services and resources, and vision enhancement and adaptive technology.

An online course entitled "Low Vision in Older Adults: Foundations for Rehabilitation" is the result of collaboration between the AOTA and SightCare, a program of The

Jewish Guild for the Blind. The courses in the Mult-E-Skills program are ACVREP approved.

The American Foundation for the Blind (AFB) (www.afb.org) is one of the best resources for information in assistive technology. *AccessWorld* is a quarterly publication that offers critical reviews. The journal of visual impairment and blindness published by the AFB is dedicated exclusively to publishing information on low vision and blindness. The AFB also publishes several textbooks on low vision and blindness rehabilitation and education.

Formal University-Based Graduate Education

Some occupational therapists may prefer more formal, university-based graduate education. Two excellent programs designed for occupational therapists are now available to meet this need and are listed in Table 21-1. Both programs offer a certificate or master's degree in low vision rehabilitation.

The Occupational Therapy College at Salus University (www.salus.edu) prepares occupational therapists to work with clients with vision disorders. The programs leads to a post-graduate doctorate in Occupational Therapy with a specialty in vision rehabilitation. The program allows an occupational therapists to specialize in either visual impairment in the elderly, vision rehabilitation after acquired brain injury or vision rehabilitation in the pediatric population. This 18-motnh program is a hybrid program with most of the courses online, but two, 5-day on-campus sessions.

The University of Alabama, Birmingham Department of Occupational Therapy offers a graduate certificate program in low vision rehabilitation (www.uab.edu/shp/ot/low-vision-rehabilitation-graduate-certificate). This program is designed for occupational therapists with bachelors, masters, or doctorate degrees. It consists of 17 credit hours of specialized courses in low vision rehabilitation. Students take 11 credits of core courses designed to provide a foundation necessary to deliver low vision rehabilitation services, 4 credits of elective courses to address specific aspects of intervention in greater depth, and a 2-credit course in advanced application. All of the courses are offered online through a web-based curriculum. The curriculum is designed with the working occupational therapist in mind. Coursework emphasizes practical application of the information taught. Students can enroll in the certificate program or combine completion of the certificate program with a postprofessional master's degree in occupational therapy. Students completing the certificate program need to complete an additional 10 credits of coursework and 6 credits of research to receive the postprofessional master's degree. Coursework for the postprofessional degree is also online.

Thus, many educational opportunities are available for an occupational therapist who would like to become involved in low vision education. It is simply a matter of deciding on one's learning style and researching some of the available options.

CERTIFICATION

Certification in low vision therapy is not required at this time for occupational therapists. Any registered/licensed occupational therapist is able to provide low vision rehabilitation and bill for these services. In Chapter 1, we discussed the various professionals involved in low vision rehabilitation of adult clients. These include occupational therapists, low vision therapists, vision rehabilitation therapists (formerly rehabilitation teachers), and orientation and mobility (O&M) specialists. Of these three groups, only occupational therapists are licensed and function as independent service providers in the Medicare system and other commercial medical insurance programs. Vision rehabilitation therapists, low vision therapists, and O&M specialists often work for state agencies, private organizations, the Veteran's Administration, and school systems. Currently the services of these professionals are not reimbursed by Medicare, Medicaid, or most private insurance.

Although occupational therapists do not require certification to practice low vision rehabilitation, it is a desirable goal for the following reasons:

- Certification demonstrates that the therapist has advanced skills low vision rehabilitation.
- Certification may be required in the future by insurers for reimbursement, even for occupational therapists.

Academy for Certification of Vision Rehabilitation and Education Professionals

Currently there are two active certification programs for low vision therapy. The first is a certification process run by ACVREP, which was established in January 2000. It is an independent and autonomous legal certification body governed by a volunteer Board of Directors. ACVREP's mission is to offer professional certification for vision rehabilitation and education professionals in order to improve service delivery to persons with vision impairments. Although ACVREP does not release data on how many occupational therapists are certified, it is likely that many of the between 400 and 500 who are certified low vision therapists are occupational therapists.

The ACVREP certification program that is appropriate for occupational therapists is called the Certified Low Vision Therapist (CLVT). To be eligible to take the written certification test, candidates must meet the eligibility criteria listed on their website (www.acvrep.org). Candidates passing a 100-item written examination receive certification that is valid for a 5-year period. Certified low vision therapists must go through a recertification process every 5 years. To be recertified, an individual must demonstrate that he or she has maintained continuing professional competence in the field of vision rehabilitation and education, much like the requirements for occupational therapy certification. Acceptable activities include continuing education, professional experience, publications and presentations, and professional service. Full details of all requirements can be obtained from the ACVREP website.

The advantages of ACVREP certification are:

- The guidelines for the examination and study program have been developed by experienced professionals in the field. The applicant must have his or her study program reviewed and a multiple choice examination must be passed to insure that the occupational therapist has the requisite knowledge base for competent practice.

- The organization will help applicants locate and arrange for clinical supervision. Although some direct supervision is necessary, most of the 360 hours of clinical practice may be supervised by a certified therapist off-site.

- Certification allows the occupational therapist to join, rather than compete, with the professionals who have been providing low vision and blindness rehabilitation services long before the recent increase in occupational therapy practitioners in the field.

- ACVREP meets the standards set by the National Certification Commission.

American Occupational Therapy Association Certification

In 2006, the AOTA initiated a Specialty Certification in Low Vision (SCLV). The purpose of this new specialty certification is to provide a framework for professional development that is specifically geared to occupational therapy. Whereas ACVREP is an entry level certification, because 5 years' experience is required, SCLV can be considered certification of advanced competency so both ACVREP and AOTA certification is recommended. Through its Specialty Certification programs, AOTA provides formal recognition for those who have engaged in a voluntary process of ongoing, focused, and targeted professional development. The program is voluntary and certification is not required for practice.

The process for Specialty Certification is self-directed. There is no test involved; rather, certification is based on peer review of the candidate's professional development portfolio and a series of narrative reflections covering the following topics[5]:

1. Performs an individualized occupational therapy low vision evaluation to identify factors that may facilitate, compensate for, or inhibit use of vision in occupational performance.

2. Develops and implements an individualized occupational therapy low vision intervention plan in collaboration with the client and relevant others that reflects the client's priorities for occupational performance.

3. Recognizes immediate and long-term implications of psychosocial issues related to vision loss and modifies therapeutic approach and occupational therapy service delivery accordingly.

4. Advances access to occupational therapy services and advocates for policies, programs, and products that promote engagement in occupations by persons with low vision.

OTHER PROFESSIONS AND INTERPROFESSIONAL ISSUES

It is important that occupational therapists have a firm understanding of the history of low vision in the United States (see Chapter 1). Vision rehabilitation therapists and O&M specialists have been in low vision rehabilitation for many more years than occupational therapists. With the inclusion of low vision as a disability under Medicare guidelines in the early 1990s, occupational therapists became much more involved in low vision rehabilitation and this created controversy. The primary basis for this controversy is that the impetus for occupational therapy's entrance into the low vision arena was not a change in education and preparation of its practitioners; rather, it was purely based on reimbursement issues. Thus, other vision rehabilitation therapists have raised questions about the qualifications, education, and clinical experience of occupational therapists in the area of low vision. For example, Lambert[6] raised the following concerns about occupational therapists:

1. They may be unfamiliar with the various disciplines in the field, and thereby fail to appropriately refer clients for other needed services.

2. They have inadequate knowledge or specialized training in low vision.

3. Clinics may favor occupational therapy in the delivery of low vision services, even though more disability-specific professionals may be the most appropriate providers.

Similar concerns were raised by Orr and Huebner in 2001,[7] when they expressed their unease about occupational therapists' lack of specialized knowledge base and skills needed to work with the low vision population.

Others have argued that there are a number of important reasons why occupational therapists should play a primary role in low vision rehabilitation[2,8]:

1. Although the elderly comprise the majority of the low vision population, they are the most underserved by existing state, charitable, and private programs. Because of the lack of availability of services and treatment through the blindness system, rehabilitation may be delayed and these individuals are likely to become socially isolated, depressed, and dependent. Involvement of occupational therapists through the healthcare system provides significantly greater access to low vision rehabilitation for the elderly.[8]

2. Two-thirds of older persons have at least one other chronic condition, in addition to low vision, that limits their independent functioning. Occupational therapists are already primary providers for older clients with other chronic conditions.[2,8] Occupational therapists are trained in the physical, cognitive, sensory, and psychological aspects of disability and aging, and therefore, may be the natural choice of professionals to work with older persons whose limitations in ADL are a result of a combination of deficits.[2]

3. Occupational therapists are more evenly distributed throughout the United States than O&M specialists and vision rehabilitation therapists, who tend to be located in larger metropolitan areas. Low vision services can be more widely disseminated through the healthcare delivery system.[2]

Occupational therapy as a profession, as well as individual therapists, have reacted in a positive way to this debate. In the past 15 years, many occupational therapists have gained the knowledge base and clinical skills necessary to provide excellent care to clients requiring low vision rehabilitation. This has been accomplished through a variety of learning formats, including independent study, continuing education courses, clinical internships, and university-based training. In addition, many occupational therapists have completed the certification process run by the ACVREP.

Occupational therapists active in low vision rehabilitation may work closely with vision rehabilitation therapists and O&M specialists in various clinical settings. As occupational therapists become involved, it is critical to be aware of the history of low vision rehabilitation in the United States, the various professions involved, and some of the sensitivities and important political issues described above.

PRACTICE OPPORTUNITIES

There are many potential practice opportunities available for occupational therapists who wish to become involved in the field of low vision rehabilitation. These opportunities range from employment in acute, subacute and outpatient rehabilitation settings, assisted living facilities, offices of ophthalmologists and optometrists, and home health agencies. Occupational therapists can provide services as independent providers as well. The underlying essential ingredient to finding these opportunities is to know where to look for patients with low vision. Based on the information about prevalence and incidence of low vision, we know this means looking for patients who are 65 years of age and older. These patients are found in nursing homes, assisted living facilities, and rehabilitation settings. The ophthalmologists most likely to see patients with low vision are the retinal, cataract, and glaucoma specialists. Optometrists with a specialty practice in low vision, of course, are also likely to be good resources for patients with low vision. Documentation and billing requirements for eye doctors and rehabilitation facilities are significantly different. In the eye-care settings, the rehabilitation therapist must generally have their own provider numbers and be able to design correct documentation forms for use in the facility. Sample documentation forms are provided in the online appendix (www.routledge.com/9781617116339).

Home-Based Treatments

A wonderful private practice opportunity for occupational therapists is providing low vision evaluation and rehabilitation in the client's home. To function in this capacity, the occupational therapist must first enroll as a private practitioner in Medicare and obtain a Medicare provider number. Information about becoming a provider and an application are available at: www.cms.gov/ (search for "provider enrollment"). Once a provider number is obtained, the therapist is able to perform both evaluation and treatment services and bill Medicare. Although often difficult, provider numbers can be obtained from private insurance companies so private insurers can be billed as well. The essentials of the billing and documentation process required for Medicare will be reviewed later in this chapter. In this mode of practice the occupational therapist can work as a private practitioner on a per diem basis for a home-health care agency and bill through the facility or as a private practitioner. A practitioner using their own provider numbers, must have an office address for billing while providing care in the client's home. In either case the therapist must market the low vision service to other professionals who are likely to encounter elderly clients with low vision. Such professionals include ophthalmologists (primarily retinal, glaucoma, and cataract specialists), low vision optometrists, geriatricians, large eye hospitals, and other rehabilitation therapists such as physical therapists, speech-language pathologists, other occupational therapists, recreational therapists, and social workers.

We have provided a sample brochure and introductory letter in the online appendix (www.routledge.com/ 9781617116339). These documents can be used to develop these relationships with other professionals.

Nursing Homes

Research has shown that a high percentage of nursing home residents are visually impaired. For example, Horowitz[9] conducted a study of a 250 bed, long-term care facility and found that 23% of the residents were visually impaired. Vision loss among nursing home residents complicates many of the care-related tasks for providers of nursing home services, and interferes with the clients' ability to engage in ADL.[10]

Thus, there is a significant need for occupational therapists who currently work in nursing homes to become involved in low vision rehabilitation in order to care for a large percentage of their clients.

Other Medical Rehabilitation Settings

We know that the two most common causes of low vision are macular degeneration and diabetic retinopathy. Older people with cardiovascular disease and diabetes make up a significant percentage of the patients in traditional medical rehabilitation facilities such as hospitals, acute and sub-acute inpatient services, outpatient and home-care services. These are the same people who are likely to have macular degeneration and low vision. In addition, many patients admitted to rehabilitation hospitals with stroke or traumatic brain injury may experience significant vision impairment, which also falls into the category of low vision impairment. Thus, occupational therapists working in these settings have an opportunity to establish a low vision service within such rehabilitation departments. Development of such a service helps to insure that there are therapists with appropriate clinical ability and that clients receive appropriate and timely treatment. Occupational therapists may practice in outpatient and home health services associated with rehabilitation hospitals, enabling reimbursement from private insurers as well as Medicare and Medicaid. A medical rehabilitation facility is an excellent starting point for developing a specialized low vision practice because billing and documentation services are provided by the employer, referrals come from within the facility and the therapist is able to treat other conditions as they build a low vision practice.

Retirement/Assisted Living Communities

Opportunities also exist in assisted living communities because of the aging population that live in such facilities. The basic underlying theme when looking for the population that is likely to need low vision care is to find older adults. An occupational therapist can arrange to make educational presentations about low vision and low vision rehabilitation in assisted living communities. Providing such education and helping people better understand what can be accomplished in spite of permanent vision loss can be quite important for people. Many individuals do not even seek care because they have simply been told by previous professionals that there is not much that can be done. The occupational therapist can develop a working relationship with an ophthalmologist and/or a low vision optometrist. People seeking more information or additional care for their visual impairment can be referred to an eye care professional for an evaluation. If low vision rehabilitation is required, the eye care professional can then refer the client to the occupational therapist for such care. This care would be provided by the occupational therapist as an independent provider.

Community-Based Agencies

Until the late 1990s, most of the low vision rehabilitation in the United States was provided within the service delivery system that has been called the "blindness system" (see Chapter 1). This system is also sometimes referred to as the educational rehabilitation model, or the nonmedical vision rehabilitation system.[11] This system is a comprehensive nationwide network of services consisting of state, federal, and private agencies serving children and adults with blindness and low vision.[12] Because of limited public funds to support these services, however, only a limited percentage of people requiring low vision rehabilitation are able to receive these services in community-based, state, or federally-funded agencies. This scarcity of resources has led some vision rehabilitation agencies to hire occupational therapists to provide services.[7] The advantage is that occupational therapists can be reimbursed by Medicare, while vision rehabilitation therapists and O&M specialists cannot. Thus, there may be opportunities for occupational therapists in these agencies. Occupational therapists working in these agencies would generally be salaried employees.

Low Vision Optometrist

A non-conventional opportunity would be to become affiliated with a low vision optometrist. They design and prescribe low vision devices (eg, optical, nonoptical, electronic) and make recommendations about lighting, contrast, and other environmental factors that influence vision.

Although low vision optometrists should ideally work closely with low vision therapists, this may not always be the case. Some low vision optometrists are not fully aware of the capabilities of occupational therapists. Thus, once an occupational therapist identifies a low vision optometrist in the area, one challenge may be to educate this eye care professional about the role of occupational therapy in low vision rehabilitation.

A second challenge is trying to locate a qualified low vision optometrist. The profession of optometry does not recognize "specialties." Therefore, any optometrist can provide low vision services, regardless of his or her experience in this area. However, the American Academy of Optometry Low Vision Section has a Diplomate program for interested optometrists. To become a Diplomate in Low Vision, an optometrist must pass a written test, an oral examination, and a practical low vision examination. Currently, there are few (under 100) practicing Low Vision Diplomats worldwide (www.aaopt.org). A current list of optometrists that have successfully completed this process can be found at the website for the American Academy of Optometry.[13] The American Optometric Association also has a Low Vision Section. Although there is no testing program required to become a member of this section, optometrists that have joined are likely to have a strong interest in the area of low vision. Some low vision optometrists have completed a residency program, while others have chosen to specialize in this area and have acquired additional knowledge and clinical skills through continuing education and independent learning. Currently, there are about 1000 members in the low vision section of the American Optometric Association. With experience and advanced training in optics and vision testing, an occupational therapist should be able to work in collaboration with a general optometrist or ophthalmologist.

There are two potential ways of working with the low vision optometrist. The first method would be as an employee. The low vision optometrist would refer patients to the occupational therapist working in his or her practice. The therapist would evaluate and provide treatment in the doctor's office. The office would bill and be reimbursed for the therapist's services and provide an hourly salary to the occupational therapist. Another scenario would be for the low vision optometrist to refer patients to an occupational therapist functioning as an independent provider. In this case, the therapist would not provide services in the doctor's office. Rather, he or she would need an office and also could provide services in the client's home. In either case, the occupational therapist would require registration as an independent provider. In some states, not all private insurers recognize occupational therapists as independent providers. In these situations, occupational therapists may work for and bill through agencies or outpatient rehabilitation services.

Ophthalmologist

Perhaps the most effective way of finding clients who require low vision rehabilitation is to work with an ophthalmologist. Ophthalmologists are physicians who specialize in the diagnosis and treatment of eye disease by completing a residency in ophthalmology. Many ophthalmologists also complete a fellowship program to further specialize in an area of ophthalmology. A number of specialty areas exist, including specialists in cataract, glaucoma, retina, cornea, pediatric ophthalmology, and neuro-ophthalmology. Ophthalmologists most likely to treat clients with low vision are the retinal, glaucoma, and cataract specialists. Since most patients who have low vision have retinal problems or loss of vision due to glaucoma, these are the types of specialists with whom the occupational therapist should develop relationships. Doctors in these offices examine a high percentage of patients with various retinopathies on a daily basis. A very high percentage of their patients require further care. Unfortunately, many ophthalmologists do not refer for low vision rehabilitation.[14] Occupational therapists can identify these ophthalmologists and arrange a visit, at which the therapist can educate the physician about his or her capabilities, and the potential advantages for the patients in the practice. There is no specific subspecialty of low vision in the profession of ophthalmology but a few ophthalmologists specialize in low vision. The primary areas of interest and responsibility of the ophthalmologist are the diagnosis and treatment of eye disease. Treatment modalities generally involve the use of medication and surgery. Thus, clients often see the ophthalmologist first because of a perceived significant change in vision. The ophthalmologist attempts to restore normal visual function by treating the eye disease. In some cases this fails, or in other cases the vision can never be restored to normal and the client is now faced with permanent low vision. It is at this point that the ophthalmologist should refer the client with low vision to other professionals for further evaluation and rehabilitation.

A similar working relationship described above for the low vision optometrist also applies to working with the ophthalmologist, although few ophthalmologists specialize in low vision rehabilitation. Thus, the occupational therapist would need advanced skills in vision evaluation and optics.

Eye Hospitals

Some large metropolitan areas in the United States have free-standing eye hospitals. A high percentage of adult patients seen at these hospitals have low vision. Many of these institutions have a low vision optometrist on staff and some may already have established low vision rehabilitation programs. If not, eye hospitals represent a potential opportunity for occupational therapists. Our recommended approach would be to use some of the evidence for the effectiveness of low vision rehabilitation reviewed in Chapter 9 in a presentation to key personnel at the hospital.

Colleges Of Optometry–Patient Care Clinics

There are 17 Colleges of Optometry in the United States and Puerto Rico. All of these colleges have large patient care clinics with a low vision service. These low vision services are used to train optometry students in all aspects of low vision care, including rehabilitation. The low vision departments are staffed by optometrists who have completed residencies in low vision and/or have many years of experience as low vision specialists. They are generally well-versed in the current trends in low vision care and research and should have an understanding of the important role that occupational therapy has begun to play in low vision rehabilitation. Some of these clinics may already employ rehabilitation therapists. Others, however, may not offer full-scope low vision care. Thus, this is a potential opportunity for an occupational therapist. The key contact person would be the Chief of the Low Vision Service at the College of Optometry. The occupational therapist would not have to convince this individual of the importance of low vision rehabilitation. Rather, the presentation would emphasize the unique contributions that occupational therapists could make in the low vision service.

MARKETING AND PUBLIC RELATIONS

Whether an occupational therapist establishes a low vision rehabilitation service in a nursing home, rehabilitation hospital, the office of an eye care provider, or starts a private practice, there will be a need for marketing and public relations to make the service grow. In the following section, we present a series of internal and external marketing and public relations ideas that could be used in a variety of practice settings. The best marketing is to provide a high quality service. Satisfied clients will report to their referring physicians and will encourage more referrals. Likewise, we find if one satisfied client comes from a retirement community for services, others often follow.

Internal Marketing

Within each practice setting, there will already be a client base that may be unaware of low vision and low vision rehabilitation. The first and least expensive method of marketing is to make current clients aware of the new low vision service.

Handouts and Brochures in Waiting Area

Most professionals utilize handouts and brochures in their waiting rooms to market various aspects of their practices. It is a matter of selecting appropriate materials to market the low vision rehabilitation aspect of your practice.

1. Handouts: Many materials are available that could be used as handouts in a waiting area. For example Lighthouse International offers a series of brochures for consumers that explain various aspects of low vision. They also offer a monthly newsletter designed for consumers called *Consumer Times: Living Better with Vision Loss*. Table 21-2 lists some other resources for consumer education.

2. Brochures: Think about developing your own brochure that explains low vision and the importance of low vision rehabilitation. An example of such a brochure is included in the online appendix (www.routledge.com/9781617116339).

Internal Mailings

If your office/hospital is computerized, you have the ability to make a selective mailing to clients by age and by diagnostic condition, such as macular degeneration, diabetic retinopathy, and diabetes. You can periodically send out information about low vision and low vision rehabilitation. Sample handouts are included in the online appendix (www.routledge.com/9781617116339).

Grand Rounds/Seminar Presentations

In most institutional settings, case conferences, grand rounds, and seminars are periodically scheduled. This is an outstanding opportunity to make the rest of the staff aware of your service, the clients you can help, and the expected outcomes.

External Marketing

In addition to marketing directly to current clients, it is important to make potential clients and other professionals aware of your service. We refer to this as external marketing.

Speaking Engagements

One of the best marketing tools available is to present educational information in a seminar/workshop format. Few people take advantage of this opportunity, however, because of discomfort with public speaking. Suggested audiences include groups of older adults, consumers with low vision, families of consumers with low vision, civic

TABLE 21-2: SAMPLE RESOURCES FOR CONSUMER EDUCATION		
COMPANY/VENDOR	**DESCRIPTION**	**CONTACT INFORMATION**
National Eye Institute	• Information about diseases and services with an empathetic approach • Videos, recorded narratives and downloadable pdf brochures • English and Spanish	www.nei.nih.gov/lowvision
American Foundation for the Blind	• Information on conditions with emphasis on adaptive performance strategies • Online sharing for professions and consumers • Information in English and Spanish	www.afb.org www.visionaware.org
Lighthouse International	• Information about underlying diseases • Simulations of vision loss • Emphasis on enhancing vision versus recovering performance.	www.lighthouse.org/about-low-vision-blindness

organizations, churches, and synagogues. We suggest that instead of waiting for an invitation from an organization, that the occupational therapist take the initiative and contact potential organizations. Active organizations include the macular vision research foundation (www.mvrf.org), and local chapters of the American Council for the Blind (www.acb.org).

Establish a Working Relationship with Other Professionals

In addition to ophthalmologists and optometrists, there are many other professionals who work with older adult clients with low vision. These include other occupational therapists, physical therapists, speech-language pathologists, recreation therapists, nurses, social workers, psychologists, family physicians, neurologists, neuro-ophthalmologists, and geriatricians.

One way to cultivate a working relationship with an optometrist or general ophthalmologist with an interest or specialization in low vision is to refer clients. If other physicians or professionals refer to an occupational therapist, the occupational therapist, who must work under the prescription of a physician, may then refer the client to the optometrist or ophthalmologist.

There is no simple way to get the names and addresses of these people. You can sometimes get names and addresses from telephone directories, and from professional

organization websites on the Internet. Mailing lists can be purchased from organizations such as the AOTA and similar organizations from other fields. We have included information about occupational therapy and low vision that could be included in a letter of introduction for professionals in the online appendix (www.routledge.com/ 9781617116339)that could be used to initiate contact. The goal is to develop true inter-referral relationships with a group of professionals that share an interest in the care of clients with low vision. The AFB has their Directory of Services which is an extensive listing of agencies and individuals providing low vision rehabilitation. For eligibility requirements for listing visit, www.afb.org.

BILLING, INSURANCE, AND MEDICARE ISSUES

Reimbursement Sources

The impetus for occupational therapy's involvement in the area of low vision rehabilitation was the 1991 amendment by the Health Care Financing Administration (HCFA) that first allowed Medicare coverage for licensed healthcare professionals to provide low vision rehabilitation. Medicare is currently the main source of reimbursement for low vision rehabilitation for occupational therapists in private practice. Other potential reimbursement sources are HMOs, private insurance companies, state agencies for the blind and visually impaired, and private paying clients. Other insurers pay for low vision rehabilitation delivered by occupational therapists working for hospitals, acute and sub-acute medical rehabilitation settings, outpatient and home care. A specialist in low vision rehabilitation who wishes to work independently can provide services on a per-diem basis for these agencies. In this situation, the therapist would be expected to provide the equipment necessary for evaluation and treatment.

Registration of Providers

To obtain reimbursement as medical rehabilitation, low vision rehabilitation should be provided by CMS approved professionals, currently including occupational therapists, physical therapists, speech therapists or physicians. The CMS and every medical insurance company that pays for therapy services, require that the providers or the agencies for whom they work register and have a provider number. Alternatively, CMS pays for therapy provided by approved professionals who work "incident to" a physician's professional services, or the services of a therapist who has a CMS provider number. "Incident to" services require direct supervision by the registered provider. With services provided "incident to" evaluations are not covered and are expected to be provided by the Medicare provider. To be cost-effective, the occupational therapist generally must be able to work without direct supervision. Moreover, not all insurers will pay for services provided "incident to." For this reason, unless an occupational therapist is an employee of a hospital or rehabilitation service that has institutional provider numbers, the therapist generally should have their own provider numbers from the various insurance companies that pay for services in the region where the therapist works.

MEDICARE AND LOW VISION REHABILITATION (OUTPATIENT SETTINGS)

The information we provide in this section was current when this book was published. However, it is important to understand that the CMS occasionally makes policy changes and the reader should carefully review the CMS website and seek current information about billing for low vision rehabilitation services (www.cms.gov).

The current CMS policy on low vision rehabilitation in an outpatient setting (Medicare B) states that occupational therapy is a covered service if it meets the following criteria:

1. Services must be prescribed by a physician and furnished under physician-approved plan of care.

2. Services must be performed by an occupational therapist or occupational therapy assistant under supervision of occupational therapist.

3. Services must be reasonable and medically necessary for treatment of an individual's illness (must result in significant improvement in level of function within reasonable period of time). Medically necessary is defined by the diagnostic code and rehabilitation potential.

As with other forms of rehabilitation treatment, the purpose of low vision rehabilitation restores a person's ability to perform valued activities that had been disabled by impairments resulting from specific disorders, exacerbations of an identifiable disease, or an other disorder. Activities can include self-care, homemaking, leisure, as well as activities required to maintain health and wellness. Although documentation for occupational therapy should focus on disabled activity, the occupational therapist also assists the client to build the confidence that is necessary for ongoing creative problem solving, and to establish a healthy lifestyle and quality of life. Rehabilitation appears to be more effective if it is started as soon as functional visual difficulties are identified, CMS criteria however require a moderate loss in visual acuity (less than 20/60 or 6/18) therefore does not allow for very early intervention for "mild" impairment based on visual acuity unless a field loss or central scotoma can be used to justify treatment.

There can be coverage variations among Medicare contractors, called fiscal intermediaries, which are allowed to establish local policies. Thus, it is important to check with your local Medicare fiscal intermediary before initiating any low vision rehabilitation with clients.

According to CMS, coverage of low vision rehabilitation services is considered reasonable and necessary only for patients with a clear medical need. To meet the criteria established by CMS you must demonstrate that:

1. The patient has a moderate to severe visual impairment not correctable by conventional refractive means or certain types of visual field loss.

2. The patient has a clear potential for significant improvement in function following rehabilitation over a reasonable period of time (although recent rulings have questioned this requirement).

3. Clear documentation is provided that skilled occupational therapy services were delivered throughout the time period being billed.

Before providing services, the occupational therapist must develop a written evaluation and treatment plan. The treatment plan should include:

1. An initial assessment that documents the level of visual impairment.

TABLE 21-3: FUNCTIONAL PERFORMANCE G-CODES

PERFORMANCE AREA	CURRENT STATUS (EVALUATION AND AFTER EACH 10 SESSIONS)	GOAL (ALWAYS INCLUDE)	DISCHARGE STATUS
Mobility	G8978	G8979	G8980
Self-Care	G8987	G8988	G8989
Other	G8993	G8994	G8995
Other subsequent	G8996	G8997	G8998
LEVEL OF DISABILITY SUFFIX			
CH	0% disabled		
CI	1% to 20% disabled		
CJ	> 20% to 40% disabled		
CK	>40% to 60% disabled		
CL	>60% to 80% disabled		
CM	>80% to 99% disabled		
CN	100% disabled		

2. A plan of care identifying specific observable and measurable performance goals to be fulfilled during rehabilitation.

3. A definition of specific rehabilitation services to be provided during the course of rehabilitation.

4. A reasonable estimate of when the goals will be reached and the frequency at which the services will be provided.

Periodic follow-up evaluations must be performed by the referring physician during the course of rehabilitation. These are reported in the form of G-codes (Table 21-3) that are included with the billing. A G-code indicates a percentage of disability based on a clinical evaluation, ideally standardized tests (see Chapter 8 on evaluation). Two G-codes are required at the time of initial evaluation, every 10 sessions and upon discharge, a goal G-code and a status or discharge G-code.

Currently, CMS has therapy caps on outpatient services but as of 2015 these caps can be exceeded but with a high likelihood that CMS will initially deny payment and require an appeal to insure compliance with the above requirements.

Coding Guidelines

CMS has been in the process of converting from a fee-for-service model to a pay-for-performance model of reimbursement. The Physician Quality Reporting System (PQRS) has introduced coding standards that indicate the complexity of a case (ICD-10 codes) and modifiers to procedure codes as well as outcome codes (G-codes). In the past, proper coding requires determination of the primary and secondary diagnoses and the use of ICD-10-CM codes (Table 21-4). The codes reflect the level of visual impairment and this must always be the primary diagnosis. The secondary codes reflected the actual eye disease causing the visual impairment. Coding will undergo changes with the move from ICD-9 to ICD-10 on 10/15/2015, soon after this book is published. Formal ruling has designated which ICD-9 codes can be used to justify the delivery of reimbursable occupational services. However, at the time of this book publication, such rulings had not been made for the ICD-10 codes. These new rulings are expected within a year or two of implementation. Note that the codes listed in Table 21-4 describe impairment not the underlying eye disease that led to the impairment. Disease codes may need to be included as well, although this is not clear at this time. In the past, we have found that payers did not require disease codes. Note that although all the codes marked with a 1 in Table 21-4 are listed as "billable" in the CMS document, they are not necessarily "reimbursable." Actual payment for these services under some of these codes is highly unlikely because payment has been denied in the past. The unshaded lines in Table 21-4 indicate ICD-10 codes that correspond to reimbursable ICD-9 codes in the past. We have shaded with gray all of the ICD-10 codes that have NOT had corresponding ICD-9 codes that have been reimbursable. Codes that are shaded gray should be added to the codes that are known to be reimbursable along with other impairment codes (not listed) that may reflect complicating conditions such as cognitive or physical dysfunction. We expect in the future that these added codes will reflect complications that may increase the amount paid for a course of rehabilitation.

Table 21-4: ICD-10 Codes for Low Vision Cross Referenced With ICD-9 Codes That Were Accepted by Cms in 2015 (Unshaded)

BILLABLE ICD-9 CODES	ICD-10 CODES	0 UNSPECIFIED VISUAL DISTURBANCES
	H53.10	1 Unspecified subjective visual disturbances
	H53.11	1 Day blindness
	H53.12	0 Transient visual loss
	H53.121	1 Transient visual loss, right eye
	H53.122	1 Transient visual loss, left eye
	H53.123	1 Transient visual loss, bilateral
	H53.129	1 Transient visual loss, unspecified eye
	H53.13	0 Sudden visual loss
	H53.131	1 Sudden visual loss, right eye
	H53.132	1 Sudden visual loss, left eye
	H53.133	1 Sudden visual loss, bilateral
	H53.139	1 Sudden visual loss, unspecified eye
	H53.14	0 Visual discomfort
	H53.141	1 Visual discomfort, right eye
	H53.142	1 Visual discomfort, left eye
	H53.143	1 Visual discomfort, bilateral
	H53.149	1 Visual discomfort, unspecified
	H53.15	1 Visual distortions of shape and size
	H53.16	1 Psychophysical visual disturbances
	H53.19	1 Other subjective visual disturbances
	H53.2	1 Diplopia
	H53.4	0 Visual field defects
	H53.40	1 Unspecified visual field defects
	H53.41	0 Scotoma involving central area
368.41* 368.41*	H53.411	1 Scotoma involving central area, right eye
368.41* 368.41*	H53.412	1 Scotoma involving central area, left eye
368.41 368.41	H53.413	1 Scotoma involving central area, bilateral
	H53.419	1 Scotoma involving central area, unspecified eye
	H53.42	0 Scotoma of blind spot area
368.42* 368.42*	H53.421	1 Scotoma of blind spot area, right eye
368.42* 368.42*	H53.422	1 Scotoma of blind spot area, left eye

(continued)

TABLE 21-4: ICD-10 CODES FOR LOW VISION CROSS REFERENCED WITH ICD-9 CODES THAT WERE ACCEPTED BY CMS IN 2015 (UNSHADED) (CONTINUED)

BILLABLE ICD-9 CODES	ICD-10 CODES	0 UNSPECIFIED VISUAL DISTURBANCES
368.42 368.42	H53.423	1 Scotoma of blind spot area, bilateral
	H53.429	1 Scotoma of blind spot area, unspecified eye
	H53.43	0 Sector or arcuate defects
368.47* 368.46*	H53.431	1 Sector or arcuate defects, right eye
368.47* 368.46*	H53.432	1 Sector or arcuate defects, left eye
368.47 368.46	H53.433	1 Sector or arcuate defects, bilateral
	H53.439	1 Sector or arcuate defects, unspecified eye
	H53.45	0 Other localized visual field defect
368.47* 368.46*	H53.451	1 Other localized visual field defect, right eye
368.47* 368.46*	H53.452	1 Other localized visual field defect, left eye
368.47 368.46	H53.453	1 Other localized visual field defect, bilateral
	H53.459	1 Other localized visual field defect, unspecified eye
	H53.46	0 Homonymous bilateral field defects
368.46	H53.461	1 Homonymous bilateral field defects, right side
368.46	H53.462	1 Homonymous bilateral field defects, left side
368.46	H53.47	1 Heteronymous bilateral field defects
	H53.469	1 Homonymous bilateral field defects, unspecified side
	H53.48	0 Generalized contraction of visual field
368.45	H53.481	1 Generalized contraction of visual field, right eye
368.45	H53.482	1 Generalized contraction of visual field, left eye
368.45	H53.483	1 Generalized contraction of visual field, bilateral
	H53.489	1 Generalized contraction of visual field, unspecified eye
	H53.5	0 Color vision deficiencies
	H53.50	1 Unspecified color vision deficiencies
	H53.51	1 Achromatopsia
	H53.52	1 Acquired color vision deficiency
	H53.53	1 Deuteranomaly
	H53.54	1 Protanomaly
	H53.55	1 Tritanomaly

(continued)

TABLE 21-4: ICD-10 CODES FOR LOW VISION CROSS REFERENCED WITH ICD-9 CODES THAT WERE ACCEPTED BY CMS IN 2015 (UNSHADED) (CONTINUED)

BILLABLE ICD-9 CODES	ICD-10 CODES	0 UNSPECIFIED VISUAL DISTURBANCES
	H53.59	1 Other color vision deficiencies
	H53.6	0 Night blindness
	H53.60	1 Unspecified night blindness
	H53.61	1 Abnormal dark adaptation curve
	H53.62	1 Acquired night blindness
	H53.63	1 Congenital night blindness
	H53.69	1 Other night blindness
	H53.7	0 Vision sensitivity deficiencies
	H53.71	1 Glare sensitivity
	H53.72	1 Impaired contrast sensitivity
	H53.8	1 Other visual disturbances
	H53.9	1 Unspecified visual disturbance
	H54	0 Blindness (< 20/160) and low vision (< 20/60)
369.22	H54.0	1 Blindness, both eyes
	H54.1	0 Blindness, one eye, low vision other eye
369.24	H54.10	1 Blindness, one eye, low vision other eye, unspecified eyes
369.24	H54.11	1 Blindness, right eye, low vision left eye
369.24	H54.12	1 Blindness, left eye, low vision right eye
369.25	H54.2	1 Low vision, both eyes
	H54.3	1 Unqualified visual loss, both eyes
	H54.4	0 Blindness, one eye
	H54.40	1 Blindness, one eye, unspecified eye
	H54.41	1 Blindness, right eye, normal vision left eye
	H54.42	1 Blindness, left eye, normal vision right eye
	H54.5	0 Low vision, one eye
	H54.50	1 Low vision, one eye, unspecified eye
	H54.51	1 Low vision, right eye, normal vision left eye
	H54.52	1 Low vision, left eye, normal vision right eye
	H54.6	0 Unqualified visual loss, one eye
	H54.60	1 Unqualified visual loss, one eye, unspecified
	H54.61	1 Unqualified visual loss, right eye, normal vision left eye
	H54.62	1 Unqualified visual loss, left eye, normal vision right eye
		Legal Blindness
See text	H54.7	1 Unspecified visual loss
See text	H54.8	1 Legal blindness, as defined in USA
	H55	0 Nystagmus and other irregular eye movements

(continued)

TABLE 21-4: ICD-10 CODES FOR LOW VISION CROSS REFERENCED WITH ICD-9 CODES THAT WERE ACCEPTED BY CMS IN 2015 (UNSHADED) (CONTINUED)

BILLABLE ICD-9 CODES	ICD-10 CODES	0 UNSPECIFIED VISUAL DISTURBANCES
	H55.0	0 Nystagmus
	H55.00	1 Unspecified nystagmus
	H55.01	1 Congenital nystagmus
	H55.02	1 Latent nystagmus
	H55.03	1 Visual deprivation nystagmus
	H55.04	1 Dissociated nystagmus
	H55.09	1 Other forms of nystagmus
	H55.8	0 Other irregular eye movements
	H55.81	1 Saccadic eye movements
	H55.89	1 Other irregular eye movements
* must have a billable ICD-9 condition (unshaded line) in the other eye to meet criteria.		

The therapist needs to frequently look for revisions to these codes and standards but must be careful to use credible sources as many coding apps and web sources are not frequently updated and may contain erroneous information as a result. Members of the American Occupational Therapy Association often can obtain this information in an easily understood format from www.aota.org otherwise the providers must look for publications by CMS.[16] For example, PQRS is introducing procedure code modifiers. These can be found on the AOTA (www.aota.org) or CMS websites (www.cms.gov) search for "PQRS."

The diagnostic codes that refer to "low vision" or "blindness" in Table 21-4 are based on distance visual acuity measurements that are usually provided by the referring eye care professional. If for some reason the visual acuity is not provided, the occupational therapist can use the distance acuity charts suggested in Chapter 8 to determine the visual acuity. The criteria for low vision and legal blindness are the two measures that are used for meeting the criteria for a particular ICD-10 code and these criteria are based on the old Snellen charts that did not have lines between 20/100 and 20/200. The criterion for legal blindness is one letter missed on the 20/100 line. The criterion for legal blindness based on visual efficiency of visual field loss (www.ssa.gov/disability/professionals/bluebook/2.00-SpecialSensesandSpeech-Adult.htm) can be met using a measure of visual efficiency that requires field testing equipment only available at the office of an ophthalmologist or optometrist. Extrapolating from this ruling, we use as a criterion for "low vision," one letter missed on the 10/60 line or worse. This is important because with some conditions such as macular degeneration, a person often misses only one letter on a line for several lines better than 20/70 and if one used the 3/5 criterion for acuity, they might not meet the CMS criterion for low vision. Using a criterion of 1 letter missed would establish the acuity as worse than 20/60. The older ICD-9 codes distinguished many levels of visual acuity whereas the newer ICD-10 codes designate only two level, low vision and blindness. So for the ICD-10 code for "blindness," for example, there were different ICD-9 codes for acuity 20/200 to 20/400 and 20/500 to 20/1000. Both of these codes and two others would all be included under one ICD-10 code for "blindness." In Table 21-4 we did not list all of the equivalent ICD-9 codes, only the equivalent ICD-9 code as the highest acuity that met the criterion.

REFERRALS FOR LOW VISION REHABILITATION

Medicare requires that an occupational therapist receive a referral from a physician before initiating an evaluation or low vision rehabilitation. Initially, this referral could only be issued by an ophthalmologist or other medical doctor. However, the Balanced Budget Refinements Act (P.L. 106-113) signed into law November 29, 1999, includes a technical amendment that recognizes optometrists as "physicians" for purposes of certifying a Medicare beneficiary's need for occupational therapy services under Medicare Part B. This Federal law does not, however, supersede state law. Therapists in states with broad or no referral requirements will be able to accept referrals from optometrists in 36 states. The District of Columbia and Puerto Rico have no referral requirements in either their occupational therapy statute or regulations. However, it is possible for the state occupational laws to specifically require an MD or podiatrist as a referral source, for example. In such cases, the state

TABLE 21-5: PHYSICAL MEDICINE AND REHABILITATION TREATMENT CODES USED FOR LOW VISION REHABILITATION

CODES	EVALUATIONS
97003	Occupational therapy evaluation. Billed 1 unit per procedure.
97004	Occupational therapy reevaluation. Billed 1 unit per procedure.
97530	Therapeutic activities use dynamic activities to improve functional performance. Direct patient contact is by the provider billed 1 unit per 15 minutes.
97533	Sensory integrative techniques used to enhance sensory processing and promote adaptive responses to environmental demands. Direct patient contact is by the provider billed 1 unit per 15 minutes
97535	Self-care/home management training includes ADL and compensatory training, meal preparation, safety procedures, and instructions in use of adaptive equipment. Direct patient contact is by the provider billed 1 unit per 15 minutes.
97537	Community/reintegration training includes shopping, transportation, money management, avocational activities, and/or work environment/modification analysis, work task analysis. Direct patient contact is by the provider billed 1 unit per 15 minutes.

law would have precedence and in such a state an occupational therapist could not accept a referral from an optometrist. Currently, optometrists can provide a referral to an occupational therapist in many states. To determine the regulation in your state, it is important to check with your state occupational therapy association. You can check your state law on the AOTA website (www.aota.org) by searching for the State Occupational Therapy Law Database.

OTHER MEDICARE REQUIREMENTS

Individual Rehabilitation Plan

Medicare requires an Plan of Care (POC) for each client being treated by the occupational therapist. The POC prospectively documents the treatment needed to meet reasonable, well-defined goals. The POC must be must be reviewed and signed by a physician upon initial evaluation.

Recertification/Reevaluations

Medicare also requires periodic recertification for all clients receiving low vision rehabilitation. To be recertified, the POC must be signed. The required time period varies depending on the setting. For outpatient services, a POC must be recertified every 10 sessions. Otherwise, check with the agency or rehabilitation facility for the general requirement for occupational therapists.

Documentation

The documentation requirements for vision rehabilitation therapy are identical to those required for any other condition. For every session, therapists must document that the treatment is reasonable and necessary, that skilled therapy was provided in documentation and are consistent with the procedure billing codes (Table 21-5). The therapist must provide a plan of care (POC) as well as the regular progress notes and a re-evaluation every 10 sessions, with demonstrated progress over time or evidence that lack of progress was fully explained and treatment revised as needed or evidence that skilled care was provided that prevented a decline in function. At the end of treatment a discharge summary described treatment provided and progress toward goals. Sample documentation forms are included in the online appendix (www.routledge.com/ 9781617116339).

CURRENT REIMBURSEMENT RATES FOR VISION REHABILITATION SERVICES

Medicare reimbursement has been changing. Check the CMS Website (www.cms.gov and search "Medicare therapy fee schedule").

TABLE 21-6: SUGGESTED EQUIPMENT FOR LOW VISION EVALUATION	
EQUIPMENT	**SOURCE**
MNRead Reading Test (MN Read Test)	www.precisionvision.com
LEA distance Visual Acuity Chart	www.good-lite.com www.richmondproducts.com
Veterans Affairs Low-Vision Visual Functioning Questionnaire VA LV VFQ	www.routledge.com/9781617116339
Low Vision Independence Measure (LVIM)	www.routledge.com/9781617116339
Low Vision Rehabilitation Evaluation and progress note forms	www.routledge.com/9781617116339
LEA low contrast acuity chart	www.good-lite.com www.richmondproducts.com
The Pepper Visual Skills for Reading Test (Pepper VSRT)	www.lowvisionsimulators.com
The Wand. An occluder oculomotor and field testing device	www.guldenophthalmics.com www.good-lite.com
200 Lumen flashlight and 1500 Lumen gooseneck light (see below)	Local retail outlet

Regions may differ in their documentation and billing requirements. To find your regional office for CMS consult www.cms.gov (search "CMS regional offices").

MEDICARE AND LOW VISION REHABILITATION (HOSPITAL INPATIENT AND NURSING HOMES)

Prospective Payment System

Rehabilitation services in nursing homes and hospitals are limited by a prospective payment system (PPS). In this system, patients may receive therapies only for needs that have been documented within a few days after the patient is admitted to the nursing home. Under a PPS, hospitals receive a fixed amount for treating patients diagnosed with a given illness, regardless of the length of stay or type of care received. There must be a method to insure that proper testing (visual acuity) is performed in the first few days if occupational therapy for low vision rehabilitation is to be provided.

Supplies and Equipment

Some basic equipment and supplies are necessary to start a low vision rehabilitation service/practice costing approximately $8000 to $10,000. The optical devices are generally available in a general optometric low vision practice. These are listed in Chapter 8. The table top electronic magnifier costs about $2000 and is difficult to transport but is essential as are more portable hand held devices. It is possible a local vendor may loan a EM for demonstration and training purposes. A High Definition model is recommended. Currently iPads and iPhones are highly recommended (see Chapter 14 for recommended electronic hardware and software). Apps can be obtained to use these devices as book eReaders, as well. The trial lens kits are needed to add refractive correction to stronger reading addition or to change the strength of a person's spectacle addition per orders from the collaborating eye doctor. Suggested equipment necessary for the evaluation is listed in Table 21-6 and therapy equipment is listed in the online appendix (www.routledge.com/9781617116339).

SUMMARY

Up until the mid-1990's lack of reimbursement was the major obstacle to the provision of low vision rehabilitation services. When occupational therapists were identified as possible service providers, it appeared that barrier was removed because occupational therapy was a service paid for by CMS and most medical insurance companies. Since this time low vision rehabilitation has been added to the general occupational therapy curricula, and education programs continue to be developed that enable occupational therapists to provide low vision and blindness rehabilitation as areas of specialization. ACVREP and AOTA certification is available to document competence. The major obstacle today has been in the difficulties an occupational therapist has in registering to be an independent provider for insurance companies other than CMS. Moreover, coding and documentation is very different for low vision rehabilitation than for optometry and ophthalmology services where low vision rehabilitation has been historically provided. In this chapter, we provided answers about many of the common questions and issues that occupational therapists encounter about documentation and billing requirements in any setting.. We have included information about low vision education, certification, interaction with other vision rehabilitation professionals, practice opportunities, marketing low vision services, reimbursement and coding, Medicare requirements, and recommendations for equipment and supplies.

It is our hope that many readers will use the information in this book to help meet the growing demand for low vision rehabilitation services.

REFERENCES

1. Congdon N, O'Colmain B, Klaver CC, et al. Causes and prevalence of visual impairment among adults in the United States. *Arch Ophthalmol.* 2004;122:477-485.

2. Warren M. Including occupational therapy in low vision rehabilitation. *Am J Occup Ther.* 1995;49:857-860.

3. Elliott DB, et al. Demographic characteristics of the vision-disabled elderly. *Invest Ophthalmol Vis Sci.* 1997;38:2566-2575.

4. Warren M. *Low Vision: Occupational Therapy Intervention with the Older Adult.* Bethesda, MD: American Occupational Therapy Association; 2000.

5. American Occupational Therapy Association. Specialty certification in low vision. American Occupational Therapy Association website. http://www.aota.org/education-careers/advance-career/board-specialty-certifications/low-vision.aspx. Accessed April 8, 2015

6. Lambert J. Occupational therapists, orientation and mobility specialists and rehabilitation teachers. *J Vis Imp Blind.* 1994;88:297-298.

7. Orr AL, Huebner K. Toward a collaborative working relationship among vision rehabilitation and allied health professionals. *J Vis Imp Blind.* 2001;95:468-482.

8. McGinty Bachelder J, Harkins D. Do occupational therapists have a primary role in low vision rehabilitation? *Am J Occup Ther.* 1995;49:927-930.

9. Horowitz A. Vision impairment and functional disability among nursing home residents. *The Gerontologist.* 1994;34:316-323.

10. Horowitz A, et al. Visual impairment and rehabilitation needs of nursing home residents. *J Vis Impair Blind.* 1995;88:7-15.

11. Mogk L, Goodrich G. The history and future of low vision services in the United States. *J Vis Impair Blind.* 2004;(Oct):585-600.

12. Ponchillia PE, Ponchillia SV. *Foundations of Rehabilitation Teaching With Persons Who Are Blind or Visually Impaired.* New York: American Foundation for the Blind; 1996:3-21.

13. American Academy of Optometry. Diplomate in low vision section. http://www.aaopt.org/diplomate-low-vision-section. Accessed April 8, 2015.

14. Pankow L, Luchins D. Geriatric low vision referrals by ophthalmologists in a senior health center. *J Vis Impair Blind.* 1998;92:748-753.

RESOURCES

1. Academy for Certification of Vision Rehabilitation and Education Professionals (ACVREP) www.acvrep.org/

2. AOTA Website on Low Vision. http://www.aota.org/Practice/Productive-Aging/Emerging-Niche/Low-Vision.aspx. (or search "low vision")

Financial Disclosures

Dr. Paul B. Freeman has no financial or proprietary interest in the materials presented herein.

Dr. Maxine Scheiman has no financial or proprietary interest in the materials presented herein.

Dr. Mitchell Scheiman offers continuing education courses through www.visionedseminars.com and is on the faculty of Salus University.

Debra A. Sokol-McKay has no financial or proprietary interest in the materials presented herein.

Dr. Stephen G. Whittaker offers continuing education courses through www.visionedseminars.com and receives royalties from the Pepper Visual Skills for Reading Test and The Wands, a multipurpose testing tool for visual fields and eye movement testing.

Index

abbreviations used in eye exams, 103

absorptive lenses (sunlenses), 132–133, 208, 210, 290

Academy for Certification of Vision Rehabilitation & Education Professionals (ACVREP), 4, 25, 33, 382–383

Access World, 271

accommodation, 69–71

accommodative amplitude, 69

accommodative demand, 166–167, 245

activities of daily living. *See* ADL

acuity reserve, 164, 287–288, 290, 294

ACVREP (Academy for Certification of Vision Rehabilitation & Education Professionals), 4, 25, 33, 382–383

adaptive equipment and technology, resources for, 271, 303, 307

ADL (activities of daily living), 35, 109–112. *See also* performance goals; *specific activity*

adult education theory, 145–146, 152–153

age-related macular degeneration (AMD). *See also* central visual field loss

case examples, 3–4, 17, 19–20, 151–152

depression, 79, 88

description of, 47–48

dry (nonexudative or atrophic), 13–14, 48–51, 52, 169

effect on vision, 50, 169–170

lighting requirements for, 208

prevalence, 24–25, 49

race/ethnicity, 24

risk factors, 49–50

treatment of, 50–52

wet (exudative), 14, 49–52, 169

agnosia, 183, 198–199

alexia, 6, 117, 136, 183, 193–194, 199

aligning technique, 341–342

AMD. *See* age-related macular degeneration

American Foundation for the Blind, 271, 388

American Occupational Therapy Association (AOTA), 26–27, 33, 150

American Occupational Therapy Association Certification, 383

Amsler grid, 14–15, 51–52, 63, 99–100, 129

anatomy of eye, 39–45

andragogy learning model, 145–146

angular magnification, 75, 104

anosognosia, 86–87, 183, 196

antioxidants, 52

anti-VEGF drugs, 51–52, 55

AOTA (American Occupational Therapy Association), 33, 150, 383

AOTA Certification, 26–27

Apple devices and apps, 205, 218, 254, 257, 268, 305–307, 311–313, 317, 336, 361, 364, 367, 375

appliances, marking and use of, 214, 216–217, 315–316

aqueous humor, 40, 56

arts and crafts, 267–268, 326–329
assisted living communities, 385
assistive devices and technology, resources for, 271, 303, 307
astigmatic lenses, 68
astigmatism, 9, 71
atrophic age-related macular degeneration, 13–14, 48–51, 52, 169
attention problems, 87–88, 196
auditory labeling devices, 216–218, 305–306, 313

bar magnifiers, 230, 248
bathing, 303
bathrooms, 206, 215
Beck Depression Inventory (BDI), 89
bedrooms, 215
beep baseball, 333–334
behavioral activation, 79
Behavioral Inattention Test (BIT), 63, 196
bifocals. See near vision additions
biking, 332
bill paying, 284–285, 299, 312–313
binocular vision (oculomotor function)
    anatomy/physiology of, 42–43
    evaluation of, 5, 102–103, 133–135
    low vision rehabilitation, 5, 61–62, 117, 283
bioptic mount, 231–232
bioptic telescopic system (BTS), 344–345
BIT (Behavioral Inattention Test), 63, 196
blindness
    definition of, 20–22
    leading causes of, 24–25
    legal definitions of, 6, 20, 22, 29, 62
    overall visual field loss, 185–186
    prevalence and incidence, 22–24
blindness system, 29, 31, 33
blindsight, 183
blur interpretation, 116
board games, 324
books on tape, 256–257, 275, 286
bowling, 330–331
braille, 178, 256–257, 274–276, 286, 305–306, 310–311
brain, vision areas of, 44
brain injuries, 15–17, 43–44, 62–64, 86–87, 182, 319–320. See also peripheral visual field loss
BTS (bioptic telescopic system), 344–345
bulbar conjunctiva, 39

calendars, adaptations for, 305–306
Canadian Occupational Performance Measure (COPM), 109
cancellation test, 63
cane use. See white cane use
card games, 324
case history, 97–98

cataracts, 24, 58–60, 208
Catherine Bergego Scare (CBS), 63, 196
CCTVs (closed circuit televisions), 75, 225, 254–256, 292. See also electronic assistive devices
central fixation cue, 173–174
central scotoma, 13–15, 47–52, 54, 62–63, 99, 117. See also central visual field loss
central visual field loss
    eccentric viewing techniques, 169–177, 294–295
    evaluation of, 14–15, 63, 100–101, 118, 129–136, 162–164, 287
    eye diseases and, 47–52, 54, 62–64
    first-response interventions, 5, 13–15
    general interventions, 117
    mobility problems, 344
    optical magnification and, 250
    versus peripheral, 13, 62
    reading with, 162–164, 169–178, 283, 287–289, 294
certification in low vision therapy, 382–383
certified low vision therapists (CLVTs), 25, 28, 31–32, 352–353, 382–383
certified orientation and mobility specialists (COMs), 25, 27–28, 31–32, 34, 337, 344
certified vision rehabilitation therapists (CVRTs), 25, 27, 31–32, 34, 178
Charles Bonnet syndrome, 13, 50, 169, 182, 199
choroid, 40–41
chromatic aberration, 226, 248
cleaning, household, 318–320
clinical outcomes research, evaluation of, 154–159
clinical reasoning process, 137–138, 151–152, 259
clock face technique for central scotoma assessment, 14, 129–130
clock face technique for eccentric viewing instruction, 170–175
clocks, low vision options for, 305–306
closed circuit televisions (CCTVs), 75, 225, 254–256, 292. See also electronic assistive devices
clothing apraxia, 183
clothing care and management, 206, 216–218, 304–305, 317–318
clues, 338–339
CLVTs. See certified low vision therapists
COAST method of goal writing, 148, 150–151
coding guidelines, 138, 390–395
cognitive issues. See perceptual dysfunctions; psychosocial and cognitive issues
coin clock test, 178
colleges of optometry, 387
color identifiers, electronic, 305
color modifications, 205–207, 212
color vision testing, 99–100
communication skills, 309–311
community activities and mobility, 335–346
community-based agencies, 385

compensatory approaches, overview of, 65, 144, 146–147

compensatory scanning, 17, 64, 182, 184–185, 190–198. *See also* eccentric viewing techniques

computers. *See* electronic assistive devices

COMs. *See* certified orientation and mobility specialists

concave lenses, 68

cones and rods, 42, 48

confrontation field testing, 16–17, 100, 118, 127–129

conjunctiva, 39

consumer education, 388

continuing education courses for low vision therapists, 380–381

contrast reserve, 11, 168, 288, 290, 294

contrast sensitivity, 223. *See also* glare sensitivity
    electronic assistive devices, 250, 254, 258–259, 264–265
    first-response interventions, 5, 8, 10–12
    improving performance of optical lenses, 226–227
    interventions, 168–169, 205, 212, 282–283, 290, 294
    occupational therapy evaluation, 12, 117–118, 124–127, 162–163, 168–169, 286–287
    optometric evaluation, 101

contrast threshold, 11, 162–163, 168, 286–288

control, loss of, 84–85

convergence insufficiency, 43, 62, 133–135

convex lenses, 67–68

cooking, 206, 315–317

COPM (Canadian Occupational Performance Measure), 109

cornea, 39–40

cortical blindness. *See* cortical visual impairment

cortical visual impairment 184, 199

craft activities, 267–268, 326–329

cranial nerves, 42

critical print size, 8–9, 10, 117, 122–123, 246, 286

cultural reactions to vision loss, 82–83

CVRTs. *See* certified vision rehabilitation therapists

cycling, 332

cylindrical lenses, 68

darts (game), 325

demyelinating disease, 60–62

denial, 80–82, 116, 145–146, 185, 196

depression, 79, 88–90

depth of focus, 225–226

diabetes, 347–378
    AADE7 strategies, 352, 359–376
    blood glucose levels, 363–366, 369, 373
    complications of, 349–351
    demographics, 54, 347–348
    effect on vision, 54, 348–349
    electronic assistive devices, 267, 358–359, 361, 364–365, 367, 370–372, 374
    evaluation of, 355–357
    foot care, 373–374
    general intervention strategies, 357–359

low vision therapist, role of, 352–353, 354

medication adaptations, 366–373
    injections, 368–373
    oral, 367
    with potential for affecting blood glucose, 369
    with potential for causing hypoglycemia, 368

resources, 376–377

self-management education, 351–352

self-management team and their roles, 352–355

sick days, 373–374

diabetic retinopathy, 24, 53–55, 208, 348–350, 354, 362, 373

Digit-Eyes, 218

dining rooms, 214–215

diopters, 73, 167

diplopia (double vision), 42–43, 61–62, 133–135

disability, definition of, 21, 33

disability glare, 208–209

discomfort glare, 208

diseases. *See* eye diseases

disorder, definition of, 21, 33

distance education courses for low vision therapists, 381–382

document readers (or scanners), 256, 275

dog guides, 337

dressing, adaptations for, 206, 216–218, 304–305, 317–318

driving, 13, 22, 81–82, 88, 196, 344–346

dry age-related macular degeneration, 13–14, 48–51, 52, 169

dynamic functional vision fields, 188

eating out/at a restaurant, 306–308, 335–336

eccentric viewing, assessment of, 129–132

eccentric viewing techniques, 169–177, 294–295

education and certification in low vision therapy, 380–383

elderly population, 23–24, 32, 57, 59, 72–73

electronic assistive devices, 253–277
    case studies, 253–254
    computer systems, 268–276. *See also specific type of device*
    accessories for, 258, 276–277
    client equipment and skills, 271–272
    evaluation of, 276
    instruction for, 276
    restricted visual fields, 294
    screen magnification, 256, 272–274, 292
    therapist equipment and skills, 269–271

for diabetic management, 267, 358–359, 361, 364–365, 367, 370–372, 374

electronic magnifiers, 260–268
    accessories for, 258, 276–277
    CCTVs, 75, 225, 254–256, 292
    handheld, 230, 233, 255, 292
    important properties of, 262, 264–265
    instruction for, 263, 265–268
    overview, 224, 233, 254–256, 260–261

for skin inspections, 267–268

ergonomics, 258, 264, 276–277

evaluation of, 257–260

glare sensitivity and, 250, 254, 258–259, 264–265

instruction for use of, 260, 263, 265–268, 276

for labeling, 216–218, 305, 313

overview, 75–76, 153–154, 254–257

resources for, 271

success-oriented approach, 259–260, 263

types of, 255

for writing, 266–267, 299

emmetropia, 70

emotional volatility, 88, 196

enlargement ratio, 75, 165–168, 244–247

environmental factors, 203–218

evaluation of, 109, 137, 203–204, 222–223

interventions, 153

color and brightness, 205–207, 212

contrast enhancements, 205, 212

factors that can be modified, 204

labeling and marking, 216–218, 303, 305, 313–316, 359

lighting and glare, 206–213

magnification, 204–206, 222–224

by room, 214–216

visual clutter, 184, 199, 212–214

EP. *See* equivalent power

EPIC Continuum of Adaptation from Visual to Nonvisual, 302

EPIC Framework, 301–302, 310, 324, 336, 338, 352

epidemiology, 22–24

equipment, adaptive, resources for, 271, 303, 307

equipment for low vision evaluation, 137, 396

equivalent power, 76, 167–168, 244–246

equivalent viewing distance, 76, 167, 245

e-readers, 233, 292–293

ER. *See* enlargement ratio

ergonomics, 175

electronic assistive devices, 258, 264, 276–277

leisure activities, 241, 326

magnification strategies, 236, 238, 241

reading, 296

ETDRS letter acuity chart, 8, 22, 119–120

ethnicity, 23–24, 83

evaluations. *See* first-response interventions; occupational therapy evaluation; optometric low vision evaluation

evidence-based practice, 154–159

expectations, patient, 84

extinction procedure, 128

exudative age-related macular degeneration, 14, 49–52, 169

eye anatomy and physiology, 39–45

eye diseases, 47–66. *See also* age-related macular degeneration

cataracts, 24, 58–60, 208

demyelinating disease, 60–62

diabetic retinopathy, 24, 53–55, 208, 348–350, 354, 362, 373

glaucoma, 24, 55–58, 208, 249–250

leading causes of low vision, 24–25, 47

lighting requirements for, 208

eye health evaluation, 103–104

eye hospitals, 386–387

eye muscles, 42

eye teaming. *See* binocular vision

eyeball, 39–40

eyelids, 39–40

family reactions to vision loss, 82–83

farsightedness, 9, 67–71, 98–99, 101–102, 248

field cuts. *See* homonymous hemianopsia

field expansion devices, 191, 194–198, 250–251

field of view, 76–77, 225–226

figure-ground deficits. *See* visual clutter

financial management, 206, 284–285, 298–299, 311–313, 320–321

fine motor control impairment, 223, 250

first-response interventions, 3–18

case examples, 3–4, 17

models of care, 3–4

for reading problems, 282–283

visual impairment, types of

contrast sensitivity, 8, 10–12

oculomotor function, 283

overview, 4–6

visual acuity, 6–10

visual field disorders, 12–17, 283

writing strategies, 298

fishing, 330

flip-up additions, 227–228, 291

focal distance of a lens, 73–74

focusing power of a lens, 73

font characteristics, 284–285

food

eating out/at a restaurant, 306–308, 335–336

meal preparation, 206, 214, 310, 313–317

shopping for, 319–321

foundational skills and therapeutic activities, 161–179

fovea, 41

frustration tolerance, 88, 223

full-field microscopes, 227–228, 236–238, 247–248, 291

functional reserve, 118–119

functional vision evaluation. *See* occupational therapy evaluation

games, 324–325

gardening, 329

G-codes, 109, 111, 390

Geriatric Depression Scale (GDS), 89, 116, 137

glare sensitivity, 55, 58

absorptive lenses for, 132–133, 208, 210, 290

contrast sensitivity and, 10–12
electronic assistive devices and, 250, 254, 258–259, 264–265
improving performance of optical lenses, 226–227
intervention strategies, 168–169, 206–213, 282–283, 290
glaucoma, 24, 55–58, 208, 249–250
goals, 84, 108, 115–116, 147–153, 221–222, 358
golf, 330–331
grading activities, 223–224
graduate education for low vision therapists, 381–382
Gray Oral Reading Series (GORT), 136
grocery shopping, 319–321
grooming, 267, 303–304

half-eyes, 227–228, 291
hallucinations, 13, 15, 17, 50, 85–86, 182, 199
hallways, 215
handheld magnifiers, 224, 228–230, 233–234, 238–240, 248, 255, 291–292, 317–318
handicap, definition of, 21, 34
health history, 115
hemianopsia, 15–17, 43–44, 62, 64, 128–129, 182, 186–187
heteronymous field loss, 16, 129
hiking, 333
history of low vision, 29–33
home health care practice opportunities, 384–385
home management, 309–322
   communication skills, 309–311
   financial management, 206, 284–285, 298–299, 311–313, 320–321
   housekeeping tasks, 317–319
   meal preparation, 206, 214, 310, 313–317
   shopping, 319–321
home mobility techniques, 340–343
home movie watching, 329
home study courses for low vision therapists, 381–382
homonymous field loss, 15–17, 43–44, 62, 64, 128, 182, 186–187
housekeeping, 318–320
hue, definition of, 206
human sighted guides, 339–340
hygiene, 303–304
hyperopia, 9, 67–71, 98–99, 101–102, 248

IADLs (instrumental activities of daily living), 109–112. *See also* specific activity
ICD codes, 138, 390–394
illuminance, definition of, 206-207
impairment, definition of, 21, 33
independence, definitions of, 150
independent mobility techniques, 340–343
individualized education plan (IEP), 150, 260
individualized treatment plan, 150–152
instrumental activities of daily living. *See* IADLs
interviewing clients, 108–109, 112–115

inverse square law, 169, 211
iPads/iPhones. *See* Apple devices and apps
iris, 40–41

kitchens, 206, 214. *See also* meal preparation
knitting, 324, 327
Knowles, Malcolm, 145

labeling and marking, 359
   appliances, 216–217, 315–316
   auditory devices, 216–218, 305–306, 313
   bathing, 303
   clothing, 216–218, 305
   commercial and homemade, 217
   food, 313–314
labels, reading, 267, 320
landmarks, 338–339
laser tag, 188–189, 192
laundry care, 317
laundry rooms, 216
LEA tests, 117, 129
   for lighting and contrast sensitivity, 12, 124–127
   resources for, 137
   vision function tests, overview of, 118
   for visual acuity at a distance, 120–121
legal blindness, 6, 20, 22, 29, 62
leisure activities, 206, 267–268, 323–330
lens of eye, 40
lenses
   corrective, interacting with handheld magnifier, 238
   improving performance of, 226–227
   optics of, 73–77
   types of, 67–68
letter contrast sensitivity test, 8, 12
life events, 84
life stage, 83–84
light meters, 210–211
light reflectance value (LRV), 212
Lighthouse International, 388
lighting, 50, 223. *See also* glare sensitivity
   comparison of sources, 213
   diabetes and, 54–55, 58, 357–358
   evaluation of, 8, 12, 124–127, 168–169, 207, 210–211
   intervention strategies, 168–169, 206–213, 282–283
   magnification strategies, 226, 234–242
   requirements for clients with eye diseases, 208
   room versus task lighting, 211
   terminology, 206–207
linguistic alexia. *See* alexia
living rooms, 215
localization, 176, 235, 267, 298
loupes, 227–228, 236–238, 247–248, 291, 318
low vision
   definition of, 20–22
   history of, 29–33

leading causes of, 24–25
prevalence and incidence, 22–24
related to functional problems, 22
Low Vision Independence Measure (LVIM), 109, 111–112, 137
low vision rehabilitation
    definition of, 20
    general approaches, 152–154
    general concepts, 145–152
    history of, 29–33
    models of care, 3–4, 33–36, 143–145, 151, 219–224, 243
    occupational therapists, 344
        establishing a specialty practice, 379–397
        historical involvement of, 32–33
        importance for, 19–20
        interprofessional issues, 31–33, 383–384
        role of, 25–27, 35–36
    overview of areas of treatment, 144
    professionals and their roles, 25–29, 34–36, 145, 151, 219–224, 243, 344
    research, evaluation of, 154–159
low vision therapists. *See* certified low vision therapists (CLVTs)
lumens, 206–207
luminance, definition of, 206–207
lux, 125, 206
LuxIQ, 125–126, 210–211
LVIM (Low Vision Independence Measure), 109, 111–112, 137
LVRCA (Low Vision Reading Comprehension Test), 135–136, 164, 289

macula, 42, 47–48
macular degeneration. *See* age-related macular degeneration
macular edema, 53, 349
MagnaFlyer computer program, 175–176
magnification, 219–251
    advanced concepts/techniques, 243–249
    basic principles, 220–243
    calculating changes in, 243
    case examples, 221–224
    collaborative models of care, 219–224, 243
    definition of, 74–76, 165, 244
    devices. *See also* electronic assistive devices; specific device
        fine motor control and, 223, 250
        instruction on use, 224, 233–243, 266–267, 296–298
        for leisure activities, 326
        movement/motion sickness, 226
        optical aberrations, 226–227
        positioning, 225–226
        selecting, 223–224
        special considerations for, 247–249
        for telephone use, 311
        types and properties of, 224, 227–233, 290–294
    environmental factors, 204–206, 222–224
    evaluation of needs, 104–105, 117, 123–124, 223
    field of view, 76–77, 225–226
    manufacturers' methods of calculating, 247
    methods of achieving
        angular, 75, 104
        electronic. *See* electronic assistive devices
        equivalent power, 76, 167–168, 244–246
        overview of, 224–226, 244–247
        relative size and distance, 10, 74–75, 104, 165–167, 204–206, 244
    optics of lenses, 73–77
    restricted visual fields, 175–178, 223, 249–251
magnifying glasses. *See* handheld magnifiers
MAR (minimum angle of resolution), 165
marketing, 387–388
MARS chart, 124–127
meal preparation, 206, 214, 310, 313–317
medical necessity, 150–151
medical rehabilitation settings, 385
Medicare, 23, 33, 62, 107
    coding guidelines, 138, 390–395
    converting outcomes into G-codes, 109, 111, 390
    coverage for low vision rehabilitation, 31–32, 388–396
    diabetes, 354–355
    low vision, definition of, 21
    medical necessity, definition of, 150–151
    primary diagnosis, 138, 390
medication, adaptations for, 206, 367
memory impairment, 85–86, 250
metamorphopsia, 51
microperimeters, 101, 129
microscopes, full-field, 227–228, 236–238, 247–248, 291
minimum angle of resolution (MAR), 165
Minnesota Low-Vision Reading Test. *See* MNREAD
minus lenses, 68
MNREAD (Minnesota Low-Vision Reading Test), 9, 117, 121–123, 137, 162, 210
mobility. *See* orientation and mobility
models of care, 3–4, 33–36, 143–145, 151, 219–224, 243
money identification and handling, 311–312, 320–321
Morgan Low Vision Reading Comprehension Test (LVRCA), 135–136, 164, 289
movement/motion sickness, 226
movie watching at home, 329
movie watching in theaters, 336
multiple sclerosis (MS), 60–62
muscles of the orbit, 42
music, 330
myopia, 9, 68, 70, 99, 101–102, 247–248

National Eye Institute, 388
National Library Service (NLS), 275, 312
near vision additions, 7, 9, 69, 76, 102, 166–167, 224, 227–228, 234, 236–238, 244–245, 247–248, 291
nearsightedness, 9, 68, 70, 99, 101–102, 247–248
needlework, 318–319, 327
neglect. *See* spatial neglect
NEI VFQ-25, 111
night blindness, 58, 185
NLS (National Library Service), 275, 312
nonexudative age-related macular degeneration, 13–14, 48–51, 52, 169
nonoptical assistive devices and techniques, 10, 154, 216, 218, 256–257, 274–276, 305–306, 313. *See also* specific activity
nonvisual reading options, 256–257, 275, 285–286
nonvisual senses, learning to use, 178, 192
nursing homes, 385
NVO glasses. *See* microscopes, full-field
nystagmus, 5, 134–135

objective refraction techniques, 72
occupational history, 115
occupational performance, 109–112
occupational profile, 112–116
occupational therapists, 344
   education/training for low vision therapy, 380–383
   establishing a low vision specialty practice, 379–397
   historical involvement in low vision therapy, 32–33
   importance of low vision therapy for, 19–20
   interprofessional issues, 31–33, 383–384
   models of care, 3–4, 33–36, 143–145, 151, 219–224, 243
   refractive disorders, significance of, 72–73
   role of, 25–27, 35–36
occupational therapy evaluation, 107–140
   functional vision evaluation, 116–137
      central visual field, 14–15, 63, 118, 129–136, 162–164, 287
      contrast sensitivity, 12, 117–118, 124–127, 162–163, 168–169, 286–287
      environmental factors, 109, 137, 203–204, 222–223
      glare sensitivity, 132–133
      lighting, 8, 12, 124–127, 168–169, 207, 210–211
      magnification needs, 117, 123–124, 223
      oculomotor screening, 133–135
      overview, 117–119
      peripheral visual field, 16–17, 63, 127–129, 188–189
      reading assessment/reading speed, 117, 135–136
      resources for equipment, 137, 396
      spatial neglect, 63, 196
      visual acuity, 7–9, 119–123, 162–163, 286
   interviewing clients, tips for, 108–109, 112–115
   occupational history, 115
   occupational performance, 109–112
   occupational profile, 112–116

overview, 108–109
primary diagnosis, 138
rehabilitation potential, assessment of, 137–138
Occupational Therapy Practice Framework, 20, 26, 107, 109, 115, 150
oculomotor function
   anatomy/physiology of, 42–43
   evaluation of, 5, 102–103, 133–135
   low vision rehabilitation, 5, 61–62, 117, 283
offices, 215
older population, 23–24, 32, 57, 59, 72–73
online courses for low vision therapists, 381–382
ophthalmologists, 25–26, 34, 145, 151, 219–224, 243, 353, 386
optic ataxia, 183
optic disc, 41
optical character recognition, 268
optical devices. *See also* electronic assistive devices; magnification
   accommodation, 69–71
   diabetic management, 358–359
   field expansion devices, 191, 194–198, 250–251
   field of view, 76–77, 225–226
   improving lens performance, 226–227
   lenses, optics of, 73–77
   lenses, types of, 67–68
   refractive disorders, 9, 70–73
optimizing vision, 145–146
optometric low vision evaluation, 97–105
   abbreviations used in, 103
   binocular vision, 102–103
   case history, 97–98
   color vision, 99–100
   components of, 98
   contrast sensitivity, 101
   eye health, 103–104
   magnification, 104–105
   refraction, 101–102
   visual acuity, 98–99
   visual/mobility field testing, 100–101
optometrists, 25–26, 34–35, 145, 151, 219–224, 243, 353–354, 385–386
orbit of the eye, 39–40, 42
orientation and mobility, 337–346
   certified specialists, 25, 27–28, 31–32, 34, 337, 344
   screening tool for, 338
   techniques for, 338–346
outdoor recreation and sports, 330–334

painting, 327
palinopsia, 199
patient care clinics, 387
patient case history, 97–98
patient expectations, 84
patient goals, 84, 108, 115–116, 147–153, 221–222, 358

pedagogy learning model, 145-146

Pepper Test, 109, 112, 118, 135–136, 137, 163–164, 196, 289

perceptual dysfunctions, 4, 6, 117–118, 181–184, 198–199, 223. *See also* spatial neglect

performance goals, 108, 115–116, 147–153, 221–222, 358

peripheral visual field loss, 181–201. *See also* perceptual dysfunctions

    basic functions of peripheral vision, 184–185

    versus central field loss, 13, 62

    evaluation of, 16–17, 63, 100, 127–129, 188–189

    eye diseases and, 54, 56–58, 62–64

    first-response interventions, 5, 15–17

    mobility problems, 343–344

    optical magnification and, 249–251

    overall visual field loss, 185–186

    overview, 181–184

    prevalence and risk factors, 63

    reading with, 186–187, 191–194, 283, 287–288, 294–295

    spatial neglect, 62–64, 181, 183, 195–198

    treatment for, 5, 117

        compensatory scanning, 17, 64, 182, 184–185, 190–198

        field expansion devices, 191, 194–198, 250–251

        remediation, 190

    unilateral visual field loss, 186–188

    visual pathways, 43–44, 62

peripheral warning system, 184–185, 192, 196

personal organizers, 256–257, 275–276

personality, patient, 84–85

phoria, 43

phoropters, 72, 101

photophobia. *See* glare sensitivity

photoreceptors, 42, 48

physiology, 39–45

pink eye, 39

plus lenses, 67–68

power in diopters, 167

preferred retinal loci (PRL), 170

presbyopia, 7, 9, 69, 166, 244–245

primary diagnosis, 138

print reading systems, 275

prisms, 191, 194–198, 250–251

problem-solving therapy, 89

protective techniques, 341–343

psychosocial and cognitive issues, 79–93, 116. *See also* perceptual dysfunctions

    cognitive impairment, 85–88

    depression, 79, 88–90

    factors affecting adjustment to vision loss, 80–85

    optical magnification and, 85, 87, 223, 250

    problem-solving therapy, 89

    success-oriented approach, 80

public relations, 387–388

pupil, 40

pursuits, 41

puzzles, 325

quadrantopia, 62, 129, 131, 186–187

race, 23–24

randomized clinical trial (RCT), 154–159

reading, 281–298. *See also* braille

    acuity tests, 7–9, 117–118, 121–123, 135–136, 162

    case examples, 281–282, 284, 288–289, 295–296

    evaluation of, 283–290

    first-response interventions, 282–283

    instructions for magnification devices, 266–267, 296–298

    interventions for meeting requirements of, 283, 290–294

    labels, 267, 320

    lighting needs for, 211–212, 282–283

    nonvisual options, 256–257, 275, 285–286

    performance, assessment of, 164, 289–290

    with scrolled text, 163, 175–176, 235, 288, 295

    speed/rate, 9, 117, 121–123, 135–136, 285, 289–290

    as therapeutic activity, 162, 177, 191

    typical print sizes and acuity requirements, 284

    with visual field loss

        central, 162–164, 169–178, 283, 287–289, 294

        peripheral, 186–187, 191–194, 283, 287–288, 294–295

        using eccentric viewing, 169–177, 294–295

        without eccentric viewing, 177–178

    visual requirements for, 287–290

reading glasses. *See* near vision additions

recordings for the blind, 256–257, 275

recordkeeping, 312–313

recreation and sports activities, 330–334

referrals for low vision rehabilitation, 388, 394–395

refractive errors, 7, 9, 70–73, 101–102

rehabilitation teachers. *See* vision rehabilitation therapists

relative scotoma, 130, 162, 169, 172

relative size and distance magnification, 10, 74–75, 104, 165–167, 204–206, 244

remediation, 164, 190, 196–198

research on low vision rehabilitation, 154–159

restaurants, eating in, 306–308, 335–336

retina, 41–42, 47–48

retinitis pigmentosa, 208, 249–250

retinoscopes, 72

retirement communities, 385

retracing technique, 175

rods and cones, 42, 48

room familiarization, 342–343

saccades, 41, 161, 169–170, 176, 184

saturation, definition of, 206

scanning techniques, 235–236, 268. *See also* compensatory scanning

scheduling, adaptations for, 305–306
sclera, 39
scope of practice, 344
scotoma, 13. *See also* central visual field loss
screen readers, 256, 269–270, 274–275, 292, 311
scrolling, reading by, 163, 175–176, 235, 288, 295
self-awareness and insight, 86–87
self-care, 267–268, 303–306
self-concept, 84–85
Self-Reported Assessment of Functional Vision Performance (SRAFVP), 111–112
sewing, 318–319, 327
shopping, 319–321
showering, 303
sighted guides, 339–340
signature guides. *See* typoscopes
simultagnosia, 183
skiing, 332–333
skimming, 268
skin inspections, 267–268
SKREAD test, 117–118, 121–123, 135–136, 137, 162–163
smart phones, 233, 271–272, 293, 299, 311–312. *See also* Apple devices and apps
smear, 264
Snellen notation, converting to, 120
social workers, 25, 28–29, 34
sound, learning to use, 178, 192
spatial neglect, 62–64, 181, 183, 195–198
speech recognition software, 271
sports and recreation activities, 330–334
sports events, 336
spot reading, 152, 163–164, 285
spotting techniques, 235, 267
squaring off technique, 341
SRAFVP (Self-Reported Assessment of Functional Vision Performance), 111–112
stages of acceptance, 80–82
stair climbing, 215–216, 342
stand magnifiers, 224, 230–231, 234, 240–241, 248, 291, 318
starburst glare, 209, 258–259
static functional vision fields, 189
steady eye technique, 175, 177
stereopsis test, 103
strabismus, 43, 102–103, 133–135
subjective refraction techniques, 71–72
success-oriented approach, 80, 223–224, 259–260, 263
sunlenses (absorptive lenses), 132–133, 208, 210, 290
swimming, 332

tablet computers, 233, 257, 268, 271–272, 292, 299
tangent screen
    eccentric viewing training, 171–175
    resources for, 137
    visual field loss evaluation, 118, 130–132, 189

targeting games, 325
task analysis, 222–223
task versus room lighting, 211
teachers of the visually impaired (TVI), 25, 28
telemicroscopes, 224, 232, 234, 242–243, 249, 317–318
telephone use, 311
telescopes, 185, 224, 231–233, 234, 241–242, 249, 250
television watching, 329
tennis, 332
text-to-speech technology, 254–256, 260, 268, 269–270, 272, 274–276, 292, 306
theater events, 336
therapeutic activities and foundational skills, 161–179
timekeeping, 206, 305–306
touch, sense of, 178
tracing, 235–236
tracking, 235
trailing technique, 341, 343
Trails Test, 196
travel, 337
treatment strategy, overview of, 143–160
Tuttle and Tuttle's stages of coping, 80–82
TVI (teachers of the visually impaired), 25, 28
typing instruction programs, 271
typoscopes, 211, 250, 290, 294, 298

Useful Field of View Test, 196
unilateral neglect (or inattention). *See* spatial neglect

vertical reading, 193, 294–295
Veteran Administration outcome measure (VA LV VFQ-48 and VFQ-24), 111–112, 137
vision rehabilitation therapists, 25, 27, 31–32, 34, 178
visors, 227–228, 236–238
visual acuity, 117
    definition of, 7
    first-response interventions, 5, 6–10
    occupational therapy evaluation of, 7–9, 119–123, 162, 286
    optometric evaluation of, 98–99
    refractive error assessment, 71–72
visual arts, 327
visual clutter, 184, 199, 212–214
visual field disorders. *See also* central visual field loss; peripheral visual field loss
    definition of, 12–13, 62
    first-response interventions, 5, 12–17, 283
    mobility problems, 343–344
    occupational therapy evaluation of, 118, 127–136
    optical magnification and, 223, 249–251
    optometric evaluation of, 100–101
    overview, 12–17, 62–64
visual inattention, 62–64, 195–198
visual neglect. *See* spatial neglect
visual pathways, 43–44

vitreous humor, 40
Voice Over, 268, 272, 311
volunteerism, 336–337

Warren, Mary, 32, 380
wet age-related macular degeneration, 14, 49–52, 169
where and what systems, 44, 182–183
white cane use, 185, 337, 343

woodworking, 327–329
working distance, 69–70
World Health Organization (WHO), 20–21, 33–34
Worth 4-dot test, 103
writing patient goals, 147–150
writing strategies, 266–267, 294, 298–299, 309–311, 319–320